Biomedical Equipment

Use, Maintenance, and Management

Joseph J. Carr

Prentice Hall, Upper Saddle River, NJ 07458

Preface

A generation ago, medical equipment consisted of a few respirators, a blood pressure cuff, and a lot of low-technology tools and instruments found in and about the hospital. But starting in the 1960s, and accelerating in the 1970s and 1980s, medical equipment was designed in ever-increasing numbers. The hospital, the physician's office, and even the ambulance have become centers of high-technology excellence. Doctors, nurses, ancillary medical personnel, and all others concerned with modern medicine have become electronics technologists as well as being skilled in their own fields.

In the early 1970s new skilled positions started showing up in hospitals to repair, adjust, operate, and manage this new technology. At least three different skill levels are found:

First, one finds operating personnel. Sometimes called *monitoring technicians* or *cardiovascular technicians* or *instrumentation technicians*, these people actually operate the equipment on a day-by-day basis. A specially trained (sometimes self-trained) nurse usually supervises the operators.

Second, one finds that equipment breaks down and needs repair, it needs preventative maintenance, and it needs a special skill to take care of it. These functions are performed by a *biomedical equipment technician* (BMET). Certification is available for these people from the Association for the Advancement of Medical Instrumentation (AAMI) and is based on a combination of education and practical work experience.

Third, there is now the *biomedical engineer* or *clinical engineer*. Although some groups so narrowly define these occupations as to make them different, it is generally accepted at the hospital level that they are the same person. AAMI also offers certification as a clinical engineer. These people tend to be the managers and responsible professionals who manage the biomedical equipment repair shop.

Several readers were in mind when this book was prepared. First are the users who need an introduction to the field of biomedical instrumentation. For this person there is introductory material. Then there is also the newly hired electronics or mechanical technician who is not yet familiar with this field of biomedical instrumentation. For that person this book is a self-training resource. Then there is the operating technician (monitoring tech, etc.) who must learn something about the operation of the equipment as well as failure modes.

Joseph J. Carr, MSEE
Certified Clinical Engineer
Annandale, VA

1

Introduction to Biomedical Equipment

The field of biomedical equipment technology is relatively new compared with some technologies (being almost nonexistent only 30 years ago), but nonetheless encompasses a wide variety of different devices at various levels of technology used in a variety of applications within both clinical medicine and research. Although clinical and research instruments are often quite different, this book covers them both based on their similarities rather than their differences.

EXAMPLES OF BIOMEDICAL EQUIPMENT

Nearly everyone in clinical medicine is intimately involved with both electronic and mechanical devices. Although some may not know it, they are also involved in a considerable way with computerized instruments because many devices contain "transparent" internal computers. Some instruments are quite sophisticated, while others are mundane.

In some cases, the mundane function has been technologized and made easier (in many ways) or better by using electronic or electromechanical technology. For example, consider the intravenous fluids pump shown in Figure 1-1. The "IV" was traditionally a bottle of fluid that was gravity fed into a tubing set that is inserted into the patient's arm or leg veins. There was a regulator and an on-off clamp, but no technology. Many companies offer IV pumps that use electronics and mechanics to pump the fluid. This method offers alarm functions for "out of fluid" and air bubbles in the line, as well as allowing a fixed dosage to be administered.

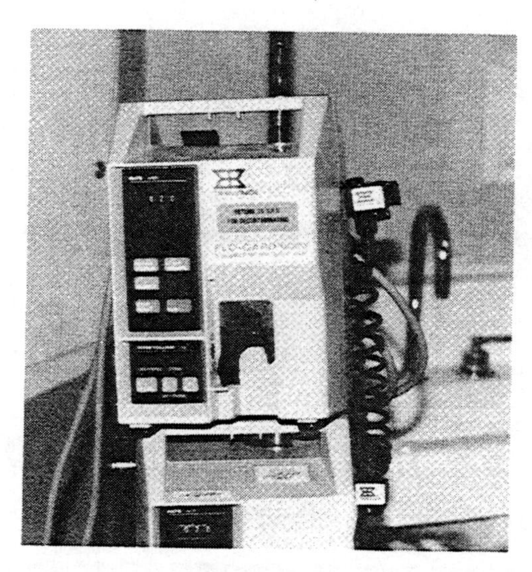

FIGURE 1-1

Nearly everyone who watches television medical shows knows about defibrillators (Figure 1-2). They are the instruments that are used to "jump start" heart attack victims who are trying to die. These instruments are found throughout the hospital, the city or county emergency medical service, and even in some doctor's

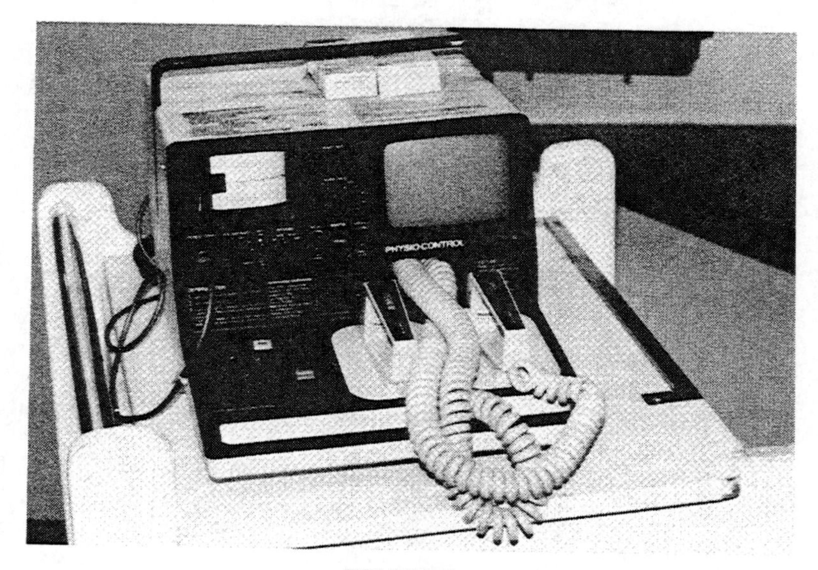

FIGURE 1-2

offices and outpatient clinics. For both the medical personnel and the biomedical equipment personnel, the defibrillator represents a significant part of the work.

Medical instrumentation also includes large-scale, computerized central monitoring systems in the operating room, coronary care unit (CCU), and intensive care unit (ICU). These systems are discussed in detail in Chapter 8. Again, much of the biomedical equipment technician's and monitor technician's work involves these central monitoring systems. See Figure 1-3.

There are also a large number of instruments that are highly specialized. For example, the device in Figure 1-4 is a thermograph, that is, an infrared television monitor. An outgrowth of certain military technology, these infrared monitors are used for a variety of clinical purposes where surface heat on the skin might be an indicator. An oximeter is shown in Figure 1-5. This instrument noninvasively monitors the level of oxygen saturation in tissues.

At one time, the amount of equipment within the hospital was limited, so manufacturers' service departments were almost universally used as the sole service resource. But today, most hospitals of moderate size or larger have their own biomedical engineering department. These in-house staffs perform troubleshooting and repair service on "down" equipment—bringing it back into service in a short period of time. They also perform preventative maintenance chores that are required both for institutional licensure and accreditation, as well as the necessities of defending oneself against lawsuits involving supposedly failed equipment.

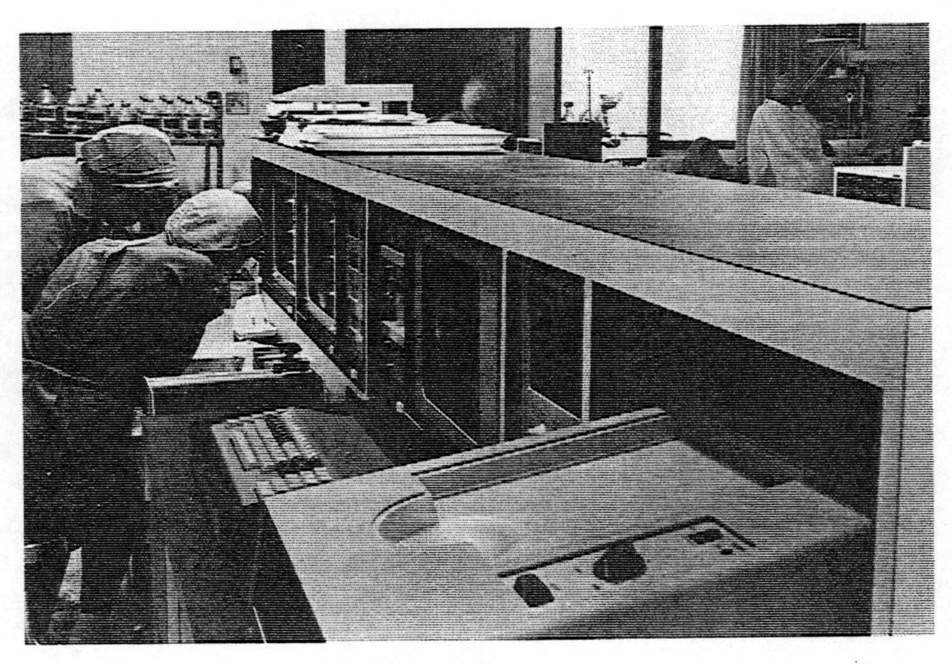

FIGURE 1-3

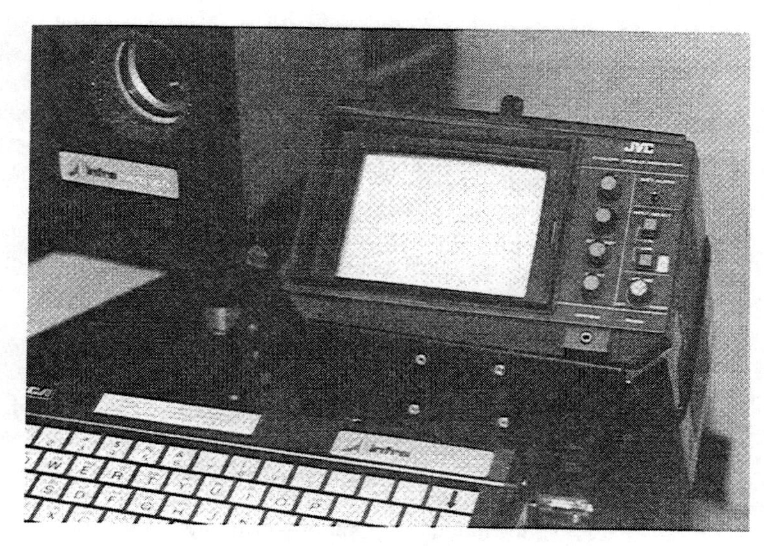

FIGURE 1-4

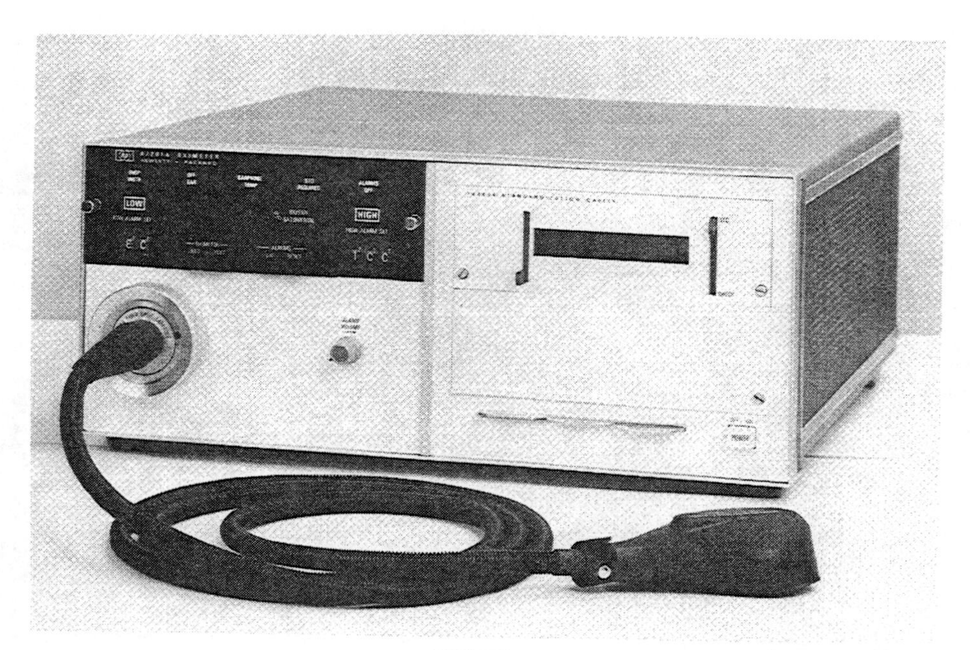

FIGURE 1-5

While the situation was once quite simple, the modern instrumentation and medical device scene is complex and not easily grasped in its entirety. Today, the hospital is equipped to the rafters with a large variety of very complex—often computer-based—medical devices. As a result, there is a need for both device literacy on the part of the medical and nursing staffs, but also specific training on the part of the technical staff that takes care of the devices.

Starting in May 1976, the U.S. Food and Drug Administration (FDA) began regulating medical devices in a manner not dissimilar to its regulation of drugs. Part of the impetus that brought Congress to pass the Medical Device Act of 1976 was a failure of many devices to provide either effective treatment or safe operation. Today, before a manufacturer can market a new product it must be submitted to the FDA for marketing approval. The maker must demonstrate that the device is safe and effective for the intended purpose and that the labeling is adequate for a qualified user to understand the operation, applications, and limitations of the device.

In the rest of this book you will be introduced to medical devices in greater detail than is possible in a simple overview chapter. For those readers who are only dimly aware of the central concepts of electronics, Chapter 2—on basic electronics—is offered as an introduction or "cultural literacy" effort.

2

Sensors for Biomedical Devices

Most medical electronic instruments require some sort of input signal that is, often as not, either generated in some form of sensor device (e.g., blood pressure) or acquired by a special-purpose electrode (e.g., ECG). In the several chapters of this book we will examine specific forms of biomedical transducers, sensors, and electrodes. Before beginning that discussion, however, it is useful to understand some basic definitions and concepts regarding these devices.

A *sensor* is any device that either acquires, or generates, an electrical signal that represents some physical phenomenon (e.g., pressure, bioelectric potentials, temperature, gas flow). The overall general class of sensors includes *electrodes* (such as the electrocardiograph electrodes) and *transducers* (such as a blood pressure sensor or rectal temperature sensor).

There is often an ambiguity regarding the use of the words *sensor* and *transducer*. A transducer, in our present context, is a data acquisition device that converts energy from one form to another for the purposes of diagnostic measurement, data collection, monitoring, or control. It serves to provide input signal to the electronic instrument, so the form of energy "converted to" is always electrical. Thus, a transducer is a device that converts energy from some physical parameter of interest to medical personnel (e.g., force, pressure, temperature, and flow) to an electrical potential or current that is either proportional to the applied physical parameter or somehow otherwise correlated to it.

But the word *transducer* also properly applies to certain output devices, such as the loudspeaker used in audio equipment, radios, and televisions, or the PMMC galvanometer in strip-chart recorders. In the context of this book, however, the output transducer is not applicable, so for simplicity's sake we limit definition (somewhat artificially) to those devices that provide input signals to instruments.

Because our definition of transducer is limited to those devices that provide input signals to electronic instruments, we can state that transducers are all sensors. Also included in the general category of sensors, however, are metallic electrodes (the ECG example) and any other device that picks up electrical signals for input to the instrument. For purposes of consistency, the word "sensor" will be used here unless some reason to use another word exists. In general, a sensor is a device that acts as a "sense organ . . . for electronic processing."[1]

TRANSDUCTION

In the class of sensors that are also transducers it is necessary to understand the linked concepts of *transduction* and *transducible property*. A transducible property is a characteristic of the physical event that is singularly able to represent that parameter and can be transformed into an electrical signal by some device or process. In an example given by Geddes and Baker,[2] we find that carbon dioxide (CO_2) absorbs electromagnetic wavelengths of 2.7, 4.3, and 14.7 microns. Although water also absorbs 2.7-micron radiation to a small degree, it is possible to make an infrared (IR) sensor that will respond to either 4.3 or 14.7 microns, or all three wavelengths, to measure CO_2 content of a gas such as air. End tidal CO_2 monitors, used in respiratory therapy, intensive care, and anesthesia, use infrared sensors. Transduction is the process of converting the transducible property into an electrical signal that can be input to an instrument.

PASSIVE VERSUS ACTIVE SENSORS

Another ambiguity found in discussions of biomedical sensors is the distinction between *passive sensors* and *active sensors*. Unfortunately, competing texts use exactly opposite definitions of these terms! This text adopts the form that is used by most people in the medical instruments field, which is also consistent with usage in other areas of electronics.

An *active sensor* is one that requires an external AC or DC electrical source to power the device. An example of the active sensor is the resistive strain gauge blood pressure sensor that requires a +7.5-V DC regulated power supply to operate. Without that external excitation potential, there is no output from the sensor.

A *passive sensor*, on the other hand, is one that provides either its own energy or derives its energy from the phenomenon being measured. An example of a passive sensor is the thermocouple (which is often used to measure temperature in research settings).

It is unfortunate that some textbook authors invert these definitions, but if the foregoing definitions are accepted, you will be consistent with the most common usage.

SENSOR ERROR SOURCES

Sensors, like all other devices, suffer from certain errors. In order to maintain consistency, an error is defined as the "difference between the measured value and the true value."[3] While the full range of possible errors is beyond the scope of this book, it is possible to break them into five basic categories: *insertion errors, application errors, characteristic errors, dynamic errors,* and *environmental errors*.

Insertion errors This class of error occurs when the act of inserting the sensor into the system is being measured. This problem arises with electronic measurements, indeed all measurements. For example, when measuring the voltage in a circuit one must be certain that the inherent impedance of the voltmeter is very much larger than the circuit impedance; otherwise circuit loading will occur—and the reading will be in significant error. Possible sources of this form of error include using a transducer that is too large for the system (e.g., pressures), one that is too sluggish for the dynamics of the system, or one that self-heats to the extent that excessive thermal energy is added to the system. Nineteenth-century British physicist Lord Kelvin formulated a "first rule of instrumentation" to the effect that "the measuring instrument must not alter the event being measured."

Application errors These errors are operator caused, that is, the proverbial "cockpit trouble" referred to by airplane mechanics. Again, far too many of these errors are possible, so we must settle on a couple of illustrative examples. One error seen in temperature measurements is either incorrect placement of the probe or erroneous insulation of the probe from the measurement site. This problem often occurs in clinical medicine when the sanitary cover over the probe of a digital thermometer is not properly seated. Other examples seen in blood pressure sensor applications include failure to purge the system of air and other gases ("bubbles in the line") and incorrect physical placement of the transducer (above or below the heart line) so that a positive or negative pressure head is erroneously added to the correct reading.

Characteristic errors This category is that which is most often meant when discussing errors without otherwise qualifying the term. These errors are those that are inherent in the device itself, that is, the difference between the ideal published characteristic transfer function of the device and the actual characteristic. This form of error may include a DC offset value (i.e., a false pressure head), an incorrect slope, or a slope that is not perfectly linear.

Dynamic errors Many sensors are characterized and calibrated in a static condition, that is, with an input parameter that is either static or quasi-static in nature. Many sensors are heavily damped, and so will not respond to rapid changes in the input parameter. For example, thermistors tend to require many seconds to respond to a step-function change in temperature. That is, a thermistor in equilibrium will not jump immediately to the new resistance on an abrupt change in temperature. But rather, the device will change slowly toward the new value. Thus, if an attempt is made to follow a rapidly changing temperature with a sluggish sensor, the output waveform will be distorted and therefore contains error. The issues to confront in respect to dynamic errors include response time, amplitude distortion, and phase distortion.

Environmental errors These errors are those which are derived from the environment in which the sensor is used. They most often involve temperature, but may also include vibration, shock, altitude, chemical exposure, or other factors. These factors most often affect the characteristic errors of the sensor, so are often lumped together with that category in practical application.

SENSOR TERMINOLOGY

Sensors, like other areas of technology, include their own terminology that must be understood before they can be properly applied. In the next section are some of the most common terms.

Sensitivity The sensitivity of the sensor is defined as the slope of the output characteristic curve (Y/X in Figure 2-1), or more generally, it is the *minimum input of physical parameter that will create a detectable output change*. In some sensors, the sensitivity is defined as the input parameter change required to produce a standardized output change. In still others, it is defined as an output voltage change for a given change in input parameter. For example, a typical blood pressure transducer may have a sensitivity rating of 10 μV/V/mmHg (millimeters of mercury); that is, there will be a 10-μV output voltage for each volt of excitation potential and each mmHg of applied pressure.

Sensitivity error The sensitivity error (shown as a dot-dash curve in Figure 2-1) is a departure from the ideal slope of the characteristic curve. For example, the pressure transducer discussed may have an actual sensitivity of 7.8 μV/V/mmHg instead of 10 μV/V/mmHg.

Range The range of the sensor is the maximum and minimum values of applied parameter that can be measured. For example, a given pressure sensor may have a range of −400 mmHg to +400 mmHg. Alternatively, it is often the case that the positive and negative ranges are unequal. For example, a certain medical blood pressure transducer is specified to have a minimum (i.e., vacuum) limit of −50 mmHg (Y_{min} in Figure 2-1) and a maximum (pressure) limit of +450 mmHg (Y_{max} in Figure 2-1). This specification is common, incidentally, and is one reason why doctors and nurses often destroy blood pressure sensors when attempting to draw blood through an arterial line without being mindful of the position of the fluid stopcocks in the system. A small syringe can exert a tremendous vacuum on a closed system!

Dynamic range The dynamic range is the total range of the sensor from minimum to maximum. That is, in terms of Figure 2-1, $R_{dyn} = Y_{max} - (-Y_{min})$.

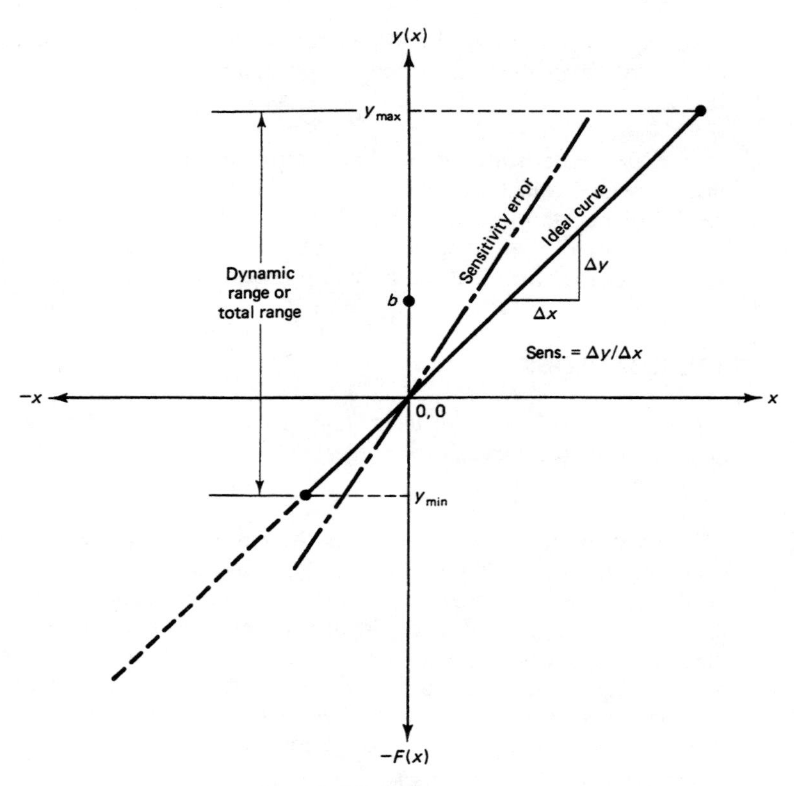

FIGURE 2-1

Precision The concept of precision refers to the degree of *reproducibility* of a measurement. In other words, if exactly the same value were measured a number of times, an ideal sensor would output exactly the same value every time. But real sensors output a range of values distributed in some manner relative to the actual correct value. For example, suppose a pressure of 150 mmHg, exactly, were applied to a sensor. Even if the applied pressure never changes, the output values from the sensor would vary considerably. Some subtle problems pop up in the matter of precision when the true value and the sensor's mean value are not within a certain distance of each other (e.g., the 1-σ range of the normal distribution curve).

Resolution This specification is the smallest detectable incremental change of input parameter that can be detected in the output signal. Resolution can be expressed as either a proportion of the reading (or the full-scale reading) or in absolute terms.

Accuracy The accuracy of the sensor is the maximum difference that will exist between the actual value (which must be measured by a primary or good secondary standard) and the indicated value at the output of the sensor. Again, the accuracy can be expressed as either a percentage of full-scale or in absolute terms.

Offset The offset error of a transducer is defined as the output that will exist when it should be zero, or alternatively, the difference between the actual output value and the specified output value under some particular set of conditions. An example of the first situation in terms of Figure 2-1 would exist if the characteristic curve had the same sensitivity slope as the ideal, but crossed the Y axis (i.e., output) at b instead of zero. An example of the other form of offset is seen in the characteristic curve of a pH electrode shown in Figure 2-2. The ideal curve will exist only at one temperature (usually 25°C), while the actual curve will between the Min. Temp. and Max. Temp limits depending on the temperature of the sample and electrode.

Linearity The linearity of the transducer is an expression of the extent to which the actual measured curve of a sensor departs from the ideal curve. Figure 2-3 shows a somewhat exaggerated relationship between the ideal, or least squares fit,

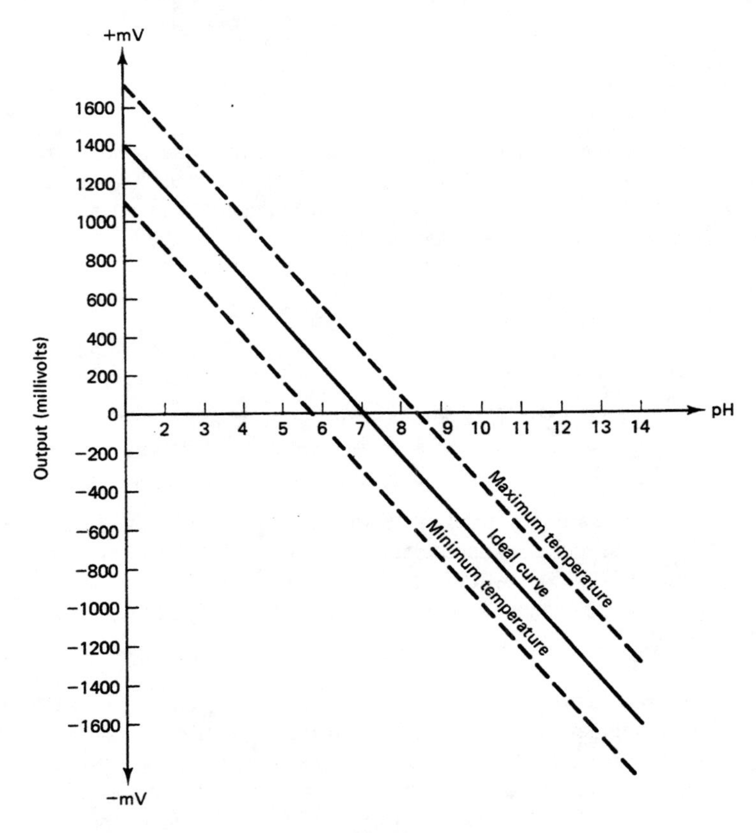

FIGURE 2-2

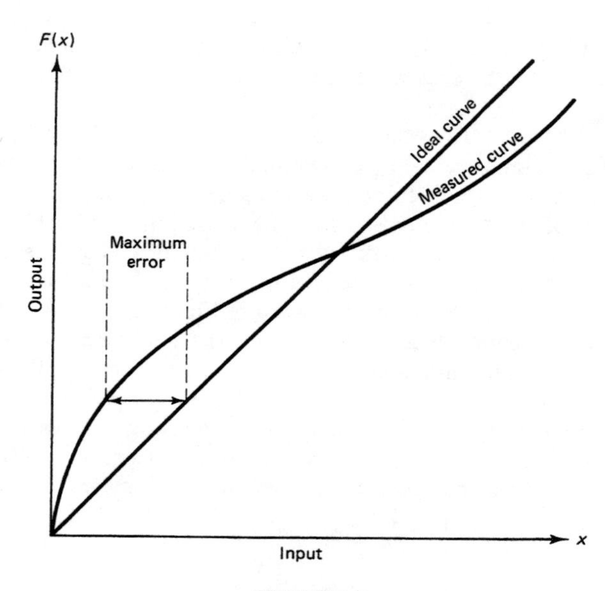

FIGURE 2-3

line and the actual measured or "calibration" line. (Note: In most cases, it is the static curve that is used to determine linearity, and this may deviate somewhat from a dynamic linearity.) Linearity is often specified in terms of *percentage of nonlinearity,* which is defined as

$$\text{nonlinearity}(\%) = \frac{D_{in(max)}}{In_{f.s.}} \times 100 \tag{2-1}$$

Where

$\text{nonlinearity}(\%)$ = the percentage of nonlinearity
$D_{in(max)}$ = the maximum input deviation
$In_{f.s.}$ = the maximum, full-scale input

The static nonlinearity defined by Equation 2-1 is often subject to environmental factors, including temperature, vibration, acoustical noise level, humidity, and so forth. It is important to know under what conditions the specification is valid—and departures from those conditions may not yield linear changes of linearity (pun not intended).

Hysteresis A transducer should be capable of following the changes of the input parameter regardless of which direction the change is made; hysteresis is the measure of this property. Figure 2-4 shows a typical hysteresis curve. Note that it matters from which *direction* the change is made. Approaching a fixed input value (e.g., point B in Figure 2-4) from a higher value (e.g., point P) will result in a different indication than approaching the same value from a lesser value (point Q or

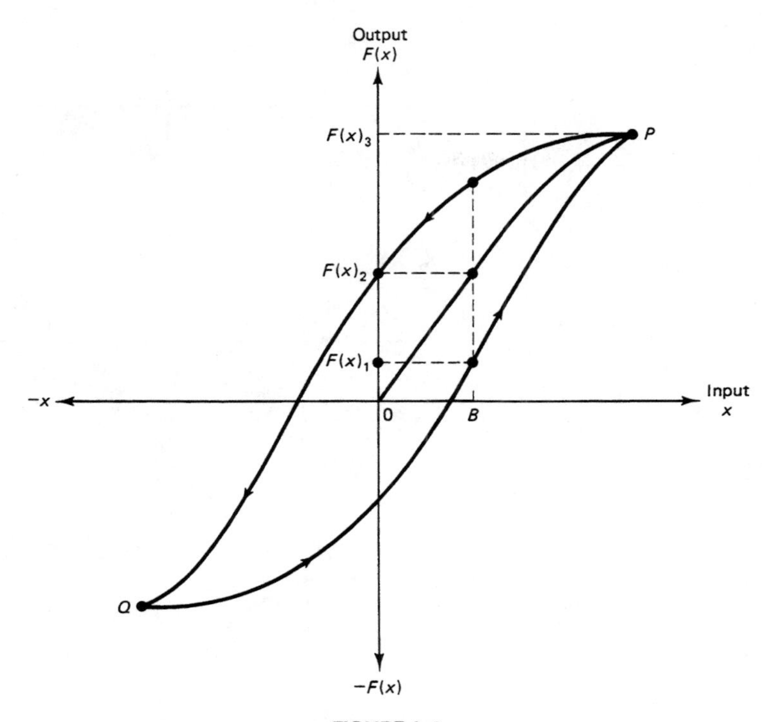

FIGURE 2-4

zero). Note that input value B can be represented by $F(X)_1$, $F(X)_2$, or $F(X)_3$, depending on the immediate previous value—clearly an error due to hysteresis.

Response time Sensors do not change output state immediately when an input parameter change occurs. But rather, it will change to the new state over a period of time, called the response time (T_r in Figure 2-5). The response time can be defined as the *time required for a sensor output to change from its previous state to a final settled value within a tolerance band of the correct new value*. This concept is somewhat different from the notion of the *time constant* (T) of the system. This term can be defined in a manner similar to a capacitor charging through a resistance and is usually less than the response time.

The curves in Figure 2-5 show two types of response time. In Figure 2-5A the curve represents the response time following an abrupt positive going step-function change of the input parameter. The form shown in Figure 2-5B is a decay time (T_d to distinguish from T_r, for they are not always the same) in response to a negative-going step-function change of the input parameter.

Dynamic linearity The dynamic linearity of the sensor is a measure of its ability to follow rapid changes in the input parameter. Amplitude distortion characteristics, phase distortion characteristics, and response time are important in deter-

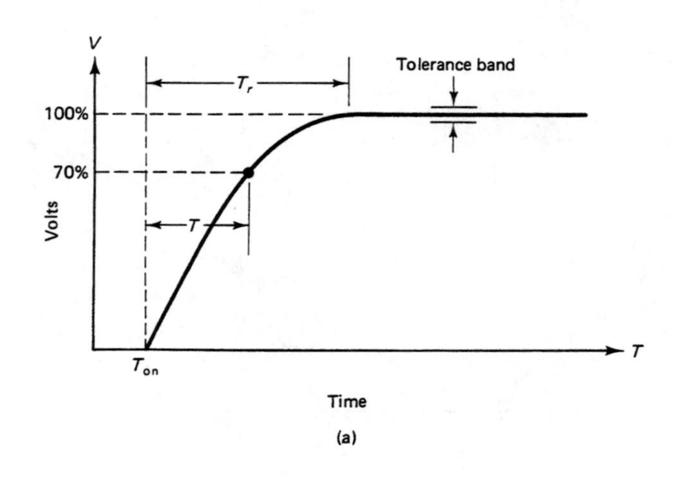

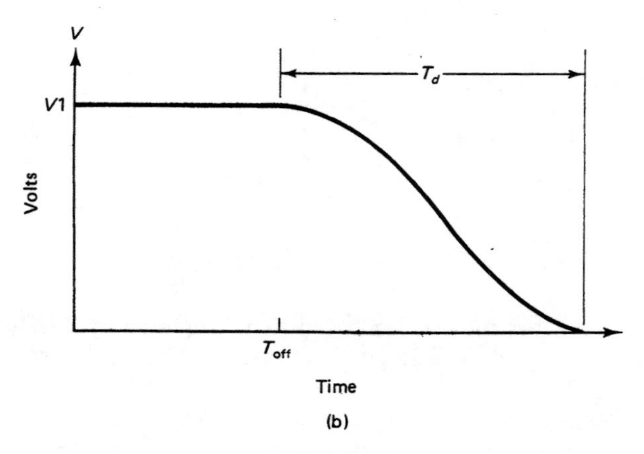

FIGURE 2-5

mining dynamic linearity. Given a system of low hysteresis (always desirable), the amplitude response is represented by

$$F(X) = aX + bX^2 + cX^3 + dX^4 + eX^5 + \cdots + K \qquad (2\text{-}2)$$

In Equation 2-2, the term $F(X)$ is the output signal, while the X terms represent the input parameter and its harmonics, and K is an offset constant (if any). The harmonics become especially important when the error harmonics generated by the sensor action fall into the same frequency bands as the natural harmonics produced by the dynamic action of the input parameter. All continuous waveforms are represented by a Fourier series of a fundamental sine wave and its harmonics. In the case of any nonsinusoidal waveform (including time-varying changes of a physical parameter), there will be harmonics present, which can be affected by the action of the sensor.

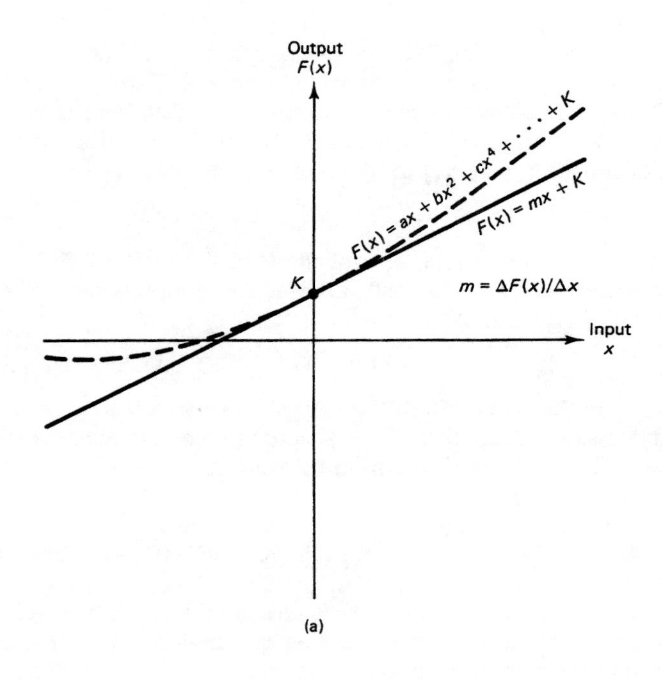
Output
F(x)
F(x) = ax + bx² + cx⁴ + . . . + K
F(x) = mx + K
K
m = ΔF(x)/Δx
Input
x

(a)

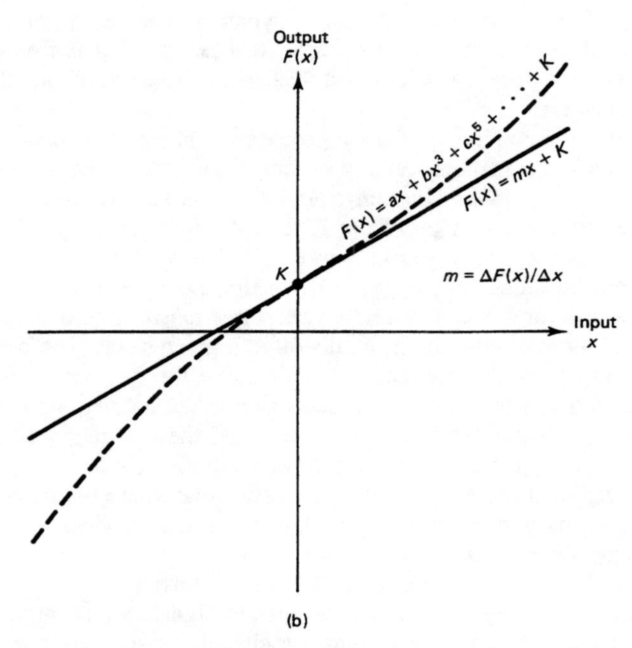
Output
F(x)
F(x) = ax + bx³ + cx⁵ + . . . + K
F(x) = mx + K
K
m = ΔF(x)/Δx
Input
x

(b)

FIGURE 2-6

The nature of the nonlinearity of the calibration curve (Figures 2-6A and 2-6B) tell something about which harmonics are present. In the case of Figure 2-6A, the calibration curve (shown as a dashed line) is *asymmetrical,* so only *odd* harmonic terms exist. Assuming a form for the ideal curve of $F(X) = mX + K$, Equation 2-2 becomes for the symmetrical case

$$F(X) = aX + bX^2 + cX^4 + \cdots + K \tag{2-3}$$

In the other type of calibration curve (Figure 2-6B), the indicated values are *symmetrical* about the ideal $mX + K$ curve. In this case, $F(X) = -F(-X)$, and the form of Equation 2-2 is

$$F(X) = aX + bX^3 + cX^5 + \cdots + K \tag{2-4}$$

In the section to follow we will take a look at some of the tactics and signals processing criteria that can be adapted to biomedical applications to improve the nature of the data collected from the sensor.

TACTICS AND SIGNALS PROCESSING FOR IMPROVED SENSING

The selection of sensors and the circuits that are connected to them can go a long way toward ensuring that the data acquired will accurately represent the physical phenomenon or event being detected.

For proper operation in a dynamic input environment, the sensor selected should have a flat response curve, that is, one that is free of amplitude distortion, phase distortion (which almost invariably causes amplitude distortion), "ringing," or resonances.

An implication of these problems concerns the *frequency response* of the sensor and its signals processing system. Figure 2-7A shows a perfectly linear system in which the gain[4] is constant over the entire spectrum of frequencies, that is, in an ideal theoretical system from "DC to daylight" and beyond. But real systems do not have such characteristics. Figure 2-7B shows the type of frequency response that might be found on real systems. In this example, the gain is flat between two frequencies, and over this region the performance is similar to the ideal case. But beyond these points, the gain falls off at a given slope. The breakpoint that defines the flat region is, by convention, taken to be the frequencies (F_L and F_H) at which the gain falls off to 70.7 percent of its gain in the flat region. These points are known as the −6-dB points in voltage systems and the −3-dB points in power systems.

When the frequency response is not entirely flat, one can expect to find phase distortion. Figure 2-7C shows the situations where the phase shift of the system is a linear function of frequency (solid line) and also where it is a nonlinear function of frequency (dashed line).

We can see the effects of phase distortion in a somewhat simplistic sense in Figure 2-8. Figure 2-8A is the applied signal, for example, the output of an ideal sensor in response to step-function changes of the measured input parameter. If the signals processing electronics and the sensor mechanism itself are perfectly ideal,

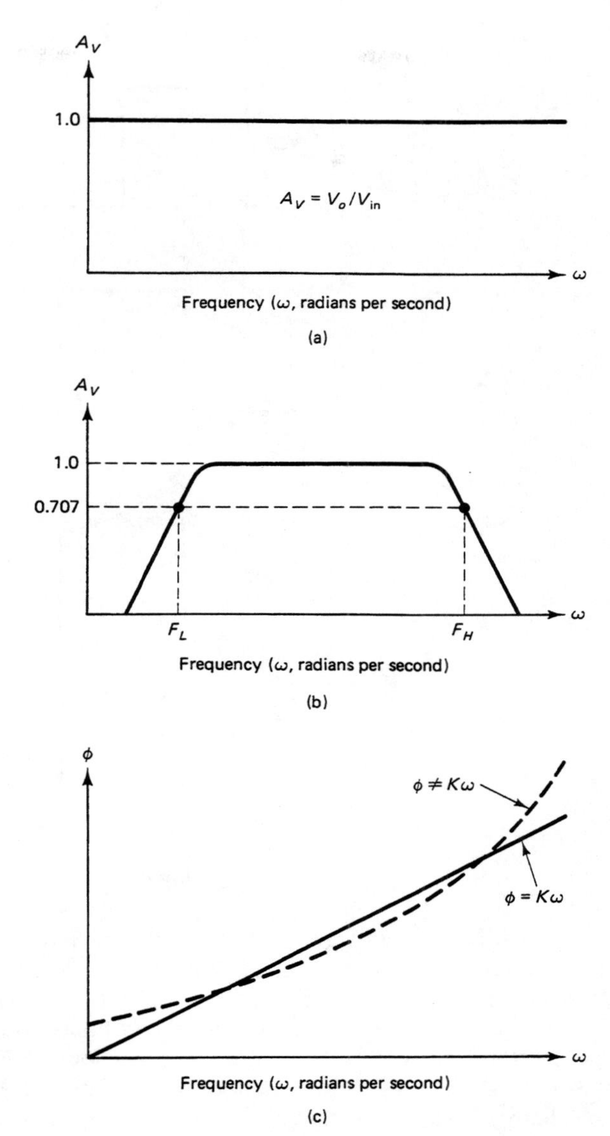

FIGURE 2-7

then the only effect of the change will be displacement in time (t), as shown in Figure 2-8B. There will be no distortion of the shape of the wave. But in the presence of phase distortion, the wave will not only be time displaced, but also distorted. Figures 2-8C and 2-8D show two forms of distortion that can occur with phase nonlinearity.

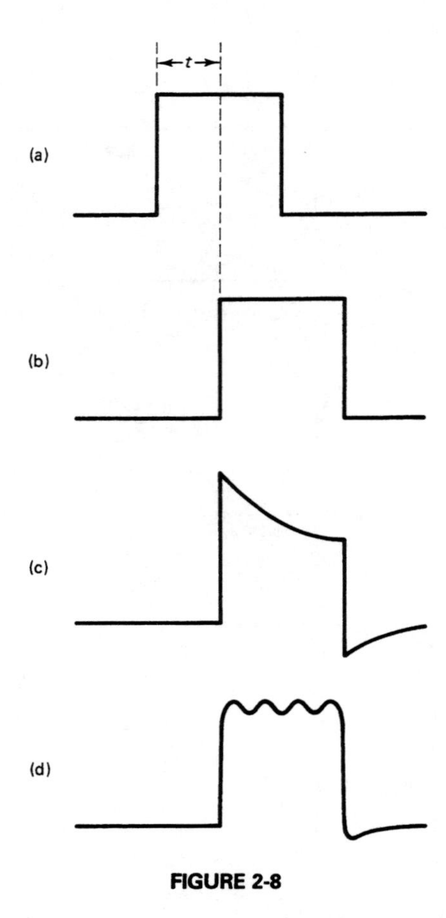

FIGURE 2-8

A slightly different view of the same phenomenon is shown in Figures 2-9 and 2-10. Consider a system in which the bandwidth can be varied across several limits, represented by curves *a*, *b*, and *c* in Figure 2-9. Curve *c* represents the most restrictive of the three possibilities because it sharply limits both low- and high-frequency response, while curve *a* is the least restrictive. Note in Figure 2-10 the various responses to the three bandwidths represented in Figure 2-9.

These curves can be simulated by examining the response to square waves in RC filter networks. In fact, one of the problems that one must consider when using electronic filters is the effects of the −6-dB points on the applied waveform.

One might erroneously assume from the foregoing discussion that the instrument designer should select amplifiers with as wide a bandwidth as possible. That is not the case, however, because bandwidth can cause other problems at least as severe as those that are solved. Noise, for example, is proportional to bandwidth. It is possible to eliminate the problems of noise, plus certain input signal problems

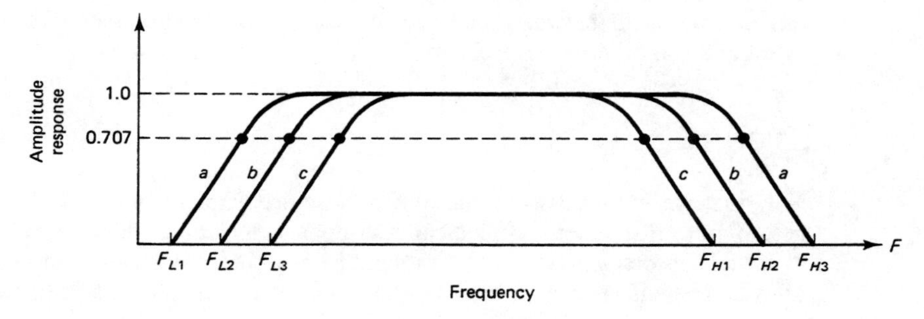

FIGURE 2-9

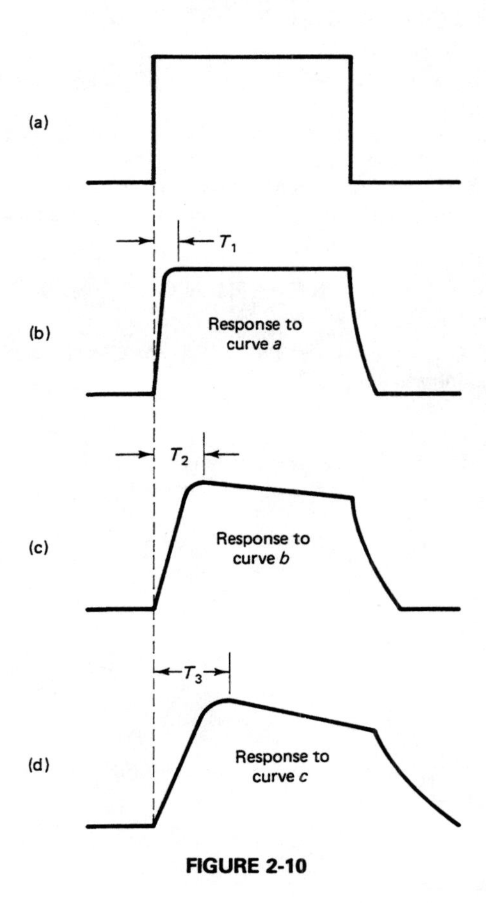

FIGURE 2-10

such as ringing or resonances by proper selection of the frequency response cutoff points. Thus, the selection of amplifier bandwidth and phase distortion characteristics is a trade-off between the need to make a high-fidelity recording of the input event and the other other problems that can occur in the system.

CONCLUSION

Now that we've discussed some of the basic problems of biomedical sensors, let's get down to discussions of medical instruments, including those in which examples of actual sensors are used. The treatment here is not exhaustive—indeed such would fill a number of very large books—but is intended, instead, to be representative.

RECOMMENDATIONS FOR FURTHER READING

1. Richard S. C. Cobbold. *Transducers for Biomedical Applications*. New York: John Wiley, 1974.
2. L. A. Geddes and L. E. Baker. *Principles of Applied Biomedical Instrumentation*. New York: John Wiley, 1968.
3. Joseph J. Carr and John M. Brown. *Introduction to Biomedical Equipment Technology*. New York: John Wiley, 1981. Acquired and republished by Prentice Hall (1989).

REFERENCES AND NOTES

1. L. A. Geddes and L. E. Baker, *Principles of Applied Biomedical Instrumentation* (New York: John Wiley, 1968).
2. Ibid.
3. Ibid.

4. Gain is defined as the ratio of the output function to input function. Because voltage gain (A_v) is used here for illustration purposes, the gain is V_o/V_{in}.

3

Medical and Laboratory Oscilloscopes

The *cathode ray oscilloscope* (CRO), also called either *oscilloscope* or simply *'scope,* is an instrument that uses a beam of electrons to "paint" a light picture on a phosphorous screen. If vertical (*Y*) and horizontal (*X*) directions each represent a different signal, then the pattern traced on the CRO viewing screen represents the relationship between the two signals. This principle is used in medical instruments such as the *vectorcardioscope*. Although differences exist between clinical medical, research laboratory, and medical instrument service shop oscilloscopes, the similarities are so great as to make it best to examine all forms in the same chapter.

Briefly restated, an oscilloscope is an instrument which uses a cathode ray tube (CRT), a device similar to a television picture tube, to display a voltage waveform. The waveform might be amplitude versus time, or it might be a complex thing that compares two amplitudes. The CRT is designed such that a beam of electrons from an "electron gun" will strike the phosphor-coated viewing screen (Figure 3-1), leaving a spot of light wherever the beam strikes. The beam can be deflected either magnetically or electrostatically, but for service, workbench, and laboratory-type oscilloscopes used in electronics, only electrostatic deflection is used. Television receivers (and some medical patient monitor 'scopes) use a magnetic deflection CRT in which a "yoke" electromagnet around the electron path in the neck of the CRT forms the controlling magnetic field. The frequency response and nonlinearity of magnetic

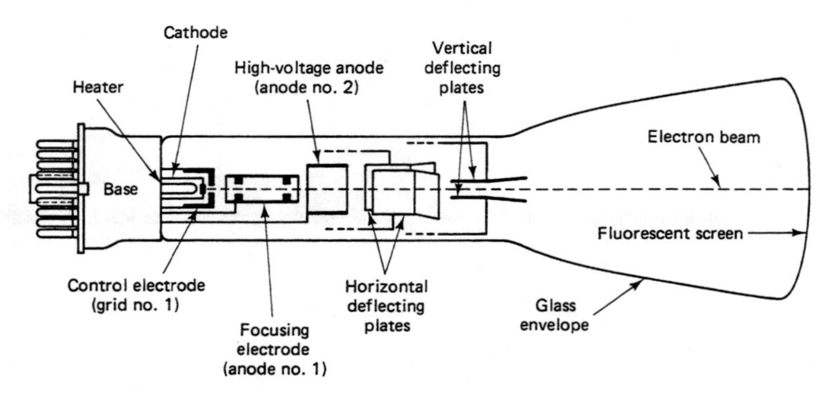

FIGURE 3-1

deflection makes it unsuitable for oscilloscope use at frequencies above a couple hundred hertz.

Electrostatic deflection CRTs use a pair of *deflection plates* (as in Figure 3-1) to deflect the electron beam in the vertical and horizontal directions. Figure 3-2 shows how the beam on the screen of the CRT moves under different situations. In Figure 3-2A the beam is centered, which fact indicates that the voltages across the deflection plates are balanced (or zero). The beam is traveling straight down the neck of the CRT and striking the screen in the center. In Figure 3-2B, however, the vertical plates remain balanced, while the horizontal plates are unbalanced such that the left side is now more positive (or less negative) than the right side; thus, the beam (and light spot) is yanked to the left. Similarly, in Figure 3-2C we see the situation where the horizontal plates are balanced or zero, and the vertical plates are unbalanced. In this case the top vertical plate is more positive (or less negative) than the bottom plate. In Figures 3-2D and 3-2E we see situations where both sets of plates are unbalanced, so the beam is deflected up and to the right in Figure 3-2D and down and to the right in Figure 3-2E.

If a sawtooth waveform is applied between the horizontal deflection plates, then the beam will sweep left to right, forming a time base (Figure 3-3). If a time-varying input signal is applied across the vertical plates, then the electron beam will trace the waveshape on the CRT screen.

Similarly, instruments called "X-Y oscilloscopes" apply input signals to both horizontal and vertical deflection plates to form a vector pattern that allows us to discern the relationship between them. Such diagrams are called "Lissajous patterns" (see Figure 3-4). Color TV repair shops, cable TV operators, and TV broadcast studios use X-Y 'scopes, as do medical instrument manufacturers.

You can measure audio frequencies with the Lissajous pattern. The ratio of the number of loops along the vertical and horizontal sides of the pattern tell you the relationship between frequencies applied to vertical and horizontal inputs (Figure 3-4).

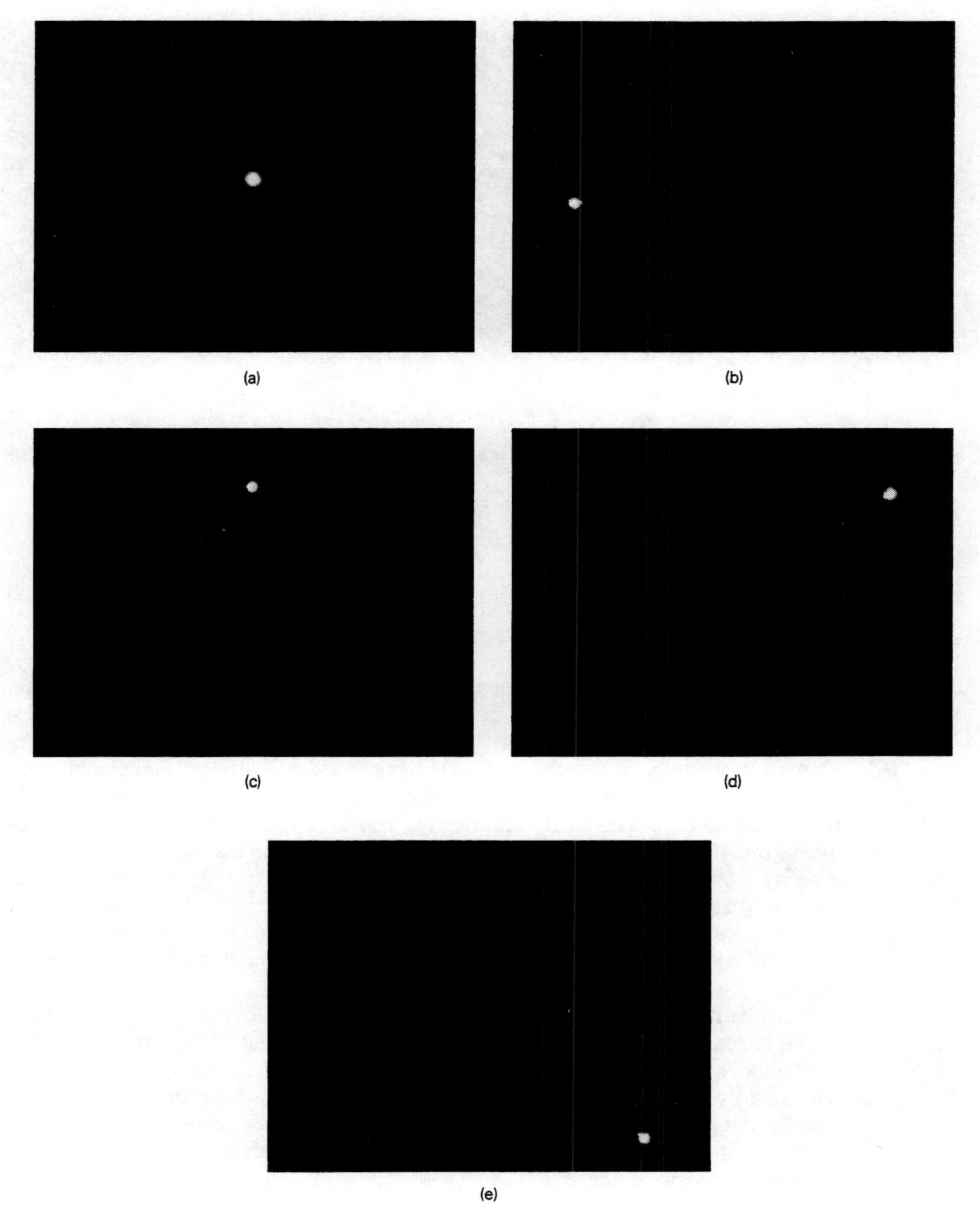

FIGURE 3-2

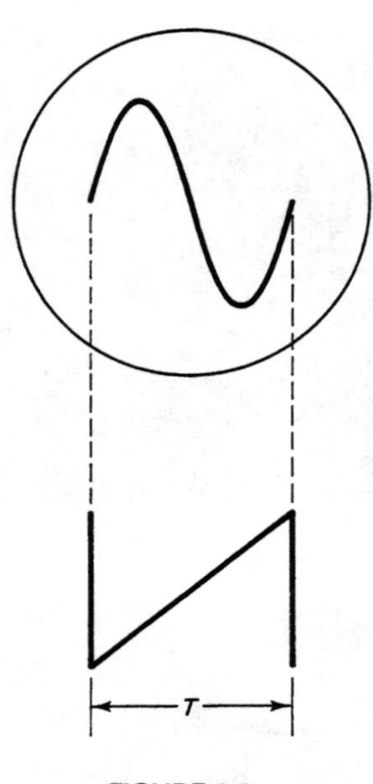

FIGURE 3-3

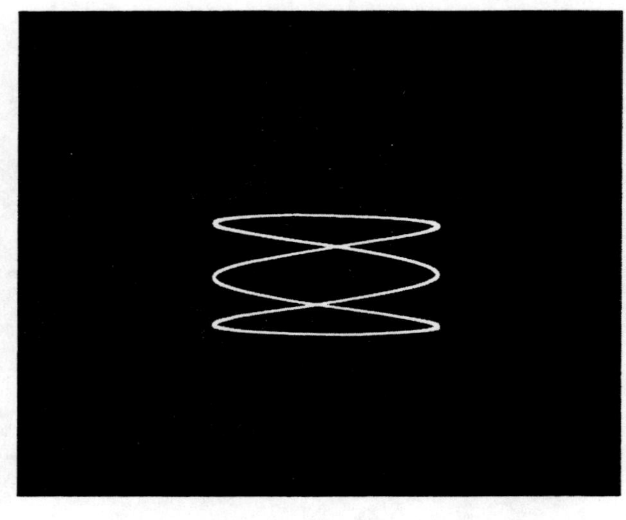

FIGURE 3-4

SOME OSCILLOSCOPE EXAMPLES

At one time only a few service shops could afford a high-performance oscilloscope. Today, however, nearly all users have their choice of good-quality, high-frequency, models that vary from cheap to backbreaking in cost. Even top-name 'scopes are no longer extremely out of reach when you compare the cost of other equipment.

Figure 3-5 shows a low-cost oscilloscope intended for service shop applications. Like all modern oscilloscopes, this one is a triggered sweep model. This means that the beam does not start to sweep left to right across the CRT screen until a signal is present in the amplifier. By controlling the sweep triggering point we can control what part of the waveform is examined. Note that the CRT screen on the left side of the instrument has a graticule grid inscribed on the face. The divisions (usually 1 cm each) are used to measure voltages and times, which we will discuss more later.

Older model oscilloscopes were not triggered sweep. In those models, the horizontal deflection of the beam was asynchronous with respect to the input signal. The horizontal sweep controls were calibrated roughly in units of frequency, that is, the number of times per second the beam swept left to right. Such instruments are of limited usefulness today. Most of them have a low-frequency vertical amplifier bandwidth, so therefore cannot display many of the signals that are of interest to the modern electronics enthusiast.

The CRO in Figure 3-5 is a *dual trace* model. These instruments were once rare and expensive and only available in the highest-priced model lines. But today

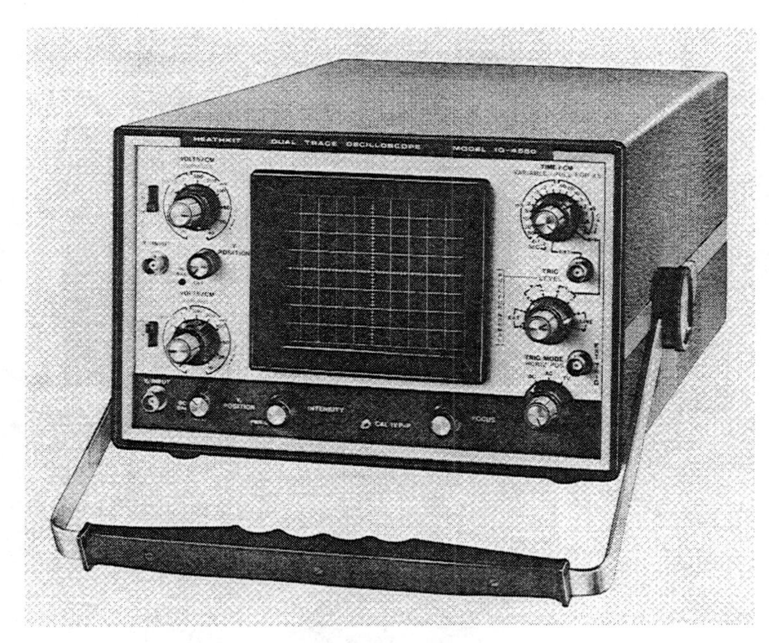

FIGURE 3-5

manufacturers can offer dual trace models in their most modest lines, so the instruments are now quite common. There are two separate vertical inputs on these CROs, so two separate signals can be viewed simultaneously against the same time base (Figure 3-6). The two *position* controls can be adjusted to either superimpose (Figure 3-6A) or separate the two input signals (Figure 3-6B). Dual-trace capability is extremely useful for examining the time relationship between two signals, or comparing them with each other on a point-by-point basis. Another application is in troubleshooting. For example, dual trace CROs can be used to examine the input and output signals of a circuit to determine which is malfunctioning.

Vertical bandwidth is a specification of much interest in selecting an oscilloscope. At one time, high-frequency vertical amplifiers were available only in the costliest engineering laboratory-grade instruments. For example, in the mid-1960s one expected to pay $4000 for a 35-MHz, two-channel oscilloscope (and those were $4000 before inflation). But today, we can buy 35-MHz 'scopes for less than $1000 and 100-MHz models are only about $2300. As a general rule, valid for most cases, select a model with as high a vertical bandwidth as you can afford. It is difficult to go wrong with too much vertical bandwidth, but too little can cost you capability.

Of course, even though domestic and imported models make it easy to obtain performance at low cost, it is still possible to spend big bucks for a really fine laboratory-model oscilloscope.

Now we will briefly describe typical controls found on a modern oscilloscope and give you some insight as to how they function. Keep in mind that not all 'scopes

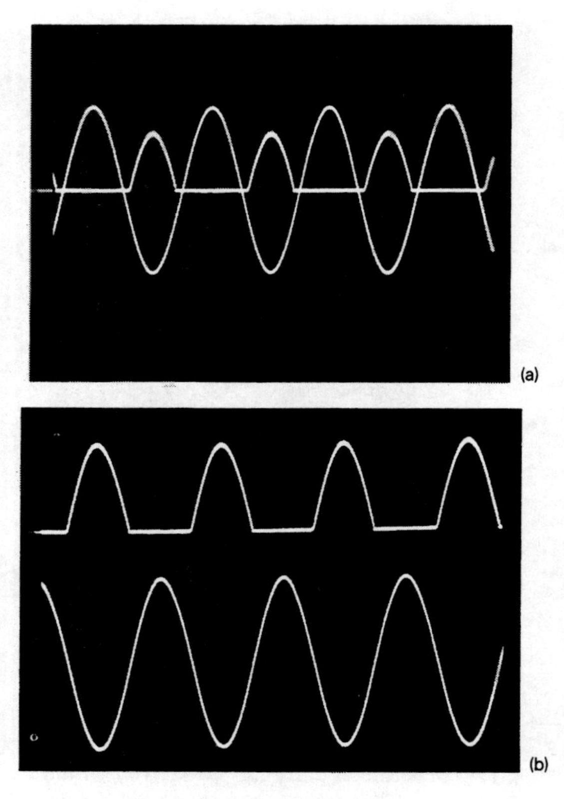

FIGURE 3-6

have all of the controls, especially some of those in the specialized triggered sweep system that the selected model offers. Also, on some models the same controls may carry slightly different names on the labels, but function pretty much the same. We will divide the controls into the following groups: *control, vertical, horizontal,* and *triggering*.

CONTROL GROUP

The controls group (some of which may appear on the rear of the 'scope), Figure 3-7, includes the on-off (power), intensity, focus, astigmatism, illumination, trace rotation, beam finder, and internal calibration signals. These controls operate as follows:

On-off/power The power control turns the instrument on and off; it is the AC main power switch (or battery switch in portable models). In some 'scopes, the on-off switch is part of another control (usually *intensity*), similar to the on-off

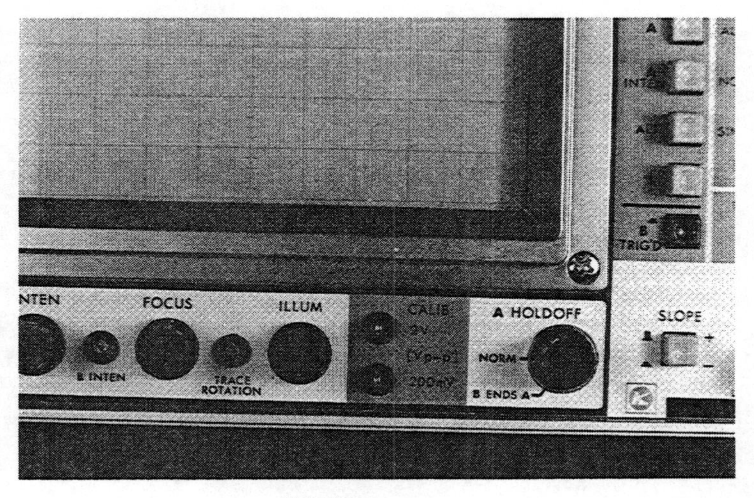

FIGURE 3-7

switch on a radio being ganged to the volume control. In other 'scopes, perhaps on most modern models, the on-off switch is a separate entity. Although on older models it may have been a toggle or rotary switch, on most 'scopes today it is a push-button switch.

Intensity The intensity control controls the brightness of the CRT beam. As a general rule, keep the intensity control just high enough to see the entire waveform comfortably. If the same waveform is expected to remain on the CRT screen for a long time (or there is no waveform), then keep the intensity low in order to prevent burning of the CRT phosphor.

Focus This control adjusts the size of the electron beam spot on the CRT screen. It is often interactive with the astigmatism control.

Astigmatism This control adjusts the "roundness" of the CRT spot, and is often interactive with the focus control. A good way to adjust the astigmatism control is to set it for a uniform line thickness when the CRT is swept horizontally (but no signal is present in the vertical channel). On many 'scopes, the astigmatism control is a screwdriver adjustment available on either the front or rear panel, while the focus control is knob adjustable on the front panel.

Illumination The illumination control adjusts a lamp that lights up the graticule lines inscribed on the CRT screen. At the lowest settings of this control no light appears on the graticule. Care must be used with this control when photographing the CRT screen, as the graticule lighting can overexpose the ASA 3000 film typically used in 'scope cameras.

Trace rotation Also called *trace align* on some models, this screwdriver adjustment compensates for the effects of local magnetic fields on the CRT trace. This control is adjusted so that the CRT beam is horizontal with respect to the graticule.

Beam finder This control disconnects the horizontal and vertical inputs, so that the beam collapses to a spot of higher intensity than the original trace. It helps the operator locate the beam, which may be off the screen at times.

Calibration The calibration control provides a standard signal to calibrate the vertical amplifier controls. Typically, such signals are 400 or 1000 Hz, either 1 volt or 2 volts peak to peak. In some cases it is a sine wave, in others a square wave. In the model shown in Figure 3-7, the 1000-Hz squarewave has both 2-V and 200-mV levels.

VERTICAL GROUP

The vertical group controls the vertical position of the beam, amplification factor and input selection of the oscilloscope. Controls in this group (Figure 3-8) include *input, input selector, position, step attenuator, vernier (variable) attenuator,*

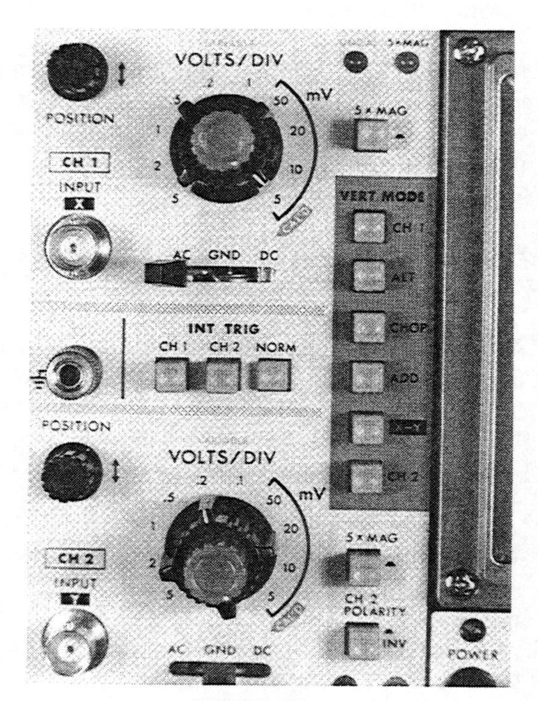

FIGURE 3-8

ground, 5X magnification, channel-2 polarity, and *vertical mode*. Also shown in Figure 3-8 is an internal trigger selector (INT TRIG), which is technically part of the trigger control group (its purpose is to select the channel that supplies the triggering signal).

Input connector The input connector is the point at which signal is applied from the external world to the oscilloscope vertical amplifier. In the model shown in Figure 3-8 the input connector is a coaxial BNC-style chassis-mounted connector. This form of connector by that means synchronizes the depolarization of the ventricle muscle cells. This contraction occurs when the ventricles are about full and forces blood out of the ventricles into circulation. From the right ventricle, blood is forced into the lungs (to take on oxygen) and then into the left atrium where the process is repeated. Blood forced out of the left ventricle goes to body circulation.

Physicians and scientists use a vector system to examine the heart biopotentials from a system of surface electrodes. In the classical ECG system, the physician will record differential signals that use the right leg (RL) as the common reference point (see Figure 4-4A). Electrical signal vectors are picked up at points such as the chest (six different points), left arm (LA), right arm (RA), and left leg (LL). In addition, certain modern computer-based recording systems look at an XYZ coordinate system that looks at vectors that run from head to toe, center of chest to center of back, and left flank to right flank.

Figure 4-4B shows the classical vector system used in ordinary ECG recording (disregarding the XYZ system and chest leads V1–V6). This illustration is a frontal view showing the axis and directions of the six major nonchest vectors. In medical terminology, these vectors are called "leads." In a moment we will examine the details of acquiring these signals electronically. But first, let's look at a typical lead I ECG signal in order to appreciate a little about what is going on.

Figure 4-4C shows the lead I ECG signal with the various signal as the standard on modern oscilloscopes. On older 'scopes, the input connector might be an SO-239 female UHF coaxial connector or even a pair of five-way binding posts spaced on 0.75-in. centers. Because most modern probes and 'scope accessories are now BNC-equipped, owners of older models usually opt to buy either an SO239-to-BNC or post-to-BNC adapter (as appropriate).

Input selector This switch is marked "AC-GND-DC" and is used to select the coupling of the input connector to the input of the vertical amplifier. The "DC" setting means that the connector is DC (direct current) coupled to the amplifier input; the "AC" setting means that a blocking capacitor is in series with the connector center conductor (hence only AC signals will pass—DC is blocked); in the "GND" setting, the input of the vertical amplifier is shorted to ground and the input connector center conductor is open circuited ("GND" does *not* ground the input connector, which would short-circuit the signal source!).

Position The position controls move the electron beam up and down on the CRT face. On a dual-trace 'scope, the two vertical position controls are normally used to prevent overlapping of the two traces (and resultant confusion). Otherwise, the control can be used to position precisely the trace over the graticule markings for amplitude measurements. It is common practice, for example, to set the AC-GND-DC input selector to "GND" and then use the position control to set the straight-line trace over either the bottommost or center graticule line, which then becomes the zero-volts reference point.

Step attenuator The sensitivity of the oscilloscope amplifier is a measure of its gain, and is expressed in terms of the voltage required to deflect the CRT beam a specified amount, that is, volts/division (or volts/cm). The step attenuator (see close-up in Figure 3-9) is a resistor/capacitor voltage divider that allows the instrument to accommodate higher potentials that would otherwise overdeflect the CRT beam. Each position of the step attenuator is calibrated in volts or millivolts per division (V/div or mV/div). The actual peak-to-peak voltage measure of the input signal is made by noting how many CRT screen divisions the signal occupies, and then multiplying that figure by the sensitivity factor in volts per division. For example, suppose a sine wave signal occupies 5.6 divisions peak to peak when the step attenuator is set to 0.2 V/div. The peak-to-peak voltage is (5.6 div) × (0.2 V/div) = 1.12 volts (i.e., 1120 mV).

Vernier attenuator This variable control is concentric to (in the center of) the step attenuator and allows continuously variable adjustment of the sensitivity factor (hence also trace vertical size). The calibration of the step attenuator is valid only when the vernier attenuator is in the CAL'D (also called CAL) position, which on most 'scopes is detented for easy location. When the vernier control is not in the

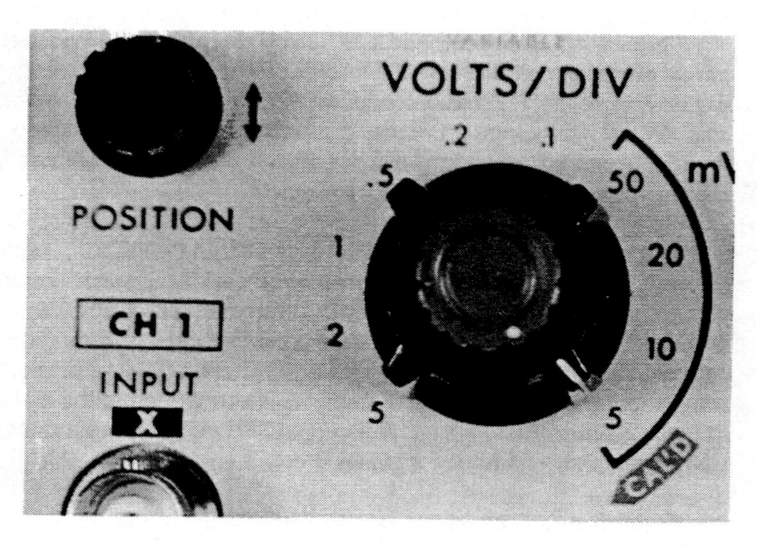

FIGURE 3-9

CAL'D position, a red UNCAL lamp on the front panel warns the operator that the step attenuator settings are not to be trusted.

Ground This ground jack is connected to the chassis ground at the input of the vertical amplifiers. It can be used to provide a proper "star" ground in order to eliminate (or prevent) ground loop errors.

5× Mag The 5× magnification control increases the sensitivity factor by five times, which means that all the volts-per-division and millivolts-per-division calibrations must be divided by 5. For example, when volts/div knob is in the 50-mV/div position and the "5× MAG" button is pressed, a "5× MAG" light turns on to warn the operator, and the sensitivity increases fivefold (i.e., 10 mV/div in the example case). This feature is especially useful when dealing with low-level signals that are ordinarily below the threshold of the normal settings, so effectively doubles the number of available sensitivity factors.

Channel-2 polarity The polarity control inverts the channel-2 vertical signal when pressed. If left unoperated, the polarity of the signal on the screen from channel 2 is normal. This control allows us to have a pseudodifferential input on a single-ended 'scope (see ADD control following).

Vertical mode This control forms a subgroup that includes the following: CH1, ALT, CHOP, ADD, X-Y, and CH2 submodes. These are as follows:

CH1, CH2 Selects the single-channel mode. When "CH1" is pressed, the 'scope operates as a single-channel model and displays only the channel-1 signal. When "CH2" is pressed, only the channel-2 signal is examined.

ALT, CHOP These are dual-channel modes. There is only one electron beam in the CRT, and it must be shared between the channels. In the ALT mode, the channel-2 trace does not start until the channel-1 sweep is finished. In other words, the 'scope alternates between the two signals. In the CHOP mode, the electron beam is switched back and forth rapidly between channel-1 and channel-2. The input signal must have a frequency that is very much less than the chopping frequency.

Add The signals are combined into one, with the resultant amplitude being the algebraic sum of the two channels (CH1 + CH2). If the CH2 polarity control is pressed, then the inputs become pseudodifferential and the summation is CH1 − CH2.

X-Y In this mode the internal oscilloscope time base is disconnected and the instrument becomes a vectorscope. Channel 1 becomes a horizontal ("X") input, while channel 2 is the vertical ("Y") input. In this mode, the oscilloscope can be used for modulation measurements, color TV Lissajous patterns, and so forth.

HORIZONTAL GROUP

The horizontal control group (Figure 3-10A) determines the horizontal deflection and sweep characteristics. These controls consist of *sweep time, sweep vernier, horizontal position, 10× MAG,* and *sweep mode*. These are as follows:

Sweep time This is the main horizontal timing control and is used to determine the amount of time required per division to sweep the beam across the CRT face left to right. The calibration of this control is in units of time per division (sec/div, mS/div, or μS/div). The period of a signal can be determined from this control and the number of divisions occupied by one cycle of the signal. For example, if exactly one cycle of a sine wave occupies 6.2 divisions of the horizontal graticule, and the switch setting is 2 mS/div, then the period of the signal is (6.2 div) × (2 mS/div) = 12.4 milliseconds. Because frequency is the reciprocal of period, we can calculate the frequency as $F = 1/T = 1/0.0124$ sec = 80.65 Hz.

Sweep vernier This is a continuously variable time control that allows us to interpolate between step-time settings. The step-time settings are accurate only when the vernier is in the CAL'D position. The vernier is ganged to the step attenuator, and is thus concentric to and in the center of that control.

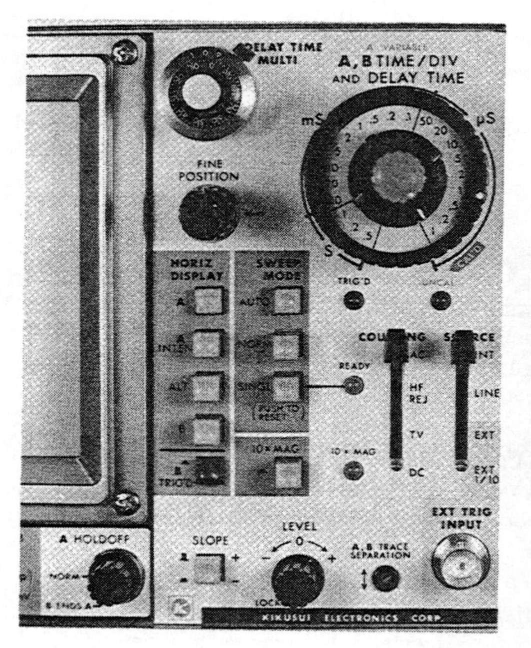

(a)

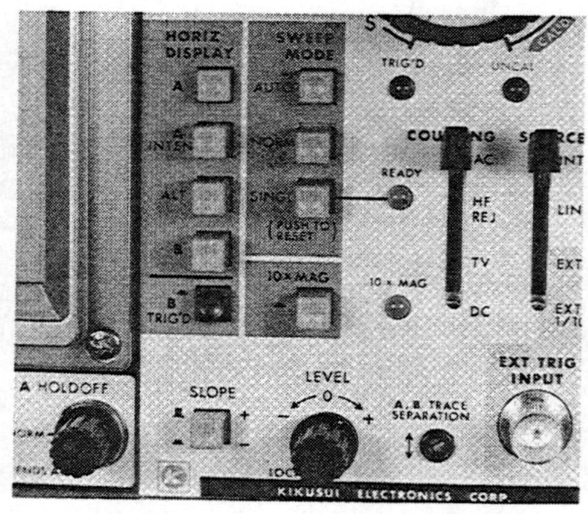

(b)

FIGURE 3-10

Horizontal position The horizontal (or "fine") position control moves the trace left and right on the CRT screen. Like the equivalent vertical control, the horizontal position control is used to place key features right over graticule points for purposes of precision measurement.

10× MAG The 10× magnification control speeds up the sweep ten times. For example, if the time/div sweep control is set to 10 mS/div, then the 10× MAG control would force it to become 1 mS/div.

Sweep mode The sweep mode control selects automatic (AUTO), normal (NORM), and single-sweep (SINGLE) submodes. In the AUTO mode, the sweep will periodically retrigger even if no signal is present in the vertical amplifier. The NORM mode requires a vertical signal to begin sweeping the CRT, and the screen will remain blank otherwise. In the SINGLE mode, the CRT beam will sweep only once. Two means of operation are noted. If there is a periodic signal present, pressing the button in the AUTO position will force one sweep to take place. If the NORM mode is selected, then the SINGLE button will reset the circuit, which will sweep only after a valid input signal is received.

TRIGGER GROUP

The triggered-sweep oscilloscope is considerably more useful than the old untriggered forms. The triggered-sweep 'scope will not allow the CRT beam to sweep across the screen unless a signal is in the vertical amplifier to trigger the sweep generator. Some models also allow delay-time triggered-sweep function. That is, the sweep will not actually begin until some preset time after the triggering event occurs. The trigger group of controls is also shown in Figure 3-10A along with the horizontal controls. The controls include *trigger level* ("*level*"), *slope, source, coupling, external trigger input,* and a *horizontal display* selector. In addition, some models (such as in Figure 3-10A) also have a time-delay vernier control. Keep in mind that the sweep mode, which we discussed under the horizontal controls, is also part of the trigger group (Figure 3-10B), as is the CH1-CH2-NORM switch shown along with the vertical group controls.

Trigger level The trigger-level control determines the minimum amplitude vertical signal required to trigger the horizontal sweep. Figures 3-11A and 3-11B show the effect of this control. Both traces were taken moments apart with the same signal input to the same oscilloscope. The only difference in these displays was the setting of the level control (see Figure 3-11A). The range of the control runs from negative, through zero, to positive voltage values.

Slope This control determines whether the trigger occurs on a negative-going or a positive-going edge of the input waveform. In Figures 3-11A and 3-11B

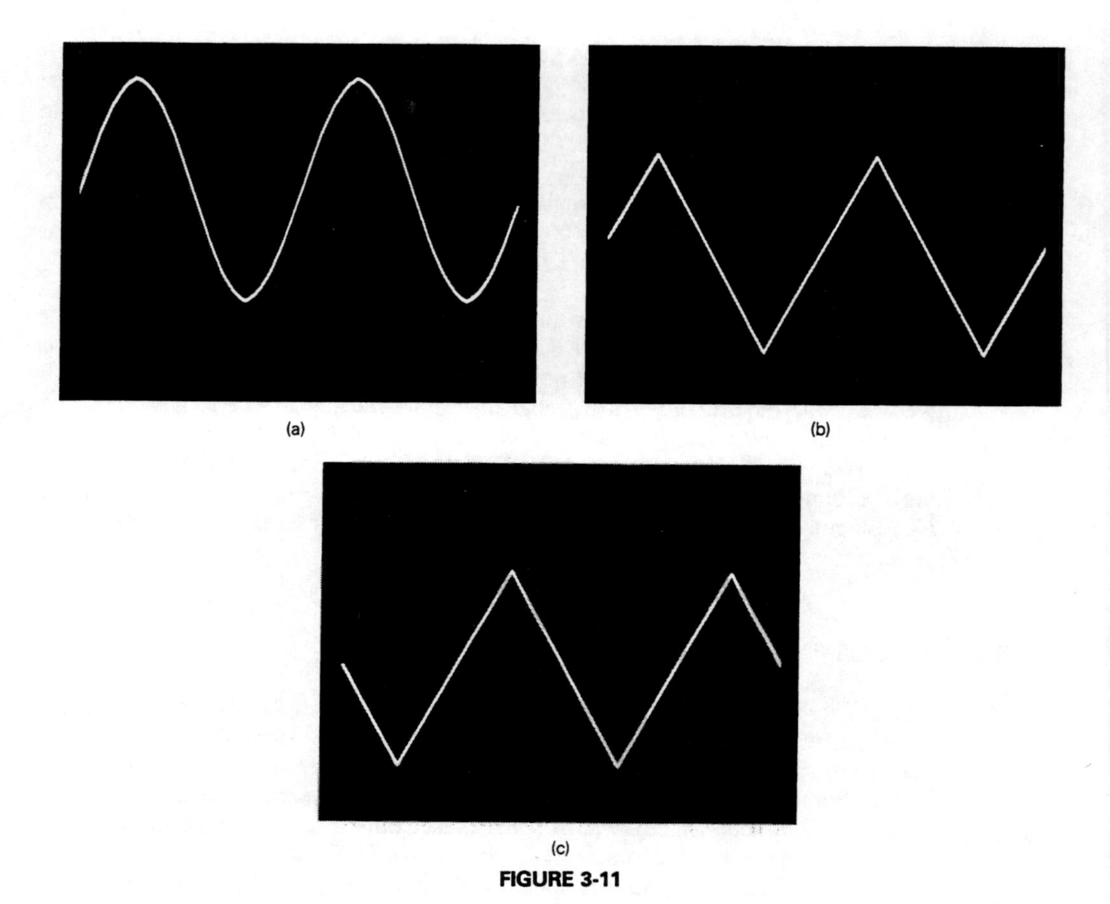
(a) (b) (c)

FIGURE 3-11

the slope control is set to the "+" position, so the triggering occurs on the positive-going edge of the sine wave. In Figure 3-11C, on the other hand, we see exactly the same signal with the level control set as it was in Figure 3-11B and the slope control changed to "−." Note that the triggering now occurs on the negative-going slope of the waveform.

Source The source control selects the source of the signal applied to the triggering circuits. The selections are INT, LINE, EXT, and EXT/10. The INT is the internal selection, which means that the source is selected by the CH1/CH2/NORM switch in the vertical section. For example, with the source control in INT and the other switch in CH1 position, the signal in the CH1 vertical amplifier will cause triggering. The LINE selection means that the 60-Hz AC line will cause triggering, a feature useful in some measurements. The EXT means that the signal applied to the external trigger input (EXT TRIG INPUT) will trigger the sweep circuits. Again, some useful measurements are possible with this feature. The EXT/10 is the same as EXT, but a 10:1 attenuator is in place.

Coupling The coupling control allows us to tailor the triggering, and has selections of AC, HF REJ, TV, and DC. The AC and DC are self-explanatory and are similar to the same markings on the vertical selector switch. The HF REJ uses a low-pass filter at the input of the trigger circuit that rejects high frequencies. This system will, for example, allow us to trigger on the modulation of a modulated RF carrier while ignoring the RF signal. Some 'scopes also have a LF REF, which is similar except that the filter is a high-pass filter. The TV selection allows us to sync to the horizontal/vertical frequencies used in television sweep systems. Some models have separate TV VER and TV HOR selections.

External trigger input An input connector that provides the trigger circuit with an external signal for special-purpose syncing and triggering. Some 'scopes also have a TRIG GATE function on this connector in certain switch selections (or a separate TRIG GATE—trigger gate—output). That feature produces a short-duration pulse for synchronizing external circuits to the sweep system.

Time delay The time-delay control allows us to program a short delay between the triggering event selected according to the level and slope controls, and the actual onset of the sweep. Using this control we can view small segments of the waveform while using the main signal as the trigger event.

Horizontal display The HORIZ DISPLAY is a switch bank (Figure 3-10B) that allows certain submodes. Not all 'scopes have this feature, even though it is very useful. Figure 3-12 shows the operation of certain features of this selector. When button "A" is pressed, the 'scope operates as any triggered sweep 'scope operates. But in the A INTEN mode, we see a trace such as in Figure 3-12A. Note the segment of the waveform that is intensified. The position of this intensified segment is a function of the time-delay control, while the length of the intensified portion is a function of the delay-time control that is concentric with the time/div control. We can use this mode to designate a small segment of the waveform for a closer look. When the "B" switch is pressed, that portion of the waveform is displayed, as in Figure 3-12B. A slightly different function is shown in Figure 3-12C, which is the trace that results when the ALT button is pressed. In this case, we see both the main waveform and the time-delayed "close-up" portion. A screwdriver "A-B separation" control allows us to either separate or superimpose these waveforms.

Figure 3-13A shows the most basic form of input probe for oscilloscopes. Here we see a length of shielded cable, usually coaxial cable, with a BNC (banana plugs or PL-259 on older instruments) on one end and a pair of alligator clips on the other end. This method works well for signals with frequencies from DC up to a certain point, and for many readers, this probe set is all that is required. But there is a problem that must be recognized. The cable has capacitance on the order of 20 pF per

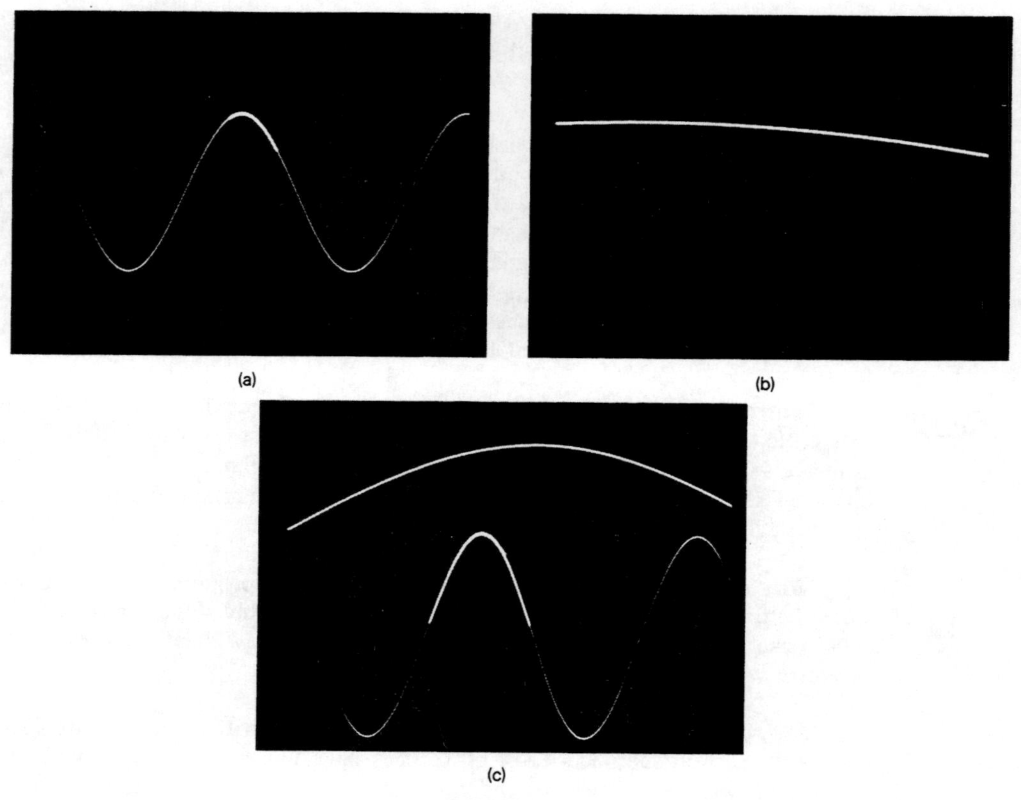

FIGURE 3-12

foot. The input impedance of a typical oscilloscope is a 1-megohm resistance shunted with a 20-pF capacitance. If the cable is 3 ft long, then it has a capacitance of 3 × 20 pF, or 60 pF, which when added to the natural input capacitance results in 80-pF shunting 1 megohm. The RC network thus created has a low-pass filter characteristic that rolls off −6 dB/octave above a −3-dB frequency of

$$F = \frac{1}{2\pi RC}$$

$$F = \frac{1}{(2)(3.14)(10^6 \text{ ohms})(8 \times 10^{-11} \text{ farads})} \tag{3-1}$$

$$F = \frac{1}{0.0005} = 1990 \text{ Hz}$$

This probe will load down any high-frequency circuit that it is used to measure, so is not the best solution. And the fundamental frequency need not be anywhere near the cutoff frequency for there to be problems. Nonsinusoidal signals are

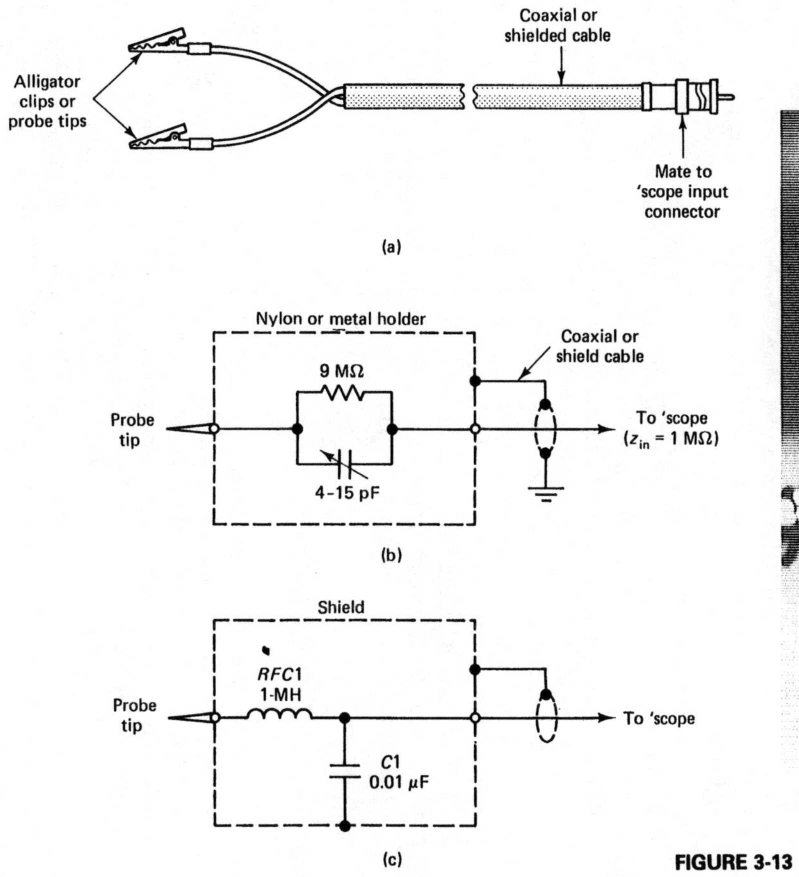

Alligator clips or probe tips
Coaxial or shielded cable
Mate to 'scope input connector
(a)
Nylon or metal holder
9 MΩ
4–15 pF
Probe tip
Coaxial or shield cable
To 'scope (z_{in} = 1 MΩ)
(b)
Shield
RFC1
1-MH
C1
0.01 μF
Probe tip
To 'scope
(c)

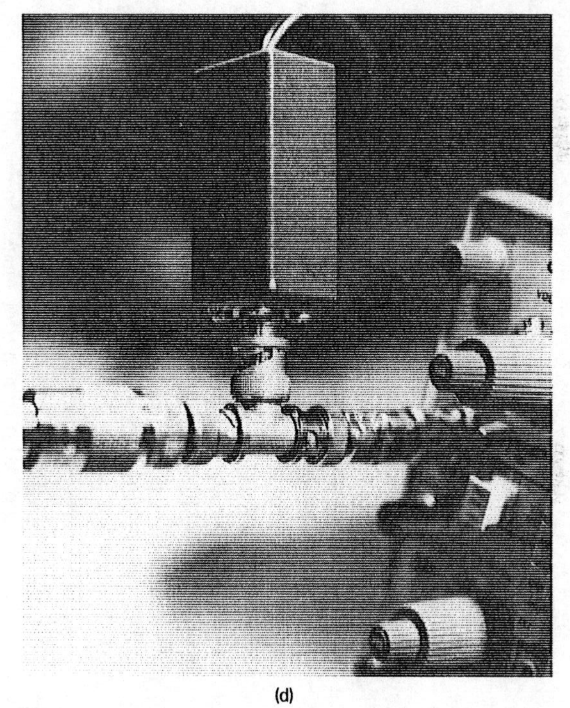

(d)

FIGURE 3-13

made up of a collection of sine waves consisting of a fundamental plus harmonics. Thus, a 100-Hz fast-risetime square wave is made of a 100 Hz sine wave plus even harmonics up to the zillionth or so. The low-pass filter effects of the probe in Figure 3-13A will roll off the higher harmonics and round off the shoulders of the square wave.

The answer to the frequency response problem is to use a low-capacitance probe, two examples of which are shown in Figures 3-13B and 3-13C. The probe in Figure 3-13B is the standard 10 : 1 ratio probe. The output signal of this probe is one-tenth the input signal. If the resistors used are precision types, then the scale factor on the 'scope vertical attenuator is multiplied by 10. For example, when the vertical attenuator is set to 0.5 volts/cm, the actual scale factor is 5 volts/cm.

In all three types of low-capacitance probe the capacitor is adjusted to flatten the frequency response. In most cases a fast-risetime 1000-Hz square wave is applied to the input of the probe when it is connected to the 'scope. Adjust the capacitance to show as square a square wave on the screen of the 'scope as possible.

Another problem is the matter of isolation from external fields. The classical problem is taking a look at a waveform in the presence of an interfering electromagnetic field. The classical approach to this problem is insertion of an RF choke in series with the 'scope probe. Figure 3-13C shows a probe that can be used on electrosurgery machine and radio transmitter measurements. The 1-millihenry (1-mH) RF choke suppresses the RF that is present on the probe when it is in the presence of a radio field.

A problem that exists on the probe in Figure 3-13C is the matter of self-resonance. All RF chokes, indeed all inductors, have a certain amount of capacitance between windings and a stray capacitance to ground. These capacitances interact with the inductance of the coil to make either (or both!) series or parallel resonances, and that spells trouble in some cases.

A different kind of oscilloscope input device is shown in Figure 3-13D. Certain RF and computer measurements require special adapter devices to make the oscilloscope work. This particular adapter is a device used in time domain reflectometry, a method for "doping out" coaxial cable transmission lines such as those used to interconnect the elements of the receiver and antenna system of the cardiac telemetary system in a hospital.

MAKING MEASUREMENTS ON THE 'SCOPE

The standard oscilloscope display (Figure 3-14) is calibrated in two axes: vertical and horizontal. The horizontal axis is calibrated in units of time, that is, typically time per division (most modern 'scopes use the centimeter as the division). The vertical axis is the amplitude (usually voltage) of the applied signal. The graticule shown in Figure 3-14 has two forms of divisions on the screen. The major divisions are each 1 cm, while the minor divisions are 0.2 cm each. These minor divisions are inscribed only on the center vertical and horizontal axes. In the example of Figure 3-14, the vertical displacement is approximately 4.4 divisions, and the horizontal is 3.25 divisions.

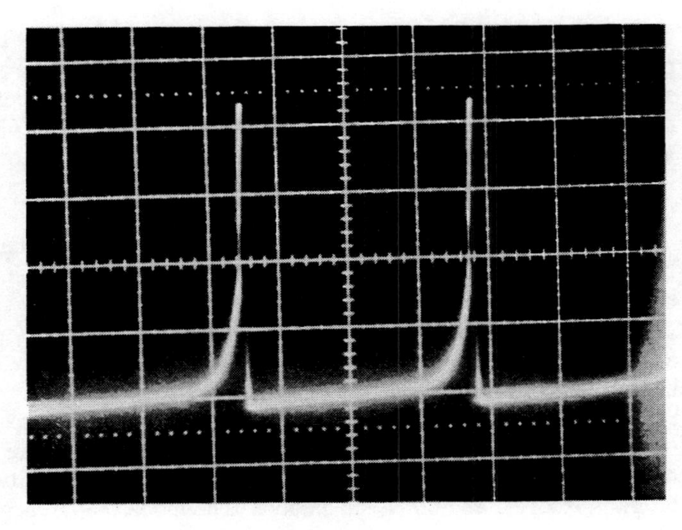

FIGURE 3-14

Medical oscilloscopes used in ECG and similar applications are often calibrated in units of distance and time. For example, the standard external lead ECG is usually calibrated at 25 millimeters per second (25 mm/sec). Other instruments will be calibrated at 50 mm/sec or 100 mm/sec. Some multipurpose models have all three calibrations.

The graticule on many medical 'scopes is inscribed with millimeter marks, and the major divisions represent 5 mm each. This calibration makes it easy to measure ECG feature parameters.

A newer form of oscilloscope now on the market is intended for use with computer graphics displays. These 'scopes are often calibrated in the units being measured, distance, or some other physical parameter. The computer will inscribe the CRT screen with a calibrating scale or will directly label the features as to calibration.

MEDICAL OSCILLOSCOPES

In the sections to follow we will take a closer look at oscilloscopes designed specifically for medical applications. There are three types of 'scope typically found in the medical world.

First, there are the straight analog "bouncing ball" models. The nickname "bouncing ball" comes from the fact that the beam of light seems to bounce as the ECG waveform parades across the 'scope face. These 'scopes are medical variants of the straight oscilloscope discussed earlier so will not be covered further. While the medical models tend to have magnetic deflection of the CRT electron beam (via a CRT neck yoke), they are otherwise very similar.

The phosphor on the CRT screen is also a bit different. The regular 'scope will probably use a P1 or P4 phosphor. These phosphor mixtures are relatively fast, so fade immediately after the electron beam passes a point. This feature is desirable for the laboratory user, but for slow waveforms such as the ECG, arterial pressure, or EEG, the fast-fading light beam does not allow examination of the entire waveform. For these reasons, a P7 or similar "long-persistence" phosphor is usually selected by the 'scope designer.

The standard long persistence phosphors have an interesting property. The light emitted is a mixture of yellow, green, and violet-blue colors. The standard unfiltered display looks "violetish" to most people (especially under fluorescent lighting). But if a filter is used over the CRT screen, then either green or yellow colors are emitted. But these colors are a bit dimmer (especially the yellow) than the unfiltered versions.

The second type of 'scope used in medical applications is the analog storage 'scope. These instruments use trickery inside the CRT to store the signal on the face of the CRT for a long period of time. These instruments are used in older vectorcardiogram 'scopes, and other applications. The modern approach, however, is to use a digital storage oscilloscope. These are the so-called "nonfade" 'scopes seen in medicine (of which we'll see more later).

Analog Storage Oscilloscopes

On a regular oscilloscope the input waveform must be periodic for the display to remain stable on the screen. Further, each repeated cycle must be identical to the previous cycle. But in medical oscilloscopes, the waveform might be periodic, aperiodic, or episodic. In addition, in cases where there is a periodic rhythm (as in ECG), the successive waveforms might not be identical (and the differences may be clinically significant). In all these cases a single event or feature might pass too rapidly to be viewed properly on a bouncing ball display unless the 'scope is equipped with a *storage* feature. There are two basic forms of storage 'scope: analog and digital. In this section we will take a look at the analog form.

The analog storage 'scope uses a special CRT and is shown in block diagram form in Figures 3-15A and 3-15B. A storage 'scope retains the image on the screen for a period of time before it eventually fades out. In the class of instruments using special CRT designs there are several subclasses that operate on slightly different principles. Figure 3-16 shows three different types of storage CRT.

The two types of CRT shown in Figures 3-15A and 3-16B depend for operation on a phosphor screen in which individual particles of phosphor are insulated from each other. In the case of Figure 3-16A the phosphors lie in the same plane to form *target dots,* while the other type (Figure 3-16B) uses layers of scattered particles of increasing weights. A special *flood gun* in the CRT emits high-energy electrons that excite the phosphors. The phosphor particles struck by these electrons take on a charge of 150 to 200 volts, but unenergized particles remain at zero volts. When electrons from the main electron gun have preenergized certain phosphors, forming an image on the CRT screen, these phosphors attract more flood gun elec-

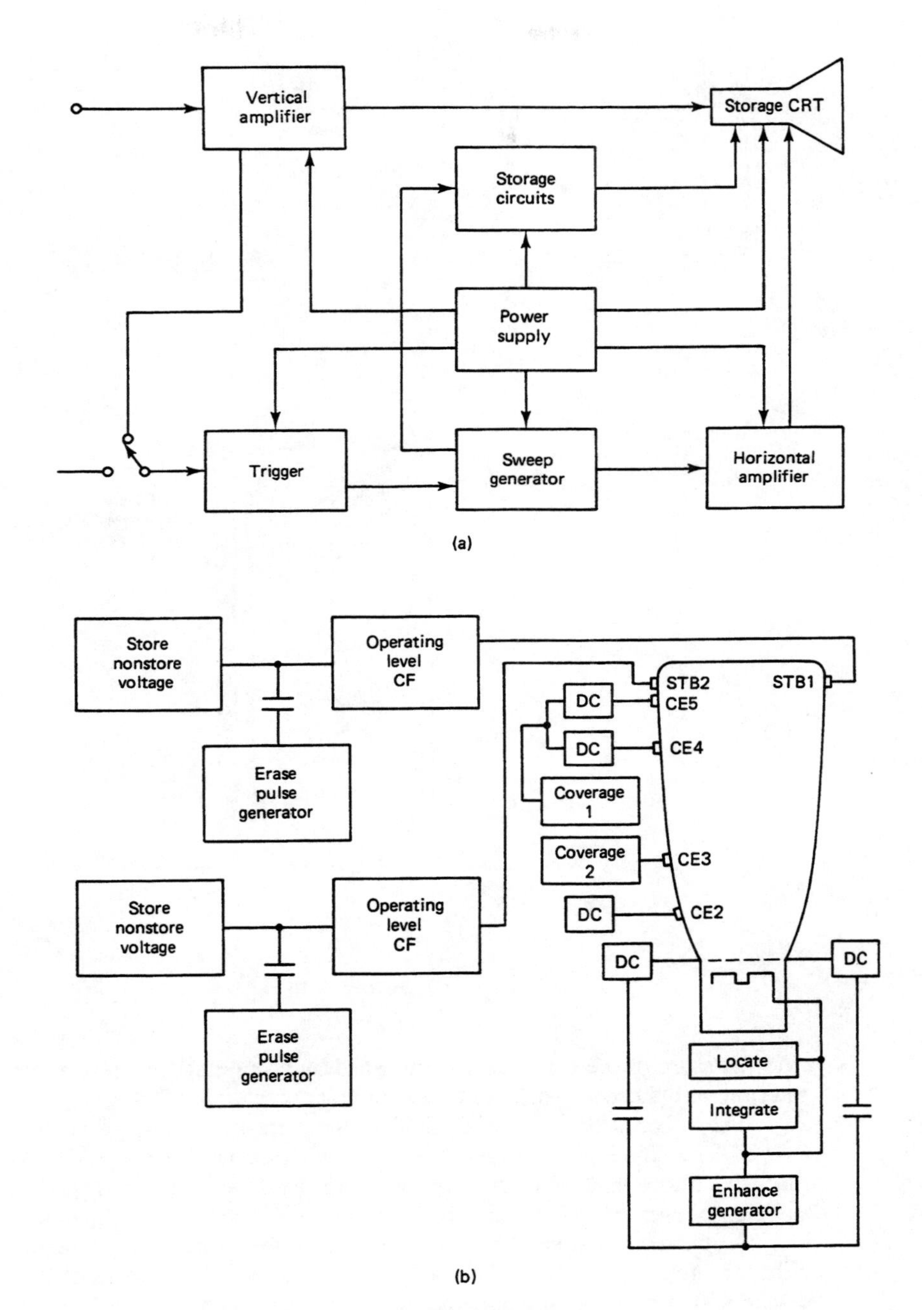
Vertical amplifier
Storage CRT
Storage circuits
Power supply
Trigger
Sweep generator
Horizontal amplifier
(a)
Store nonstore voltage
Operating level CF
Erase pulse generator
Store nonstore voltage
Operating level CF
Erase pulse generator
STB2
STB1
DC
CE5
DC
CE4
Coverage 1
Coverage 2
CE3
DC
CE2
DC
DC
Locate
Integrate
Enhance generator
(b)

FIGURE 3-15

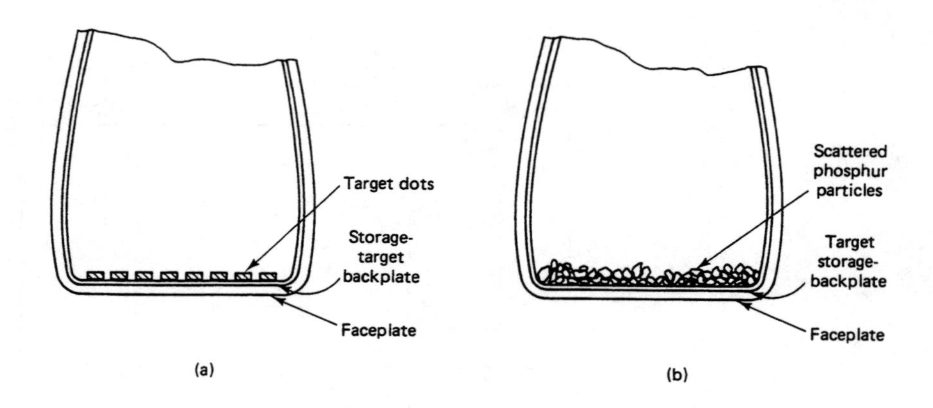

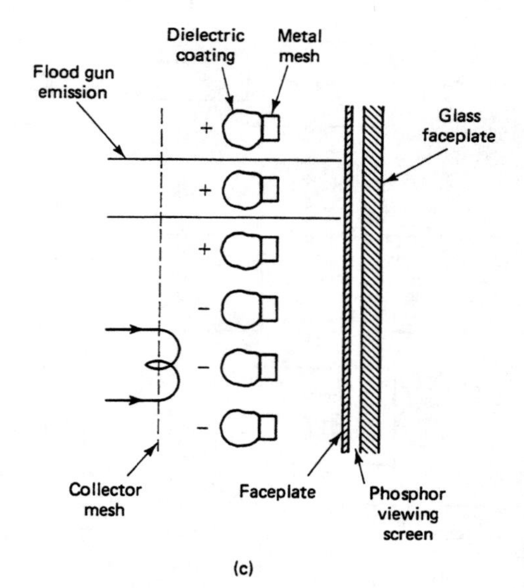

FIGURE 3-16

trons. Erasure of the screen is accomplished by grounding the phosphor screen, thus returning all phosphor particles to a zero volts potential.

The other type of special CRT is the wire-mesh variety shown in Figure 3-16C. The flood gun charges one mesh so that no further electrons can pass through, although the *write gun* or *main gun* electrons will pass through if sufficiently energetic (a function of the high accelerator anode voltage).

A *split-screen* storage oscilloscope allows the operator to store waveforms in either the top or bottom half of the screen. If both halves are turned on, then the device will store waveforms in any portion of the screen. This feature allows subsequent waveforms (for example, a before and after condition) to be examined together even though separated in time.

Some storage 'scopes, which find wide application in medical electronics, have a feature called *variable persistence,* which allows the operator to vary the length of time that the image will remain on the screen.

NONFADE MEDICAL OSCILLOSCOPES

The traditional form of oscilloscope uses a beam of electrons to sweep the screen, writing the analog waveform as it is deflected. Even with long-persistence phosphors, however, the trace vanishes from the CRT shortly after it is written onto the screen. The type of CRO is usually called a bouncing ball display in the jargon. To the medical personnel using the bouncing ball display, it is very difficult to evaluate waveform anomalies because the trace fades too rapidly.

The analog storage oscilloscope is a partial solution to the problem for some research applications, but it is generally not suited to monitoring and other clinical applications. A problem with the analog storage 'scope is that the trace tends to "bloom" out and become fuzzy a few minutes after it is taken—or if circuit conditions are not exactly right.

The solution to these problems is the *digital storage oscilloscope,* also called the *nonfade oscilloscope* in the jargon. CRT storage systems are not used in most medical 'scopes because, at the low frequencies involved, the digital types offer a better display at competitive prices. Also, the digital type of nonfade display does not bloom when the display is either old or erased. While most earlier nonfade 'scopes used discrete digital logic (as do many today), modern computer techniques (which are all but ubiquitous in medicine now) offer an easy approach to the nonfade display.

Two different formats are commonly used: *parade* or *erase bar* (see Figure 3-17). The waveform marches across the screen from right to left. The newest data, which is being written in real time, appear in the upper-right-hand corner of the screen. The light beam bounces up and down at a fixed horizontal point in response to the vertical waveform; it does not move along the time base as it does in regular

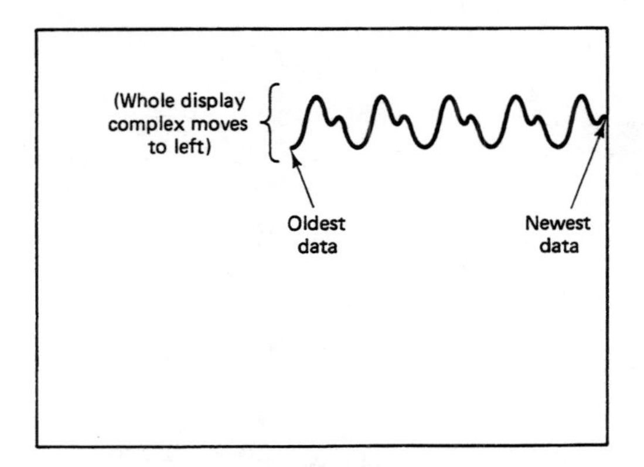

FIGURE 3-17

analog 'scopes. The waveform is nicknamed the "parade" display because the oldest data march across the screen seemingly leading a parade of waves.

In the erase bar format (Figure 3-18), a nonfade 'scope, the beam of light travels left to right (it is not stationary as on parade models). There is an erase bar (i.e., a dark region) traveling ahead of the beam that obliterates the oldest data so that the new data can be written onto the CRT screen.

There are two basic forms of digital circuit for nonfade oscilloscopes. Figure 3-19 shows a complex form that uses a regular computer memory, as might be found in a personal computer. The signal is applied to the input amplifier and is scaled to match the dynamic range of the analog-to-digital converter (A/D). The A/D converter is used to convert the analog voltage to an equivalent binary word. For example, in a unipolar system with a 0- to +10-volt range, the binary word 00000000 might represent 0 volts, while 11111111 might represent +9.96 volts (it is not possible to get exactly to +10 volts if zero is to be represented properly).

The output of the A/D is stored first in a short-term "scratch pad" memory. The contents of the scratch pad memory are periodically dumped to the main display memory. The rate of transfer from the scratch pad to the main memory is done at a rate faster than the eye can see (typically 40 to 80 times per second). The memory is scanned via a signal from the control logic section, and output in sequence to a digital-to-analog converter (DAC) that forms the signal that is applied to the oscilloscope vertical amplifier.

The horizontal sweep signal should be a sawtooth waveform. This signal is formed by a DAC that is driven by a binary counter. As the clock causes the counter to increment through its range, the output of the DAC ramps upward. When the counter overflows, however, the DAC output snaps back to zero so the process can start anew.

The type of nonfade 'scope depicted in Figure 3-19 can store an immense amount of waveform data. In fact, it can also transfer that data to a computer or to a long-term magnetic media such as a floppy disk, tape, or main disk. But in simpler instruments a different form of nonfade 'scope might be used.

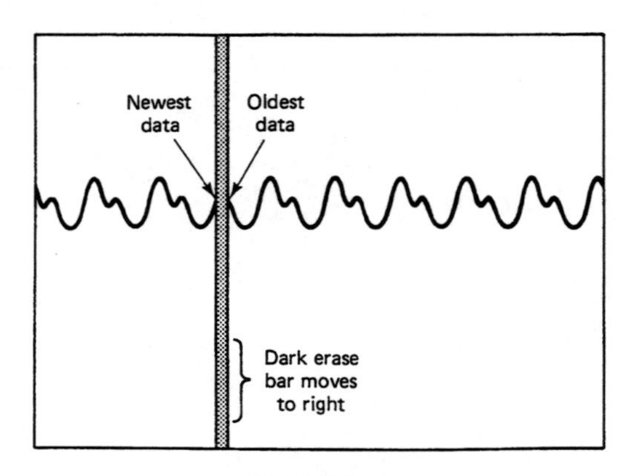

FIGURE 3-18

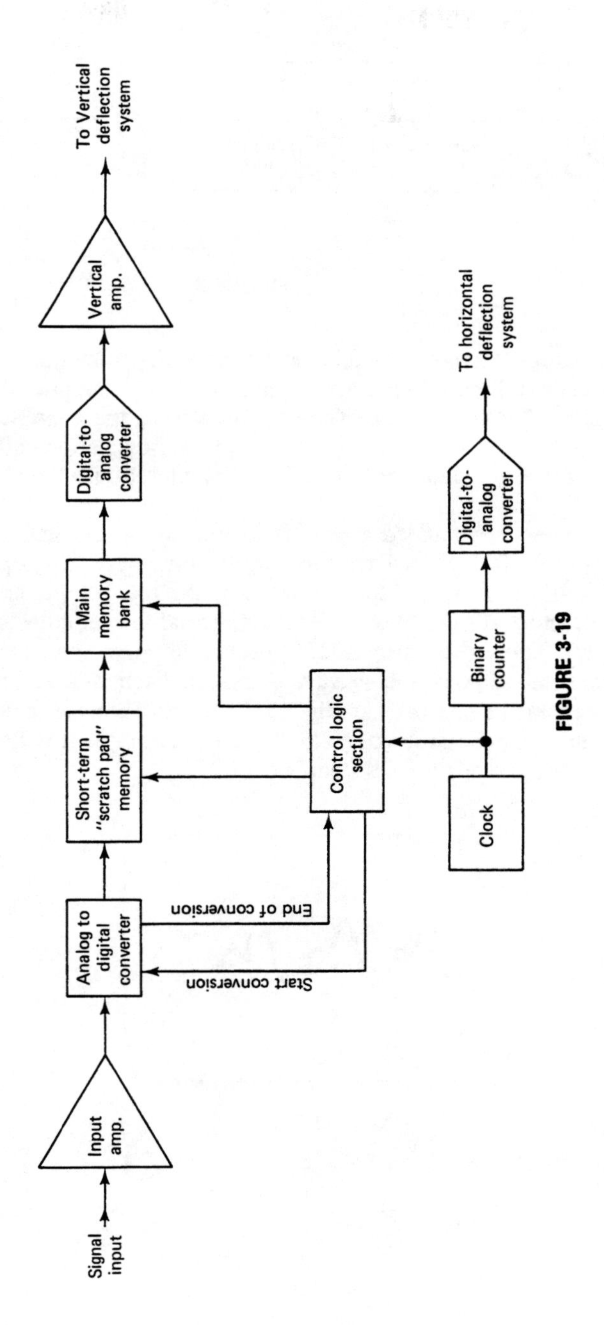
Signal input
Input amp.
Analog to digital converter
Short-term "scratch pad" memory
Main memory bank
Digital-to-analog converter
Vertical amp.
To Vertical deflection system
End of conversion
Start conversion
Control logic section
Clock
Binary counter
Digital-to-analog converter
To horizontal deflection system

FIGURE 3-19

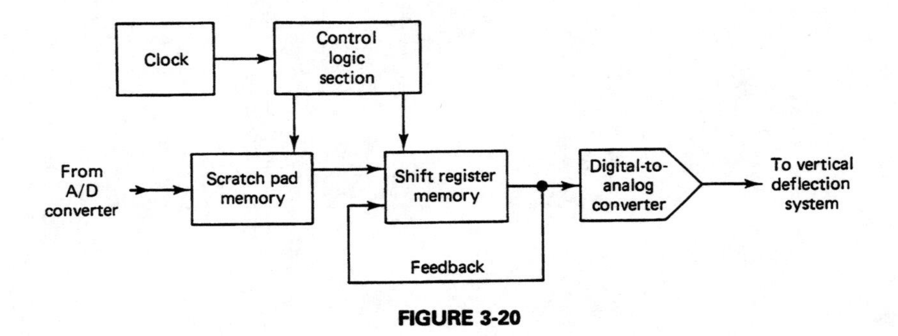

FIGURE 3-20

The simple form of nonfade 'scope system is shown in Figure 3-20. The system is similar to Figure 3-19, but the main memory is replaced with a *recirculating shift register*. The data are updated by outputting the contents of the scratch pad memory to the input of the recirculating shift register periodically. Between updates, however, the output data are fed back and reentered into the shift register, preserving the image.

Computers have added a new dimension in the medical instruments industry, and medical oscilloscopes have fared well with these developments. Figure 3-21 shows a form of graphics display for a computer that can be used for medical applications (Hercules, CGA, EGA, VGA, and special format graphics protocols are used extensively). The screen of the CRT is broken into a matrix of tiny square or rectangular zones called *picture elements,* or *pixels*. Each storage location in the digital memory represents one pixel on the CRT screen. The pixel can be lighted to an intensity defined by the protocol (6 to 32 shades of gray). It is lighted by the electron beam as it raster scans the CRT surface.

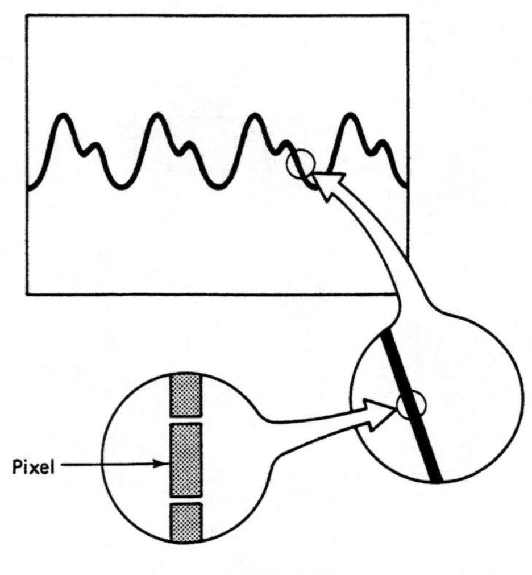

FIGURE 3-21

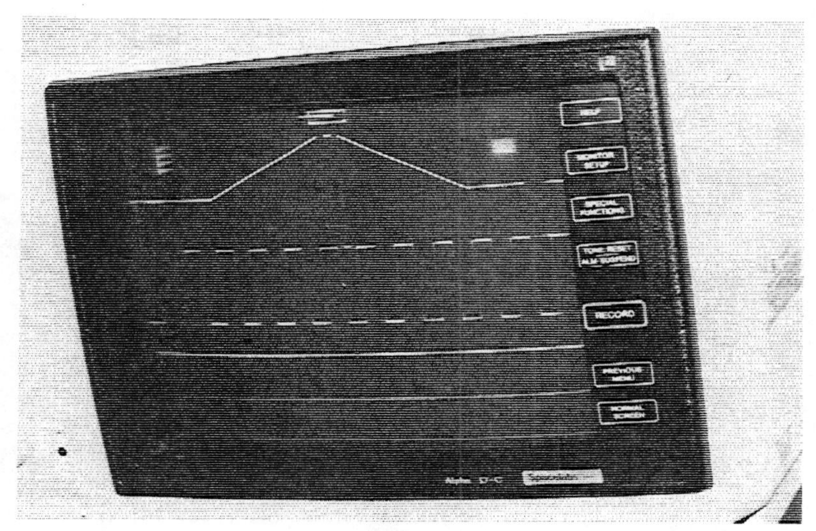

FIGURE 3-22

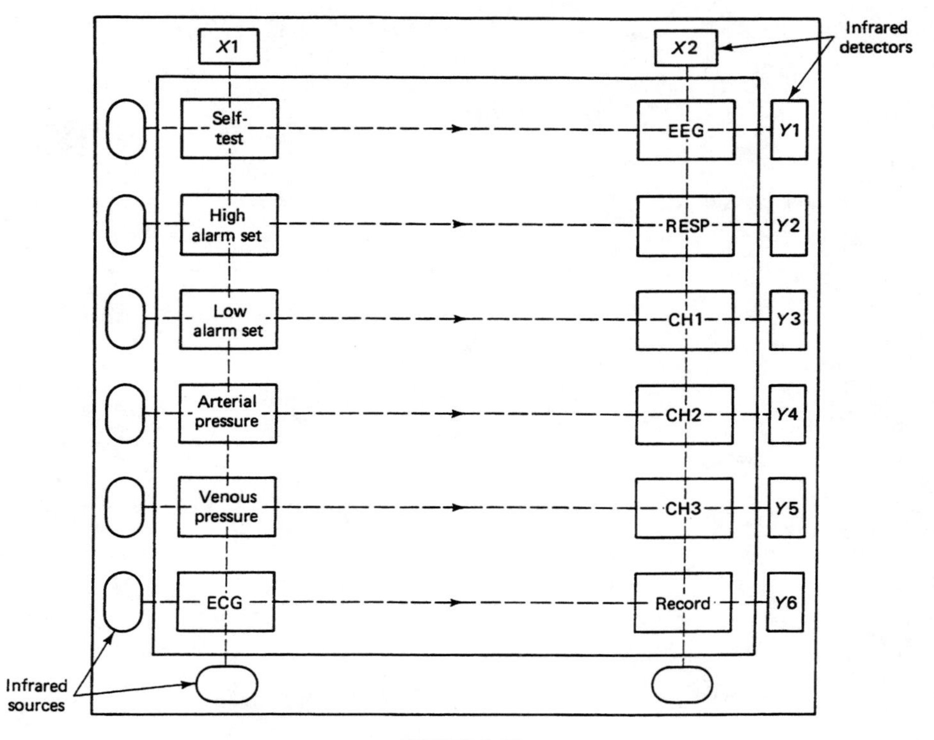

FIGURE 3-23

Figure 3-22 shows a typical medical monitor 'scope used in an intensive care unit. The pattern on the screen is the self-test pattern that comes on the screen either on operator initiation or at turn/on. This type of monitor is used in a computer-based system that actually forms the image.

The monitor of Figure 3-22, like certain other displays, uses a "touch screen" method for the selector "switches." Figure 3-23 shows how most such 'scopes operate. Positioned along the edges of the display are a series of infrared sources (light-emitting diodes, LEDs, operating in the IR region), and infrared detectors. The IR light is invisible to the naked eye, so is not seen by the operator. The function labels are either painted onto the CRT by the computer (as in Figure 3-23) or affixed to the edge as in Figure 3-22. When the operator touches the screen over any label, his or her finger interrupts one vertical and one horizontal beam, causing a unique pattern. For example, suppose all detector outputs are at binary LOW when the IR reaches the detector. The X outputs X1-X2 are L-L, and the Y outputs Y1-Y2-Y3-Y4-Y5-Y6 are L-L-L-L-L-L. And then someone touches the SELF-TEST label. In this case, X1 and Y1 are both interrupted and their respective outputs go HIGH. Thus, the patterns become H-L and H-L-L-L-L-L. The internal computer recognizes this as an operator command to branch to the SELF-TEST software stored in program memory.

4

ECG and EEG Signals: Where Do They Come From?

In most emergency medical instruments the acquisition and processing of electrical signals constitutes a large part of instrumentation design. Such devices are used also by others in biology, physiology, biochemistry, and certain aspects of psychology. In this chapter we will discuss where these signals come from, why they are important, and some of the problems encountered in monitoring them.

BIOELECTRICAL PHENOMENA

Biophysical signals are directly derived from electrical activity of the body at the cell level. Examples are the electrocardiograph (ECG), which measures heart activity, the electroencephalograph (EEG), which measures brainwave activity, and the electromyograph (EMG), which measures skeletal muscle activity. These signals have their origin in the electrical properties of the cell.

The human body is constructed from the basic building blocks called cells. Each body is composed of a number of different types of cells. The human body is believed to contain 75 trillion individual cells, of which about 25 trillion are red blood cells. The types of cells vary considerably as to size, shape, construction, and properties according to their function. Cell size varies from 200 nanometers (1 nm = 10^{-9} m) to several centimeters (cm). The ostrich egg is a single cell that reaches 20 cm (1 cm = 10^{-2} m) in size. Most cells in the human body fall into the range 0.5 to 20 micrometers (1 μm = 10^{-6} m).

The cell can be viewed as a closed body in which internal material (cytoplasm and, in some, a nucleus) is separated from the surrounding body fluid by a cell wall membrane (Figure 4-1). The key to cell bioelectricity is in the fact that the cell wall is a *semipermeable membrane*. That is, its structure is such that it is permeable (i.e., will pass) only certain ions, and no others. As a result of a sodium-potassium phenomenon associated with this membrane, the concentration of ions inside and outside the cell are different.

The job of the sodium-potassium pump is to force sodium outside the cell and potassium inside the cell. Because the rate of sodium pumping is two to five times the rate of potassium pumping, the net result is a cell interior that is largely potassium (K) ions and an external environment that is largely sodium (Na) ions. The difference in ionic concentration produces an electrical membrane potential (voltage) across the cell wall (again, see Figure 4-1).

The normal potential of the cell with respect to its environment is between −70 and −90 millivolts (mV). This variation is somewhat dependent on the cell and its situation, but also indicates some disagreement among the various authorities on cell structure. A mathematical expression called the "Nernst equation" governs cell potential. Readers who wish to follow up and learn more than is necessary here may consult any elementary college-level physiology textbook.

A cell at rest is said to be "polarized." That is, the concentration of ions is such as to make the interior of the cell much more negative than the exterior (the cell floats in a sea of salty intercellular fluid). Certain types of cell can be stimulated in certain ways (dependent upon function and type) that change polarity. When stimulated the cell becomes "depolarized." During the depolarization period the character

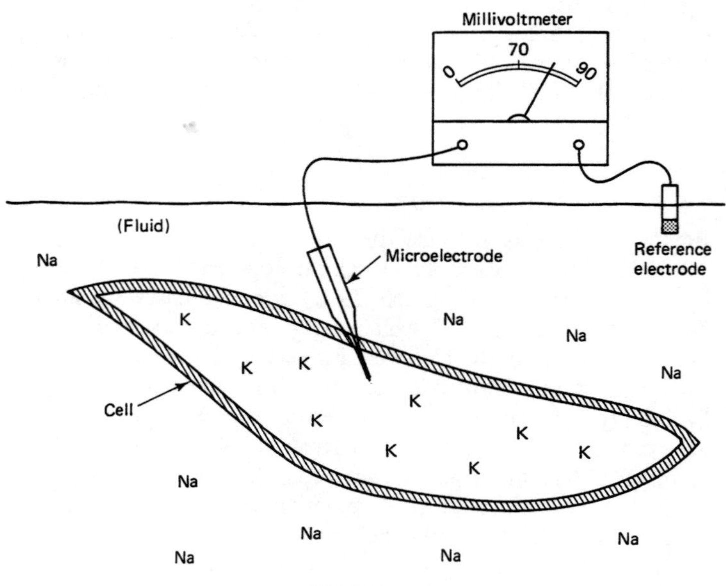

FIGURE 4-1

of the cell membrane changes radically; the change forces potassium out of the cell and allows sodium inside. The depolarization phenomenon lasts typically for several milliseconds. During this period, the change of ionic concentrations forces a change in membrane potential from −70/90 mV to +20/40 mV. This latter potential is called the *action potential* (Figure 4-2).

The duration of the action potential is typically 1.5 to 4 milliseconds (mS). During most of this time the cell cannot be retriggered by repeated episodes of the stimulus. This segment is called the *refractory period*. The membrane potential need not return all the way to its resting potential before retriggering is possible, so the refractory period is measured from initiation of the stimulus until the potential again reaches the retriggering threshold (a little above the resting potential, or about −60 mV in Figure 4-2).

The action potential phenomenon is analogous to a light with a timer. On some automobiles a headlight timer is used to permit the user to light up an area after he or she gets out of the car. A button is pressed (stimulated or triggered), the light comes on (action potential), and then the light goes back to the resting "off" condition.

The "all or nothing" operation of the cell action potential explains why restimulation does not cause an increase in the intensity of a phenomenon. For example, if you stub your toe, pain sensation results from depolarization of the right sensor cells. But if you immediately restub your toe before the refractory period expires, the second injury is not felt as an increase in pain. An increase in pain is felt only if some or all of the pain sensors have completed their refractory period.

Conduction of the action potential signal occurs by two mechanisms. *Ohmic conduction* occurs through tissue because the action potential is an electrical poten-

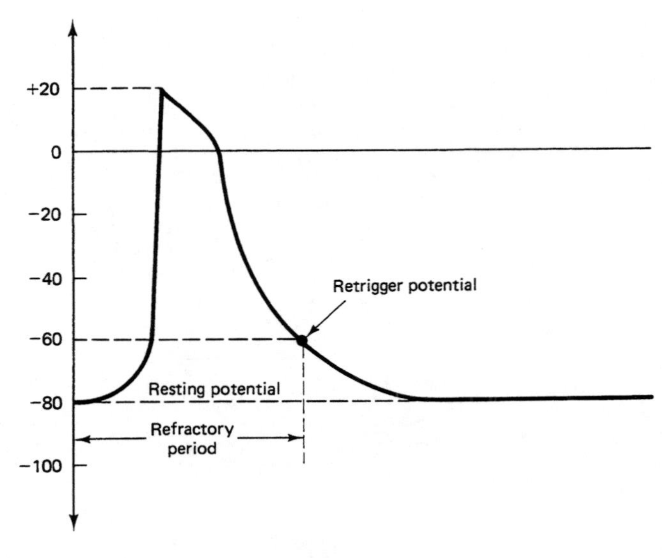

FIGURE 4-2

tial difference—like a small battery—acting on electrically conductive tissue in accordance with Ohm's law. This phenomena is also called *ionic conduction*. Ionic or ohmic conduction results in very low signals at a distance because the electrical energy is integrated over the body area. Thus, a large action potential in the heart muscle diminishes to a weak 1-mV signal at the surface. Another means of conduction is found in nerve cells and certain other cases. This type of conduction results from the successive depolarization of adjacent cells. In other words, the depolarization of one cell forces the spontaneous depolarization of the adjacent cell. By this same means, the action potential is propagated over a relatively long distance without being diminished. Each successive cell depolarization effectively reconstitutes the pulse amplitude.

By way of example, let's take a look at a well-known biopotential: the electrocardiogram ("ECG," or "EKG" after the German spelling). The ECG signal is the surface view of the averaged cell action potentials from the heart (which is a muscle). Figure 4-3 shows a highly simplified schematic of the heart. Notice that the heart consists of four chambers that together form a dual two-chamber pump. Each pump (right and left) consists of an atrium (input chamber) and ventricle (output chamber).

Blood returning from the body circulatory system is a low pressure of 2–4

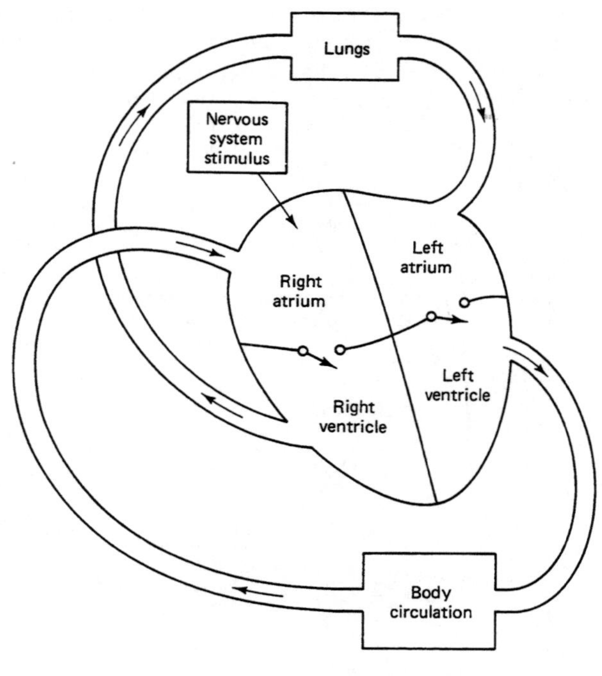

FIGURE 4-3

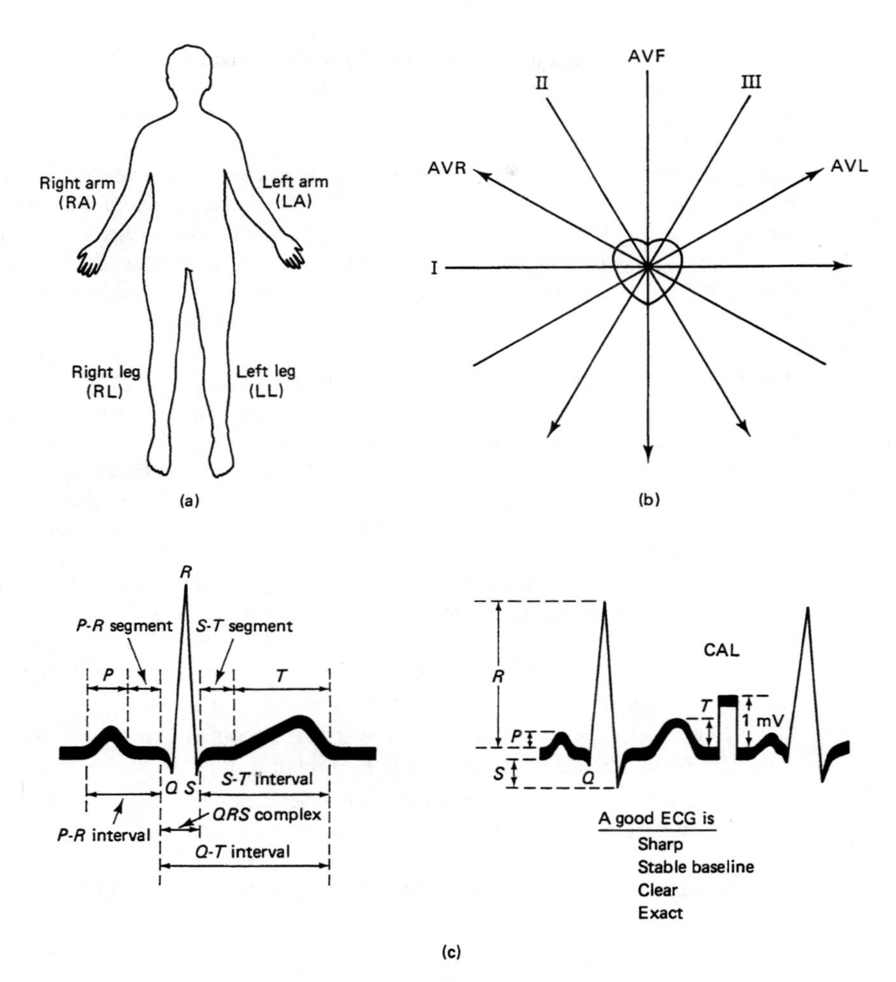

FIGURE 4-4

millimeters of mercury, mmHg. Note: The modern scientific unit for pressure is the torr, but medicine persists in the archaic unit mmHg;—1 torr = 1 mmHg—and is drawn in the right atrium. When the pressure of returned blood builds up to a certain critical point, a valve between upper and lower chambers opens and allows the blood to enter the lower chamber (or "ventricle"). The pressure on the blood inside the atrium is increased to the point where the valve opens by a gentle contracting action that starts in the upper-right atrium from a nervous system stimulus and then spreads across the upper portion of the heart. This same electrical stimulation travels along an internal conduction system faster than through other tissue, designations used in medicine to denote the segments. Interestingly, the timing of the ECG signal within each waveform is essentially constant (by point of reference the QRS "spike" complex takes about 40 mS), and only the number of waveforms per minute changes with heartrate. The P-wave corresponds to the firing of the atria, which begins pumping blood through the heart. The QRS segment is the major feature of the waveform because it represents the deep contraction of the ventricles as they force blood into the circulatory system. The T-wave corresponds to a refractory period when the cells of the heart muscle repolarize to be able to fire again. The trained physician is able to diagnose the type, site, and extent of heart disease from evaluation of the ECG and other clinical factors. In one of the waveforms of Figure 4-4C we see a 1-mV calibration pulse as a comparison of amplitudes.

As a person interested in things electrical you may have heard from time to time that short-duration electrical shocks, such as discharge from a high-voltage capacitor, will kill some victims and not others. A principal reason for this difference is that an electrical shock that occurs during the T-wave segment, when the heart is repolarizing, often causes fatal ventricular fibrillation, while shocks at other times do not—the difference is a matter of a few milliseconds of bad luck.

Figures 4-5 through 4-7 show the three major recording configurations for ECG signals. The set of leads (I, II, and III) shown in Figure 4-5 constitute what medical people call the *Einthoven triangle*. These *bipolar limb leads* are recorded as follows (in all cases RL is the reference electrode):

Lead I. LA is connected to the amplifier's noninverting (+) input, while the RA is connected to the amplifier's inverting (−) input.
Lead II. LL is connected to the amplifier's noninverting (+) input, while the RA is connected to the inverting (−) input.
Lead III. LL is connected to the amplifier's noninverting (+) input, while the LA is connected to the inverting (−) input.

In these schemes, the RL serves as the reference point and the amplifier mea-

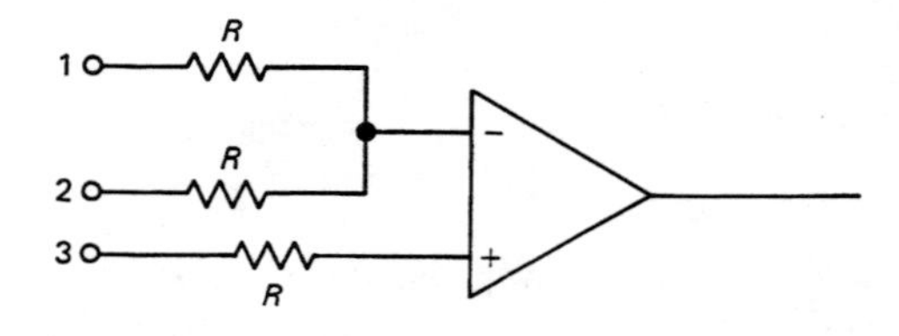

	Inputs		
Lead	1	2	3
AVR	LA	LL	RA
AVL	LL	RA	LA
AVF	LA	RA	LL

Augmented limb leads

FIGURE 4-5

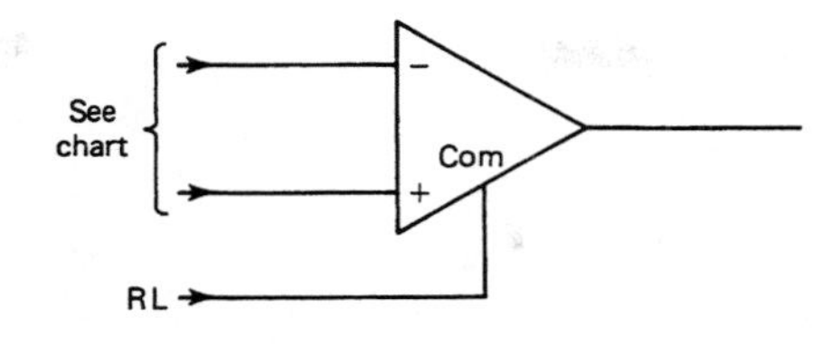

Lead	+Input	−Input
I	LA	RA
II	LL	RA
III	LL	LA

FIGURE 4-6

sures a differential voltage across two limbs (the unused limb electrode in each case is shorted to the RL).

Figure 4-6 shows the "augmented limb leads," also called the "unipolar limb leads." In this type of recording, the noninverting (+) input of the biophysical amplifier is independent, while the inverting (−) input sees the summation of two the other two limb signals. The chart in Figure 4-6 shows the connection scheme. The augmented limb leads are designated AVR, AVL, and AVF.

Lead AVR. RA is connected to the noninverting (+) input of the amplifier, while LA and LL are summed at the inverting (−) input.

Lead AVF. LL is connected to the noninverting (+) input of the amplifier, while LA and RA are summed at the inverting (−) input.

Lead AVL. LA is connected to the noninverting (+) input of the amplifier, while LL and RA are summed at the inverting (−) input of the amplifier.

The *unipolar chest leads* are measured with an electrode on any six locations on the chest applied to the noninverting (+) input (see Figure 4-7), and the other limb electrode signals summed at the inverting (−) input. The summed signals form what clinicians are pleased to call the "indifferent electrode."

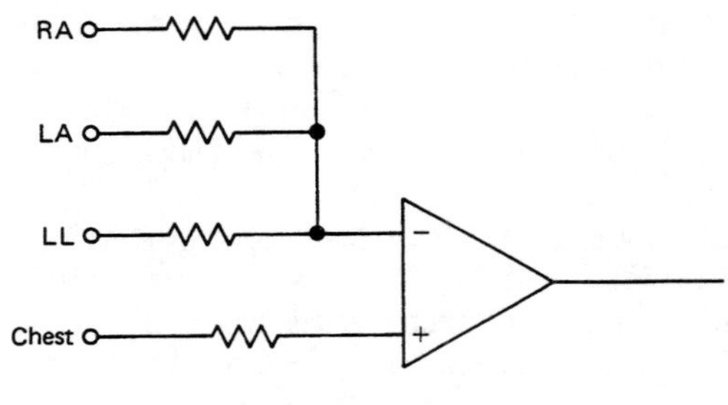

FIGURE 4-7

5

Bioelectric Amplifiers

Bioelectrical signals acquisition (EKG, EEG, EMG, etc.) requires amplifiers with special specifications. For example, the input circuitry of an ECG amplifier requires a high internal impedance between the amplifier's input terminals (typically well over 1 megohm), a LEAD selector switch (if required), a 1-mV calibration source, and a means for protecting the amplifier against high-voltage electrical transients that occur during defibrillation. This latter requirement applies especially to emergency medical equipment where the patient may require repeated high-voltage jolts (>2500 volts) from a defibrillator during resuscitation attempts.

In emergency medicine, as well as those research applications involving human subjects, the biopotentials amplifier must be electrically isolated from the AC power lines for reasons of patient safety. This requirement usually means that an isolation amplifier stage is used in the "front end" of the equipment. The reason for the isolation amplifier is that certain patients are at risk from minute electrical currents that would pass through their bodies unnoticed in normal situations. But when the body is invaded, as in surgery or certain other medical procedures, currents as low as 20 μA are thought to be harmful—thus leakage from the AC power lines can be extremely dangerous.

The standard frequency response of the amplifier used in making diagnostic grade recordings of ECG signals is 0.05 Hz to 100 Hz, while emergency medical and bedside monitoring instruments are often bandwidth limited to 0.05 to 45 Hz, or so. The reason for this difference is that in monitoring situations the higher-frequency response makes muscle artifact more severe—ruining the recording by making it difficult to read. By filtering out the higher frequencies, we gain a smoother and more useful waveform, but only at the cost of losing certain subtle diagnostic features. For example, the notch in the descending portion of the R-S segment that indicates partial heart block is all but obliterated by the filtering effect in monitoring-grade instruments.

Other biophysical signals will have somewhat different frequency response requirements. For example, the EEG (brainwave) signal is mostly sinusoidal. The amplifier must retain the low-frequency response of the ECG amplifier, but can cut the high-frequency response to 30 or 40 Hz. The EMG (skeletal muscle) signals, on the other hand, often have higher-frequency components, so a 1000-Hz amplifier is generally specified for EMG. It is not usually a good idea to make the frequency response of any data acquisition system significantly wider than needed because noise introduced can create recording artifacts.

Figure 5-1 shows a typical ECG/biophysical amplifier used in both clinical and research applications. This unit plugs into a bedside or laboratory mainframe. Note the various controls. The input connector is a five-pin female jack that accepts the four limb electrodes, a chest electrode, and a shield. The LEAD switch selects which of the three ECG leads (I, II, or III) is displayed. The ECG DIAG/MON/PULSE switch is a filter selector. This type of control is often missing on clinical amplifiers, except those intended for catheterization laboratories and other specialized uses. The SENS control is a display amplitude control, and can be used to calibrate the display to the 1-mV internal calibration signal.

Modern biopotentials amplifiers, whether isolated or nonisolated, are usually based on the integrated circuit (IC) operational amplifier device. Most operational amplifiers have differential inputs (Figure 5-2); that is, there are two inputs (−IN and +IN) that each provide the same amount of gain, but have opposite polarities. The inverting input (−IN) of the operational amplifier provides an output that is 180 degrees out of phase with the input signal. In other words, a positive-going input signal will produce a negative-going output signal, and vice versa. The noninverting input (+IN) produces an output signal that is in phase with the input signal. For this type of input, a positive-going input signal will produce a positive-going output signal. We will use these properties to understand biopotentials amplifiers, most of which are differential models.

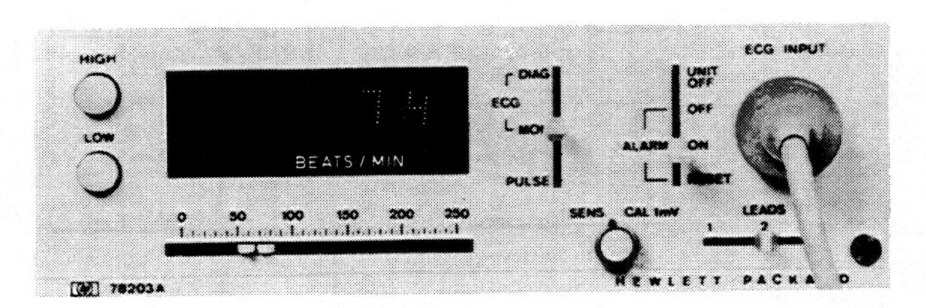

FIGURE 5-1

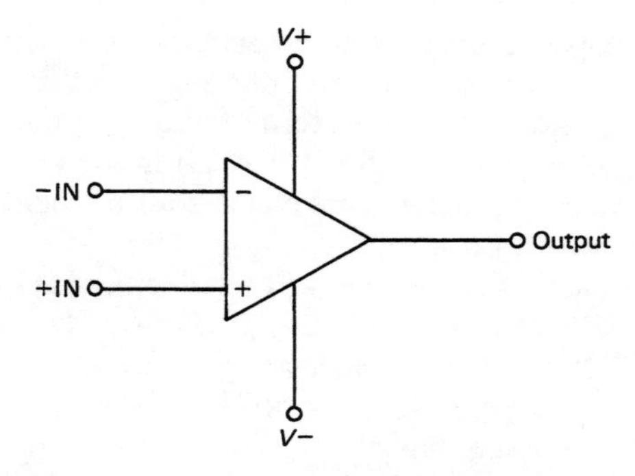

FIGURE 5-2

INPUT SIGNAL CONVENTIONS

Figure 5-3 shows a generic differential amplifier with the standard signals applied. Signals VI and V2 are single-ended potentials applied to the −In and +In inputs, respectively. The *differential input signal,* V_d, is the difference between the two single-ended signals: $V_d = (V2 - V1)$. Signal V_{cm} is a *common mode signal*; that is, it is applied equally to both −In and +In inputs. These signals are described further in the paragraphs that follow.

Common mode signals A common mode signal is one which is applied to both inputs at the same time. Such a signal might be either a voltage such as V_{cm} or a case where voltages V1 and V2 are equal to each other and of the same polarity (i.e., V1 = V2). The implication of the common mode signal is that, being applied equally to inverting and noninverting inputs, the net output voltage is zero. Because the two inputs have equal but opposite polarity gains for common mode signals, the net output signal in response to a common mode signal is zero.

The differential amplifier cancels common mode signals. An example of the usefulness of this property is in the performance of the differential amplifier with re-

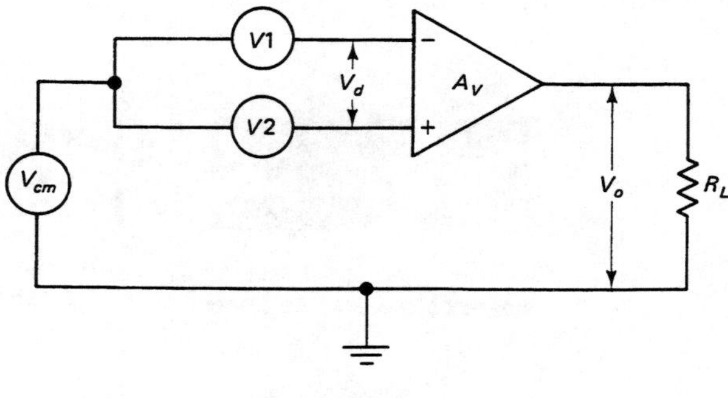

FIGURE 5-3

spect to 60-Hz hum pickup from local AC power lines. These signals are easily able to obscure weak ECG and EEG signals, so this property of differential amplifiers is quite handy. Almost all input signal cables for practical amplifiers will pick up 60-Hz radiated energy and convert it to a voltage that is seen by the amplifier as a genuine input signal. In a differential amplifier, however, the 60-Hz field will affect both inverting and noninverting input lines equally, so the 60-Hz artifact signal will disappear in the output. This feature of common mode signals is used to good advantage in ECG/EEG amplifiers, but only if the wires connecting the patient to the amplifier are approximately equal in length, and the electrodes are designed (and attached) in such a manner that the patient impedances are balanced between the two inputs.

The practical operational differential amplifier will not exhibit perfect rejection of common mode signals. A specification called the *common mode rejection ratio* (CMRR) tells us something of the ability of any given op-amp to reject such signals. The CMRR is usually specified in decibels (dB) and is defined as

$$\text{CMRR} = \frac{A_{vd}}{A_{cm}} \tag{5-1}$$

or, in decibel form,

$$\text{CMRR}_{\text{dB}} = 20 \log \left(\frac{A_{vd}}{A_{cm}}\right) \tag{5-2}$$

where

CMRR = the common mode rejection ratio in decibels
A_{vd} = the voltage gain to differential signals
A_{cm} = the voltage gain to common mode signals

In general, the higher the CMRR, the better the operational amplifier. Typical low-cost devices have CMRR ratings of 60 dB or more.

Differential signals Signals V1 and V2 in Figure 5-3 are each (by themselves) single-ended signals. The total differential signal seen by the operational amplifier is the difference between the two single-ended signals:

$$V_d = \text{V2} - \text{V1} \tag{5-3}$$

The ouput signal from the differential operational amplifier is the product of the differential voltage gain and the difference between the two input signals (hence the term "differential" amplifier). Thus, the transfer equation for the operational amplifier is

$$V_o = A_v(\text{V2} - \text{V1}) \tag{5-4}$$

Example

A DC differential amplifier has a gain of 2000. Calculate the output voltage if V1 = 2.006 and V2 = 2.003.

Solution:

$$\begin{aligned} V_o &= A_v(\text{V2} - \text{V1}) \\ &= (2000)(2.003 \text{ V DC} - 2.006 \text{ V DC}) \\ &= (2000)(-0.003 \text{ V DC}) = -6 \text{ V DC} \end{aligned}$$

DIFFERENTIAL AMPLIFIER TRANSFER EQUATION

The basic circuit for the simplest DC differential amplifier is shown in Figure 5-4. This circuit uses only one IC operational amplifier, so is the simplest possible configuration. Later you will see additional circuits that are based on three operational amplifier devices. In its most common form the circuit of Figure 5-4 is balanced such that R1 = R2 and R3 = R4.

The output voltage (V_o) is the product of the difference between single-ended input potentials V1 and V2 and the differential voltage gain (V_{vd}) of amplifier A1. The differential input voltage (V_d) is

$$V_d = \text{V2} - \text{V1} \tag{5-5}$$

If A_{vd} is the differential voltage gain, then

$$V_o = V_d A_{vd} \tag{5-6}$$

Assuming that R1 = R2 and R3 = R4, Equation 5-6 resolves to

$$V_o = \frac{\text{R3}}{\text{R1}}(\text{V2} - \text{V1}) \tag{5-7}$$

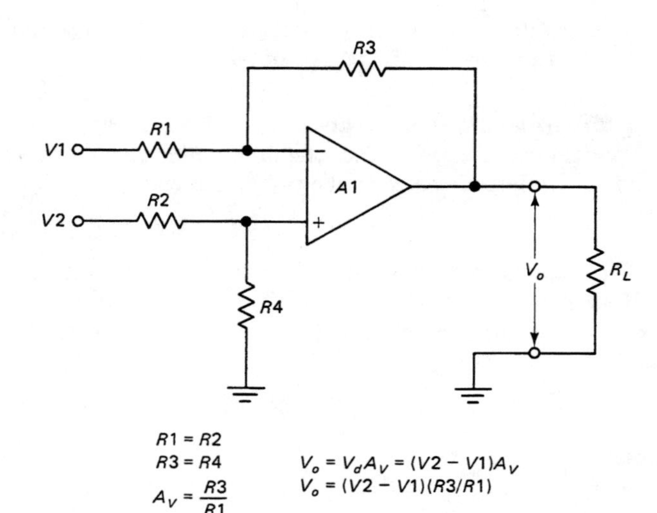

FIGURE 5-4

In this case, A_{vd} is R3/R1 and V_d is (V2 − V1). The standard transfer equation for the single op-amp DC differential amplifier is

$$V_o = V_d A_{vd} \tag{5-8}$$

$$= V_d \frac{R3}{R1} \tag{5-9}$$

COMMON MODE REJECTION

Figure 5-5 shows two different situations; Figure 5-5A shows a single-ended amplifier, while Figure 5-5B shows a differential amplifier in a similar situation. In these circuits a noise signal, V_n, is placed between the input ground and the output ground. This noise signal might be either AC or DC noise. In Figure 5-5A we see the case where the noise signal is applied to a single-ended input amplifier. The input signal seen by the amplifier is the algebraic sum of the two independent signals: $V_{in} + V_n$. Because of this fact, the amplifier output signal will see a noise artifact equal to the product of the noise signal amplitude and the amplifier gain, $-A_v V_n$. Now consider the situation of a differential amplifier depicted in Figure 5-5B. The noise signal in this case is common mode, so is essentially canceled by the common mode rejection ratio. Of course, in nonideal amplifiers the actual situation is that the input signal, V_{in}, is subject to the differential gain, while the noise signal, V_n, is subject to the common mode gain. If an amplifier has a CMRR of 100 dB, for example, the gain seen by the noise signal will be 100 dB down from the differential gain.

Consider a practical example. A standard ECG amplifier has a differential voltage gain of 1000. An ECG signal is typically 1-mV peak, so the output signal from the amplifier will be (1 mV) × 1000 = 1000 mV = 1 volt. If the CMRR is 120 dB, then the actual gain seen by the common mode signal is 120 dB lower than the differential gain. Because 120 dB is a ratio of 1,000,000 : 1, the common mode gain will be 1000/1,000,000 or 0.001. Now suppose that the 60-Hz common mode input signal is 10 mV (a reasonable value for 5-ft electrode wires). The 60-Hz signal component in the output of the amplifier is the product of the common mode signal voltage and the common mode gain, or in this case 10 mV × 0.001, or 0.01 mV. The output signal from the ECG signal is 1000 mV, so the signal-to-noise ratio in this case is 1000 mV/0.01 mV, or 100 dB. Clearly, there is a good reason to use a differential amplifier for biopotentials signals acquisition.

The common mode rejection ratio of the operational amplifier DC differential circuit is dependent principally upon two factors: first, the natural CMRR of the operational amplifier used as the active device, second, the balance of the resistors, R1 = R2 and R3 = R4. Unfortunately, the balance is typically difficult to obtain with fixed resistors. We can use a circuit such as in Figure 5-6. In this circuit, R1 through R3 are exactly the same as in previous circuits. The fourth resistor, however, is a potentiometer (see R4). The potentiometer will "adjust out" the CMRR errors caused by resistor and related mismatches.

A version of the circuit with greater resolution is shown in the inset to Figure 5-6. In this version the single potentiometer is replaced by a fixed resistor and a po-

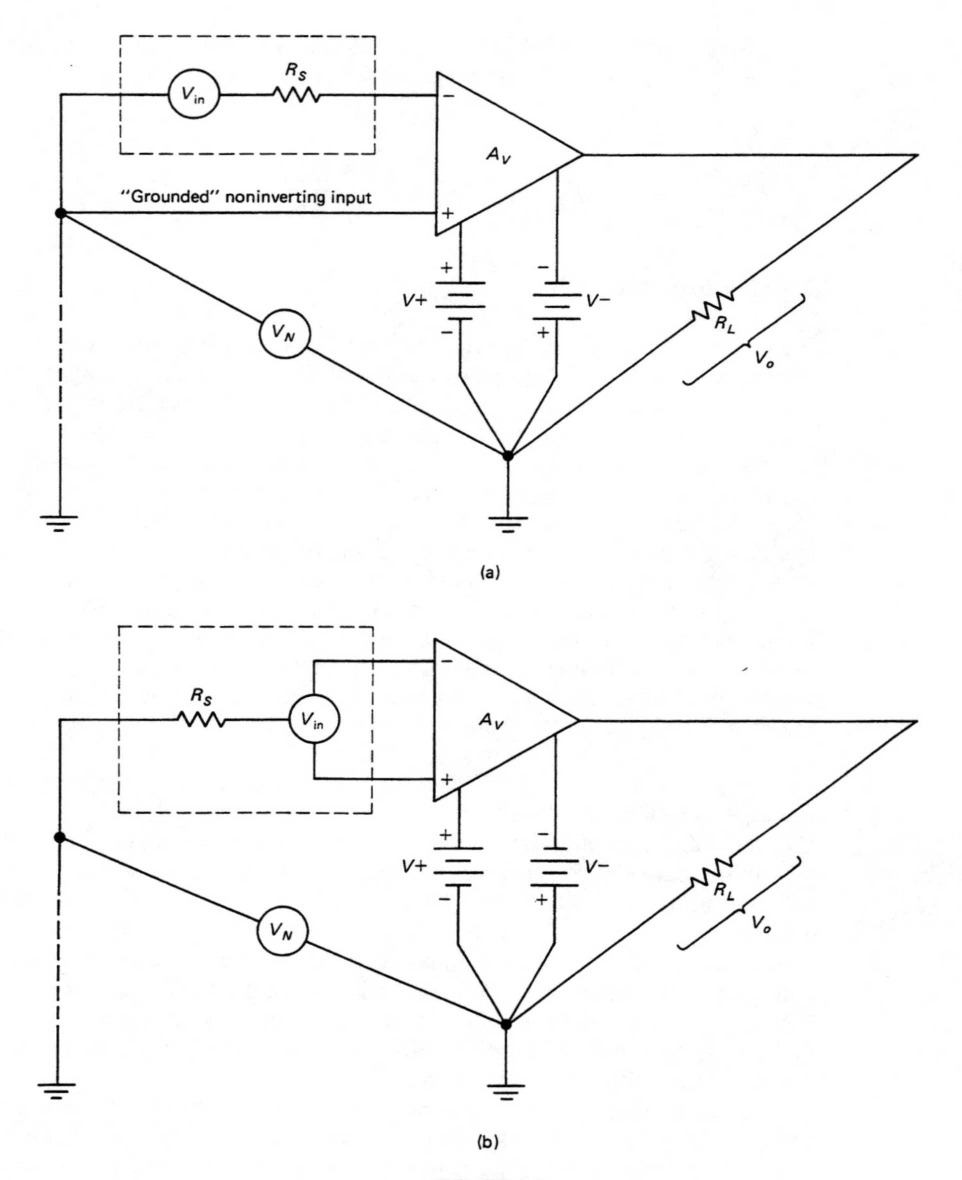

FIGURE 5-5

tentiometer in series; the sum resistance (R4A + R4B) is equal to approximately 20 percent more than the normal value of R3. Ordinarily, the maximum value of the potentiometer is 10 to 20 percent of the overall resistance.

The adjustment procedure for either version of Figure 5-6 is the same (see Figure 5-7):

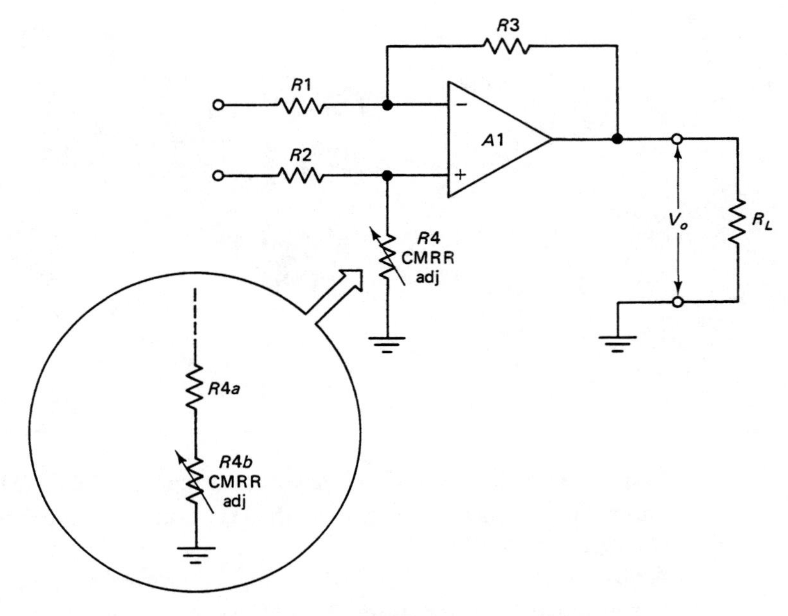

FIGURE 5-6

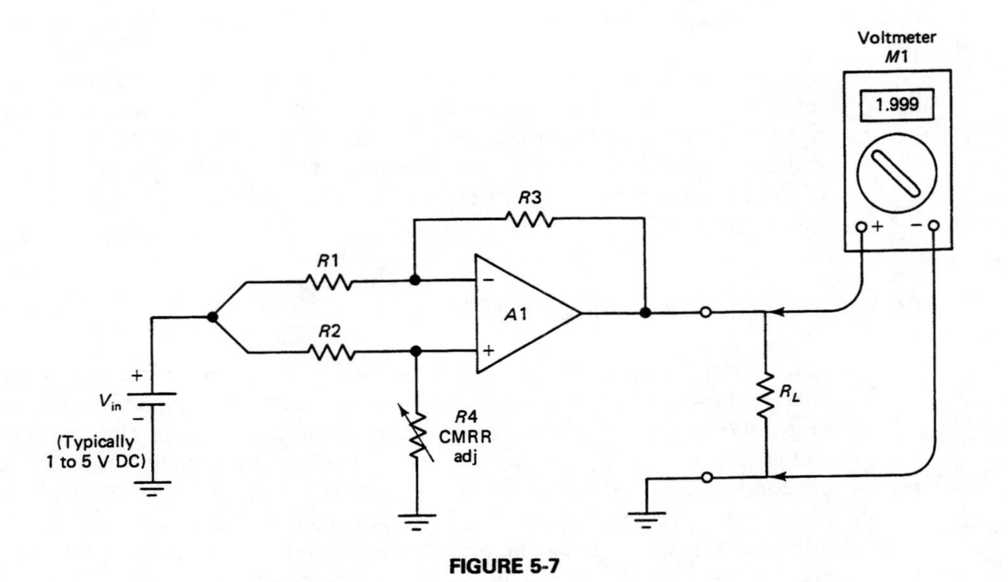

FIGURE 5-7

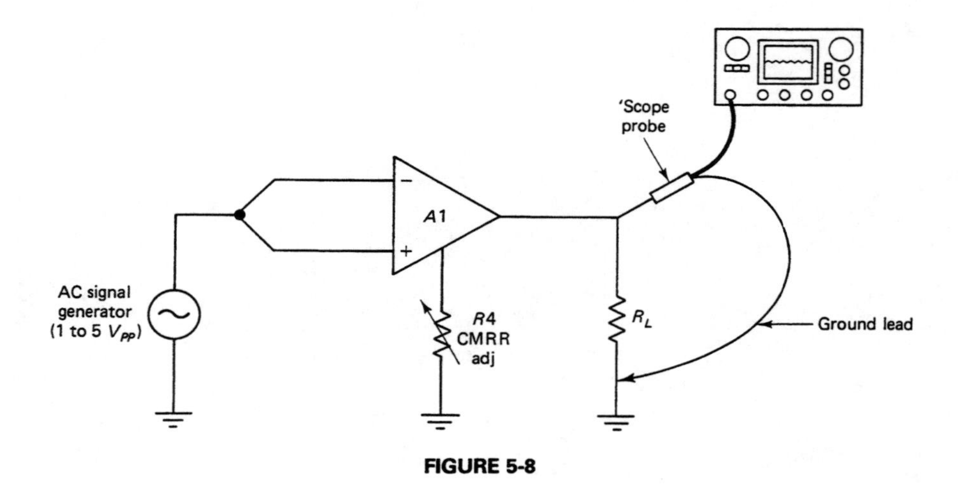

FIGURE 5-8

1. Connect a zero-center DC voltmeter to the output terminal (M1 in Figure 5-7).
2. Short together inputs *A* and *B* and then connect them to either a signal voltage source or ground.
3. Adjust potentiometer R4 (CMRR ADJ) for zero volts output.
4. If the output indicator (meter M1) has several ranges, then switch to a lower range and repeat step 3 until no further improvement is possible.
5. Disconnect the signal source, and unshort the amplifier input terminals.

Alternatively, connect the amplifier output to an audio voltmeter or oscilloscope (see Figure 5-8), and connect the input to a 1-volt to 5-volt peak-to-peak AC signal that is within the frequency range of the particular amplifier. For EMG and wideband amplifiers, a 400-Hz to 1000-Hz, 1-volt signal is typically used, while for ECG/EEG amplifiers, the frequency will be 10 Hz to 40 Hz (the signal voltage is the same, however).

DIFFERENTIAL INSTRUMENTATION AMPLIFIERS

The simple DC differential amplifier circuit is only useful for low gain applications, and for those applications where a low to moderate input impedance is permissible (e.g., 300 to 200,000 ohms). In the medical context, they are often used in instruments such as transducer amplifiers and microelectrode amplifiers, and for other applications where the signal levels are relatively high (e.g., >100 mV). Where a higher gain is required (as in ECG/EEG), then a more complex circuit called the operational amplifier instrumentation amplifier (or IA) is used. We will examine the classical three-device IA circuit, as well as several integrated circuit instrumentation amplifiers (ICIA) that offer the advantages of the IA in a single small IC package.

Some of those devices are now among the most commonly used in many medical instrumentation applications.

The simple DC differential amplifier just discussed suffers from several drawbacks. First, there is a limit to the input impedance: Z_{in} is approximately equal to the sum of the two input resistors. Second, there is a practical limitation on the gain available from the simple single-device DC differential amplifier. If we attempt to obtain high gain, then we find that either the input bias current tends to cause large output offset voltages, or the input impedance becomes too low. In this section we will demonstrate a solution to these problems in the form of the instrumentation amplifier. All these amplifiers are differential amplifiers, but offer superior performance over the simple DC differential amplifier. The instrumentation amplifier can offer higher input impedance, higher gain, and better common mode rejection than the single-device DC differential amplifier.

SIMPLE IA CIRCUIT

The simplest form of instrumentation amplifier circuit is shown in Figure 5-9. In this circuit the input impedance is improved by connecting inputs of a simple DC differential amplifier (A3) to two input amplifiers (A1 and A2) that are each of the unity gain, noninverting follower configuration (their use here is as buffer amplifiers). The input amplifiers offer an extremely large input impedance (a result of the noninverting configuration) while driving the input resistors of the actual amplifying stage

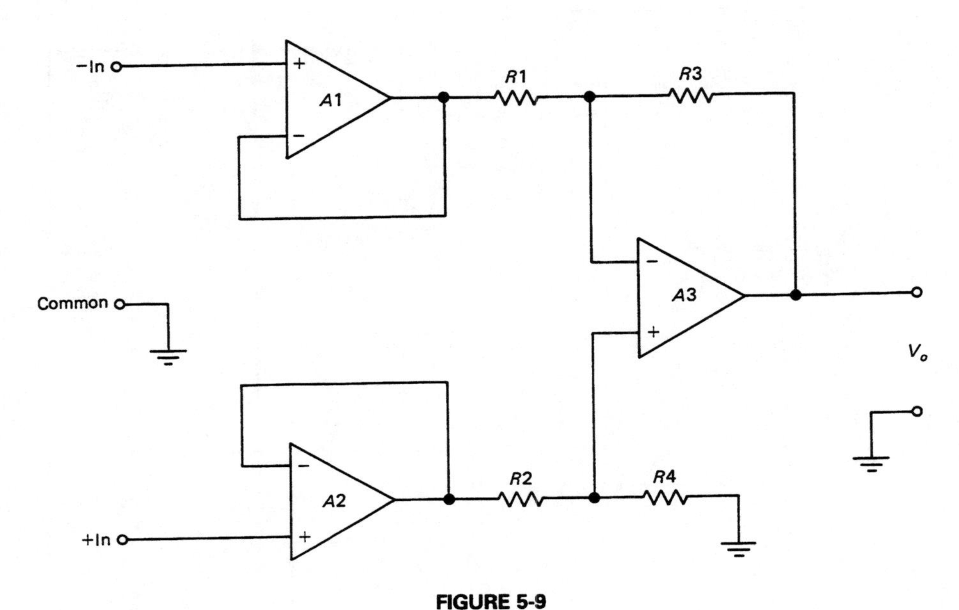

FIGURE 5-9

(A3). The overall gain of this circuit is the same as for any simple DC differential amplifier:

$$A_v = \frac{R3}{R1} \tag{5-10}$$

where A_v is the voltage gain, assuming R1 = R2 and R3 = R4.

It is considered best practice if A1 and A2 are identical operational amplifiers. In fact, it is advisable to use a dual operational amplifier for both A1 and A2. The common thermal environment of the dual amplifier will reduce thermal drift problems. The very high input impedance of superbeta (Darlington), BiMOS and BiFET operational amplifiers make them ideal for use as the input amplifiers in this type of circuit.

One of the biggest problems with the circuit of Figure 5-9 is that it wastes two good operational amplifiers. The most common form of instrumentation amplifier circuit uses the input amplifiers to provide voltage gain in addition to a higher input impedance. Such amplifier circuits are discussed in the next section.

STANDARD INSTRUMENTATION AMPLIFIERS

The standard instrumentation amplifier is shown in Figure 5-10. Like the simple circuit discussed, this circuit uses three operational amplifiers. The biggest difference is that the input amplifiers (A1 and A2) are used in the "noninverting follower with

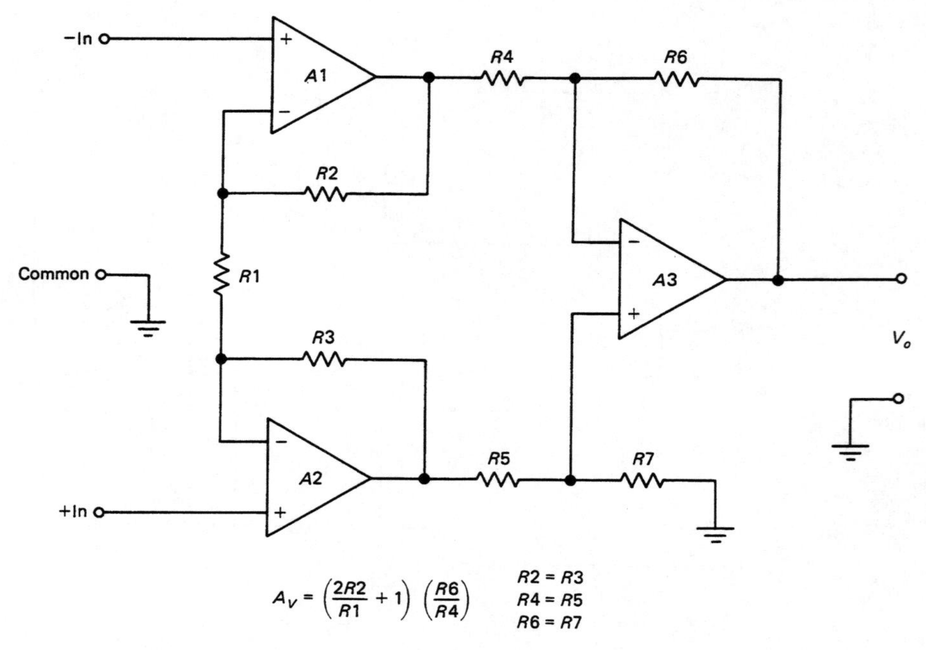

FIGURE 5-10

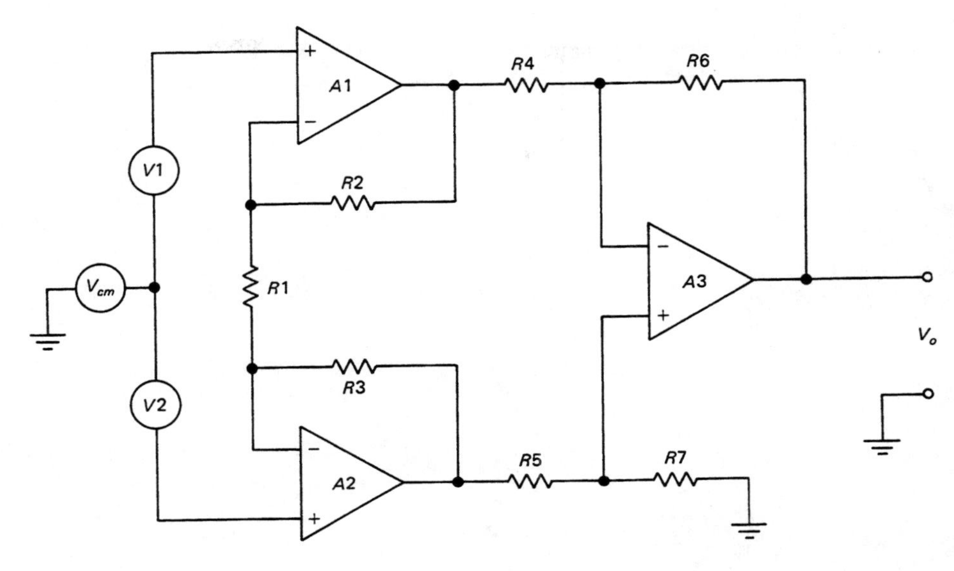

FIGURE 5-11

gain" configuration. Like the circuit of Figure 5-9, the input amplifiers are ideally BiMOS, BiFET, or superbeta input types for maximum input impedance. Again, for best thermal performance use a dual, triple, or quad operational amplifier for this application. The signal voltages shown in Figure 5-11 follow the standard pattern: voltages V1 and V2 form the differential input signal (V2 − V1), while voltage V_{cm} represents the common mode signal because it affects both inputs equally.

The transfer equation for the instrumentation amplifier is

$$A_v = \left(\frac{2\ \text{R2}}{\text{R1}} + 1\right)\left(\frac{\text{R6}}{\text{R4}}\right) \tag{5-11}$$

provided

$$\text{R2} = \text{R3}$$
$$\text{R4} = \text{R5}$$
$$\text{R6} = \text{R7}$$

GAIN CONTROL FOR THE IA

It is difficult to provide a gain control for a simple DC differential amplifier without adding an extra amplifier stage (for example, an inverting follower with a gain of 0 to −1). For the instrumentation amplifier, however, resistor R1 can be used as a gain control provided that the resistance does not go to a value near zero ohms. Figure 5-12 shows a revised circuit with resistor R1 replaced by a series circuit consisting of fixed resistor R1A and potentiometer R1B. This circuit prevents the gain from

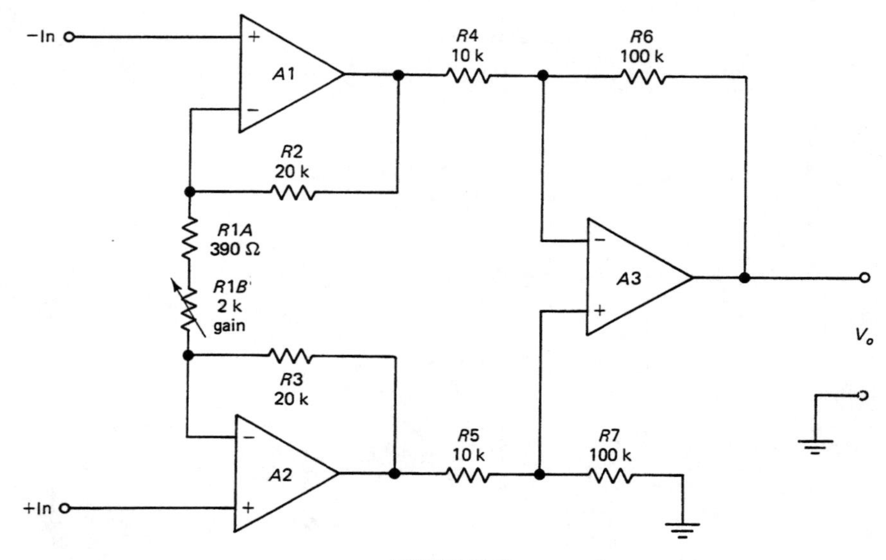

FIGURE 5-12

rising to above the level set by R1A. Don't use a potentiometer alone in this circuit because it can have a disastrous effect on the gain. Note in Equation 5-11 that the term "R1" appears in the denominator. If the value of R1 gets close to zero, then the gain goes very high (in fact, supposedly to infinity if R1 = 0). The maximum gain of the circuit by using the fixed resistor is in series with the potentiometer. The gain of the circuit in Figure 5-12 varies from a minimum of 167 (when R1B is set to 2000 ohms) to a maximum of 1025 (when R1B is zero). The gain expression for Figure 5-12 is

$$A_v = \left(\frac{2\ \mathrm{R2}}{\mathrm{R1A} + \mathrm{R1B}} + 1\right)\left(\frac{\mathrm{R6}}{\mathrm{R4}}\right) \tag{5-12}$$

or, rewriting Equation 5-12 to take into account that R1A is fixed,

$$A_v = \left(\frac{2\ \mathrm{R2}}{390 + \mathrm{R1B}} + 1\right)\left(\frac{\mathrm{R6}}{\mathrm{R4}}\right) \tag{5-13}$$

where R1B varies from 0 to 2000 ohms.

COMMON MODE REJECTION RATIO ADJUSTMENT

The instrumentation amplifier is no different from any other practical DC differential amplifier in that there will be imperfect balance for common mode signals. The operational amplifiers are not ideally matched, so there will be a gain imbalance. This gain imbalance is further deteriorated by the mismatch of the resistors. The result is that the instrumentation amplifier will respond at least to some extent to common mode signals. As in the simple DC differential amplifier, we can provide a common mode rejection ratio adjustment by making resistor R7 variable. As was true with the simple differential amplifier circuit, the CMRR ADJ control can be a fixed resistor in series with a potentiometer for best resolution.

AC INSTRUMENTATION AMPLIFIERS

What is the principal difference between "DC amplifiers" and "AC amplifiers"? A DC amplifier will amplify both AC and DC signals up to the frequency limit of the particular circuit being used. The AC amplifier, on the other hand, will not pass or amplify DC signals. In fact, AC amplifiers will not pass AC signals of frequencies from close to DC to some lower −3-dB bandpass limit. The gain in the region between near-DC and the "full-gain" frequencies within the passband rises at a rate determined by the design, usually +6 dB/octave (an "octave" is a 2 : 1 frequency change). The standard low-end point in the frequency response curve is defined as the frequency at which the gain drops off −3 dB from the full gain.

Figure 5-13 shows a modified version of the instrumentation amplifier that is designed as an AC amplifier. The input circuitry of A1 and A2 is modified by placing a capacitor in series with each op-amp's noninverting input. Resistors R8 and R9 are used to keep the input bias currents of A1 and A2 from charging capacitors C1

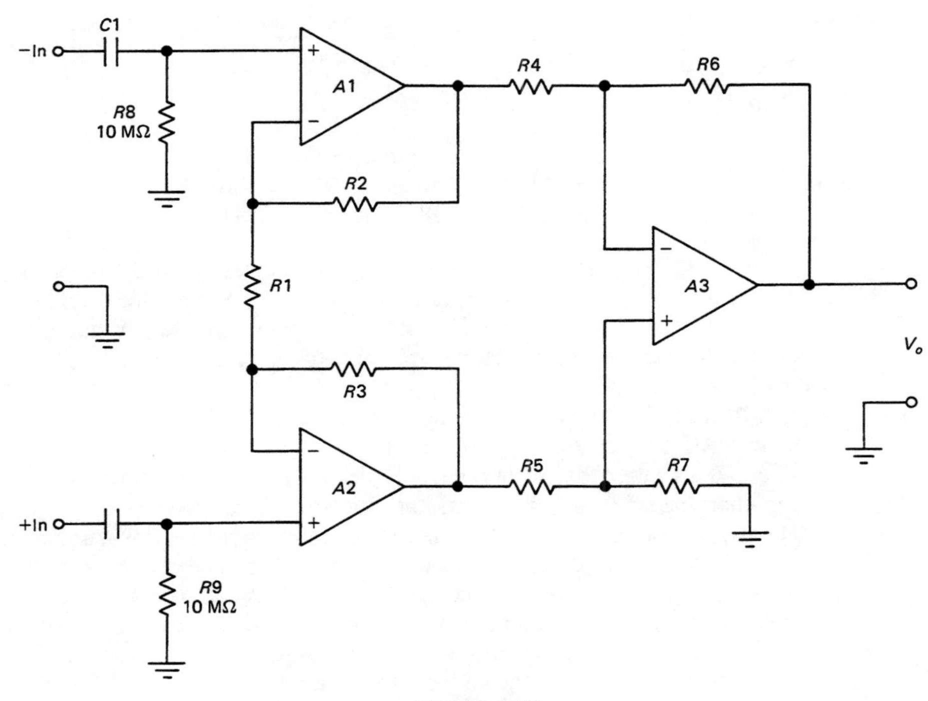

FIGURE 5-13

and C2. In some modern low-input current operational amplifiers, these resistors are optional because of the extremely low levels of bias current that are normally present.

The −3-dB frequency of the amplifier in Figure 5-13 is a function of the input capacitors and resistors (assuming that R8 = R9 = R and C1 = C2 = C):

$$F = \frac{1{,}000{,}000}{2\pi RC_{\mu F}} \tag{5-14}$$

where

F = the −3-dB frequency in hertz
R = resistance in ohms
$C_{\mu F}$ = capacitance in microfarads

The equation given here for frequency response is not the most useful form. In most practical cases you will know the required frequency response from evaluation of the application. Furthermore, you will know the value of the input resistors (R9 and R10) because they are selected for high input impedance, and are by convention either >10× or >100× the source impedance (depending upon the application). Typically, these resistors are selected to be 10 megohms. You will therefore need to select the capacitor values from Equation 5-15:

$$C_{\mu f} = \frac{1{,}000{,}000}{2\pi RF} \tag{5-15}$$

where

$C_{\mu f}$ = the capacitance of C1 and C2 in microfarads
R = the resistance of R9 and R10 in ohms
F = the −3-dB frequency in hertz

The AC instrumentation amplifier can be adapted to all the other modifications of the basic circuit discussed earlier in this chapter. We may, for example, use a gain control (replace R1 with a fixed resistor and a potentiometer) or add a CMRR ADJ control. In fact, these adaptations are probably necessary in most practical AC IA circuits.

In many instrumentation amplifier applications it is desirable to provide selectable AC or DC coupling, as well as the ability to ground the input of the amplifiers. This latter feature is especially desirable in circuits where an oscilloscope, strip-chart paper recorder, digital data logger, or computer is used to receive the data. By grounding the input of the amplifier (without also grounding the source, which could be dangerous), it is possible to set (or at least determine) the $V_d = 0$ baseline. Figure 5-14 shows a modified input circuit that uses a switch to select AC-GND-DC coupling. In addition, a second switch is provided that sets the low-end −3-dB frequency response point according to Equation 5-15. A table of popular frequency response limits is shown inset to Figure 5-14.

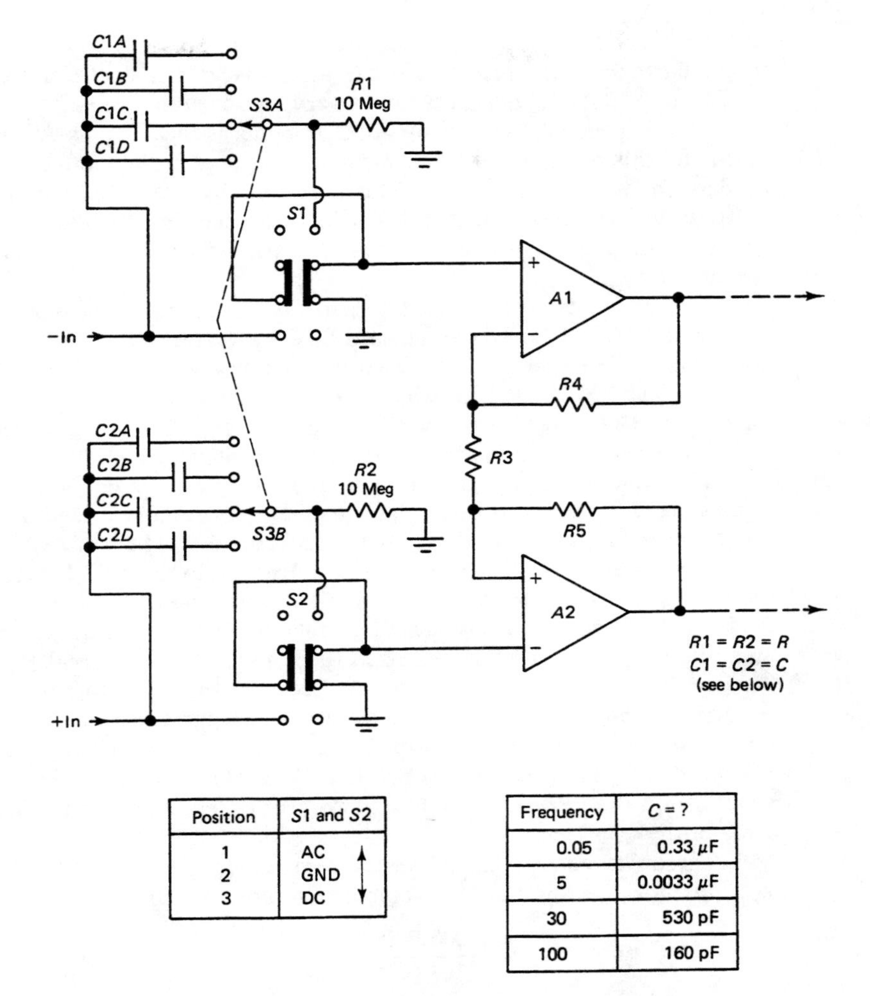

Position	S1 and S2
1	AC
2	GND
3	DC

Frequency	C = ?
0.05	0.33 μF
5	0.0033 μF
30	530 pF
100	160 pF

FIGURE 5-14

DESIGN EXAMPLE: AN ANIMAL ECG AMPLIFIER

Note: The circuit in this section is for animal use only. It should not be used for human ECGs because of electrical safety considerations. For human ECGs use an isolated amplifier.

The heart in man and animals produces a small electrical signal that can be recorded through skin surface electrodes and displayed on an oscilloscope or paper strip-chart recorder. This signal is called the electrocardiograph, or ECG, signal. The peak values of the ECG signal are on the order of 1 millivolt. To produce a 1-volt signal to apply to a recorder or oscilloscope, then we need a gain of 1000 mV/1 mV, or 1000. Our ECG amplifier, therefore, must provide a gain of 1000 or more. Furthermore, because skin has a relatively high electrical resistance (1 to 20 Ω), the ECG amplifier must have a very high input impedance.

Another requirement for the ECG amplifier is that it be an AC amplifier. The reason for this requirement is that metallic electrodes applied to the electrolytic skin produces a "half-cell potential." This potential tends to be on the order of 1 to 2 volts, so it is more than 1000 times higher than the signal voltage. By making the amplifier respond only to AC, we eliminate the artifact caused by the DC half-cell potential.

The frequency selected for the −3-dB point of the ECG amplifier must be very low, close to DC, because the standard ECG waveform contains very-low-frequency components. The typical ECG signal has significant frequency components in the range 0.05 to 100 hertz (Hz), which is the industry standard frequency response for diagnostic ECG amplifiers (some clinical monitoring ECG amplifiers use 0.05 Hz to 40 Hz to eliminate muscle artifact due to patient movements).

The typical ECG amplifier has differential inputs because the most useful ECG signals are differential in nature, and suppress 60-Hz hum picked up on the leads and the patient's body. In the most simple case, the right arm (RA) and left arm (LA) electrodes form the inputs to the amplifier, with the right leg (RL) defined as the common (see Figure 5-15). The basic configuration of the amplifier in Figure 5-15 is the AC-coupled instrumentation amplifier discussed earlier. The gain for this amplifier is set to slightly more than ×1000, so a 1-mV ECG peak signal will produce a 1-volt output from this amplifier. Because of the high gain it is essential that the amplifier be well balanced. This requirement suggests the use of a dual amplifier for A1 and A2. An example might be the RCA CA-3240 device, which is a dual BiMOS device that is essentially two CA-3140s in a single eight-pin miniDIP package. Also in the interest of balance, 1 percent or less tolerance resistors should be used for the equal pairs.

The lower-end −3-dB frequency response point is set by the input resistors and capacitors. In this case, the combination forms a response of

$$F_{\mathrm{Hz}} = \frac{1{,}000{,}000}{2\pi RC}$$

$$= \frac{1{,}000{,}000}{(2)(3.14)(10{,}000{,}000 \text{ ohms})(0.33\ \mu\text{F})}$$

$$= \frac{1{,}000{,}000}{20{,}724{,}000} = 0.048 \text{ Hz}$$

The CMRR ADJUST control in Figure 5-15 is usually a 10- to 20-turn trimmer potentiometer. It is adjusted in the following manner:

1. Short together the RA, LA, and RL inputs.
2. Connect a DC voltmeter to the output (either a digital voltmeter or an analog meter with a 1.5-volt DC scale (alternatively, a DC-coupled oscilloscope can be used, but be sure to identify the zero baseline).

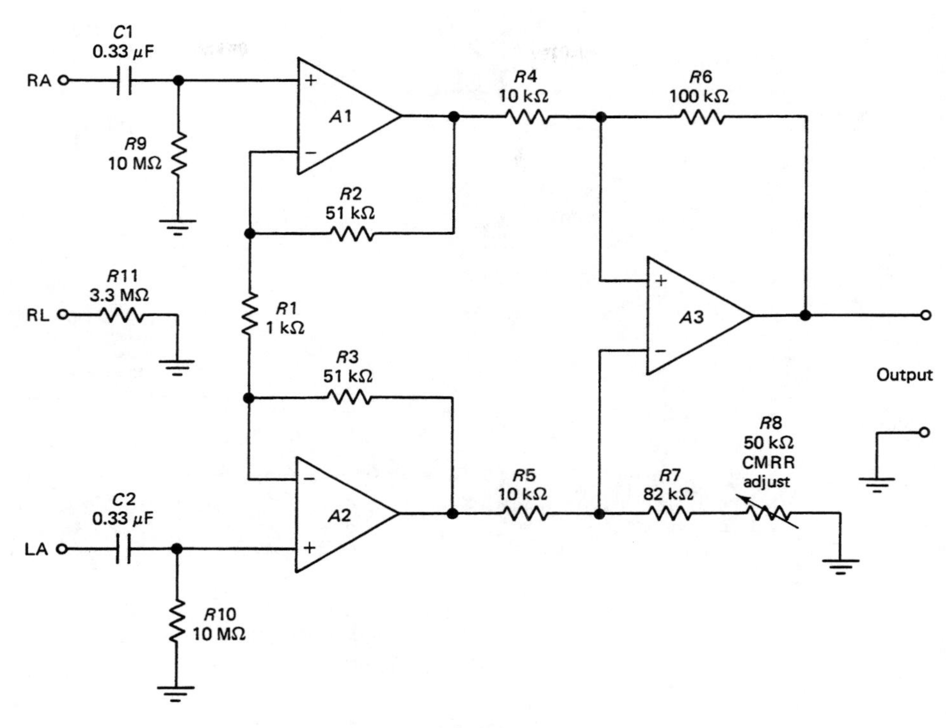

FIGURE 5-15

3. Adjust CMRR ADJUST control (R7) for zero volts output.
4. Disconnect the RL input, and connect a signal generator between RL and the still-connected RA/LA terminal. Adjust the output of the signal generator for a sine wave frequency in the range 10 to 40 Hz, and a peak-to-peak potential of 1 volt to 3 volts.
5. Using an AC scale on the voltmeter (or an oscilloscope), again adjust CMRR ADJUST (R7) for the smallest possible output signal. It may be necessary to readjust the voltmeter or oscilloscope input range control to observe the best null.
6. Remove the RA/LA short. The ECG amplifier is ready to use.

A suitable postamplifier for the ECG preamplifier is shown in Figure 5-16. This amplifier is placed in the signal line between the output of Figure 5-15 and the input of the oscilloscope or paper chart recorder used to display the waveform. The gain of the postamplifier is variable from 0 to +2; it will produce a 2-volt maximum output when a 1-millivolt ECG signal provides a 1-volt output from the preamplifier. Because of the high-level signals used, this amplifier can use ordinary 741 operational amplifiers.

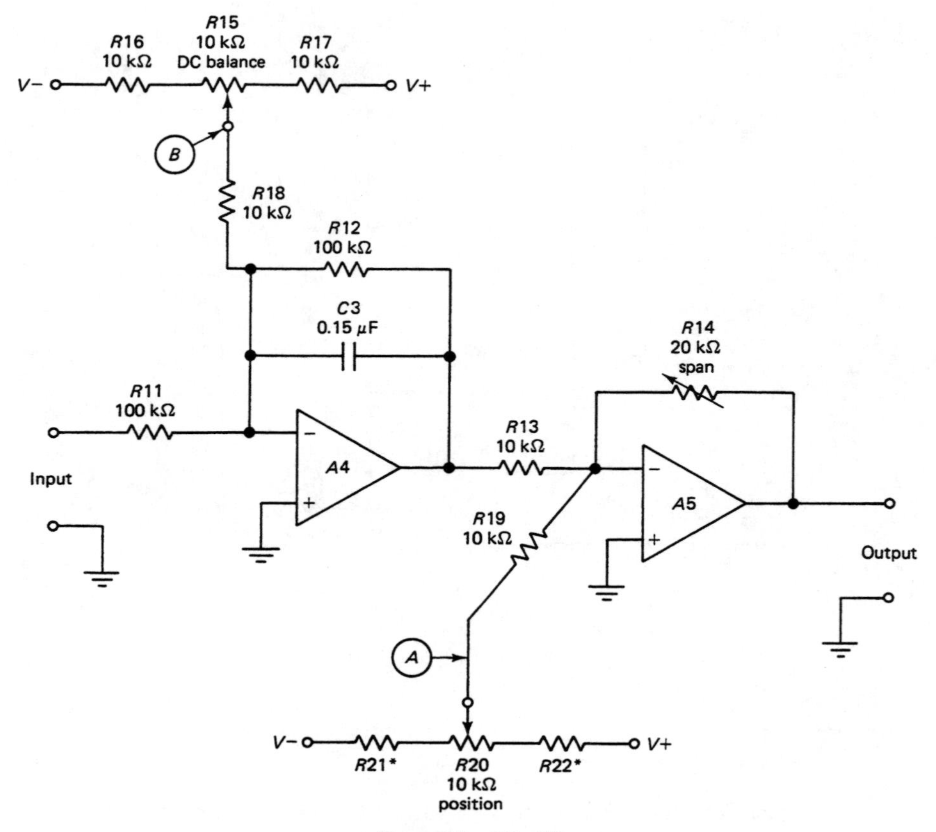

FIGURE 5-16

The frequency response of the amplifier is set to an upper −3-dB point of 100 Hz, with the response dropping off at a −6-dB/octave rate above that frequency. This frequency response point is determined by capacitor C3 operating with resistor R12:

$$F_{Hz} = \frac{1{,}000{,}000}{2\pi RC}$$

$$= \frac{1{,}000{,}000}{(2)(3.14)(100{,}000)(0.015\ \mu F)}$$

$$= \frac{1{,}000{,}000}{9420} = 106\ \text{Hz}$$

There are three controls in the postamplifier circuit: *span, position,* and *DC balance*. The span control is the 0 to 2 gain control, and the label "span" reflects instrumentation users language, rather than electronics language. The position control sets the position of the output waveform on the display device. Resistors R21 and R22 are selected to limit the travel of the beam or pen to full scale. Set these resistors so that the maximum potential at the end terminals of R20 corresponds to full-scale deflection of the display device.

The DC balance control is used to cancel the collective effects of offset potentials created by the various stages of amplification. This control is adjusted as follows:

1. Follow the CMRR ADJUST procedure; then reconnect the short circuit at RA, LA, and RL. The voltmeter is moved to the output of Figure 5-16.
2. Adjust the position control for zero volts at point "A."
3. Adjust the DC balance control for zero volts at point "B."
4. Adjust the span control (R14) through its entire range from zero to maximum while monitoring the output voltage. If the output voltage does not shift, then no further adjustment is needed.
5. If the output voltage in the previous step varied as the span control is varied, then adjust DC balance until varying the span control over its full range does not produce an output voltage shift. Repeat this step several times until no further improvement is possible.
6. Remove the RA, LA, RL short; the amplifier is ready for use.

IC INSTRUMENTATION AMPLIFIERS: SOME COMMERCIAL EXAMPLES

The operational amplifier truly revolutionized analog circuit design. For a long time, the only additional advances were that op-amps became better and better (they became nearer the ideal op-amp of textbooks). While that was an exciting development, they were not really new devices. The next big breakthrough came when the analog device designers made an IC version of the instrumentation amplifier in Figure 5-10, the integrated circuit instrumentation amplifier (ICIA). Today, several manufacturers offer substantially improved ICIA devices.

The Burr-Brown INA-101 (Figure 5-17) is a popular ICIA device. This ICIA is very simple to connect and use. There are only DC power connections, differential input connections, offset adjust connections, ground, and an output. The gain of the circuit is set by

$$A_{vd} = (40k/R_g) + 1 \tag{5-16}$$

The INA-101 is basically a low-noise, low-input-bias current integrated circuit version of the IA of Figure 5-10. The resistors labeled R2 and R3 in Figure 5-10 are internal to the INA-101, and are 20 Ω each; hence, the "40 k" term in Equation 5-16.

Potentiometer R1 in Figure 5-17 is used to null the offset voltages appearing at the output. An offset voltage is a voltage that exists on the output at a time when it

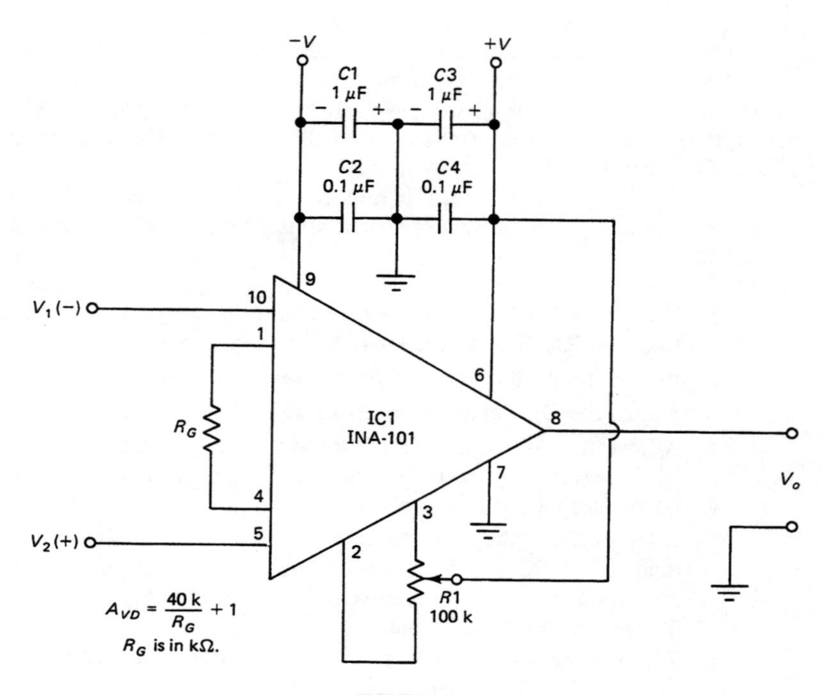

FIGURE 5-17

should be zero (i.e., when V1 = V2, so that V1 − V2 = 0). The offset voltage might be internal to the amplifier or a component of the input signal. DC offsets in signals are common, especially in biopotentials amplifiers such as ECG and EEG and chemical transducers such as pH, pO_2, and pCO_2.

Another ICIA is the LM-363-xx device shown in Figure 5-18; the miniDIP version is shown (an eight-pin metal can is also available), while a typical circuit is shown in Figure 5-19. The LM-363-xx device is a fixed gain ICIA. There are three versions of the LM-363-xx enumerated according to gain:

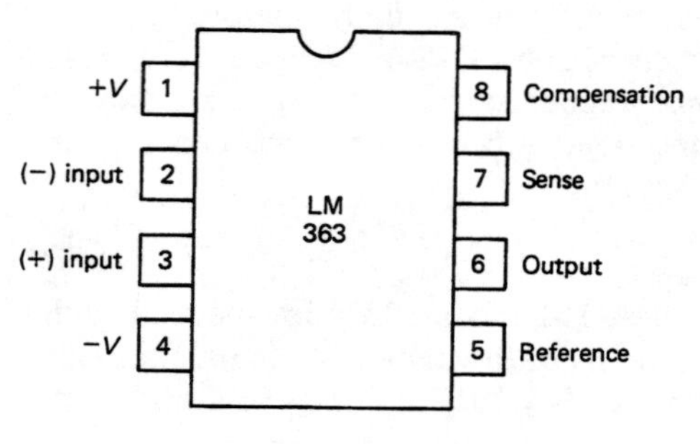

FIGURE 5-18

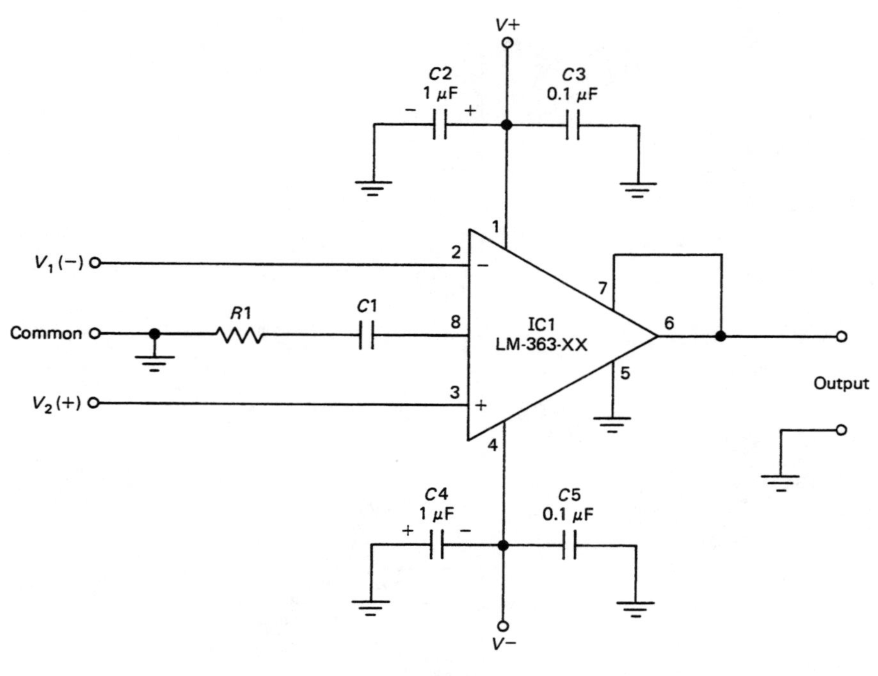

FIGURE 5-19

DESIGNATION	**GAIN (A_v)**
LM-363-10	×10
LM-363-100	×100
LM-363-500	×500

The LM-363-xx is useful in places where one of the standard gains is required and there is minimum space available. Two examples spring to mind. The LM-363-xx can be used as a transducer preamplifier, especially in noisy signal areas; the LM-363-xx can be built onto (or into) the transducer to build up its signal before sending it to the main instrument or signal before sending it to the main instrument or signal acquisition computer. Another possible use is in biopotentials amplifiers. Biopotentials are typically very small, especially in lab animals. The LM-363-xx can be mounted on the subject and a higher-level signal sent to the main instrument.

A selectable gain version of the LM-363 device is shown in Figure 5-20; the 16-pin DIP package is shown. A typical circuit is shown in Figure 5-21. The type number of this device is LM-363-AD, which distinguishes it from the LM-363-xx devices. The gain can be ×10, ×100, or ×1000, depending upon the programming of the gain setting pins (2, 3, and 4). The programming protocol is as follows:

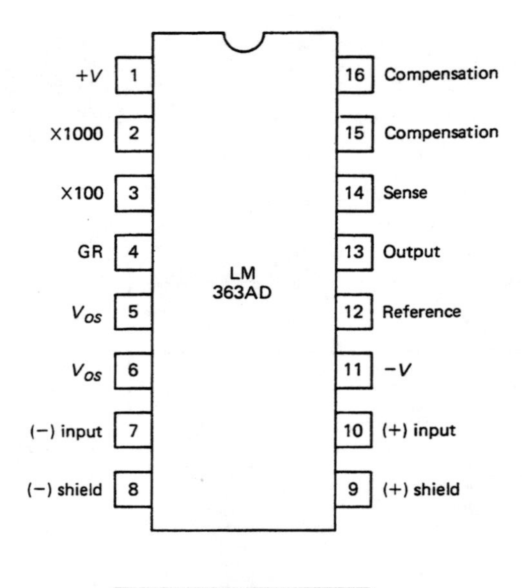

Programming	
Gain	Jumper pins
×10	(all open)
×100	3, 4
×1000	2, 4

FIGURE 5-20

GAIN DESIRED	JUMPER PINS
×10	(all open)
×100	3, 4
×1000	2, 4

Switch S1 in Figure 5-21 is the gain select switch. This switch should be mounted close to the IC device, but is quite flexible in mechanical form. The switch could also be made from a combination of CMOS electronic switches (e.g., 4066).

The DC power supply terminals are treated in a manner similar to the other amplifiers. Again, the 0.1-μF capacitors need to be mounted as close as possible to the body of the LM-363-AD.

Pins 8 and 9 are guard shield outputs. These pins are a feature that makes the LM-363-AD more useful for many instrumentation problems than other models. By outputting a signal sample back to the shield of the input lines, we can increase the common mode rejection ratio. This feature is used a lot in bipotentials amplifiers and in other applications where a low-level signal must pass through a strong interference (high-noise) environment. Guard shield theory will be discussed shortly.

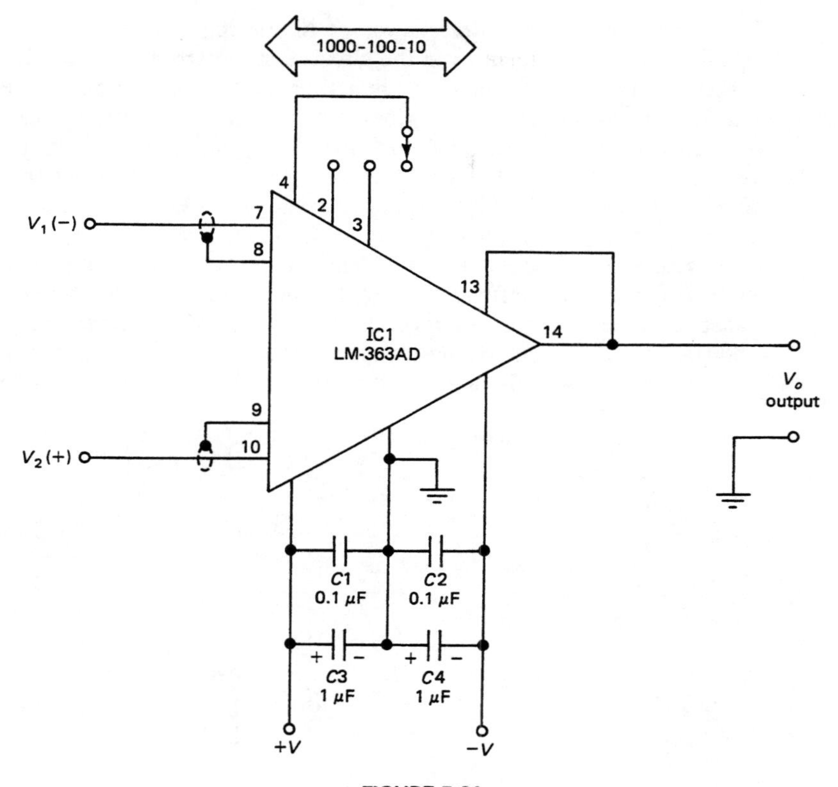

FIGURE 5-21

The LM-363 devices will operate with DC supply voltages of ±5 volts to ±18 volts DC, with a common mode rejection ratio of 130 dB. The 7 nV/$\sqrt{\text{Hz}}$ noise figure makes the device useful for low-noise applications (a 0.5-nV model is also available).

GUARD SHIELDING

One of the properties of the differential amplifier, including instrumentation amplifiers, is that it tends to suppress interfering signals from the environment. The common mode rejection process is at the root of this capability. When an amplifier is used in a situation where it is connected to an external signal source through wires, those wires are subjected to strong local 60-Hz AC fields from nearby power line wiring. Fortunately, in the case of the differential amplifier, the field affects both lines equally, so the induced interfering signal is canceled out by the common mode rejection property of the amplifier.

Unfortunately, the cancellation of interfering signals is not total. There may be, for example, imbalances in the circuit that tend to deteriorate the CMRR of the amplifier. These imbalances may be either internal or external to the amplifier circuit. Figure 5-22A shows a common scenario. In this figure we see the differential amplifier connected to shielded leads from the signal source, V_{in}. Shielded lead wires offer some protection from local fields, but there is a problem with the standard wisdom regarding shields: it is possible for shielded cables to manufacture a valid differential signal voltage from a common mode signal!

Figure 5-22B shows an equivalent circuit that demonstrates how a shielded cable pair can create a differential signal from a common mode signal. The cable has capacitance between the center conductor and the shield conductor surrounding it. In addition, input connectors and the amplifier equipment internal wiring also exhibits capacitance. These capacitances are lumped together in the model of Figure 5-22 as

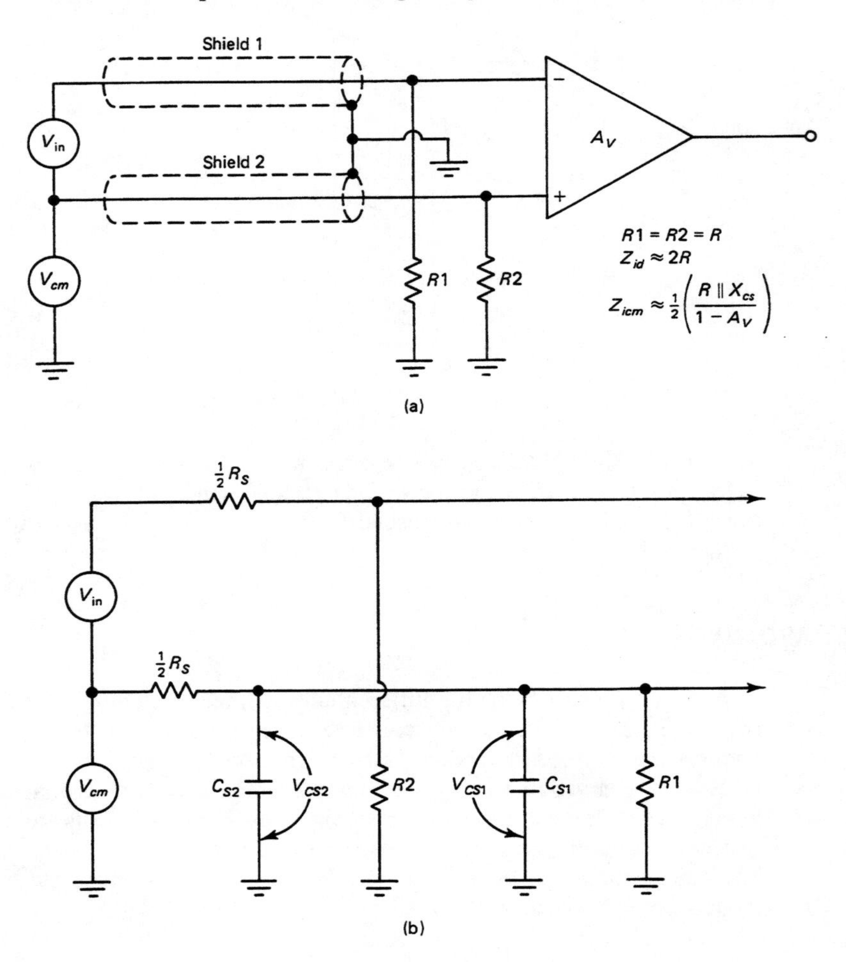

FIGURE 5-22

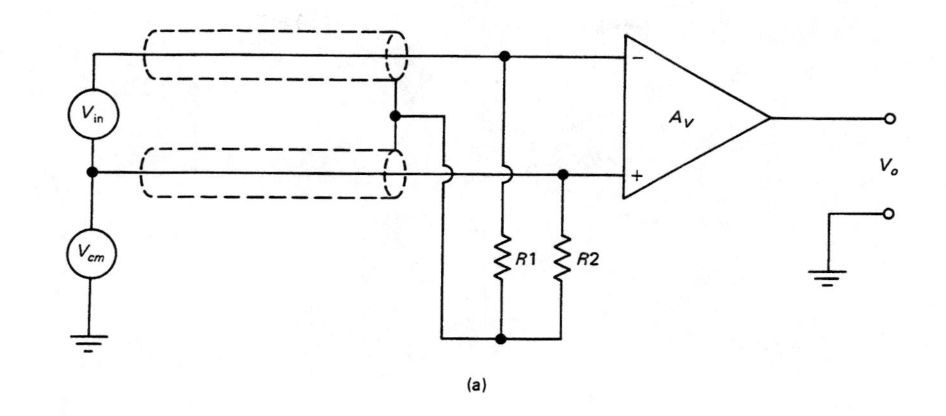

(a)

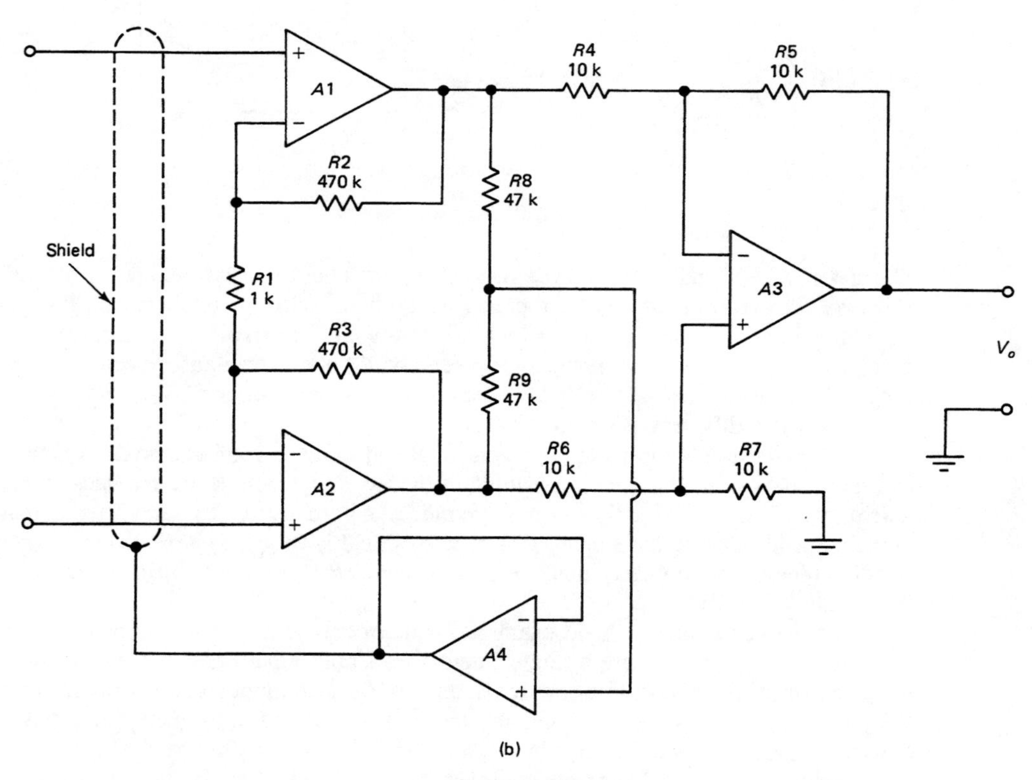

(b)

FIGURE 5-23

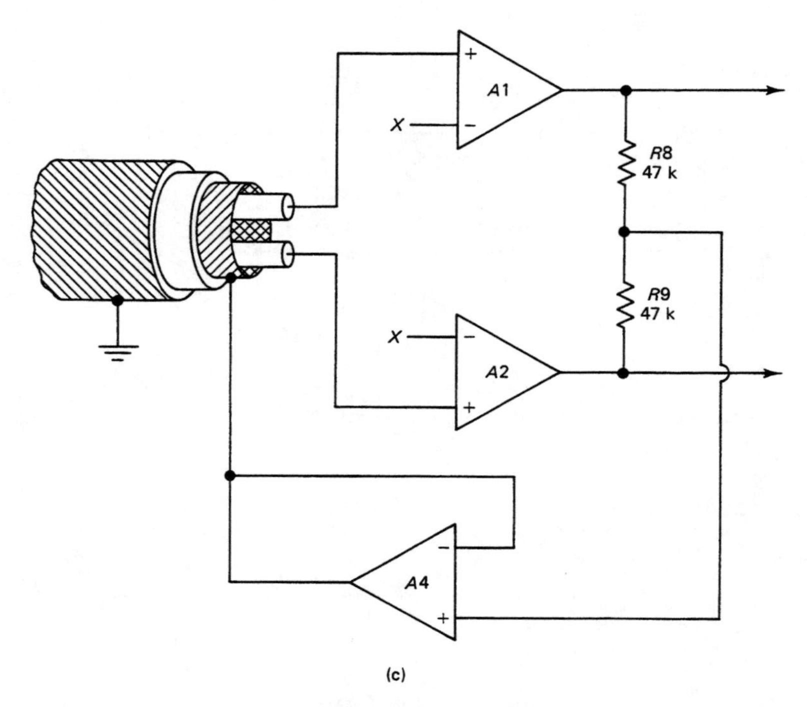

FIGURE 5-23 (continued)

C_{S1} and C_{S2}. As long as the source resistances and shunt resistances are equal, and the two capacitances are equal, there is no problem with circuit balance. But inequalities in any of these factors (which are commonplace) create an unbalanced circuit in which common mode signal V_{cm} can charge one capacitance more than the other. As a result, the difference between the capacitance voltages, V_{CS1} and V_{CS2}, is seen as a valid differential signal.

A low-cost solution to the problem of shield-induced artifact signals is shown in Figure 5-23A. In this circuit a sample of the two input signals are fed back to the shield, which in this situation is not grounded. Alternatively, the amplifier output signal is used to drive the shield. This type of shield is called a *guard shield.* Either double shields (one on each input line), as shown, or a common shield for the two inputs can be used.

An improved guard shield example for the instrumentation amplifier is shown in Figure 5-23B. In this case a single shield covers both input lines, but it is possible to use separate shields. In this circuit a sample of the two input signals is taken from the junction of resistors R8 and R9, and fed to the input of a unity gain buffer/driver "guard amplifier" (A4). The output of A4 is used to drive the guard shield.

Perhaps the most common approach to guard shielding is the arrangement shown in Figure 5-23C. Here we see two shields used; the input cabling is double-shielded insulated wire. The guard amplifier drives the inner shield, which serves as the guard shield for the system. The outer shield is grounded at the input end in the normal manner and serves as an electromagnetic interference suppression shield. This is the configuration of many ECG electrode cables.

ISOLATION AMPLIFIERS

There are a number of applications in which ordinary solid-state amplifiers are either in danger themselves because of a harsh environment or present a danger to the patients. An example of the former is an amplifier in a high-voltage experiment such as a biochemist's electrophoresis system, while the latter is represented by cardiac monitors and other devices used in medicine. Many of the commercial products of this type now available on the market are not, strictly speaking, integrated circuits; rather they are hybrids. Nonetheless, it is important to cover these devices in any book on medical amplifiers.

An *isolation amplifier* (Figure 5-24) has an extremely high impedance between the signal inputs and those power supply terminals that are connected to a DC power supply that is, in turn, connected to the AC power mains. Thus, in isolation amplifiers there is an extremely high resistance (order: $>10^{12}$ ohms) between the amplifier input terminals and the AC power line. In the case of medical equipment, the goal is to prevent minute leakage currents from the 60-Hz AC power lines from being applied to the patient. Current levels that are normally negligible to humans can be fatal to a hospital patient in situations where the body is invaded by devices that are electrical conductors. In other cases, the high impedance is used to prevent high voltages at the signal inputs from adversely affecting the rest of the circuitry. Modern isolation amplifiers can provide more than 10^{12} ohms of isolation between the AC power lines and the signal inputs.

Several different circuit symbols are used to denote the isolation amplifier in electronic schematic diagrams, but the one that is the most common is shown in Fig-

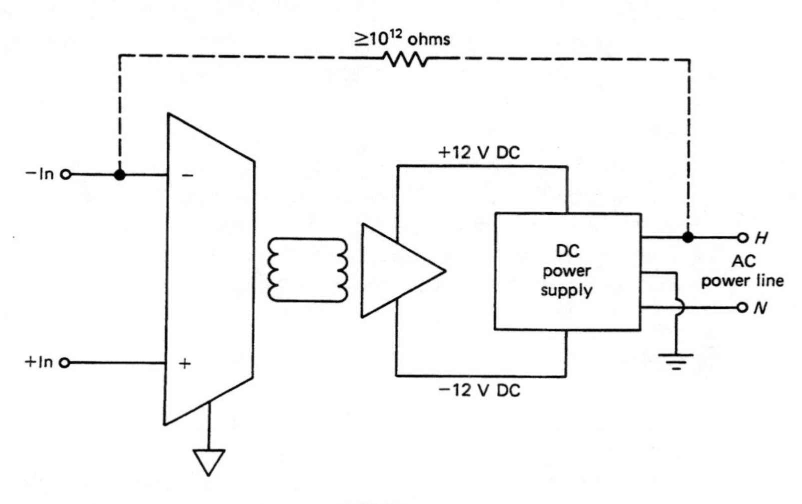

FIGURE 5-24

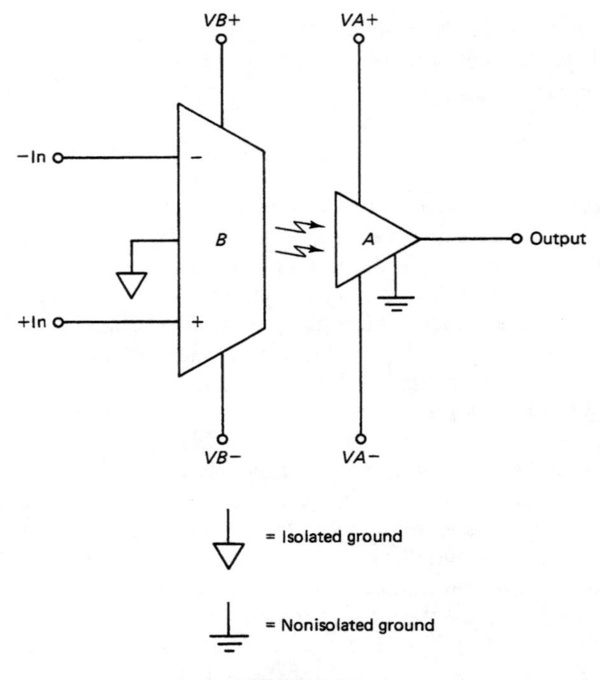

FIGURE 5-25

ure 5-25. It consists of the regular triangular amplifier symbol broken in the middle to indicate isolation between the *A* and *B* sections. The following connections are usually found on the isolation amplifier:

> *Nonisolated A side:* $V+$ and $V-$ DC power supply lines (to be connected to a DC supply powered by the AC lines), output to the rest of the (nonisolated) circuitry, and (in some designs) a nonisolated ground or common. This ground is connected to the chassis or main system ground also served by the main DC power supplies.
>
> *Isolated B side:* Isolated $V+$ and $V-$, isolated ground, or common and the signal inputs. The isolated power supply and ground are not connected to the main power supply or ground systems. Batteries are sometimed used for the isolated side, while in other cases special isolated DC power supplies derived from the main supplies are used (of which, more later).

APPROACHES TO ISOLATION AMPLIFIER DESIGN

Different manufacturers use different approaches to the design of isolation amplifiers. Common circuit approaches to isolation include *battery power, carrier operated, optically coupled,* and *current loading*. These methods are discussed in detail in the sections that follow.

Battery-Powered Isolation Amplifiers

The battery approach to isolation amplifier design is perhaps the simplest to implement, but it is not always most suitable due to problems inherent in battery upkeep. A few medical products exist, however, that use a battery-powered front-end amplifier, even though the remainder of the equipment is powered from the 110-volt AC power line. Other products are entirely battery powered. A battery-powered amplifier or instrument is isolated from the AC power mains only if the battery is disconnected from the charging circuit during use. In some battery-powered instruments used in medicine, mechanical interlocks and electrical logic circuitry prevent the instrument from being turned on if the AC power cord is still attached.

Carrier-Operated Isolation Amplifiers

Figure 5-26A shows an isolation amplifier that uses the carrier signal technique to provide isolation. The circuitry inside of the dashed line is isolated from the AC power lines (in other words, the "B" side of Figure 5-25). The voltage gain of the isolated section is typically in the range $\times 10$ to $\times 500$.

The isolation is provided by separation of the ground, power supply, and signal paths into two mutually exclusive sections by high-frequency transformers T1 and T2. These transformers have a design and core material that works very well in the ultrasonic (20-KHz to 500-KHz) region, but is very inefficient at the 60-Hz frequency used by the AC power lines. This design feature allows the transformers to easily pass the high-frequency carrier signal, while severely attenuating 60-Hz energy. Although most models use a carrier frequency in the 50-KHz to 60-KHz range, examples of carrier amplifiers exist over the entire 20-KHz to 500-KHz range.

The carrier oscillator signal is coupled through transfer T1 to the isolated stages. Part of the energy from the secondary of T1 is directed to the modulator stage; the remainder of the energy is rectified and filtered and then used as an isolated DC power supply. The DC output of this power supply is used to power the input "B" amplifiers and the modulator stage.

An analog signal applied to the input is amplified by A1 and is then applied to one input of the modulator stage. This stage amplitude modulates the signal onto the carrier. Transformer T2 couples the signal to the input of the demodulator stage on the nonisolated side of the circuit. Either envelope or synchronous demodulation may be used, although the latter is considered superior. Part of the demodulator stage is a low-pass filter that removes any residual carrier signal from the output signal. Ordinary DC amplifiers following the demodulator complete the signal processing chain.

An example of a synchronous demodulator circuit is shown in Figure 5-26B. These circuits are based on switching action. Although the example shown uses bipolar PNP transistors as the electronic switches, other circuits use NPN transistors, FETs, or CMOS electronic switches (e.g., 4066 device).

The signal from the modulator has a fixed frequency in the range from 20 KHz to 500 KHz and is amplitude modulated with the input signal from the isolated am-

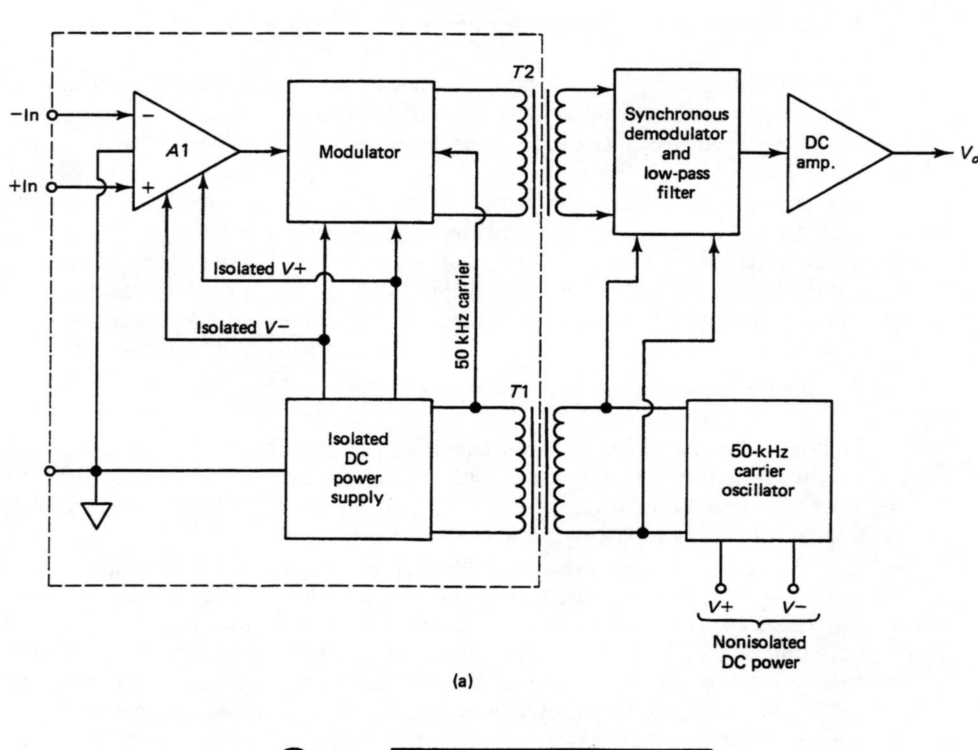

(a)

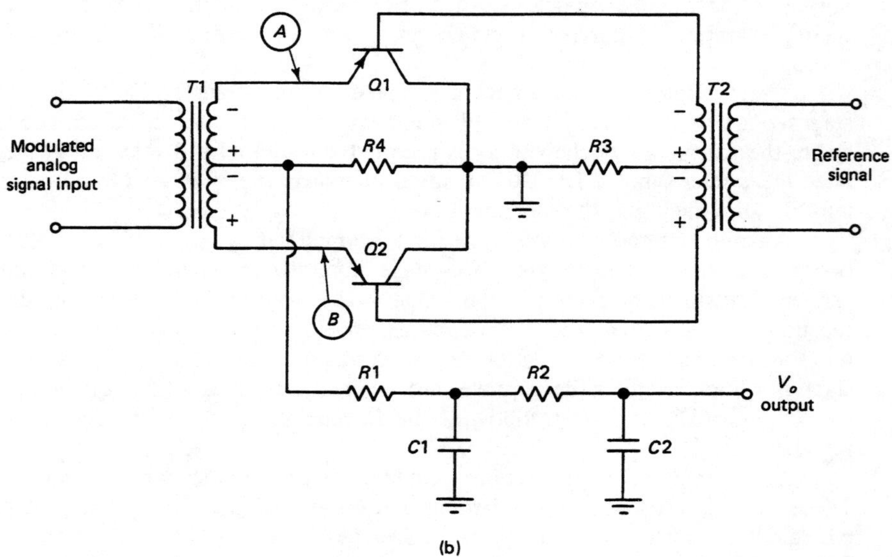

(b)

FIGURE 5-26

plifier. This signal is applied to the emitters of transistors Q1 and Q2 (via T1) in push-pull. On one-half of the cycle, therefore, the emitter of Q1 will be positive with respect to the emitter of Q2. On alternate half-cycles, the opposite situation occurs: Q2 is positive with respect to Q1. The bases of Q1 and Q2 are also driven in push-pull, but by the carrier signal (called here the *reference signal*). This action causes transistors Q1 and Q2 to switch on and off out of phase with each other.

On one-half of the cycle, the polarities are as shown in Figure 5-26B; transistor Q1 is turned on. In this condition point "A" on T1 is grounded. The voltage developed across load resistor R4 is positive with respect to ground.

On the alternate half-cycle, Q2 is turned on, so point "B" is grounded. But the polarities have reversed, so the polarity of the voltage developed across R4 is still positive. This causes a full-wave output waveform across R4, which when low-pass filtered becomes a DC voltage level proportional to the amplitude of the input signal. This same description of synchronous demodulators also applies to the circuits used in some carrier amplifiers (a specialized laboratory amplifier used for low-level signals).

A variation on this circuit replaces the modulator with a *voltage-controlled oscillator* (VCO) that allows the analog signal to *frequency modulate* (FM) a carrier signal generated by the VCO. The power supply carrier signal is still required, however. A phase detector, phase-locked loop (PLL), or pulse-counting FM detector on the nonisolated side recovers the signal.

Optically Coupled Isolation Amplifier Circuits

Electronic optocouplers (also called optoisolators) are sometimes used to provide the desired isolation. In early designs of this class, a light-emitting diode (LED) was mounted together with a photoresistor or phototransistor. Modern designs, however, use integrated circuit optoisolators that contain an LED and phototransistor inside of a single DIP IC package.

There are actually several approaches to optical coupling. Two common methods are the *carrier* and *direct* methods. The carrier method is the same as discussed in the previous section, except that an optoisolator replaces transformer T2. The carrier method is not the most widespread in optically coupled isolation amplifiers because of the frequency response limitations of some IC optoisolators. Only recently have these problems been resolved.

The more common direct approach is shown in Figure 5-27. This circuit uses the same DC-to-DC converter to power the isolated stages as was used in other designs. It keeps A1 isolated from the AC power mains but is not used in the signal-coupling process. In some designs, the high-frequency "carrier" power supply is actually a separate block from the isolation amplifier.

The LED in the optoisolator is driven by the output of isolated amplifier A1. Transistor Q1 serves as a series switch to vary the light output of the LED proportional to the analog signal from A1. Transistor Q1 normally passes sufficient collector current to bias the LED into a linear portion of its operating curve. The output of the phototransistor is AC coupled to the remaining amplifiers on the nonisolated side of the circuit, so that the offset condition created by the LED bias is eliminated.

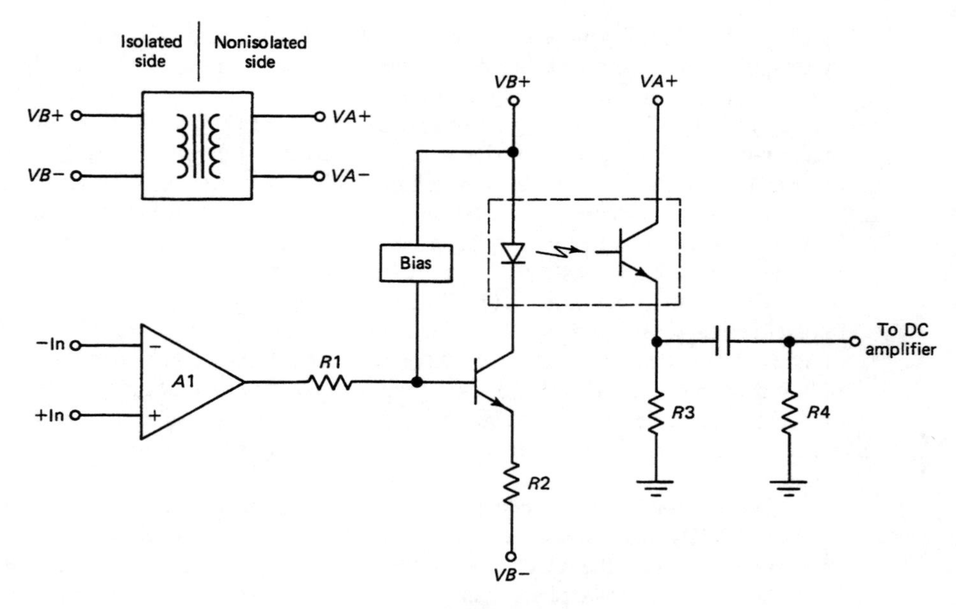

FIGURE 5-27

Although not strictly speaking an isolated amplifier by the definition used here, there is another category of optical isolation that is especially attractive for applications where the environment is too hostile for ordinary electronics. It is possible to use LED and phototransistor transmitter and receiver modules in a fiber optic system to provide isolation. A battery-powered (or otherwise isolated) amplifier will sense the desired signal, convert to an AM or FM light signal and transmit it down a length of fiber optic cable to a phototransistor receiver module. At that point the signal will be recovered and processed by the nonisolated electronics.

Current Loading Isolation Amplifier Methods

A unique "current loading" isolation amplifier was used in the front end of an electrocardiograph (ECG) medical monitor. A simplified schematic is shown in Figure 5-28. Notice that there is no obvious coupling path for the signal between the isolated and nonisolated sides of the circuit.

The gain-of-24 isolated input preamplifier (A1) in Figure 5-28 consists of a high-input impedance operational amplifier. This amplifier is needed in order to interface with the very-high-source impedance normal to electrodes in ECG systems. The output of A1 is connected to the isolated −10-volt DC power supply through load resistor R1. This power supply is a DC-to-DC converter operating at 250 KHz. Transformer T1 provides isolation between the floating power supplies on the isolated "B" side of the circuit and the nonisolated "A" side of the circuit (which are AC-line powered).

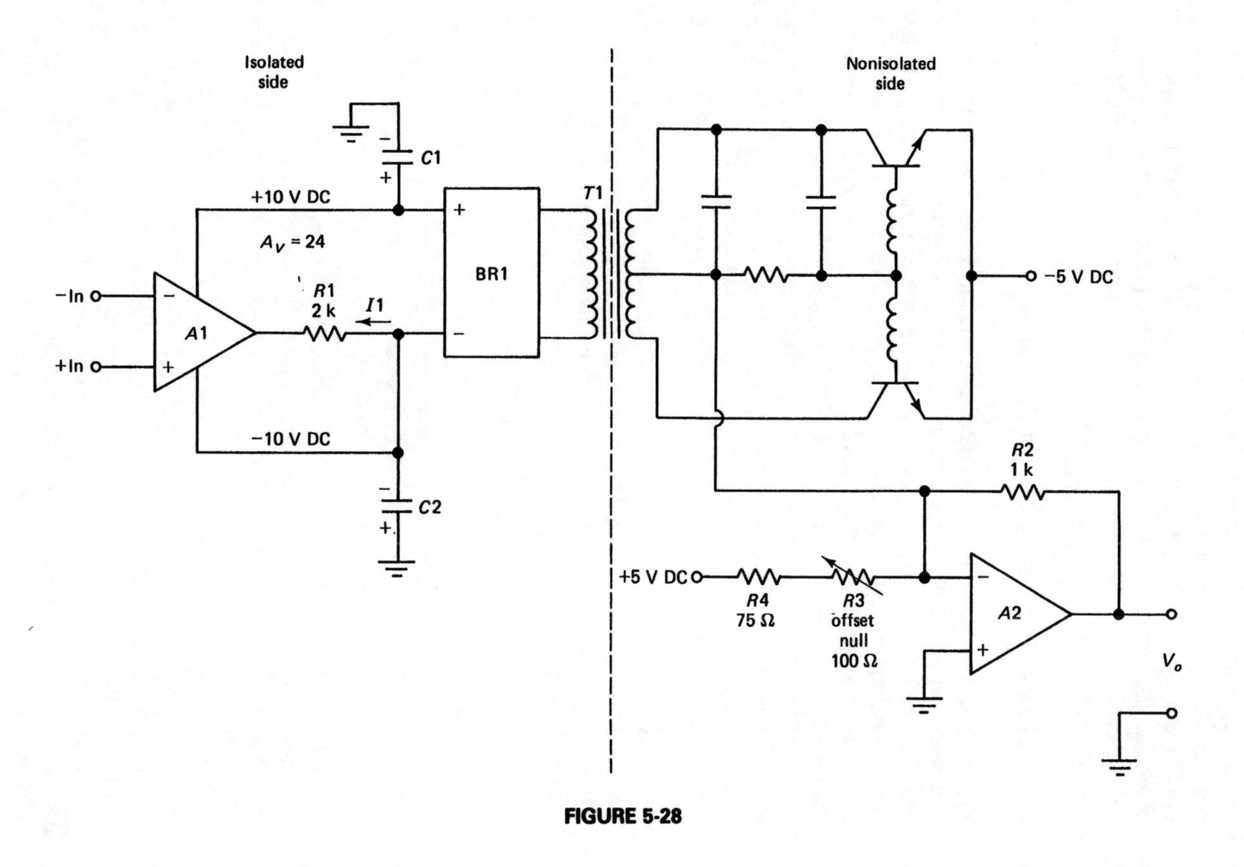
Isolated side
Nonisolated side
−In
+In
A1
+10 V DC
−10 V DC
$A_V = 24$
R1
2 k
I1
C1
C2
BR1
T1
−5 V DC
+5 V DC
R4
75 Ω
R3
offset null
100 Ω
R2
1 k
A2
V_o

FIGURE 5-28

An input signal causes the output of A1 to vary the current loading of the floating −10-volt DC power supply. Changing the current loading proportional to the analog input signal causes variation of the T1 primary current that is also proportional to the analog signal. This current variation is converted to a voltage variation by amplifier A2. An offset null control (R3) is provided in the A1 circuit to eliminate the offset at the output due to the quiescent current flowing when the analog input signal is zero. In that case, the current loading of T1 is constant—but still provides an offset to the A2 amplifier.

Design Example: Cardiac Output Computer

The problems presented by most electronic signals acquisition situations are simple compared with the problems presented in measuring human cardiac output. The principal difference is that cardiac output is usually measured using an invasive surgical technique on living humans. This type of measurement is presented here to demonstrate a data acquisition technique that for the sake of safety almost absolutely requires an isolation amplifier to interface with the signal source.

Cardiac output (C.O.) is defined as the rate of blood volume pumped by the heart. The question being asked of the C.O. measurement is, "how much blood is this person pumping per unit of time." Cardiac output is measured in units of liters of blood per minute of time (l/min). In healthy adults C.O. typically reaches a value between 3 and 5 l/min.

A quantitative measure of cardiac output is the product of the stroke volume and the heart rate. The stroke volume is merely the volume of blood expelled from the heart ventricle (lower chamber) during a single contraction of the heart. Cardiac output is calculated from

$$\text{C.O.} = V \times R \tag{5-17}$$

where

$$\begin{aligned} \text{C.O.} &= \text{the cardiac output in liters per minute (l/min)} \\ V &= \text{the stroke volume in liters per beat (l/beat)} \\ R &= \text{the heart rate in beats per minute (beat/min)} \end{aligned}$$

It is difficult, and usually impossible (except on animals in laboratory settings) to measure cardiac output directly using any technique based on Equation 5-17. The main problem is obtaining good stroke volume data without excessive risk to the patient.

The *thermodilution method* of cardiac output measurement has become the standard indirect method for measuring cardiac output in clinical settings and is also popular among laboratory scientists. Thermodilution technique forms the basis for most clinical and research cardiac output computers now on the market. One reason why thermodilution is prefered is that no poisonous injectates are used (as they are in radioopaque or optical dye dilution methods), only ordinary medical intravenous (IV) solutions such as normal saline or 5 percent dextrose in water (D_5W) are used.

The thermodilution measurement of cardiac output is made using a special hollow catheter that is inserted into one of the patient's veins, usually on the right arm (the brachial vein is popular). The catheter is multilumened, and one of the lumens has its output hole several centimeters from the catheter tip. This proximal lumen is situated so that it is outside the heart (close to the input valve on the right atrium) when the tip is all the way through the heart, resting in the pulmonary artery (Figure 5-29). Other lumens in the catheter output at the tip, so are used to measure pressures in the pulmonary artery in hemodynamic procedures. A thermistor in the catheter tip registers a resistance change with changes in blood temperature.

Most thermodilution cardiac output computers operate on a version of the following equation:

$$\text{C.O.} = \frac{(64.8) \times C(t) \times V(i) \times [T(b) - T(i)]}{\int T(b)'\,dt} \tag{5-18}$$

Note: The mathematical "integral" symbol and the "dt" in the denominator of Equation 5-18 indicates that "integration" takes place and that the result is thus the time average of temperature $T(b)'$, where

C.O. = the cardiac output in liters per minute
64.8 = a collection of other constants and the conversion factor from seconds to minutes
$C(t)$ = a constant that is supplied with the injectate catheter that accounts for the temperature rise in the portion of the outside of the victim's body
$T(b)$ = the blood temperature in degrees Celsius

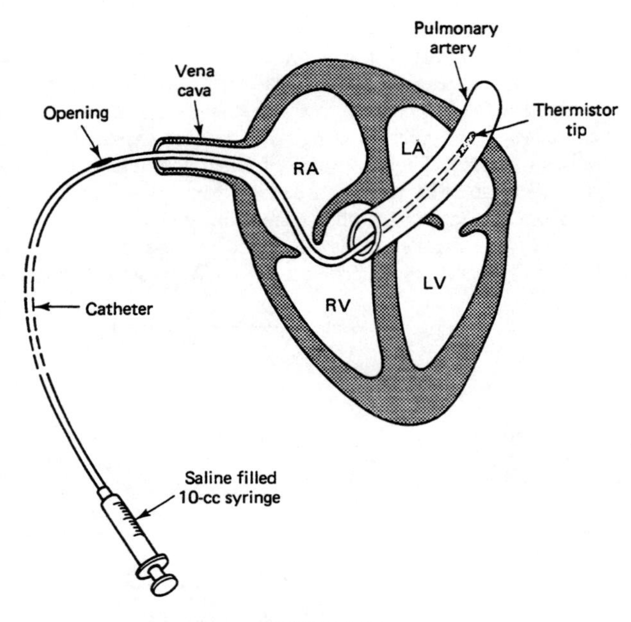

FIGURE 5-29

$T(i)$ = the temperature of the injectate in degrees Celsius
$T(b)'$ = the temperature of the blood as it changes due to mixing with the injectate

The mathematical symbol in the denominator of Equation 5-18 tells us that the temperature of the blood at the output side of the heart is integrated, that is, the computer finds the time average of the temperature as it changes.

Example

A special cardiac output computer "dummy catheter" test fixture enters a temperature signal that simulates a temperature change of 10°C for a period of 10 seconds. Find the expected reading during a test of the instrument if the following front-panel settings are entered: $C(t) = 49.6$, $T(b) = 37°\mathrm{C}$, injectate temperature $T(i)$ is 25°C, and injectate volume $V(i)$ is 10 ml.

Solution:

$$\text{C.O.} = \frac{(64.8) \times C(t) \times V(i) \times [T(b) - T(i)]}{\int T(b)'\,dt} \text{ (l/min)}$$

$$= \frac{(64.8) \times (49.6) \times (10 \text{ ml} \times 1 \text{ l}/1000 \text{ ml}) \times [(37) - (25)]}{(10°\mathrm{C})(10 \text{ sec})}$$

$$= \frac{3214 \times 0.01 \times 12}{100}$$

$$= 385.68/100 = 3.9 \text{ l/min}$$

The thermistor in the end of the catheter is usually connected in a Wheatstone bridge circuit (see Figure 5-30). The DC excitation of the bridge is critical. Either the short-term stability of this voltage must be very high, or a ratiometric method must be used to cancel excitation potential drift. In addition, it is also necessary to limit the bridge excitation potential to about 200 mV for reasons of safety to the patient (electrical leakage is especially dangerous because the thermistor is *inside the heart or pulmonary artery*). This low value of excitation voltage promotes both patient safety and thermistor stability through freedom from self-heating induced drift, even though imposing a greater burden on the amplifier design.

Figure 5-30 shows a simplified schematic of a typical cardiac output computer front-end circuit. The thermistor is in a Wheatstone bridge circuit consisting also of R1

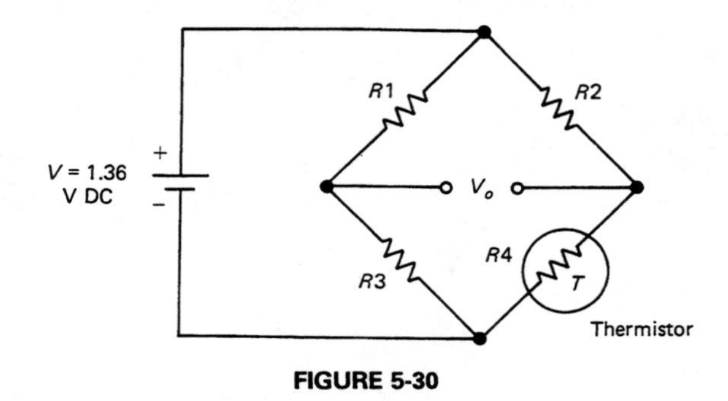

FIGURE 5-30

through R3, with potentiometer R5 serving to balance the bridge. An autobalancing or zeroing method is sometimes used for this function. Those circuits use a digital-to-analog converter (DAC) to inject a current into one node of the bridge, and that current nulls the bridge circuit to zero. The physician waits a few minutes for the thermistor to equilibrate with blood temperature (usually it is in this condition by the time it is threaded through the venous system to the pulmonary artery). The output of the bridge, depending upon the design, is typically 1.2 to 2.5 millivolts per degree Celsius, with 1.8 mV/°C being quite common. This signal is amplified approximately 1000 times to 1 volt/°C by the preamplifier. This preamplifier is an isolated amplifier for reasons of patient safety. The output of this circuit, V_o, is used in the denominator of an equation as shown earlier.

A COMMERCIAL ICIA PRODUCT EXAMPLE

Figure 5-31 shows the circuit of an isolation amplifier based on the Burr-Brown 3652 isolation amplifier device. The DC power for both the isolated and nonisolated sections of the 3652 is provided by the 722 dual DC-to-DC converter. This device produces two independent ±15-V DC supplies that are each isolated from the 60-Hz AC power mains and from each other. The 722 device is powered from a +12-V DC source that is derived from the AC power mains. In some cases, the nonisolated section (which is connected to the output terminal) is powered from a bipolar DC power supply that is derived from the 60-Hz AC mains, such as a ±12-V DC or ±15-V DC supply. In no instance, however, should the isolated DC power supplies be derived from the AC power mains.

There are two separate ground systems in this circuit, symbolized by the small triangle and the regular three-bar "chassis" ground symbol. The isolated ground is not connected to either the DC power supply ground/common or the chassis ground. It is kept floating at all times and becomes the signal common for the input signal source.

The gain of the circuit is approximately

$$\text{gain} = \frac{1{,}000{,}000}{\text{R1} + \text{R2} + 115} \qquad (5\text{-}19)$$

In most design cases, the issue is the unknown values of the gain-setting resistors. We can rearrange Equation 5-19 to solve for (R1 + R2):

$$(\text{R1} + \text{R2}) = \frac{1{,}000{,}000 - (115 \times \text{gain})}{\text{gain}} \qquad (5\text{-}20)$$

where

$$\text{R1} + \text{R2} = \text{resistors in ohms}$$
$$\text{gain} = \text{the voltage gain desired}$$

Example

An amplifier requires a differential voltage gain of 1000. What combination of R1 and R2 will provide that gain figure?

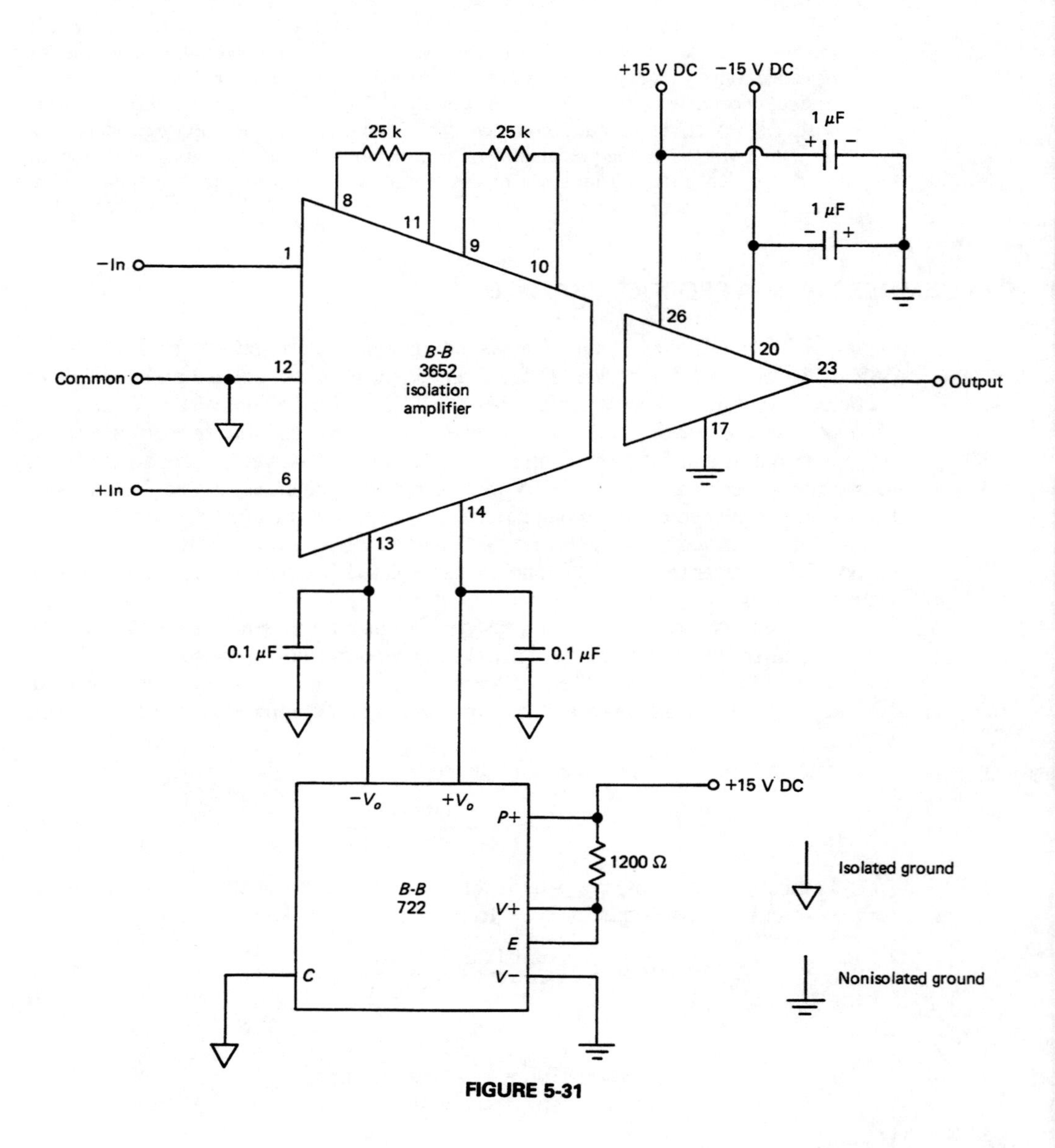

+15 V DC
−15 V DC
1 μF
+
−
1 μF
−
+
25 k
25 k
8
11
9
10
1
−In
Common
12
+In
6
B-B
3652
isolation
amplifier
26
20
23
Output
17
14
13
0.1 μF
0.1 μF
+15 V DC
−V_o
+V_o
P+
1200 Ω
B-B
722
V+
E
C
V−
Isolated ground
Nonisolated ground

FIGURE 5-31

Solution: If gain = 1000,

$$(R1 + R2) = \frac{1{,}000{,}000 - (115 \times 1000)}{1000}$$

$$= \frac{1{,}000{,}000 - (115{,}000)}{1000}$$

$$= \frac{885{,}000}{1000}$$

$$= 885 \text{ ohms}$$

In this case, we need some combination of R1 and R2 that adds to 885 ohms. The value 440 ohms is "standard" and will result in only a tiny gain error if used.

Although the isolation amplifier is considerably more expensive than common IC linear amplifiers, there are applications where these amplifiers are absolutely critical. Wherever the instrument could cause injury to a human, or wherever the environment is such that the electronics must be isolated as far as possible, the isolation amplifier is the device of choice (at least in the front end).

PROTECTED INPUT ISOLATION AMPLIFIERS

Biopotentials amplifiers used in medical applications are sometimes subjected to an intense electrical transient shock from a defibrillator (see Chapter 10). Because the physician uses the electrocardiograph monitor to see if the defibrillation attempt was successful, the biopotentials amplifiers used in the inputs of these instruments must be protected against high-voltage electrical shocks. Figure 5-32 shows several methods for protecting the amplifier input. It is unlikely that all these methods will be used in any one amplifier, but all have been (or still are) used.

Most protected biopotentials amplifiers will have current limiting resistors in series with each input line. These resistors also have the effect of voltage division. In some amplifiers a spark gap device (SG1) is used. These devices consist of a pair of electrodes in close proximity to each other inside of a glass envelope that was evacuated of air and then refilled with a partial pressure of inert gas. In some older instruments an NE-2 or NE-51 neon glow lamp served as the spark gap. Alternatively, a metal oxide varistor (MOV) device is used. These components have a high resistance

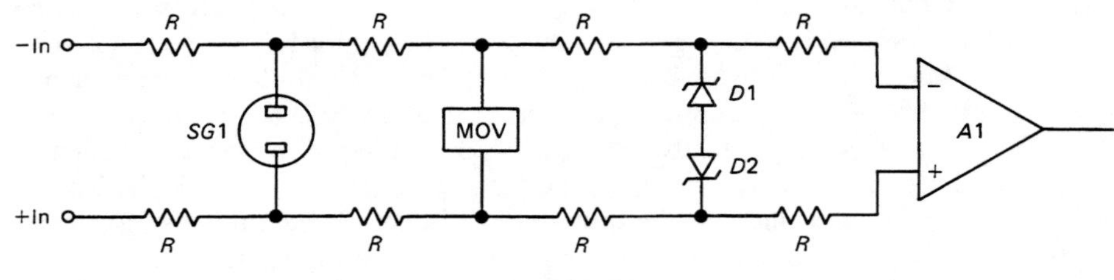

FIGURE 5-32

if the applied voltage is less than a certain threshold and a very low resistance if the voltage exceeds the threshold. Finally, there might be a pair of back-to-back zener diodes shunted across the line to clip high-voltage transients.

ACTIVE ELECTRONIC FILTERS

A frequency selective filter is a circuit that will discriminate against certain frequencies or bands of frequencies. In other words, a filter circuit will pass some frequencies and reject others. Passive filters are made of combinations of passive components such as resistors (R), capacitors (C), and inductors (L). An active filter is one based on an active device such as an operational amplifier along with passive components. In most cases, the passive components are resistors and capacitors (although a few with inductors are known).

The topic of active filters is too complex for comprehensive coverage in a single chapter, so we will just make a few observations that allow you to understand practical circuits.

FILTER CHARACTERISTICS

Filters of all types can be divided into categories based on the respective passbands. Figure 5-33 shows several popular combinations. In Figure 5-33A we see the low-pass filter. This type of filter passes all frequencies below a certain critical frequency (F_c). The breakpoint between the passband and the stopband is the point at which the gain of the circuit has dropped off -3 dB from its lower-frequency value. Above the critical frequency the gain falls off at a certain slope. The steepness of the slope is usually given in terms of decibels of gain per octave of frequency (an octave is a 2:1 change in frequency); alternatively, dB per decade (a decade is a 10:1 change in frequency) is sometimes used.

The high-pass filter frequency response is shown in Figure 5-33B. In this case, the filter circuit will pass all frequencies above the critical frequency (F_c) and reject frequencies below that point. The high-pass filter is the inverse of the low-pass filter.

A bandpass filter is one that combines both high-pass and low-pass concepts (Figure 5-33C). In this case, the filter rejects all frequencies below F1 and above F2. These frequencies are the upper and lower -3-dB points in the response; gain is compared with the midband frequency, F_c. The bandwidth is the bandpass filter is the difference $F2 - F1$. The response in Figure 5-33C is a relatively low-Q type because it has a wide bandwidth. A higher-Q circuit has a narrower bandpass, as in Figure 5-33D; it admits a smaller range of acceptable frequencies.

A notch filter, also called a stopband filter, will pass all frequencies except for those clustered around a critical frequency (see Figure 5-33E). The notch filter is used to take out a single unwanted frequency. A common use for notch filters is to remove 60-Hz interference signals from electronic instruments.

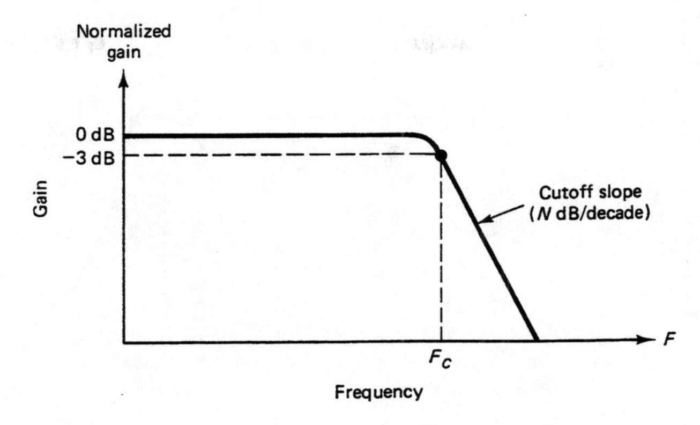

(a) Low-pass filter

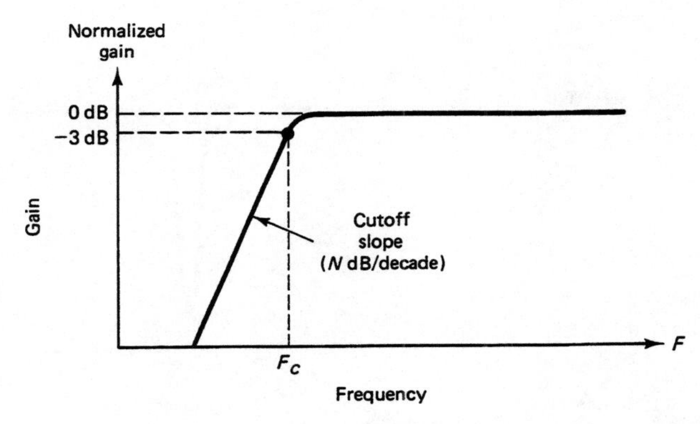

(b) High-pass filter

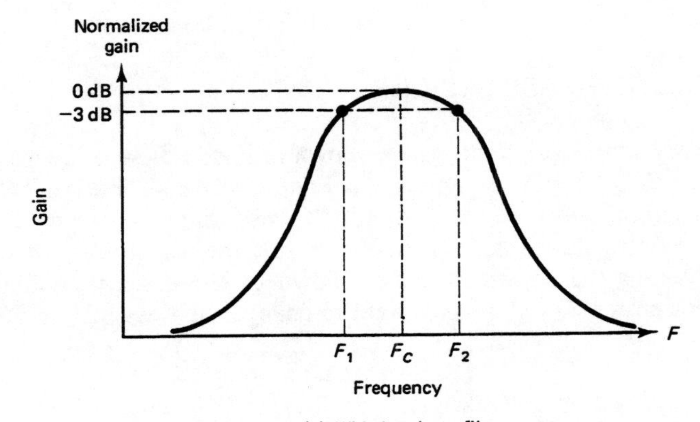

(c) Wide bandpass filter

FIGURE 5-33

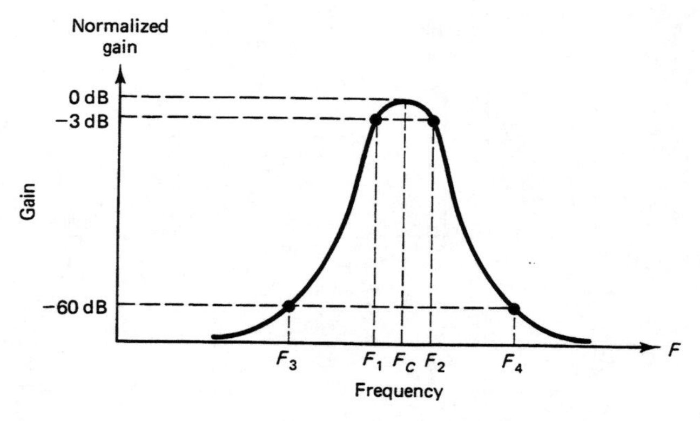

(d) Narrow bandpass filter

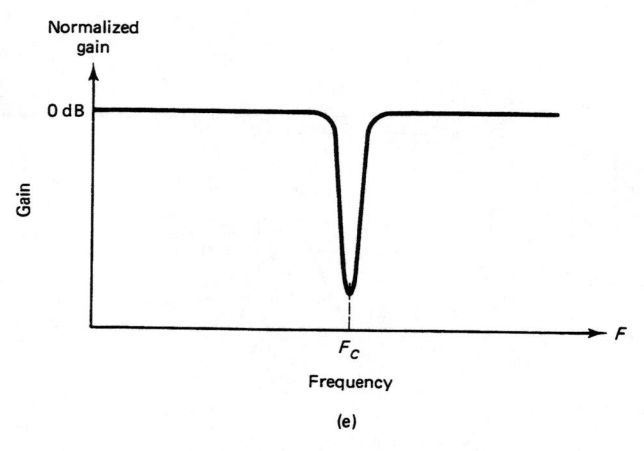

(e)

FIGURE 5-33 (continued)

HIGH-PASS/LOW-PASS DESIGNS

Very simple active filters are shown in Figure 5-34; a low-pass type is shown in Figure 5-34A, and a high-pass in Figure 5-34B. These designs are really little more than buffered versions of simple RC passive filters. The values shown in Figure 5-34 are normalized for 1 KHz. We can find the actual required values (R1′ and C1′) by dividing the strawman values shown by the desired cutoff frequency in kilohertz. For example, suppose we want to change the frequency to 60 Hz (i.e., 0.06 KHz):

$$C1' = \frac{(R1)(1\ \text{KHz})}{F}$$

$$= \frac{(0.0159\ \mu\text{F})(1\ \text{KHz})}{0.06}$$

$$= 0.265\ \mu\text{F}$$

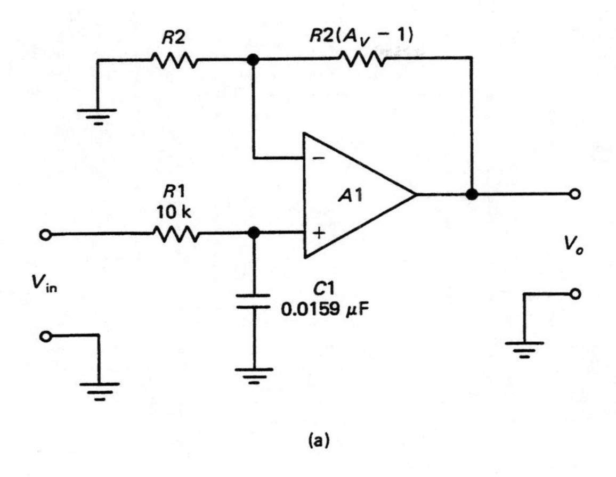

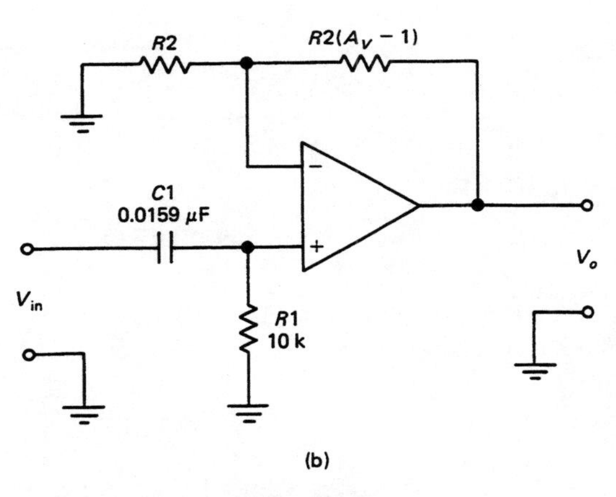

FIGURE 5-34

We must leave one of the values alone and calculate the other. In the example, 0.265 μF is not a standard value, but 0.22 and 0.27 μF are standards. Select samples of these for tolerance differences as close as possible to 0.265 μF. Custom selection of capacitors did not use to be so easy, but many modern, low-cost digital multimeters now come equipped with digital capacitor meter functions.

Practical Notch Filter

The purpose of the notch filter is to eliminate a single frequency or small band of frequencies. The most common form of notch filter in biopotentials amplifiers is to remove unwanted 60-Hz interference. Figure 5-35 shows the circuit for a common form of operational amplifier notch filter. The frequency selective element consists of a twin-tee passive notch filter network. Two of the resistors have a value *R*, while

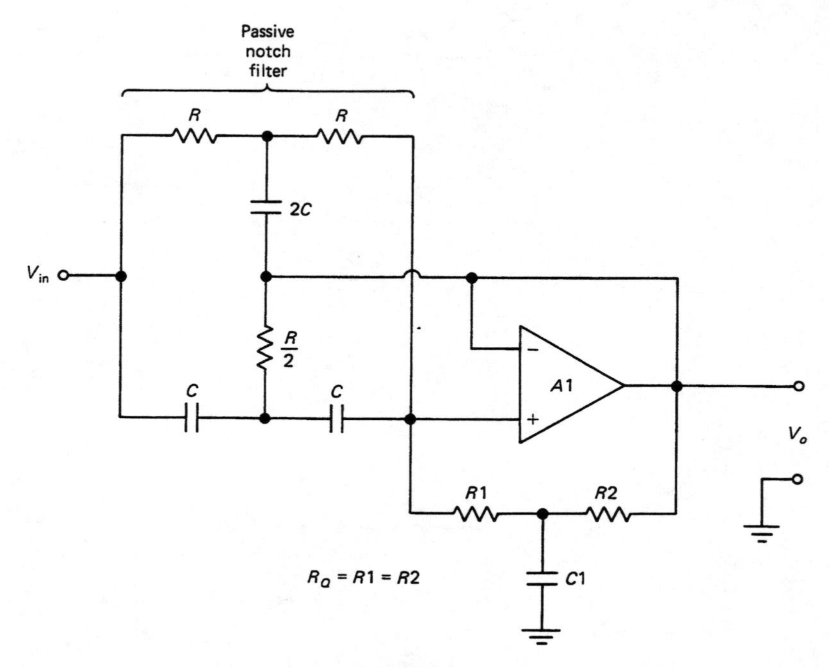

FIGURE 5-35

the other resistor has a value $R/2$. Similarly, two capacitors have a value C, while the third has a value $2C$. The values of these components have values determined by

$$F_c = \frac{1}{2\pi RC}$$

The Q of the notch filter defines its sharpness. It is the ratio of the center frequency to the bandwidth. For the circuit of Figure 5-35 the Q is a function of either

$$Q = \frac{R_q}{2R}$$

or

$$Q = \frac{C}{C1}$$

Example

Design a notch filter for 60 Hz with a Q of 5.

Solution:

1. Select a trial value of C: 0.47 μF.
2. Calculate the value of R:

$$R = \frac{1}{2\pi FC}$$

$$R = \frac{1}{(2)(3.14)(60 \text{ Hz})(0.47 \times 10^{-6} \text{ F})}$$

$$R = \frac{1}{1.77 \times 10^{-4}} = 5647 \text{ ohms}$$

Note: Unless great precision is needed, select 5.6 Ω for R because it is a standard value.

3. Select a value for $C1$:

$$C1 = \frac{C}{Q} = \frac{0.47 \text{ } \mu\text{F}}{5} = 0.094 \text{ } \mu\text{F}$$

(Actually use 0.1 μF, the nearest standard value.)

4. Select a value for R_q:

$$R_q = 2QR$$
$$= (2)(5)(5.6 \text{ k}\Omega) = 56 \text{ k}\Omega$$

The circuit of Figure 5-35 will offer notch depths of 40 to 50 dB with commonly available components and up to 60 dB if the components are selected for precise value.

INTEGRATOR AND DIFFERENTIATOR CIRCUITS

Integration and differentiation are inverse mathematical processes that are used extensively in biomedical amplifier applications. The integration process finds the area under a curve, while the differentiation process finds the instantaneous rate of

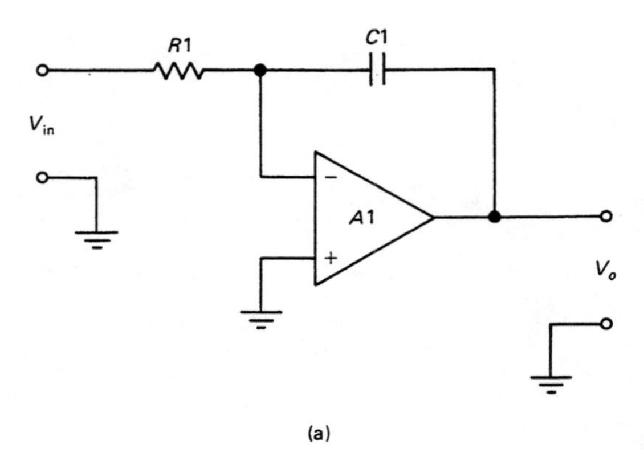

FIGURE 5-36

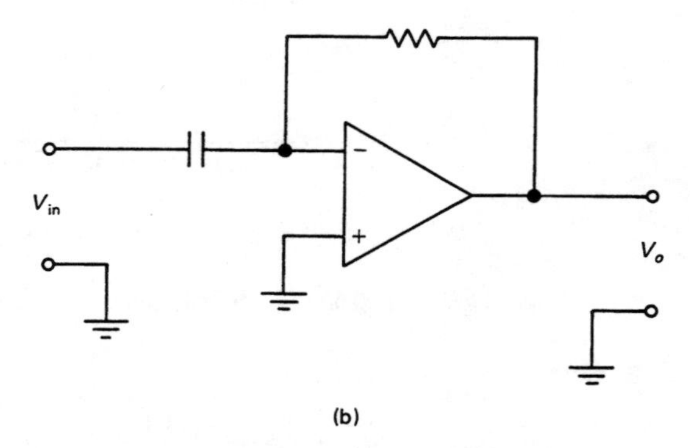

(b)

FIGURE 5-36 (continued)

change. An electronic integrator will find the time average of an applied waveform. These circuits are used in cardiac output computers (see earlier discussion) and to find the mean arterial blood pressure from the applied waveform. The differentiator finds the instantaneous rate of change with respect to time. The differentiator circuit is used in some medical and biological research applications to find the rate of change of a blood pressure waveform (dP/dt).

The integrator circuit is shown in Figure 5-36A. The circuit consists of a resistor in series with the inverting input and a capacitor in the negative feedback path. The differentiator shown in Figure 5-36B uses the same components, but in exactly the opposite roles.

6

Electrocardiograph Machines

Electrocardiographs (abbreviated *ECG* or sometimes *EKG* after the German spelling) are probably the oldest class of medical electronic instruments on the market. Their long clinical history and almost universal distribution to even the smallest doctors' offices attest to their importance in the overall scheme of things. The basic ECG machine picks up minute voltages on the surface of the patient's skin that are generated by the heart. The function of the ECG machine is to draw the waveform of that amplitude-versus-time function on a strip of special graph paper. Figure 6-1 shows such a machine.

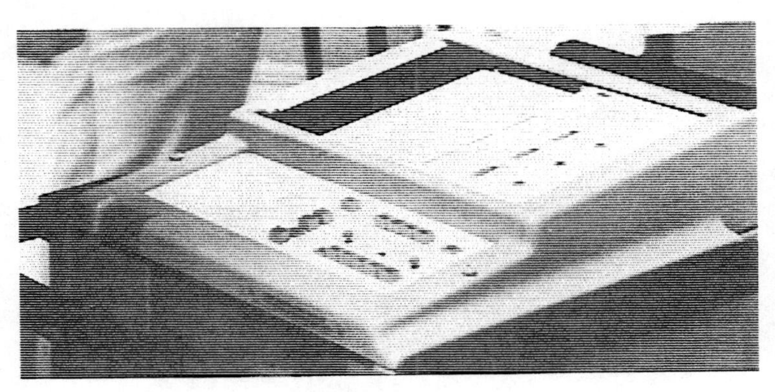

FIGURE 6-1

The weak bioelectric potentials picked up and displayed by the ECG machine are generated by the cells of the heart. These cells, as well as many other types of cells in the body, can be viewed as a form of miniature biological "battery." Under normal circumstances, both sodium (Na) and potassium (K) are found on each side of the cell wall, or membrane. In Figure 6-2 only one element is shown on each side because the normal relative concentrations of the two are so radically different. Inside the cell, for example, the fluid has a concentration of potassium that is approximately 30 times that of sodium. On the outside, on the other hand, the concentration of sodium is approximately 10 times that of potassium. These concentration gradients produce an electrical potential difference across the cell wall of about −90 millivolts (mV), with the inside being the negative reference point.

When the heart cell is stimulated, the nature of its membrane wall changes so that it becomes more permeable to sodium ions. This allows sodium ions to rush into the cell in an attempt to neutralize the imbalance in concentrations. The voltage drop across the cell wall during this period (Figure 6-3) switches rapidly from −90 mV to +20 mV. At this point the cell is said to be depolarized. The characteristics of the cell wall then change back to the prestimulus condition. During this period, called the repolarization period, the membrane potential gradient drops back to

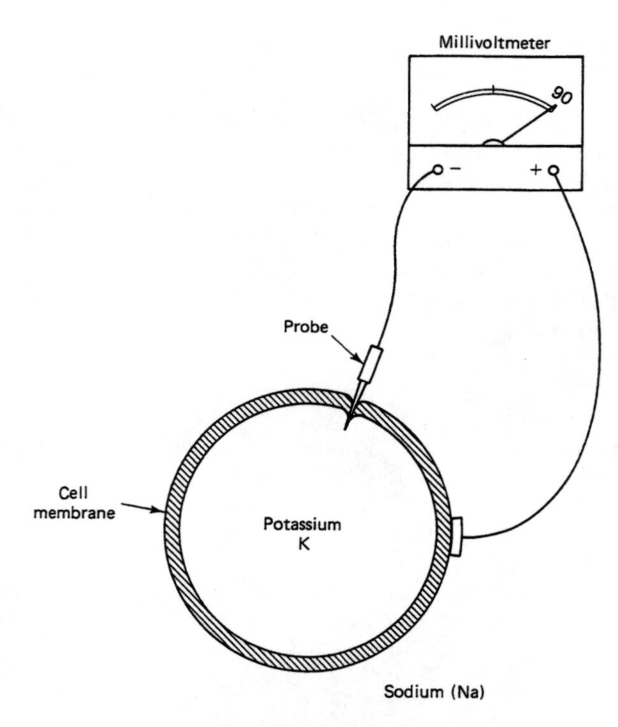

FIGURE 6-2

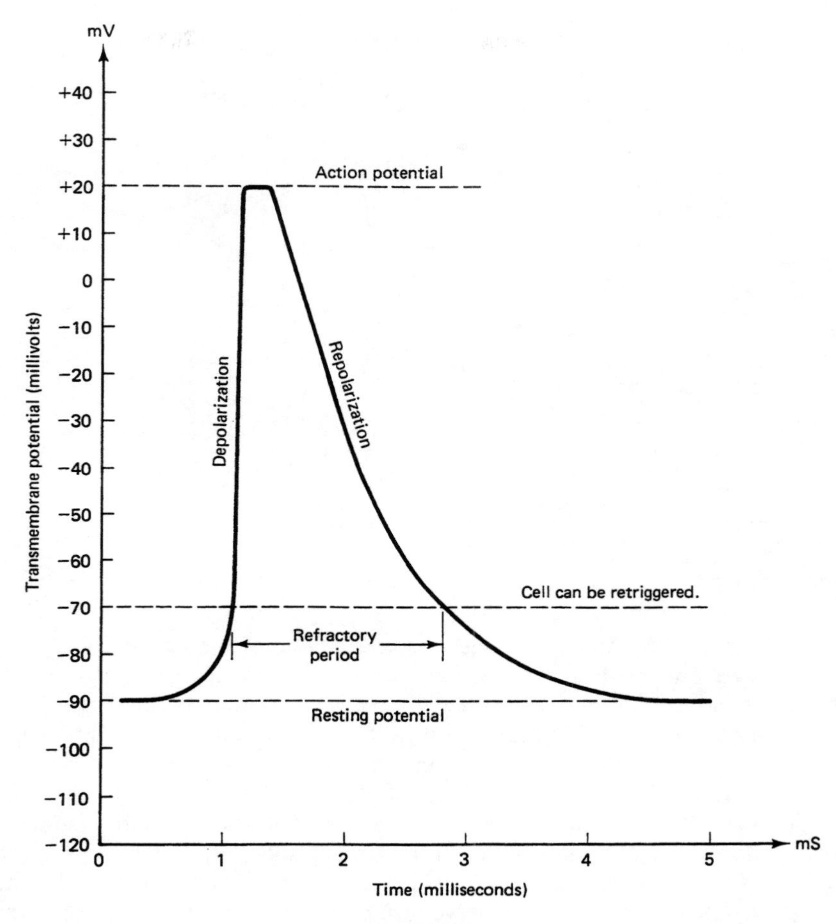

FIGURE 6-3

its −90 = mV resting level. Once the cell is triggered by a stimulus, it will go through this cycle completely and cannot be retriggered until after it is repolarized.

The cells of the heart generate an electrical current from the cell depolarizations as it beats. The vector sum of these currents can be picked up as voltage drops across various points on the surface of the skin (Figure 6-4). Different views of the heart's electrical activity result in different waveforms, and these are obtained from different points on the patient's body. Each of these views is called a *lead* in ECG terminology. The reason why so many different views of the heart's electrical activity are desired by medical staff is that it helps them diagnose disease conditions more accurately. A multiplicity of views assists them in localizing and analyzing the areas that are diseased.

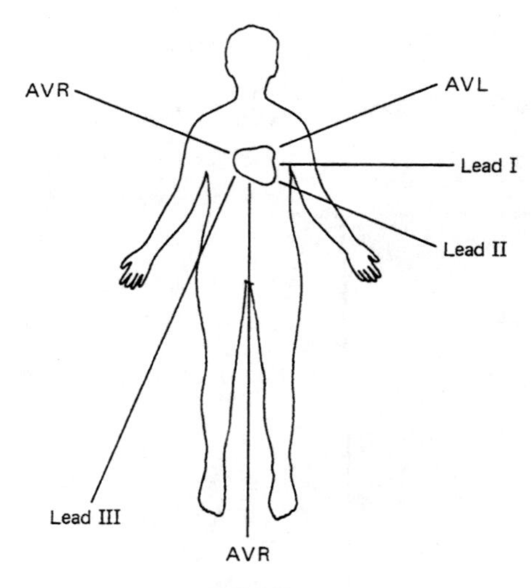

FIGURE 6-4

ECG LEADS

Figure 6-5 shows the major features of one of the classic ECG waveforms, called *lead I* in medical terminology. Here we see the major amplitude features of the waveform and the standardized alphabetical letters normally used to identify these features. The first feature, on the left, is called the *P-wave,* and it corresponds to the pumping of the atria. Following the P-wave is a sharp spike corresponding to the beating of the ventricles (i.e., the "power stroke" of the heart), and this is called the *QRS complex*. The QRS complex generally has the highest amplitude (on the order of 1 mV) of all features in the lead I display. Its major property, however, is the fast rise and fall times and rapid slope reversal. This, incidentally, indicates a high-frequency content of the waveform compared with its fundamental frequency in the

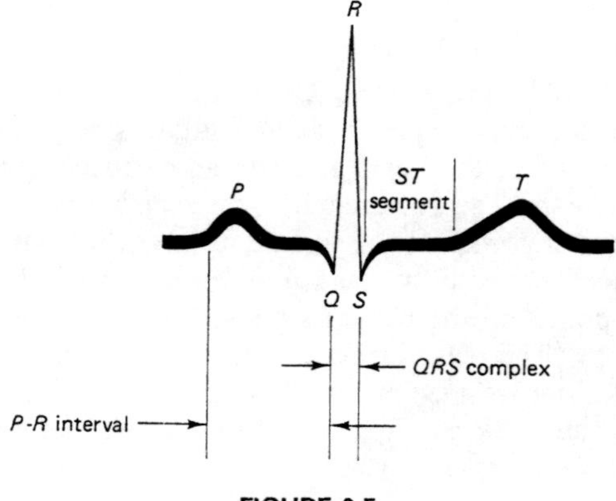

FIGURE 6-5

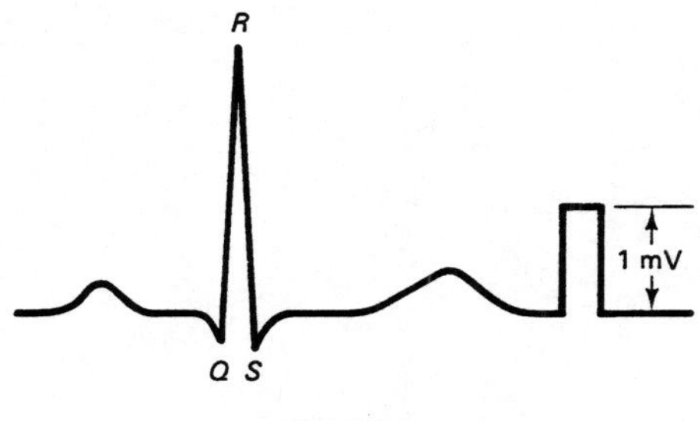

FIGURE 6-6

1 Hz region. The normally accepted frequency spectrum of the ECG waveform is 0.05 to 100 Hz (which is also the frequency response required of instruments that reproduce the waveform). The relative waveform amplitudes compared with a 1-mV calibration pulse are shown in Figure 6-6.

The basic waveform acquisition system from a typical ECG machine is shown in Figure 6-7. Wires from a patient cable are connected through a lead selector switch to the inputs of a differential amplifier. This amplifier usually has a push-pull output that is then used to drive a permanent magnet moving coil (PMMC) galvanometer pen assembly. The pen draws the vertical component of the waveform on a special graph paper that is passed under the pen tip at a fixed rate (in most cases 25 mm/sec). Figures 6-8, 6-9, and 6-10 show the common ECG leads. In all cases, the common or reference ground point is the patient's right leg.

The three simplest leads are the *bipolar limb lead,* designated I, II, and III. These are known collectively as the Einthoven triangle leads because of the triangle formed by the right arm, left arm, and left leg (against a right leg reference).

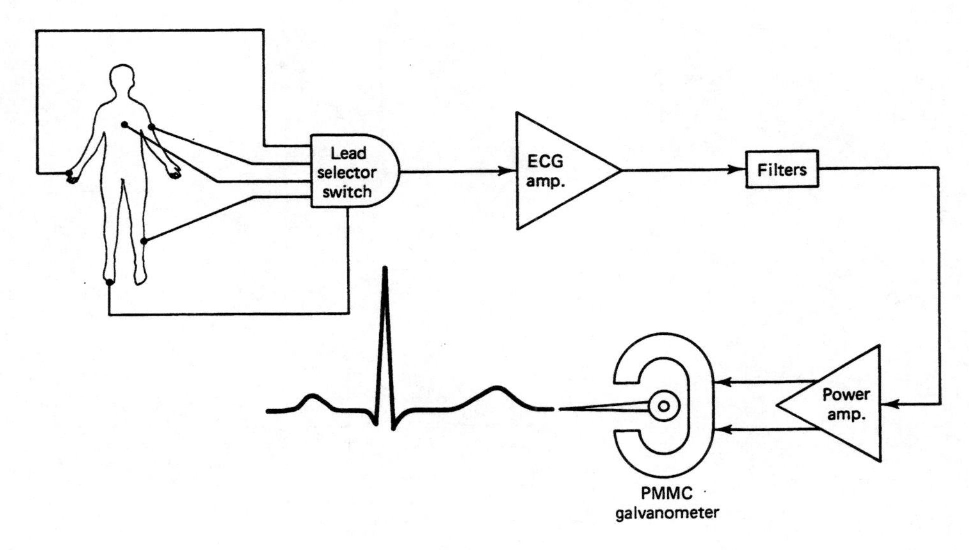

FIGURE 6-7

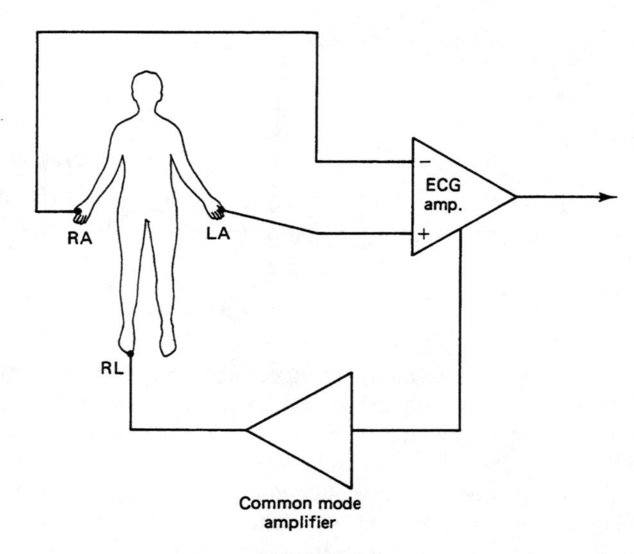

FIGURE 6-8

Three more leads are called either the *augmented* or *unipolar limb leads,* which are designated by the letters AVR, AVL, and AVF. These leads are created by summing currents from two of the limbs in a resistor network and measuring them relative to the third limb electrode.

The last set of common standard leads are the *V leads* (V1 through V6). These leads are taken by summing currents from all three limbs in a resistor network and

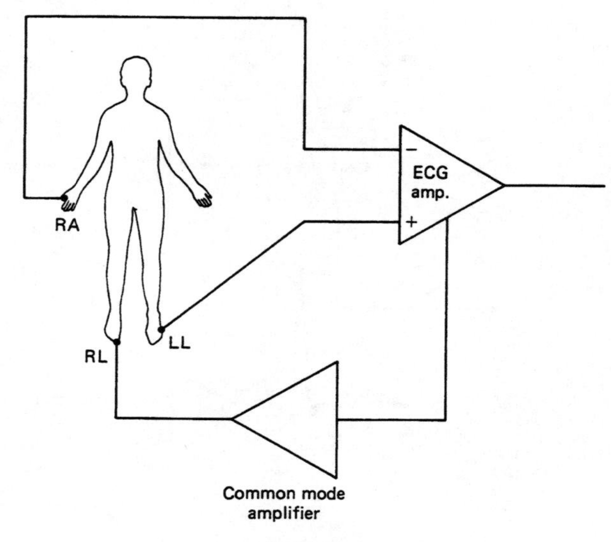

FIGURE 6-9

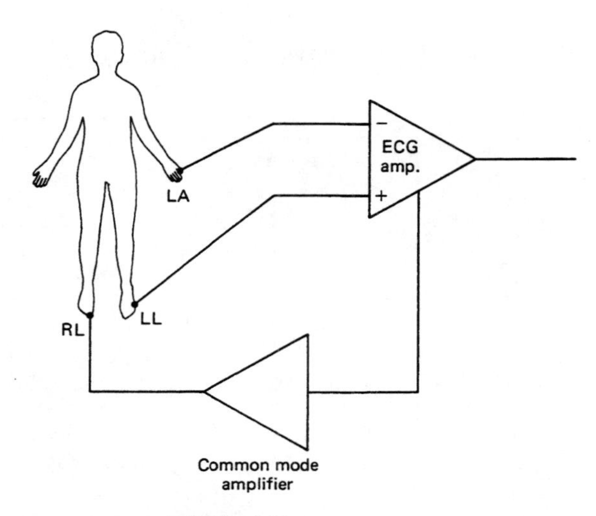

FIGURE 6-10

then measuring them against signals picked up from one of six standard positions on the patient's chest.

Each wire on an ECG patient cable is color coded so that it won't be connected to the wrong place. This color code is

RA—white
LA—black
RL—green
LL—red
Chest—brown

ECG MACHINE OPERATION

Figure 6-11 is a simplified drawing of a typical ECG machine drive mechanism. Such devices are actually part of a larger family of instruments known collectively as *strip-chart recorders* (see Chapter 18). The most common single-channel, one-trace paper used in ECG recording is 50 mm wide and is divided into 1-mm and 5-mm squares to form a kind of graph paper. The paper is usually stored in a special compartment in either roll or Z-fold form.

Three different mechanisms are used in normal clinical ECG machines, and all of them are discussed in detail in Chapter 18. The three forms are thermal writer, ink pen writer ("ink slingers"), and dot matrix writer.

In repairing ECG machines you will note that few drive motors ever go bad. In nearly eight years of servicing these machines I saw only one bad motor. However, there are a large number of idler rollers and a large (but somewhat smaller) number of drive rollers found bad in these machines. Rollers in machines located in high-use

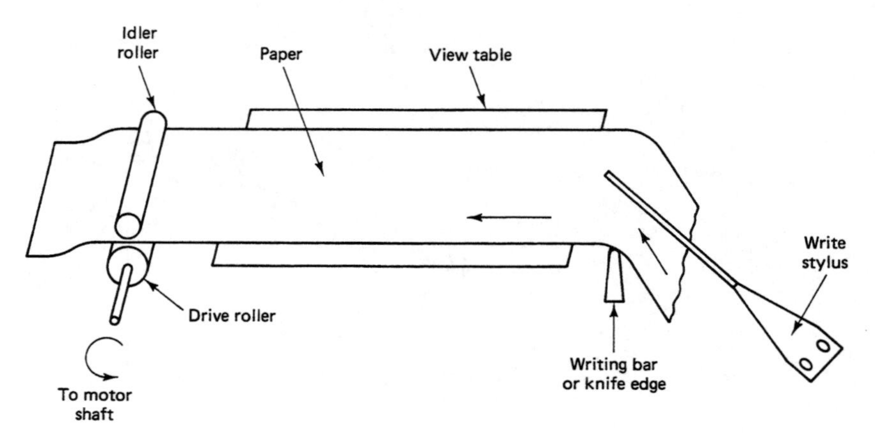

FIGURE 6-11

areas can be expected to wear out in a predictable period of time. The usual symptoms are a drive roller that seems to turn normally yet the paper moves either not at all or only haltingly.

Another common problem area is the write stylus. There are actually two types encountered in older ECG machines: ink and thermal. The dot matrix type is found on some modern machines. It is the thermal, by far, which is most frequently seen in ECG machines. Both, however, are subject to a variety of assorted faults. You can expect pens to clog with dried ink (especially if not used for several days) and thermal types to burn out. Both types of stylus are very delicate and will easily bend if allowed to slam against the high- or low-end mechanical stops or travel limits. This may occur if too high an amplitude signal is applied to the input, which is often the result of pulling the cable electrodes off the patient before turning the machine off or to an inactive condition. Expect to replace a lot of styluses.

Still another mechanical defect is poor paper tension. Normal functioning ECG machines will produce a nice clean trace. When paper tension across the knife edge is reduced, either by a machine mechanical defect or improper paper loading by the operator, the paper strip chart will be allowed to skew under the tip of the stylus and a smeared trace is produced. In fact, it is the drag of the pen on the paper surface that tends to aggravate the skewing effect. Although the fault may be either mechanical or human failure, it is very common for the nurse, doctor, or monitoring technician using the machine to complain of a worn-out or bad stylus. For the sake of doing a good job, let me hasten to admonish the new technician to examine each machine before automatically replacing the stylus.

Interfering voltages applied to the input of the ECG machine may tend to obscure the real waveform and render it unreadable. Anomalies on the tracing that represent either machine errors or voltages present but not generated by the patient's heart are called *artifacts*. Most of the time, artifacts can be easily diagnosed and corrected by the operator. In some cases, however, artifacts will be referred to an electronics person for correction. You will, therefore, see both machine defects and user errors causing various artifacts. Thus, learn to recognize and correct some of the more common ECG artifacts.

Figure 6-12A shows a reasonably clean ECG tracing with few, if any, artifacts. In Figures 6-12B and 6-12C, however, we see severe and mild muscle jitter, respectively. All of the muscles in the body are capable of producing voltages, and these will be picked up by the ECG machine just as easily as the desired voltages. The cure for this class of artifacts is usually to have the patient calm down and lie still. If this does not work and there are no errors in operation or machine faults that

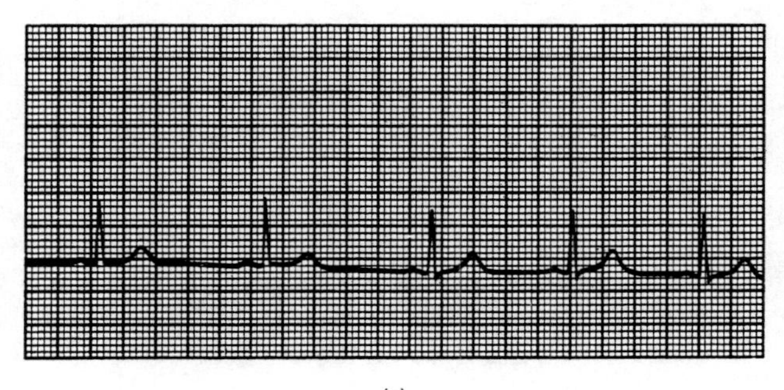

(a)

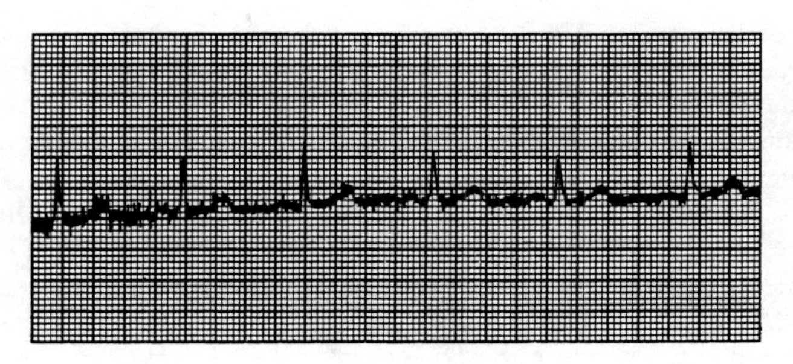

(b)

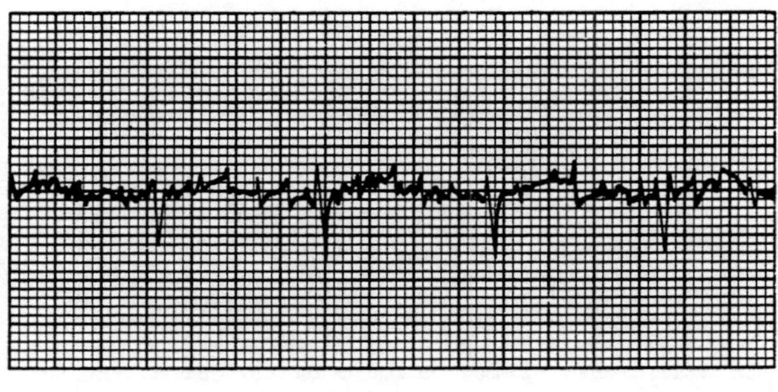

(c)

FIGURE 6-12

can be corrected, then try the internal machine filter (if any). This circuit may be labeled *filter* or *monitor/diagnostic* switch. The monitor position offers a lower −3-dB cutoff frequency and will therefore attenuate much of the noise—although at the expense of a slightly modified ECG waveform.

One cause of jitter can be operator corrected. This is a loose electrode. If the ECG paste or alchohol pad used between the patient's skin and the electrode has dried out, or if the electrode has been placed over a particularly bony area of the patient's body, then apparent muscle jitter and possibly other artifacts will increase.

Figure 6-12C also shows a wandering baseline along with the muscle artifact. This defect can also be caused by poor electrical contact with the skin. When this defect is seen, try cleaning the skin under the electrode (or slightly abrading it) and use a new alchohol swab or fresh dab of ECG paste under the electrode. Also be sure to check the electrode to see if it is free of corrosion and is clean.

Another form of common artifact is 60-Hz interference from AC power lines is shown in Figure 6-13. The electrical power lines radiate energy into all nearby conductors—and that includes the patient's body and the ECG cables. This effect can also be demonstrated somewhat more vividly to many electronics people by simply touching the input leads of an oscilloscope or audio amplifier. In the former case you will see a sine wave trace on the oscilloscope screen, while in the latter a buzz will be heard in the loudspeaker.

An ECG preamplifier, though, has two input leads that are balanced with respect to common; that is, it uses a differential input. The two inputs have an equal gain, but opposite polarity, effect on the output signal. Although each input of this pair will produce an output signal in response to a ground-referenced signal, if the same signal is applied to both inputs simultaneously then they will cancel each other out. The differential ECG amplifier produces an output signal only when a differential input signal is present. Wires feeding the ECG inputs will pick up approximately the same amount of 60-Hz signal, provided that they are of equal length and are in the same general vicinity. If the input circuits remain balanced, the preamplifier sees these signals as a common mode signal, that is, there are equal voltages applied to each input. Therefore, no 60-Hz output signal should be seen.

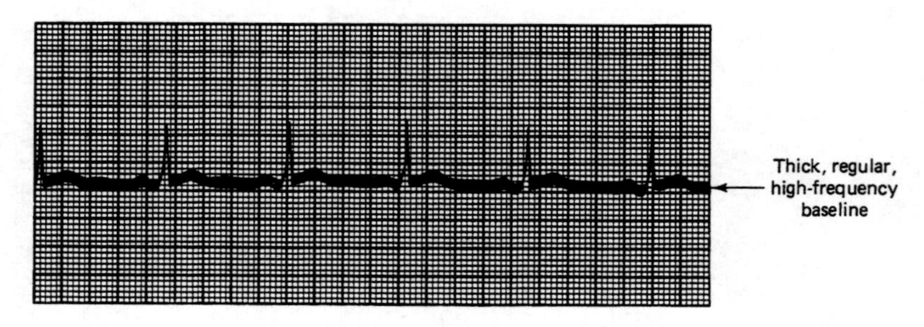

FIGURE 6-13

Several common defects tend to upset the input balance of the ECG preamplifier, and allow the 60-Hz signal to become differential. If an electrode is in poor contact with the skin, or if the skin itself is in such a condition to produce poor contact, 60-Hz interference will result. Another frequently found cause of 60-Hz interference is a broken wire in the patient cable. In a few cases, the trouble is inside the ECG machine electronics circuits. Look for broken input wires or a faulty or dirty lead selector switch. Clean it with a good contact cleaner or electronic switch degreaser and solvent. A bad input socket is often found because of the torque placed on the socket by the heavy patient cable and the abuse usual to such equipment—TLC seems reserved for patients, not medical equipment.

Diagnosing the cause of 60-Hz interference is usually pretty simple and straightforward, and can be performed rapidly. First, short together all the electrodes. If this causes the interference to disappear altogether, then suspect the connection to the patient. If it persists, then look to the cable. One means of testing the cable is to replace it with one that is known to be good; another way is to measure continuity using an ohmmeter. Keep in mind, though, that some ECG patient cables use a series resistor of between 1 K and 10 K, and so may appear to be open circuited if an inappropriate ohmmeter scale is used.

Some hospitals keep a special lamp-and-battery continuity tester that is designed to test ECG patient cables. The machine end and the individual electrode ends are all plugged into appropriate jacks. A switch is then turned to connect first one and then the other end into the test lamp circuitry. You can also keep a dummy ECG plug with all the pins shorted together so that it can be inserted into the input jack; this puts all input lines at ground potential. If 60-Hz interference still is seen, then you may suspect a defect inside the machine. In that case, incidentally, you can almost predict that one of the causes discussed earlier will be the fault. It is relatively rare, but not unheard of, for the actual electronic amplifiers to be at fault.

Do not overlook the possibility of a bad power line ground as the cause of the 60-Hz interference. All ECG machines use a three-wire power cord that has a third wire connected to the chassis ground. If the ground is broken or is not as good as it should be, then interference will result. If an ohmmeter check reveals an open or high-resistance ground to the chassis of the ECG machine, replace the power cord or plug. In most cases the break will be at the plug end of the cord immediately behind the connector, which is the major point of stress in most power cords. Also replace the plug if the blades or the ground lug appear to be worn, or even if they appear to be simply ratty.

If the power cord and plug seem to be all right, suspect a bad duplex outlet in the wall. It is often the case that a soon-to-be-bad outlet on the wall will give itself away by causing interference on ECG machines or bedside monitors. Loss of tension on the ground lug can cause this problem, as well as presenting additional problems with regard to patient safety. This condition can be easily tested by plugging the machine into another outlet that is known to be good. Another means of testing the outlet is with a special tension gauge. Have the electrician replace the AC outlet if it is found to be defective.

There are several parameters that we use to examine and evaluate the typical ECG machine. Although the actual specifications may vary somewhat from one manufacturer to another, the commonality of purpose for which they are designed makes some tests common to all instruments of that class.

Every ECG machine has a voltage calibration button used to place a 1.0-mV pulse across the differential inputs of the preamplifier. This is usually labeled "STANDARDIZE" or "1 mV." The calibration pulse is used by the operator to adjust the amplifier gain until the 1-mV signal produces a stylus deflection of 10 mm (two large squares on standard ECG paper). This button is located at a point in the circuit that will allow you to make a quick and cheap evaluation of machine performance without any additional test equipment. Simply press the calibration button and hold it for 2 seconds (Figure 6-14). The amplifier is to drop about 5 to 7 mm in this time period. Next, make a few 1-mV pulses in quick succession by pressing and releasing the button several times. Make sure the amplifier has sufficient gain to give more than the required minimum amplitude.

A somewhat more comprehensive analysis of overall ECG machine performance can be realized by using some of the more sophisticated test equipment in the electronics laboratory. Do not make the mistake of assuming that all of that high-cost test equipment is the be-all and end-all of ECG testing. You may well—in fact you will—find defects that only show up when a real, live human test subject is used as the ECG source. (ECG machine repair technicians tend to see their own ECG waveform a great deal because it makes a handy, portable "signal generator" that's with them all of the time.)

There are some tests that are important. You will need a square wave generator that is capable of producing a 1-Hz signal with an amplitude of several volts. These specifications, incidentally, are well within the range of most of the low-cost function generators on the market today. With older generators that only go down to 10 or 20 Hz, you can use digital IC logic dividers, such as the 7490 series TTL devices. A single 7490 will divide an input square wave frequency by 10, and so will produce 1-Hz output from a 10-Hz input signal.

Since few generators come with a balanced output, it may prove wise to construct a balancing attenuator pad such as that in Figure 6-15. This circuit takes the single-ended input and delivers a balanced, although greatly attenuated, output. Resistors R1 through R3 in the circuit form a voltage divider network in which output

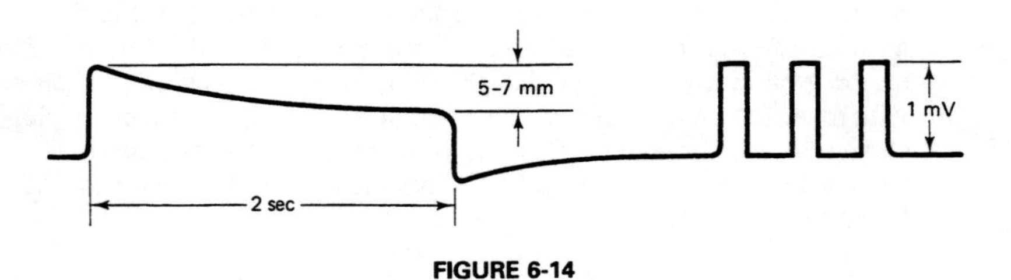

FIGURE 6-14

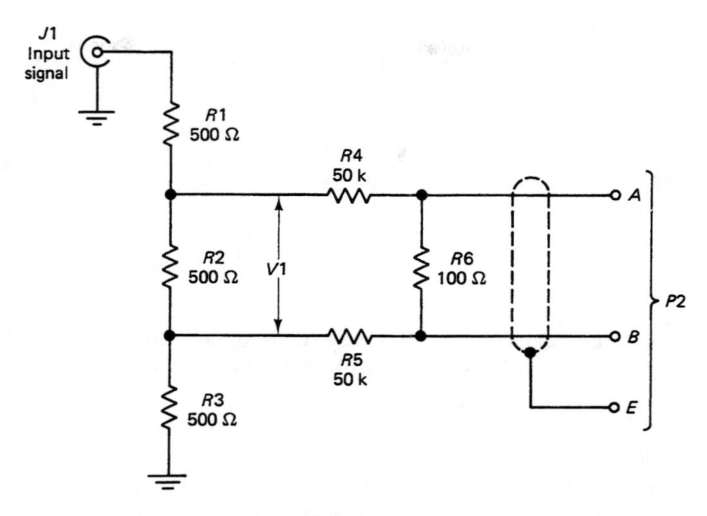

FIGURE 6-15

signal V1 will be approximately one-third the input. This output voltage is impressed across a balanced voltage divider consisting of resistors R4 through R6. This is the voltage actually delivered to the ECG machine, and it has a value of

$$V_o = \frac{\text{V1R6}}{\text{R4} + \text{R5} + \text{R6}}$$

The values listed for the resistors in Figure 6-15 will attenuate voltage V1 approximately 60 dB (1/1000), so to produce an ouput voltage of 1 mV, the input signal will be about 3 volts peak. Connector J1 can be a standard BNC type, or whatever is compatible with your signal source. Connector P2 must be compatible with the ECG input jack on your machine. In most cases this means a five-pin, size 14 AN (aka MS) connector wired in the now standard "Sanborn" ECG configuration:

AN/MS Pin	ECG Input Wire
A	Right arm (RA)
B	Left arm (LA)
C	Left leg (LL)
D	Chest (C)
E	Right leg (RL)

The pins called out in the table reflect the ECG lead I configuration.

The ECG machine can be tested in several ways using this adapter and a 1-Hz square wave. Figure 6-16 shows a pattern of square waves taken from an ECG machine tracing. Note that the pulses to the left overshoot and ring. This fault is characteristic of misadjusted damping. In a few models this is caused by adjustment of the

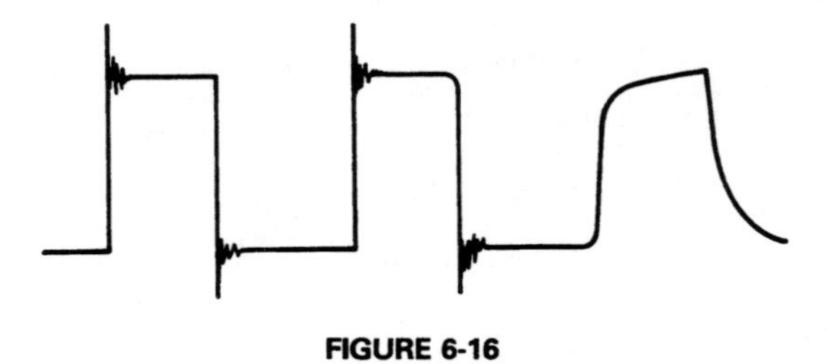

FIGURE 6-16

stylus pressure, while in most an electrical adjustment is required. In the latter case you will find a damping control somewhere on the machine: adjust it for the best possible square shape.

The square wave can also give you a rough idea of the proper frequency response in the amplifiers and galvanometer assembly. If the waveshape of the 1-Hz signal has rounded corners, suspect poor high-frequency response. Low-frequency attenuation is indicated if the top of the square wave appears to tilt. Be aware that some ECG machines have their high-frequency response intentionally limited so that muscle jitter and 60-Hz artifacts are reduced naturally. These instruments are normally used for long-term monitoring purposes rather than diagnostic ECG strips. On those machines the square wave response will always be poor, and no repair is either possible or feasible.

ECG ELECTRONICS

Figure 6-17 shows a block diagram of a common type of ECG preamplifier. The overall gain provided by stages A1 and A2 must be several thousand. Their frequency response should be 0.05 to 100 Hz. Amplifier A1 has differential inputs, for reasons already discussed and a push-pull output stage so that it can drive the differential input of amplifier A2. In machines typically found in hospitals, you can expect to see all of the well-known amplifier technologies of the past 20 years—vacuum tubes, transistors, and integrated circuits.

The frequency response at the lower end of the range is limited by capacitors C5 and C6. These will normally have a value in the 10-μF to 100-μF range in solid-state designs.

One further requirement is that amplifier A1 have a high input impedance. Since these circuits are actually no more than voltage amplifiers, you would ideally want a low source impedance (the patient) and a high input impedance. With the patient's impedance at the electrodes on the order of 10 kΩ to 50 kΩ, the amplifier would thus require a very high input impedance. The usual rule of thumb is 10 to 100 times the source impedance! In actual design practice, this is not too hard to accomplish with modern IC electronics, but at one time it was a rough specification to meet.

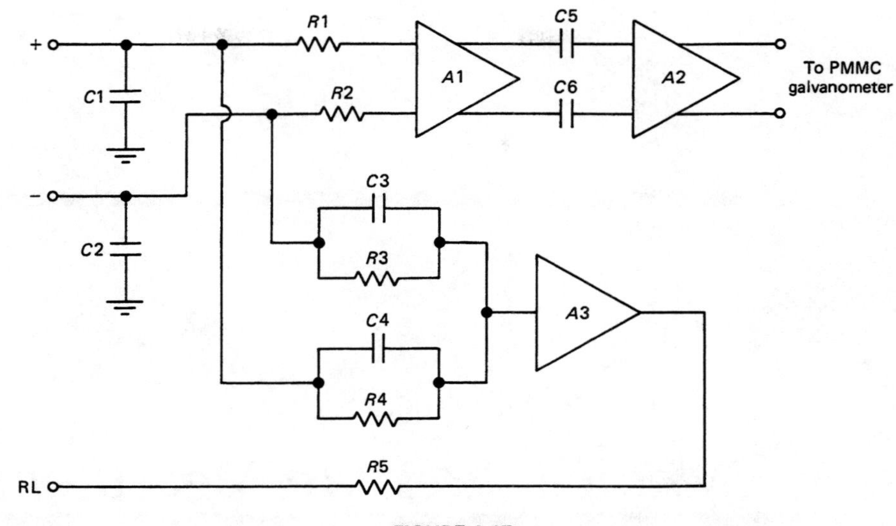

FIGURE 6-17

7

Medical Pressure Measurements

Medical clinicians measure several different forms of fluid and gas pressure. The general principles are the same for all cases, but in this chapter we will focus on blood pressure measurements because these are the most common in emergency and critical care medicine. The most common blood pressure measurement is arterial blood pressure, which is almost routinely monitored by electronic instruments in ICU, CCU, emergency room, trauma unit, or operating room. Also of interest in special cases are venous pressures, central venous pressure (CVP), intracardiac blood pressure, pulmonary artery pressure, spinal fluid pressures, and intraventricular brain pressures. The principal differences among these pressures is primarily one of range; often, the same instruments are used for all these different pressures. The medical pressure measurement system needs to be as least invasive as possible (it is, however, invasive) and sterile (to prevent infection). In addition, electrical isolation from the AC power mains needs be maintained at a higher level for purposes of patient safety.

Figure 7-1 shows a typical medical monitor that includes a pressure monitor module. Many of the features of this instrument are also incorporated in nonmedical pressure measurement instruments. In fact, medical pressures monitors are often used for nonmedical applications. The readout is a digital meter that displays the pressure in millimeters of mercury (mmHg). (Note: Medical pressures are still expressed in mmHg, where modern engineering and scientific practice uses the torr. But since 1 T = 1 mmHg, the difference is a moot point.) The display on some mon-

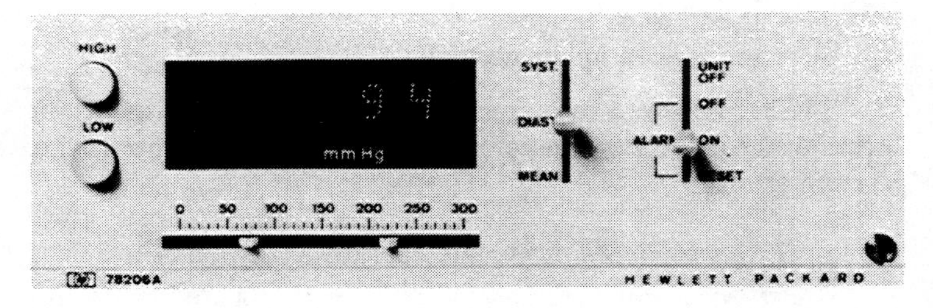

FIGURE 7-1

itors can be switched from systolic, diastolic, mean, and venous. The systolic and diastolic pressures are taken from the arterial waveform by peak and valley (inverted peak) holder circuits, respectively. The venous pressure is merely a higher gain position that allows a lower pressure to be displayed full scale. The mean pressure is merely the time average of the input pressure waveform; that is, it is the time integral of the pressure waveform.

The alarm section of the pressure monitor is used to set upper and lower limits through the use of either slide controls underneath the meter or separate knobs. Ordinarily, in analog circuits the alarm system consists of a voltage window comparator in which one control sets the lower limit and the other control sets the upper limit. In microprocessor- or microcomputer-controlled ("digital") instruments, the controls are either digital in their own right or are potentiometers connected to a reference voltage source input and an analog-to-digital (A/D) converter output. In some microcomputer-controlled models, a numerical keyboard is used to set the exact limits demanded by the operator.

The transducer connector at the input terminal is sometimes used to house certain calibrating components. Very few transducers have repeatable zero, range, and output potential from one unit to another. Thus, the maker must either provide calibrating controls on the electronic unit or normalize all transducers with calibrating components (e.g, a potentiometer output level control and Wheatstone bridge linearization resistors). The calibrating components in the transducer plug bring the output within range of the sensitivity and zero controls.

WHAT IS "PRESSURE"?

Most readers have some idea of how "pressure" is defined, but all too often we find that people have a poor idea of exactly what they are measuring in their pressure monitors. The proper definition of pressure is that it is *force per unit area.*

$$P = \frac{F}{A}$$

where

P = the pressure in newtons per square meter (N/m^2) or pascals (Pa), 1 N/m^2 = 1 Pa

F = the force in newtons
A = the area in square meters

The pressure can be increased by either increasing the applied force or by reducing the cross-sectional area over which the force operates. Alternate units for the pressure are

CGS System: dynes per square centimeter ($dyne/cm^2$)
British Engineering System: pounds per square inch ($lb/in.^2$ or psi)

When the force in any system is constant or static (that is, nonvarying), then that pressure is said to be *hydrostatic*. If the force is varying, on the other hand, the force is said to be *dynamic* or *hydrodynamic*. Physiological pressures (e.g, human arterial blood pressure) are examples of hydrodynamic pressures; the pressure head in a stoppered keg of beer, or in a toilet or commode tank, is a hydrostatic pressure—at least until the bong is popped or the flush lever is depressed.

Pascal's Principle

Pascal's principle (after French scientist/theologian Blaise Pascal, 1623–1662) governs pressures in a closed system. This physical law states that

> Pressure applied to an enclosed fluid is transmitted undiminished to every portion of the fluid and the walls of the containing vessel.

Let's consider an example. If a pressure is applied to the stoppered system (e.g., the syringe and vessel in Figure 7-2), then the same pressure is felt throughout the interior of both the syringe and the vessel. Changing the applied pressure at the rear of the plunger causes the same change to be reflected at every point throughout the interior of the system.

A physics professor I had in engineering school had an experiment that amply illustrated Pascal's principle—even though over several years it caused the first floor lecture hall stage in the science building to rot away. He had a wooden water barrel that was sealed all around, except for a hole in the top where a water hose fitting was installed. A long garden hose was snaked out the door, up the outside of the building to the fourth floor, where a graduate student was posted. The system was filled with water, and a wooden dowel snug fit to the hose at the open end on the fourth floor served as the plunger (similar in concept to Figure 7-2). On command from the professor (issued over a pair of CB walkie-talkies), the graduate student drove the dowel into the hose with great force. The force of the student's hand produced a large force per unit area (i.e., the cross-sectional area of the dowel) that was felt inside the barrel as a high pressure—causing the barrel to burst apart violently. Although the experiment forcibly illustrated Pascal's principle, the twice annual inundation of the lecture stage with water from the barrel caused the wood beneath to rot out!

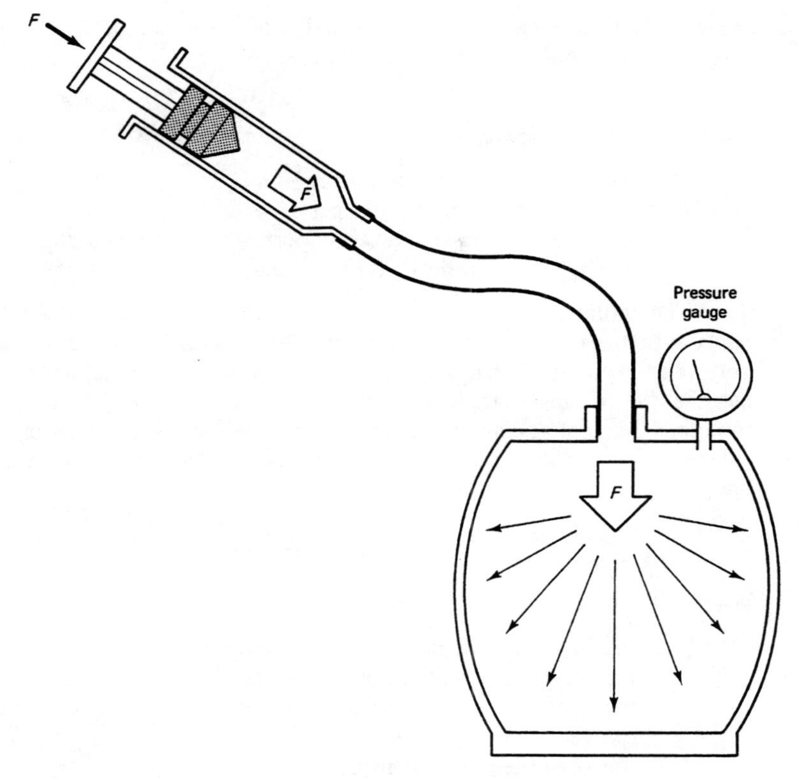

FIGURE 7-2

Pascal's principle holds true in hydrostatic systems always. In hydrodynamic systems it holds true only for quasi-static changes, that is, when a very small change is made, and the turbulence is allowed to die down before subsequent measurements are made. Pascal's principle holds approximately true for those hydrodynamic systems where the flow is reasonably nonturbulent (no true nonturbulent flow exists) and the pipe lumen is small compared with its length. The simple model holds true in those cases, however, only in the center of the flow mass but not at the pipe wall boundaries.

In physiological systems, the situation is somewhat more complicated. Unfortunately, many students in life sciences lack the mathematics background to perform proper analysis of blood flow systems. Many medical students, for example, are taught a hopelessly naive model that fails to take into account the fact that the situation is complicated by four factors: (1) the particulate nature of blood (it is not a strict fluid, but contains red cells and other material), (2) that blood vessel walls are distensible and not rigid, (3) blood viscosity changes under certain influences, and

(4) the walls are not smooth, especially in older subjects. The naive model is analogous to Ohm's law, and states that

$$P = RF$$

where

P = the pressure difference in torr (mmHg)
F = the flow rate in milliliters per second
R = the blood vessel resistance in peripheral resistance units (PRU), such that 1 PRU allows a flow of 1 ml/s under a 1-torr pressure

The actual situation in physiological blood flow systems is a lot more complex because of the factors listed. The actual vessel diameter changes (which is one way your body regulates blood pressure) both from systemic readjustments and from the fact that the beating heart forms a pulsatile pressure wave. The flow rate (and hence the other parameters) is not a simple factor like the current flow in a simple electrical resistance analogy, but rather is better (but still imperfectly) given by Poiseulle's law, which is

$$F = \frac{P \pi R^4}{8nL}$$

Where

F = the flow in cubic centimeters/second (cc/s)
P = the pressure in dynes per square centimeter
n = the coefficient of viscosity in dyne-seconds per square centimeter
R = the vessel radius in centimeters
L = the vessel length in centimeters

The study of pressure in turbulent or large lumen systems, or in the boundary area close to the pipe/vessel wall, is the subject of advanced engineering mechanics and physics courses. And, until chaotic systems were discovered, even these luminaries "faked it" in their studies. For our purposes, we may assume that Pascal's principle either holds true absolutely, or the system can be made quasi-static for measurement, discussion, or analysis purposes.

Pulsatile waves result from a cardiac pumping action that is not constant. In physiological systems, the heart of the subject animal or human beats in a manner that produces a pulse flow (which can be felt with the fingertips where arteries run close to the surface—in the wrist for example). Figure 7-3 shows the human arterial blood pressure waveform, here used as an example of pulsatile systems. There are several values which can be measured in this system:

1. Peak pressure (systolic)
2. Minimum pressure (diastolic)
3. Dynamic average (one-half peak minus minimum)
4. Average pressure (called *mean arterial pressure*)

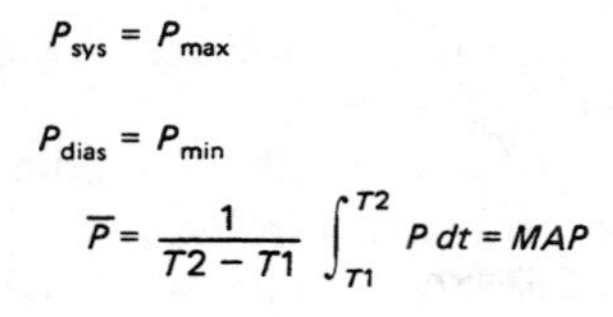

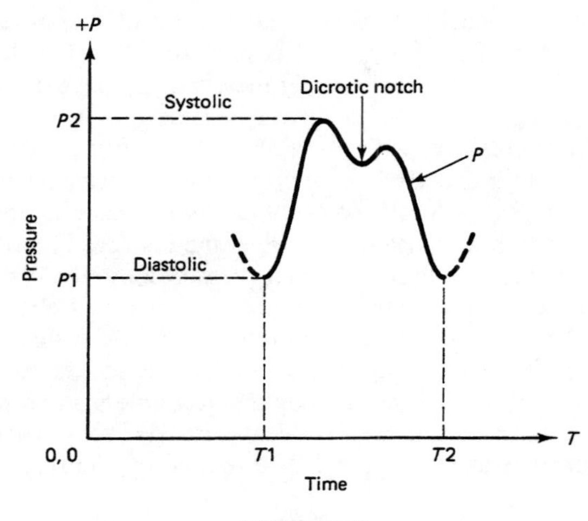

FIGURE 7-3

When one discusses "pressure" in a pulsatile system, one must also specify *what* pressure is intended! In a later section we will discuss the methods used for measuring these pressures electronically.

As biomedical engineers we have a constant problem with both clinicians and medical researchers regarding the average pressure readings on the electronic blood pressure monitors. The problem was in their definition of "mean arterial pressure" (that is, the time average). The correct definition, which is used in the design of the typical instrument, is written as a calculus expression:

$$\overline{P} = \left(\frac{1}{T2 - T1}\right) \int P\, dt$$

In medical and nursing schools, and in typical intensive care unit nursing courses, however, a synthetic (and often incorrect) definition is used (referring to Figure 7-3) because those people lack the mathematics sophistication to deal with calculus. The approximation is

$$\overline{P} = \frac{(P2 - P1)}{3} + P1$$

In medical terminology, this definition states that the mean arterial pressure (or MAP) is equal to the diastolic ($P1$) plus one-third the difference between systolic and diastolic ($P2 - P1$).

The problem faced by the biomedical engineer (and more often either the biomedical equipment technician who repairs the equipment for complaining nurses or monitoring technicians who operate the equipment) is that the synthetic definition is merely an approximation of the functional calculus definition for *healthy people!* In many sick people, however, the portion of the waveform between the dicrotic notch and time $T2$ (Figure 7-3) is very heavily damped, so the actual MAP is less than the functional MAP actually measured by the electronic instrument (try telling that to an angry nurse at a patient's bedside!).

The simple test, which is revealed by plugging values into both equations, is to place a constant pressure on the system and see what happens to the readings. In that case, $P1 = P2 =$ MAP, so all three digital readouts should be the same. In other words, to test a pressure system when the displayed MAP and your calculated MAP are different is to pump a constant pressure onto the system (or press the CAL button) and see if all three pressures are the same: diastolic, systolic, and MAP. If they differ when $P =$ constant, then there is a system fault.

The CAL button alternative works only to test the electronics. A fault in the transducer will not be revealed by this test unless a real pressure is applied.

In a later section we will deal with electronic measurement of pressures, so will want to return to Figure 7-3 to see the relationships of the various pressures.

BASIC PRESSURE MEASUREMENTS

The air forming our atmosphere exerts a pressure on the surface of the earth, and all objects on the surface (or above it). This pressure is usually expressed in atmospheres (atm), pounds per square inch (lb/in.^{2} or psi), or other pressure units. The magnitude of 1 atm is approximately 14.7 lb/in.^{2} at mean sea level.

If a pressure is measured with respect to a perfect vacuum (defined as 0 atm), then it is called *absolute pressure,* and if against 1 atm ("open air"), it is called a *gauge pressure*. Two gauge pressures, or a gauge pressure and an absolute pressure, can be measured relative to each other to form a single measurement called variously relative pressure or differential pressure. Pressures in fluid pipelines, storage tanks, and the human circulatory system are usually gauge pressures (if measured at a point) or differential pressures (if measured between two points along a length).

Figure 7-4 shows the Torricelli manometer, named after Evangelista Torricelli (Italian scientist, 1608–1647), which is used to measure atmospheric pressure. An evacuated, small lumen glass tube stands vertically in a pool of mercury. The end that is inside the mercury (Hg) pool is open, while the other end is closed. The pressure exerted by the atmosphere on the surface of the mercury pool forces mercury into the tube, forming a column. The mercury column rises in the tube until its weight (i.e., gravitational force) exactly balances the force of the atmospheric pressure. Torricelli found that a 760-mm column of mercury could be supported by at-

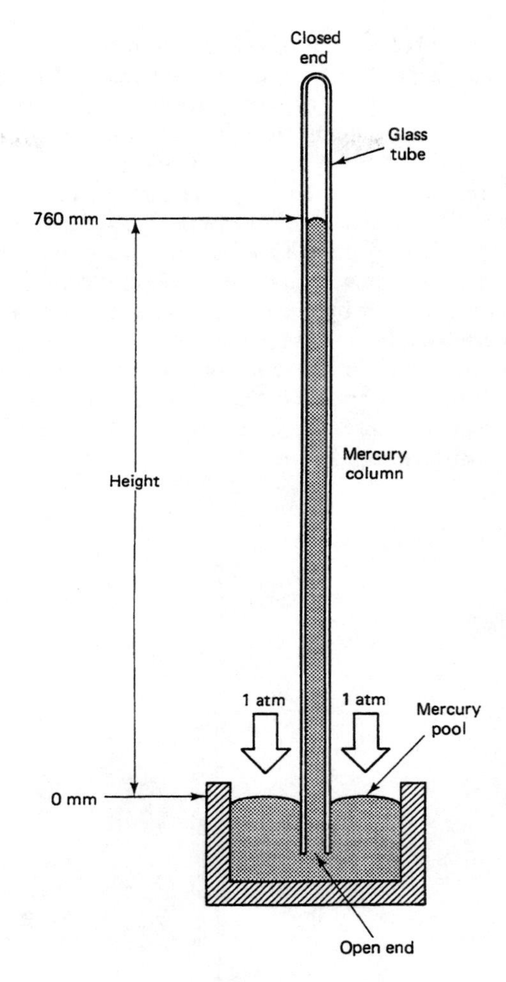

FIGURE 7-4

mospheric pressure at sea level. Thus, 1 atm is 760 mmHg (also sometimes given in weather reports and aviation in inches, that is, 1 atm = 760 mmHg = 29.92 in.Hg).

The proper units of pressure, as established by scientists in international agreement, and adopted in the United States by the *National Bureau of Standards* is the torr (named after Torricelli), where 1 torr is equal to 1 millimeter of mercury (i.e., 1 T = 1 mmHg). Workers in medicine and medical science (e.g., physiology) still use mmHg instead of the correct torr.

Gauge pressures are usually given in mmHg (or inches) above or below atmospheric pressure. A manometer is any device that measures gauge pressure, positive or negative. By convention, pressures above atmospheric pressure are signed positive, and those below atmospheric pressure are signed negative. Also by convention, negative gauge pressures are called vacuums and negative-reading manometers are called vacuum gauges (positive-reading manometers are also called pressure gauges). Both instruments are nonetheless properly called manometers, and in this chapter we will discuss both mercury and electronic manometers.

All measurements require some form of reference point, and for gauge pressures, the zero reference is a pressure of 1 atm. Even though the absolute value of the atmospheric pressure varies from one place to another, and in the same location over the space of a few hours, the zero point can be established by setting the zero scale on the indicator by opening the manometer to atmosphere.

Figure 7-5 shows a mercury manometer that is similar to those used to measure pressures and calibrate electronic pressure manometers. The open tube is connected to a mercury reservoir that is fitted with a rubber squeeze ball pump that can be used to increase pressure in the system. A valve is used to either open the chamber to atmosphere, or close it off.

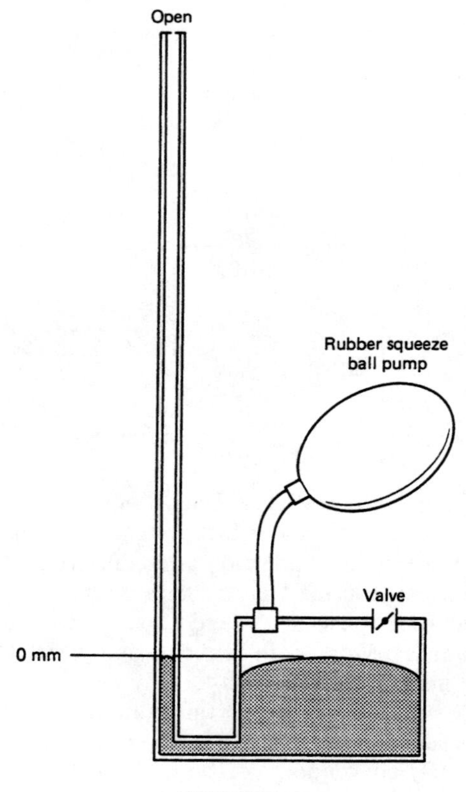

FIGURE 7-5

If the valve is open to the atmosphere, then the pressure on the chamber is equal to the pressure on the column, that is, one atmosphere. Under this condition the mercury column in the tube is at the same height as the mercury in the chamber. This point is defined as 0 mmHg. If the valve is closed, and the pressure inside the chamber is increased by operating the pump, then the mercury in the column will rise to a level proportional to the new pressure above atmospheric pressure.

If the rubber ball in Figure 7-5 is replaced with a connection to a closed pressure system other than the squeeze ball, then the mercury will rise to a level proportional to the pressure in that system. We can use this manometer as a calibrating device for medical personnel by adding a tee-connector in the line between the rubber squeeze ball and the chamber. One port of the tee goes to the rubber ball, one port goes to the chamber, and the third port goes to the transducer or other instrument being calibrated.

Gauge pressure is used for measurement purposes because it is a lot easier to be referenced at the zero point (open the manometer to the atmosphere) and can be easily recalibrated for each use (no matter where in the world the measurement is made). In addition, for most practical applications, the absolute pressure conveys no additional information content over gauge pressure. Should absolute pressure be needed, then it becomes a relatively simple matter to measure the atmospheric pressure (with a device like that in Figure 7-4) and then add that value to the pressure measured on the gauge pressure manometer of Figure 7-5.

BLOOD PRESSURE MEASUREMENT

Until 1905, the only method available for the measurement of blood pressure was to insert a Torricelli manometer tube into the vein or artery being measured, and note how far up the tube the blood flowed after a few pulses. This method is still used for some spinal fluid and central venous pressure measurements. It was pioneered in 1773 by English physician Stephen Hales, who used an open-ended glass tube in the neck artery of an unanesthetized horse (which was presumedly tied down securely!).

The modern indirect medical measurement of pressure (using the familiar blood pressure cuff) is *sphygmomanometry*. This method was pioneered in 1905 by Nicolas Korotkoff, but was not used widely until after 1935 when the Korotkoff readings were finally correlated to the Hale's method values. It wasn't until well after World War II that nurses were permitted to take blood pressure readings, being considered "doctor's work" up until that time.

Sphygmomanometry is an indirect method of measuring pressure. An inflatable cuff is placed over the patient's arm and inflated to a point where it occludes the underlying artery to a point where no blood can flow. A stethoscope placed downstream from the occlusion is used to monitor the onset of blood flow. The operator slowly releases the pressure in the cuff (3 mmHg/sec is optimum) until a series of sharp snapping "Korotkoff sounds" are heard. These occur due to the turbulence of blood under pressure breaking through the occlusion into the downstream artery. This event occurs when the cuff pressure equals the systolic pressure. The operator continues to monitor the pressure until the Korotkoff turbulence dies out, an event that occurs when the cuff pressure equals the diastolic pressure.

The modern electronic measurements consist of two types. One is an electronic version of the 1773 Hales method, in which a thin, hollow catheter is introduced into the artery, and then connected to a transducer (see Figure 7-6 for an example). The transducer outputs an electrical analog of the pressure waveform that can be directly calibrated in millimeters of mercury. The second type of electronic measurement is used by many all-electronic home-type blood pressure kits. In these instruments, a microphone (optimized for low-frequency sounds) is placed under the cuff and the pressure released. When the Korotkoff sounds are heard, the internal circuitry records the cuff pressure as the systolic, and when they disappear, it records the diastolic pressure.

Another (and related) method for measuring blood pressure indirectly is used in certain automatic bedside instruments. It was observed that the pressure inside the blood pressure cuff begins to oscillate as the decreasing cuff pressure approaches the mean arterial pressure (MAP). This phenomenon is thought by some to be an example of chaos in a physical system. ("Chaos" is a new science that is only now emerging. It's first widespread impacts were in cardiology and the type of turbulent dynamical systems represented by the blood pressure measuring system.) By monitoring this pressure variation, and noting when it peaks (at the MAP), the diastolic and systolic pressures can be calculated using a formula rearranged from either of the MAP equations given.

Other automatic blood pressure cuffs rely on either a low-frequency microphone or an ultrasonic transducer embedded in the cuff. These transducer elements are used to sense automatically the Korotkoff sounds generated by the blood spurting through the occlusion. These instruments are relatively sensitive to the positioning of the microphone or transducer over the brachial artery. Failure to read the pressure properly could be the result of improper adjustment of the cuff position.

FLUID PRESSURE TRANSDUCERS

Figure 7-6 shows a cutaway view of a typical blood pressure transducer. The body of the transducer contains the circuitry, which is separated from the fluid dome by the transducer's pressure sensitive diaphragm. This thin metallic membrane feels the pressure in the dome and is distended an amount proportional to the applied pressure. The other side of the diaphragm will either be connected to the core of an LVDT transformer or a piezoresistive Wheatstone bridge transduction element. The dome is used to contain the fluid and in most medical applications will be disposable (to prevent cross infection between patients).

There are at least two ports on the transducer dome. These ports are controlled by *stopcocks,* either built in or add on. When the stopcock is opened, then fluid flows into or out of the transducer, but when it is closed, the transducer is basically a closed system. In normal operations, one port will be connected to the system being measured, while the other port initially is open to the atmosphere. With the atmo-

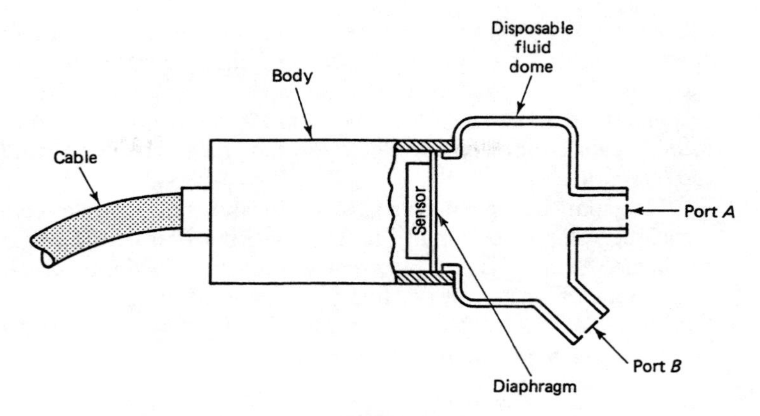

FIGURE 7-6

spheric port open, the transducer is at zero gauge pressure, so the electronic instrument it drives can be "zeroed."

Figure 7-7 shows the calibration setup for an electronic blood pressure measurement instrument. The transducer is of the sort discussed earlier, which is connected to an electronic manometer. In this test setup, the atmospheric port is connected to a regular mercury (or in low-pressure cases water) manometer. When the

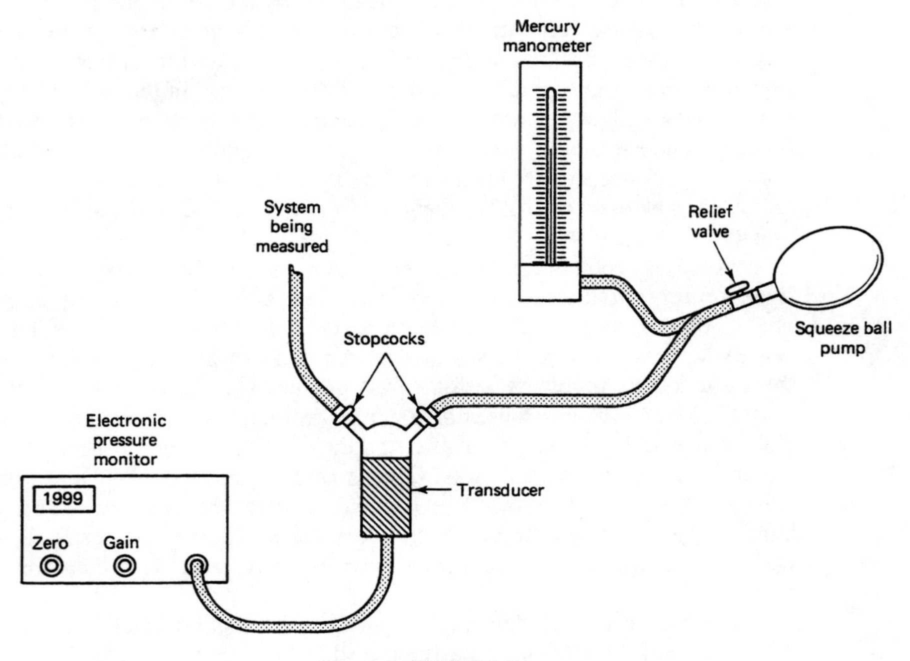

FIGURE 7-7

relief valve is open to atmosphere, the pressure monitor is set to zero. The valve is then closed, and a pressure pumped onto the system by the squeeze ball pump. In most cases, it is a good idea to set the pressure (as read on the mercury manometer) to some standard value such as 100 torr, 200 torr, and so on. You can then adjust the span or gain control on the electronic monitor to the same reading as obtained on the mercury.

In biomedical applications, it is critical that the operator be instructed in proper technique. One reason is to prevent contamination of the patient's lines, or other problems. Another is that incorrect settings of sometimes complicated stopcock arrangements can cause the system to be pumped with air—that could enter the patient as a potentially fatal air embolism: *get instruction from a medically qualified person before manipulating these units!*

FLUID MEASUREMENT SYSTEM FAULTS

The measurement of fluid pressures with electronic apparatus is not always the simple matter that it appears—unless certain precautions are observed. There are several problems that can affect the data acquired. For example, although it seems like a trivial observation, in multibranch or varying diameter systems we have to understand which pressure is being measured. One problem engineers have with medical personnel in pressure measurement situations is that the pressure measured by the instrument is not the same pressure measured by the blood pressure cuff. Typically, the blood pressure cuff measures a pressure in the upper arm, while the electronic instrument catheter is placed distal (that is, downstream) from that point. The blood pressure catheter is typically placed in the radial artery in the wrist. The problem is that these two pressures are normally different, so a nurse who accurately takes the blood pressure manually (albeit accuracy is a problem with the manual method) will normally obtain a slightly higher reading than the downstream reading—taken after the artery has branched. Also, height of the measurement site relative to the heart affects the reading.

Another problem frequently encountered is either resonance or damping of the pressure in nonstatic systems. Of course, if the pressure is a dead pressure, that is, one which does not vary or varies quasi-statically, then the problem does not exist. But if the pressure has a dynamic waveform, as in a blood pressure system, then there are certain problems with the system plumbing that can yield error.

There are several causes of damping in blood pressure systems. One is clogging of the tubing to and from the transducer. This cause is especially likely when blood enters the tubing and clots. Other forms of fluid will show the problem either due to phenomena like clotting or particulate matter blocking the sampling catheter lumen. The result of damping is to add a certain degree of inertia to the system, with a resultant loss of frequency response and peak data that are of medical significance.

Another cause of damping is purely a procedural problem. Sometimes the wrong form of tubing is used for the transducer plumbing system. The correct tubing is stiff walled. If the tubing is rubber, neoprene or some other distensible material (like IV tubing), then there will be a problem. The cause of the problem is that increases and decreases of the pressure waveform cause the tubing diameter to increase or decrease in response to the changes. Unfortunately, changing the diameter of the measurement system also changes the pressure, so the measurement interferes with the system being investigated. This problem is especially common in medical or life sciences areas because users will press various forms of medical tubing into service. Both surgical tubing and intravenous (IV) set tubing are sometimes used—erroneously—and will result in a damped waveform. The end result is an incorrect waveshape and artifactual readings.

Resonance or "ringing" (Figure 7-8A) in the system is caused mainly by two phenomena. First, there is the possibility of air or other gas bubbles in the system. It is almost impossible to rig a pressure system without having air enter the plumbing. It is, therefore, necessary to purge the system of air bubbles. Placing the transducer and plumbing in an attitude where the air can rise to the top—near a port or stopcock—and be removed will clear the system.

The second cause of resonance or ringing is improper length of tubing. Like any dynamic mechanical or electrical system, the transducer plumbing has a certain resonant frequency. If the length and diameter of the tubing is such that the system is resonant for the applied waveform, then ringing will result. Typically, a ringing system produces a jagged waveform, or one in which the peak pressure indication is substantially larger—and sharper in shape—than can be justified by the application.

All waveshapes can be represented mathematically by a "Fourier series" that lists a group of alternating current frequencies consisting of a fundamental frequency, and a collection of harmonics (integer multiples: 2, 3, etc.) or subharmonics (reciprocals of integer multiples, e.g., 1/2, 1/3, etc). For this reason, an ECG amplifier must have a frequency response of 0.05 to 100 Hz and a pressure amplifier a response of 0.05 to 85 Hz (1 Hz = 1 cycle per second). In the case of a perfect square wave, the Fourier series consists of a fundamental and an infinite series of odd order harmonics (3, 5, 7, 9, . . .). In medical applications such as pressure monitoring, however, the "ideal" square wave has harmonics only to about 85 Hz, so the edges will appear rounded (see the "ideal" square wave in Figure 7-8B). This is the wave that should result from a quick, single-stroke flushing of a blood pressure transducer with a syringe.

Note in Figure 7-8B the ringing square wave. In this case, the plumbing or some other factor has caused the high frequencies to be accentuated out of balance. This is an example of an *underdamped* system. The *damping factor* is a measure of the system response, and is given crudely by

$$DF = \frac{-\ln (B/A)}{\{\pi^2 + [\ln (B/A)]^2\}^{1/2}}$$

See Figure 7-8B for definitions of A and B.

The opposite problem, a severely *overdamped* system, is shown in Figure 7-8C. In this case, the higher frequencies are not passed, so the pressure waveform changes much more slowly than the actual applied pressure. This problem is sometimes caused by fouled pressure lines.

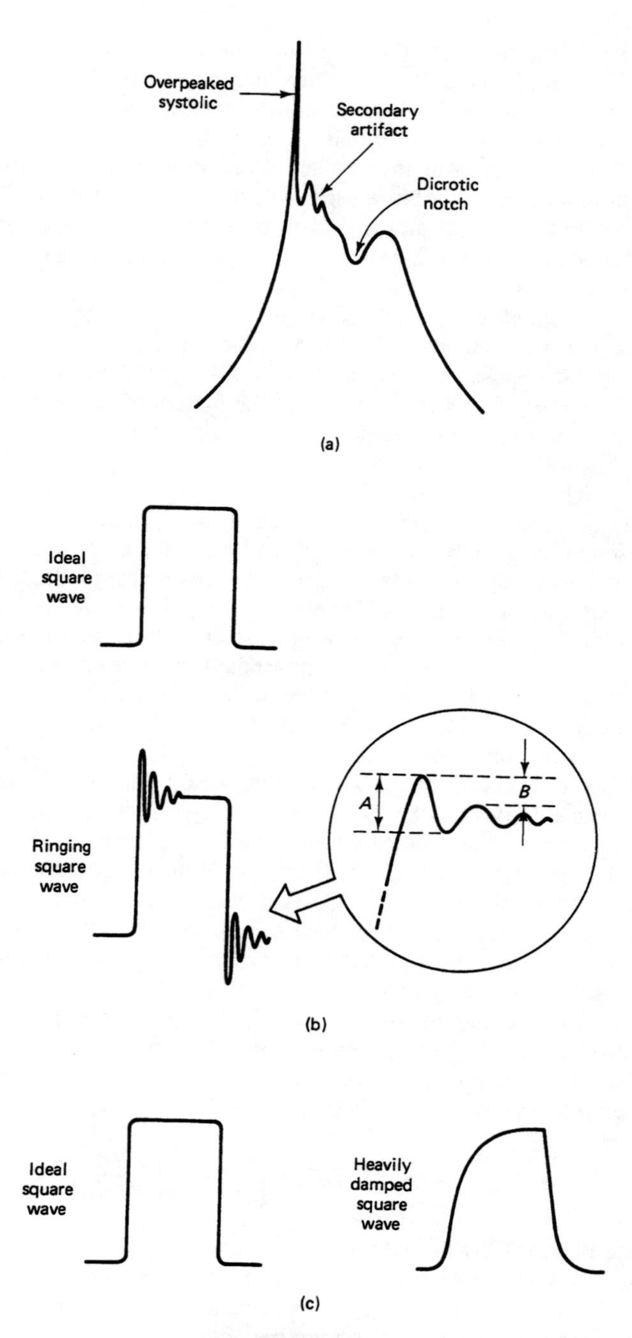

Overpeaked systolic
Secondary artifact
Dicrotic notch
(a)
Ideal square wave
Ringing square wave
A
B
(b)
Ideal square wave
Heavily damped square wave
(c)

FIGURE 7-8

Static Pressure Head

Another problem is transducer placement when the transducer is not physically part of the system being measured. When measuring the pressure at the bottom of a tank, for example, the transducer should be placed at the same height as the bottom of the tank. This line is called a *pressure datum reference line*. In the human blood pressure application, the nurse or monitoring technician should place the transducer at the level of the patient's heart—or not complain to the biomedical equipment technician that the readings are "wrong." The problem is hydrostatic pressure head differences—which are nullified by proper transducer placement.

Another example of hydrostatic pressure head problems is shown in Figure 7-9. The fluid in the tubing has weight, and so will add a pressure of its own due to

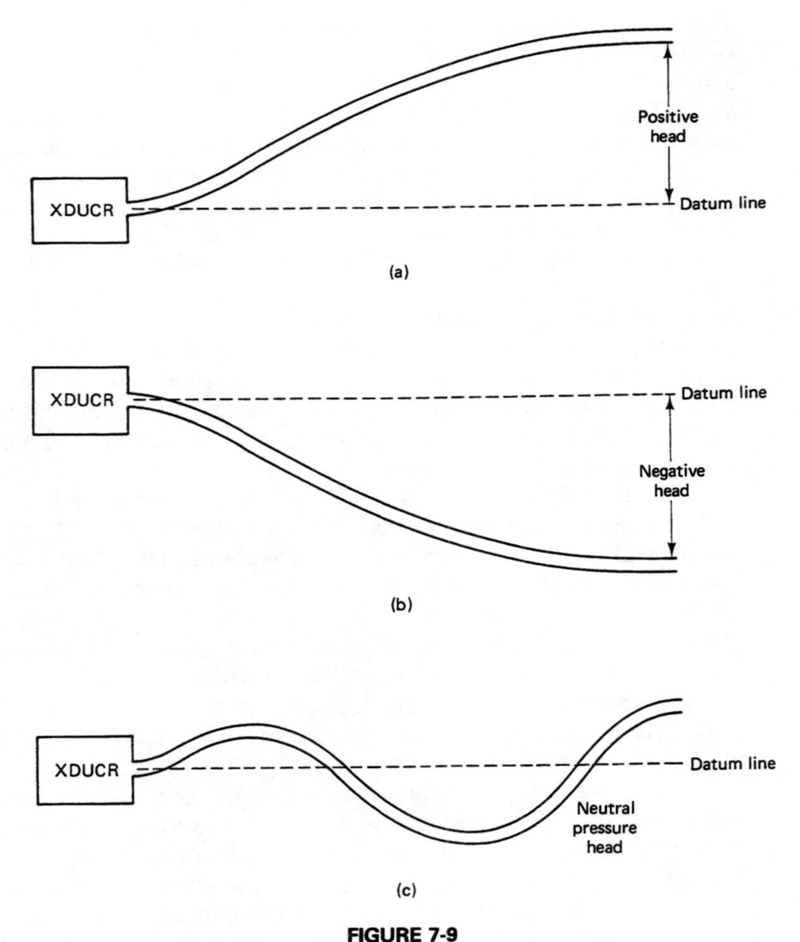

FIGURE 7-9

the force of gravity. Figure 7-9A shows a positive pressure head, in which the tubing approaches the transducer from above. Similarly, a negative pressure head (Figure 7-9B) is produced when the plumbing approaches from below. Figure 7-9C shows the proper scheme (where it can be accomplished) in which the tubing is routed equally above and below the datum reference line, so the positive and negative head cancel out each other.

In the event that you cannot place the transducer in a manner that permits a system such as Figure 7-9C, it is sometimes possible to live with the positive or negative offset or to make electronic corrections in the amplifier or processor circuits.

PRESSURE MEASUREMENT CIRCUITS

There are several basic forms of pressure amplifier circuits. Some of them are so simple that it is easy to build them from operational amplifiers or other linear integrated circuit devices. Common types include DC, isolated DC, pulsed excitation, and AC carrier amplifiers. The DC amplifiers work only with resistance strain gauge transducers or those newer forms of inductive transducer that outputs a rectified DC signal; AC carrier amplifiers work with both resistive strain gauges and inductive transformers (inductive Wheatstone bridges and LVDTs). The pulsed excitation works with resistive strain gauges, but only works with some of the inductive transducers (which depends upon the inductance, duration of the pulse, and other factors).

Regardless of the design, however, there are certain features common to all forms of pressure amplifier. Some devices are narrowly limited in range for special purposes, while others are capable of a wider range for more general applications. In cases where moderate accuracy is needed, we can rely on internal calibration methods, but where superior accuracy is a requirement, the user should calibrate the system against a mercury manometer.

When designing pressure amplifier/display systems, manufacturers provide both zero control and gain control. There are no perfect transducers on the market, and all will exhibit an offset and a gain problem. The offset is caused by errors in the strain gauges, errors in the other circuitry, and distension of the diaphragm. The gain error is caused by variations in the sensitivity of the transducer. Although some transducers contain internal circuitry (sometimes in the connector), all will exhibit to some extent both offset and gain problems. For example, I once received 12 Statham transducers (a good brand), nominally rated at a sensitivity of 5 μV/V/torr, that came with factory calibration certificates showing the real sensitivity figures were 37 to 65 μV/V/torr.

There are three approaches to standardizing the transducer for medical applications. One is to specify tightly the offset and sensitivity to the suppliers and force them to hand select or high-grade their product. Another is to provide an internal balance and sensitivity adjustment. Figure 7-10 shows a transducer with both zero offset and sensitivity trimmer potentiometers installed. The final method is to provide a "calibration factor" for the transducer (which is printed on a label on the body of the transducer) that is used to adjust the external amplifier circuitry.

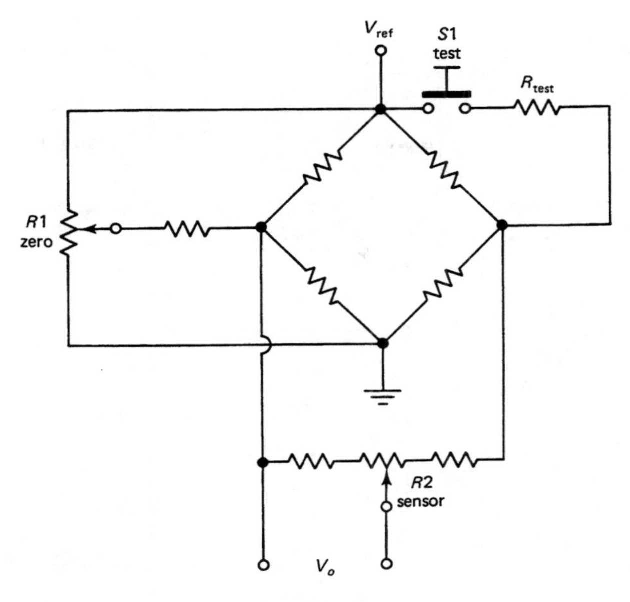

FIGURE 7-10

The calibration resistor, R_{cal}, is used to provide a standardized offset to the transducer bridge in order to mimic a specified pressure level. If the resistor is carefully chosen, then pressing the CAL button will cause the output voltage to shift an amount equal to the shift if a standard pressure is used (usually 100 mmHg for arterial transducers and 10 mmHg for venous models).

Figure 7-11 shows the simplified circuit of a DC pressure amplifier that uses the calibration factor method. The pressure amplifier (A1) is a DC amplifier, so the pressure transducer is a resistive Wheatstone bridge strain gauge. Diode D1 provides the 7.5-volt DC excitation to the transducer, and the potentials for the balance and cal factor controls. The calibration factor for the transducer will sometimes change, so it is necessary to provide a procedure for measuring the new factor:

1. The DC pressure amplifier is first calibrated with an accurate mercury manometer.
2. Set switch S1 to the operate position, open the transducer stopcock to atmosphere, and adjust R3 for zero volts output (that is, 0 torr reading on the display).
3. Close the transducer stopcock and then pump a standard pressure (for example, 100 torr, or at least half-scale). Adjust gain control R6 until the meter reads the correct (standard) pressure. Check for agreement between the meter and the manometer at several standard pressures throughout the range (for example, 50, 100, 150, 200, 250, and 300 torr). This last step is needed to ensure the transducer is reasonably linear—that is, the diaphragm was not strained by out of range pressures or vacuums.

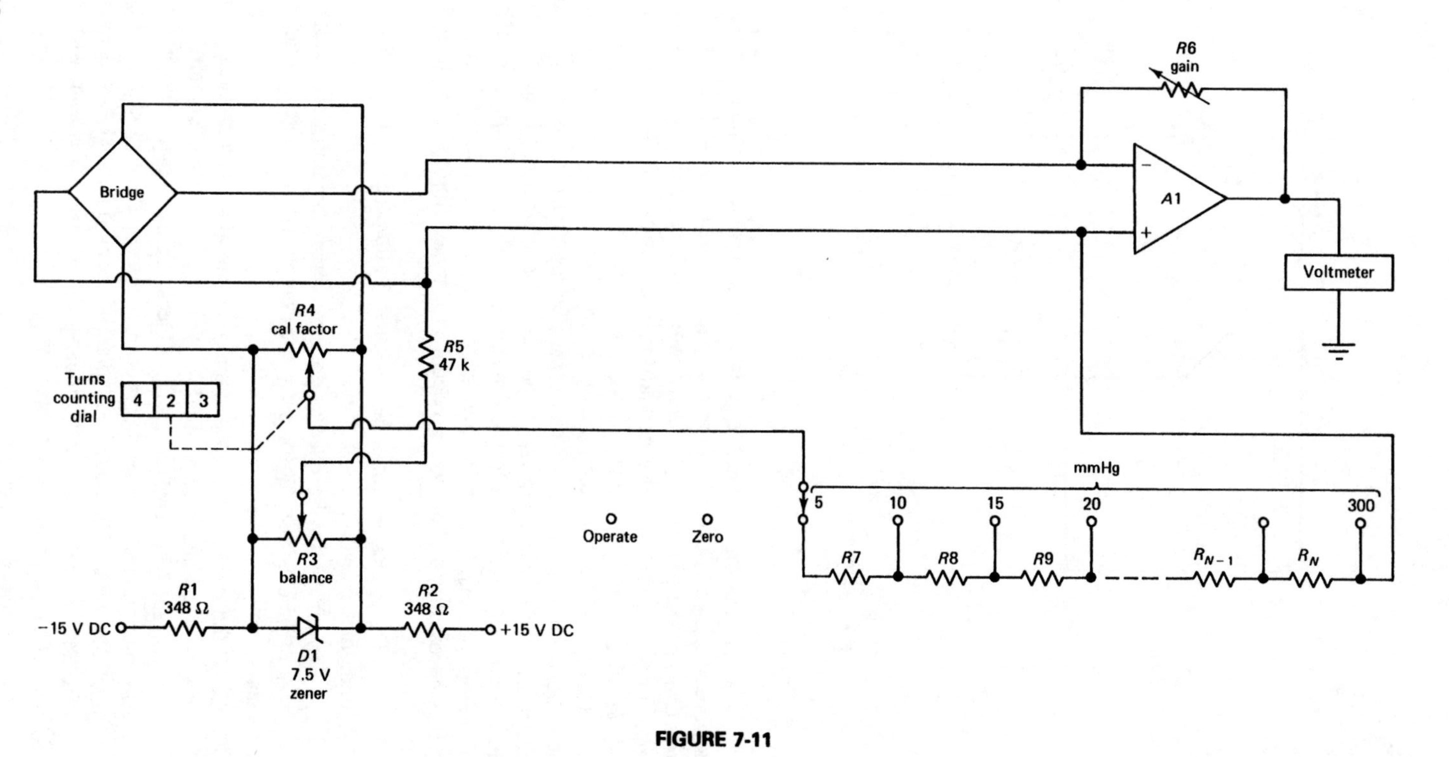
R6
gain
A1
Voltmeter
Bridge
R4
cal factor
R5
47 k
Turns
counting
dial
4
2
3
mmHg
5
10
15
20
300
Operate
Zero
R7
R8
R9
R_{N-1}
R_N
R3
balance
R1
348 Ω
R2
348 Ω
−15 V DC
+15 V DC
D1
7.5 V
zener

FIGURE 7-11

4. Turn switch S1 to the position corresponding to the applied standard pressure, and then adjust cal factor control (R4) until the same standard pressure is obtained on the meter. The cal factor control is gauged to a turns counting dial. The number appearing on the dial at the position of R4 that creates the same standard pressure signal is the calibration factor for that transducer. Record the turns counter reading for future reference.

For a period of time (usually six months), the calibration factor will need not be redetermined unless damage to the transducer occurs. The calibration factor is entered into the amplifier by turning R4 (or digitally in modern instruments). The following procedure is normally used:

1. Open the transducer stopcock to atmosphere, place switch S1 in the 0-torr (0 mmHg) position and adjust R3 for a zero volts output indication (0 torr on the display).
2. Set switch S1 to a position that is most convenient for the range of pressures to be measured. In general, select a scale that places the reading midscale or higher.
3. Set the cal factor knob to the figure recorded previously.
4. Adjust the gain control (R6) until the meter reads the standard pressure used in the original calibration.

The circuit in Figure 7-11 is an example of a DC pressure amplifier, while Figure 7-12 is a more detailed version of the actual amplifier block. Note that there are only two operational amplifiers in this circuit—there is little complex about the simple DC amplifier. Amplifier A1 is the input amplifier, and it should be a low-drift, premium model. Both gain and zero controls are provided, so the amplifier will work with a wide variety of transducers.

The excitation voltage of the transducer is determined (as a maximum) by the transducer manufacturer, with a value of 10 volts being common. In general, it is best to operate the transducer at a voltage lower than the maximum in order to prevent drift due to self-heating. Pressure amplifier manufacturers typically specify either 5 volts or 7.5 volts for a 10-volt (max) transducer.

The required amplifier gain can be calculated from the required output voltage that is used to represent any given pressure. Because digital voltmeters are used extensively for readout displays, the common practice is to use an output voltage scale factor that is numerically the same as the full-scale pressure. For example, 1 millivolt or 10 millivolts per millimeter of mercury is common. Let's assume a maximum pressure range of 400 mmHg (common on arterial monitors), if we use a scale factor of 1 mV/mmHg, when 400 mmHg is represented by 400 mV, or 0.40 volt. No further scaling of the meter output is needed.

The sensitivity and the excitation potential give us the transducer output voltage at full scale. For example, let's assume that a 400-mmHg pressure amplifier, scaled at 1 mV/mmHg is desired. What is the output voltage of the transducer if a +5-V DC excitation is applied, and the sensitivity is 50-μV/V/mmHg?

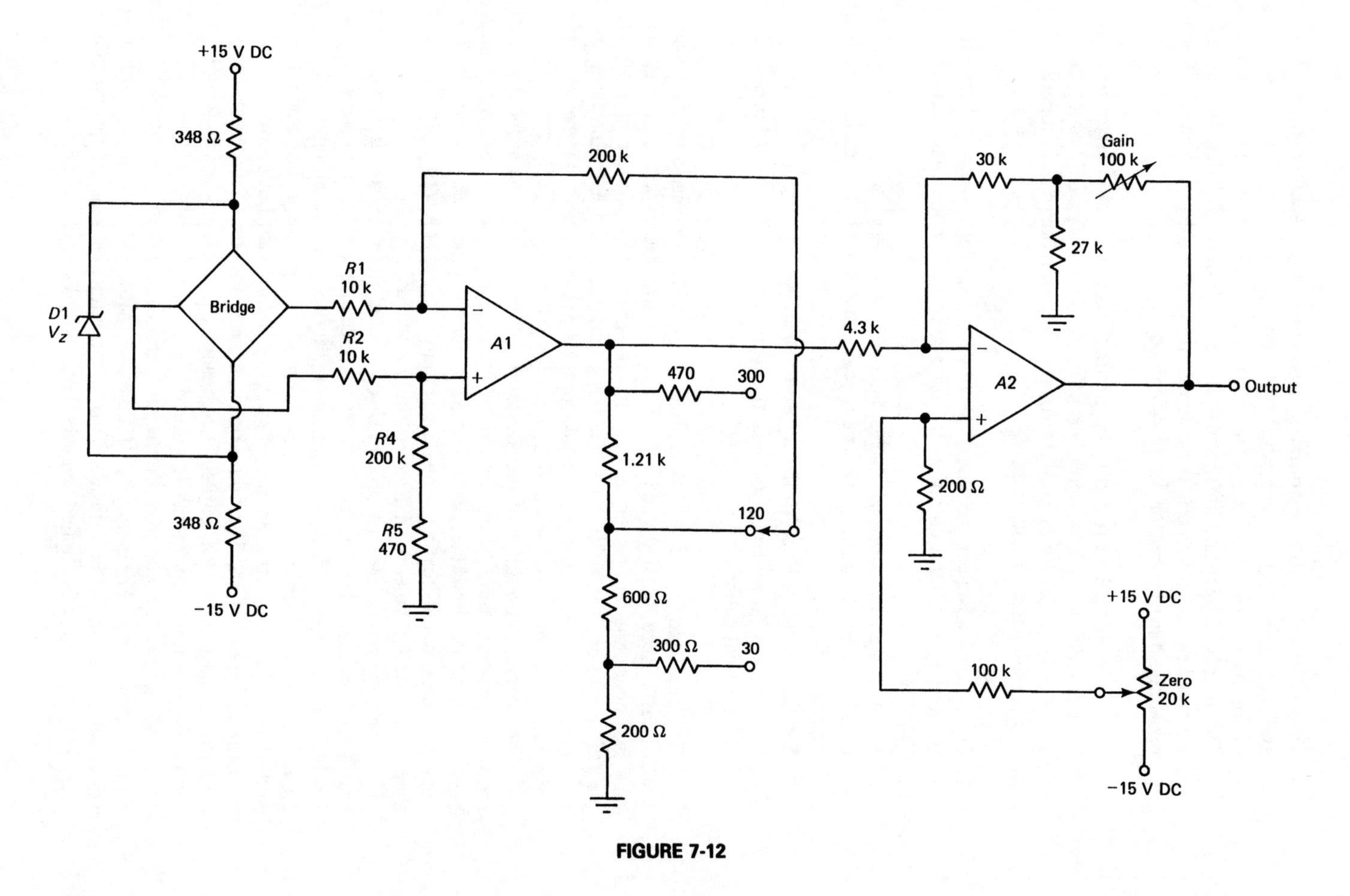
+15 V DC
348 Ω
D1
V_z
Bridge
348 Ω
−15 V DC
R1
10 k
R2
10 k
R4
200 k
R5
470
200 k
A1
470
300
1.21 k
120
600 Ω
300 Ω
30
200 Ω
4.3 k
30 k
Gain
100 k
27 k
A2
Output
200 Ω
+15 V DC
100 k
Zero
20 k
−15 V DC

FIGURE 7-12

$$V_t = \frac{50\ \mu V}{V\ mmHg} \times (5\ volts) \times (400\ mmHg)$$
$$= (50\ \mu V)(5)(400)$$
$$= 100{,}000\ \mu V$$
$$= 100\ mV$$

The output of the transducer at full scale will be 100 millivolts. This potential is the amplifier input voltage, so the gain can be calculated as:

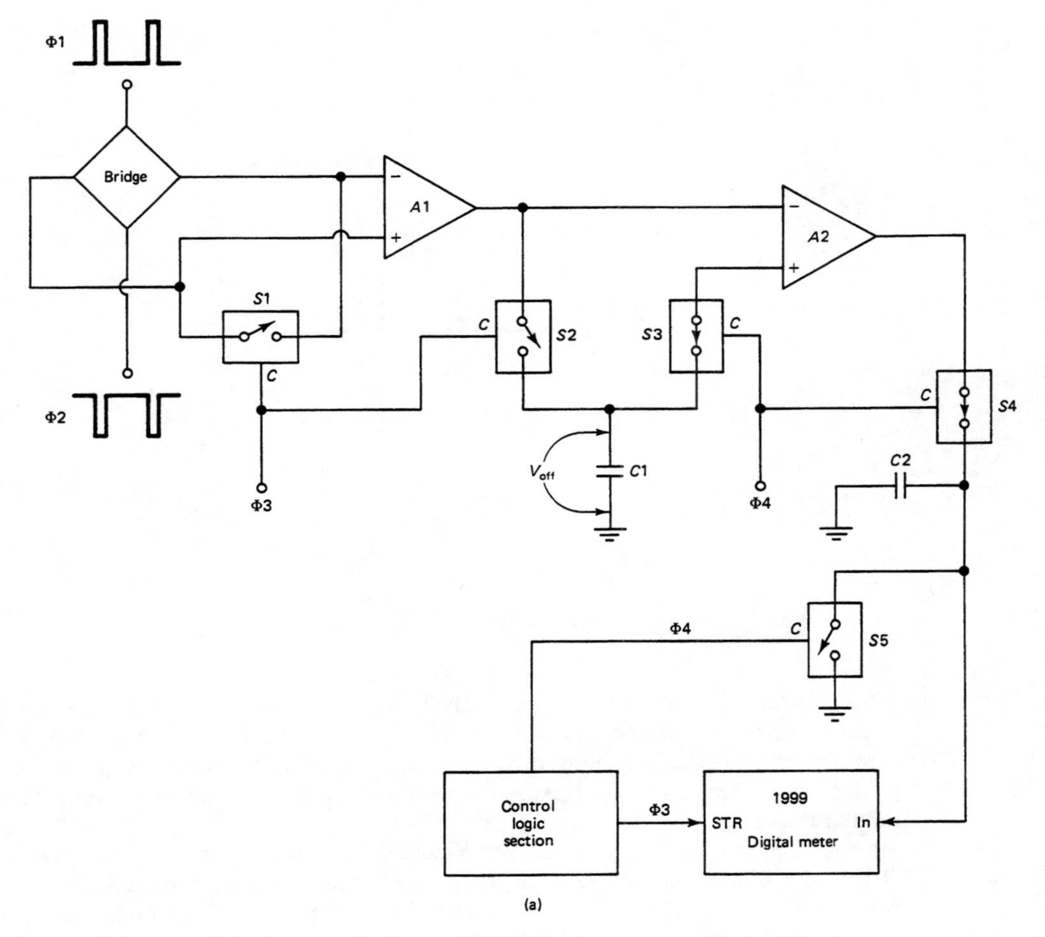

FIGURE 7-13

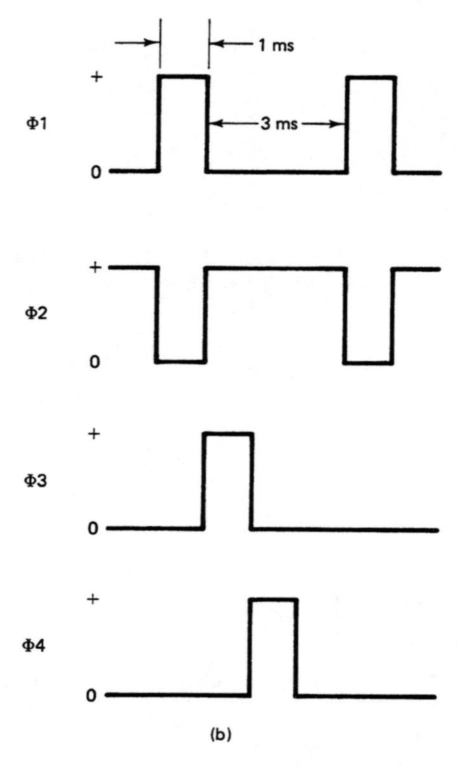

FIGURE 7-13 (continued)

$$A_v = \frac{V_o}{V_{in}}$$

$$= \frac{400 \text{ mV}}{100 \text{ mV}}$$

$$= 4$$

A variation on the DC amplifier scheme is the isolated DC amplifier. In these circuits, the input amplifier is a special isolation amplifier. These devices provide a very high impedance (10^{12} ohms or more) between the input and the DC power supply terminals. This electrical isolation is required in medical applications for patient safety reasons.

An example of a pulsed excitation amplifier is shown in Figure 7-13A. Instead of DC, the Wheatstone bridge strain gauge is excited with a short-duration biphasic pulse. This method allows the transducer to be excited to a voltage high enough to make a measurement possible, without a constant flow of current to aggravate the self-heating problem inherent in DC transducers. The pulse typically has a 1-mS duration and a 25 percent duty cycle (which translates to a 4-ms period, or a frequency

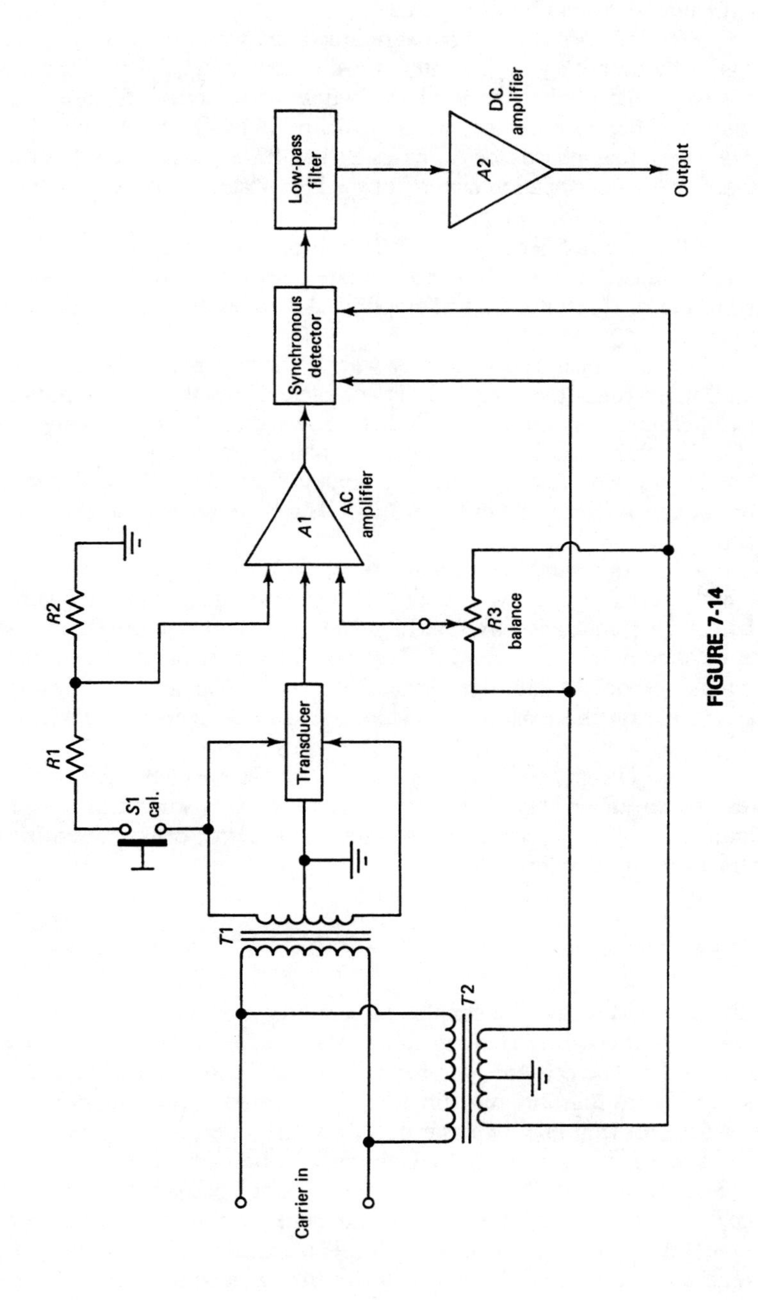
Low-pass filter
DC amplifier
A2
Output
Synchronous detector
A1
AC amplifier
R1
R2
S1 cal.
Transducer
R3 balance
T1
T2
Carrier in

FIGURE 7-14

of 250 Hz). An advantage of the short duty cycle is that operations like amplifier drift cancelation can be incorporated.

Amplifier A1 is a DC pressure amplifier, while A2 is a unity gain summation stage. The output signal indicator is a digital voltmeter that will update the display only when the strobe line is high. Switches S1 through S3 are CMOS electronic switches which close when the control line (C) is high. All circuit action is controlled by a four-phase clock. Phases P1 and P2 excite the transducer and operate the amplifier drift cancelation circuit. Phase P3 updates the display meter, and phase P4 resets the circuit following the update.

All DC amplifiers tend to drift (although modern premium IC op-amps have sharply reduced drift); that is, they create output voltage offset voltages due to thermal changes. Capacitor C1 and amplifier A2 serves as a drift cancellation circuit (see Figure 7-13A).

The transducer is excited only when P1 is high positive and P2 is high negative. At all other times the transducer is not excited, which keeps transducer self-heating to a minimum. Amplifier A1 will drift, however, because of its high gain and inherent offset voltages. The idea in this circuit is to charge capacitor C1 during the nonexcited period (during which A1 input is shorted by S1), and then add the capacitor voltage algebraically to the signal—thereby removing the amplifier drift component.

AC carrier amplifiers (Figure 7-14) use an AC signal for transducer excitation, so will operate equally well with resistive strain gauges and inductive transducers. The carrier frequencies are typically 200 to 5000 Hz, with 400 and 2400 Hz being the most common. The Hewlett-Packard 8800 series pressure carrier amplifiers, for example, produce a 2400-Hz, 5-volt RMS signal. Carrier amplifiers are probably the most stable on the market, a function of using narrow-bandwidth, heavy-feedback design.

Some cheap carrier amplifiers use simple envelope detectors to extract the pressure waveform, but all proper instruments use a variant of the circuit shown in Figure 7-14. This circuit uses a quadrature detector, or phase-sensitive detector, to extract the signal information.

PRESSURE PROCESSING

Only rarely do we need a simple pressure amplifier for dynamic measurements (the same is not true where static pressures are involved). We will want a system such as Figure 7-15. The pressure waveform, P, is the analog output of a pressure amplifier, and it is fed to four different circuits: a peak detector (maximum pressure), inverted peak detector (minimum pressure), a time integrator, and a differentiator (dP/dt).

The peak detectors and integrator can be calibrated by applying a constant value of pressure, P. But since the differentiator measures dP/dt, we need a varying signal. Typically, a square wave of the same amplitude as a standard value of the P-signal is applied, as in Figure 7-16. This signal produces an output from the differentiator (as shown) which is a linearly rising slope that can be measured.

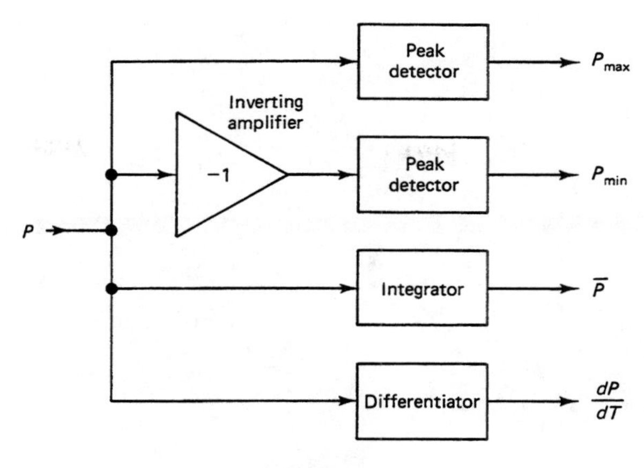

FIGURE 7-15

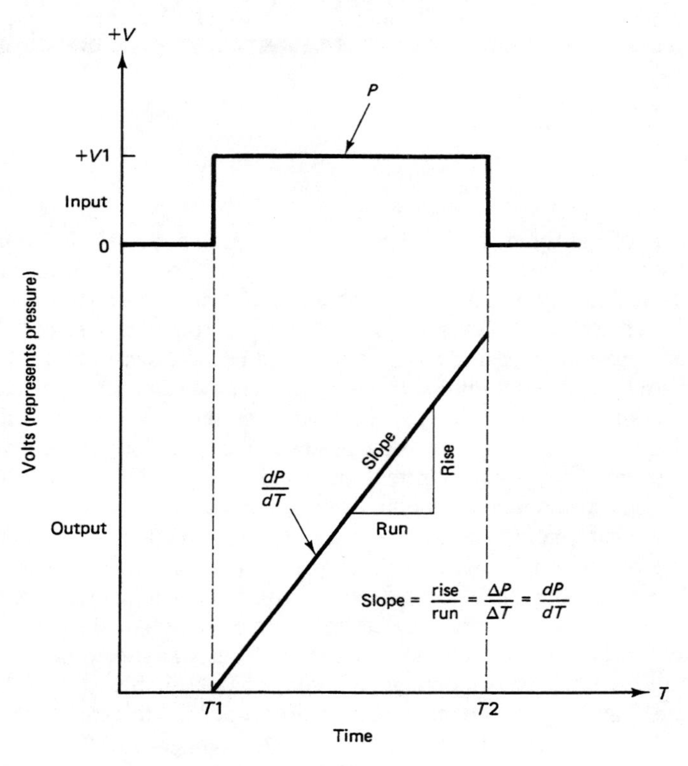

FIGURE 7-16

8

Patient Monitoring Systems

One of the things that makes modern intensive care medicine possible is the patient monitoring systems that are now available. Prior to the invention of these machines it was nearly impossible to obtain real-time information on very sick patients. "Intensive care" consisted of stationing a single private-duty nurse—without any information-gathering means other than her five senses and a blood pressure cuff—with the seriously injured trauma patient or heart patient. Private-duty intensive care nursing was the best they had at that time, but it was insufficient. The electronic patient monitoring system brought about the situation where critical patients can be clustered together in a special unit, and cared for by highly skilled specialty nurses. No one would demean the knowledge and skills of the intensive care nurse or physician, but the simple truth is that without monitoring electronics, they would be highly limited in what they could do for their patients. And what they could do (which is nonetheless considerable) would require many more members of the team than are presently needed. The information flow would simply be too limited in systems where there were no electronics. Thus, the electronic patient monitoring system both broadens the range of information available to the medical person in "real time" and reduces the numbers of people needed to care for the patient.

There are two major aspects to the standard intensive care patient monitoring system: *bedside monitors* and *central station monitors*. In some cases, the central station system is merely the slave of the bedside system and acts like a mere repeater of the same data. In other cases, the central station takes on a larger role and actually performs active determinations of patient condition. The latter form is possible because of the invention of the microprocessor chip. The so-called "personal" computer, now familiar to all, is the basis for many central monitoring systems currently in use. Because of this fact, the reader is also referred to Chapter 20. Bedside monitors also contain microprocessors, so are able to act like a computer terminal unit that has a highly specialized medical analog subsystem to provide input data.

BEDSIDE MONITORS

The bedside monitor is an electronic instrument that collects physiological data from the patient and then either displays it locally (that is, in the room) or transmits it to the central station. Most modern bedside monitors perform both functions. That is, they acquire and locally display the signal information about various physiological parameters and also transmit it to the central station. The transmission system may be either analog or digital in nature.

Figure 8-1 shows an older-style portable bedside monitor that can be used on an ad hoc basis, that is, wherever needed. These type monitors were very popular in the early days of intensive care medicine when central station systems were not widespread. They are still very popular for transporting patients and for providing

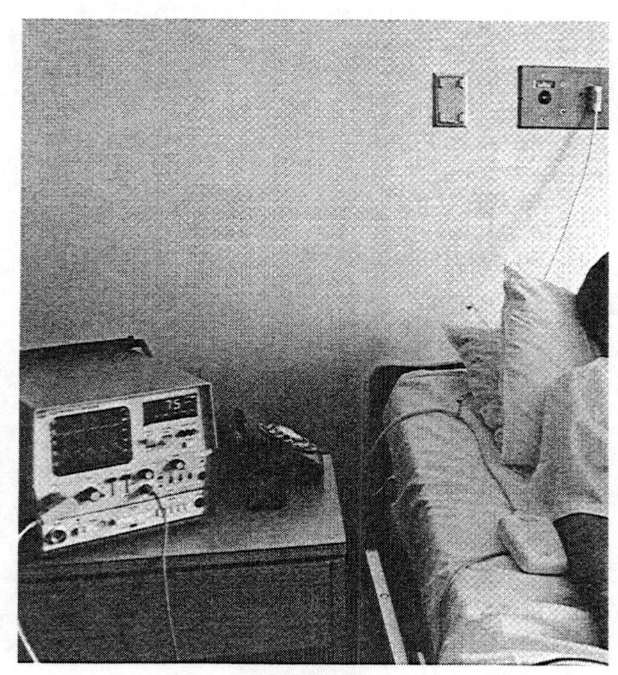

FIGURE 8-1

closer monitoring of patients who, for one reason or another, are not in the intensive care unit. Emergency departments often use portable bedside monitors when the crush of business gets too large for the regular system.

In the mid- and late 1970s patient monitoring systems became a lot more popular as the number of hospitals with formal intensive care units increased dramatically. Figure 8-2 shows a typical late 1970s modular patient monitoring system manufactured by General Electric. The analog display is a nonfade oscilloscope (see Chapter 3) that can accommodate up to four channels. The pressure monitoring unit to the right of the 'scope is set up with four different pressure modules: *systolic, diastolic, mean arterial pressure,* and *venous*. The next module over houses electrocardiograph amplifiers and a heart rate meter display. Finally, there is a control and alarm module.

The patient monitor units depicted in Figure 8-2 represented a trend away from rigidly defined "black box" models that offered only what the manufacturer thought was needed. While that type of design is still common among portable monitors, it has long since departed from the formal bedside monitor scene. The modular design still survives because it allows the manufacturer, the hospital, and indeed the individual nursing and physician staffs to custom configure a monitor for a patient's needs. For example, it may be policy to provide continuous arterial pressure and ECG monitoring for all patients. All of the bedside monitors in that unit would be equipped with these modules. Other measurements, such as venous pressure or continuous rectal temperature or EEG, on the other hand, would typically be ordered for fewer patients. The physician could order these facilities, and they could then be provided by a monitoring technician or biomedical equipment technician. The hospital would thus be spared the cost of completely equipping each bed with all functions, while still providing the functions whenever needed.

Two examples of modern bedside monitors are shown in Figure 8-3; Figure 8-3A is a Hewlett-Packard system, while Figure 8-3B is a Spacelab system. Both are equipped with four-channel oscilloscopes that can measure a variety of physiological parameters. Both units are also representative of the wall-mounted style of monitor

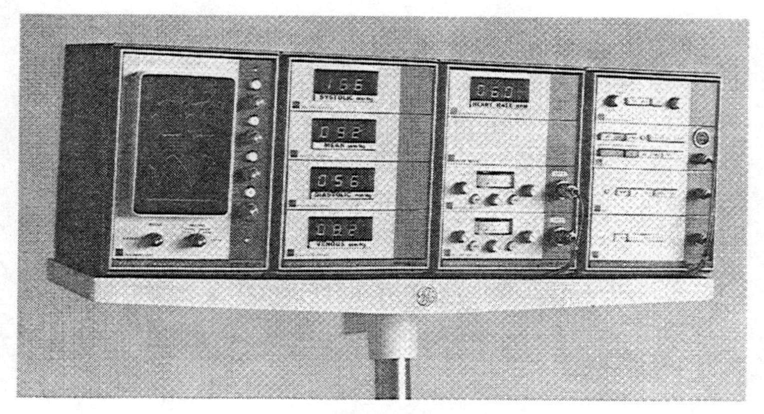

FIGURE 8-2

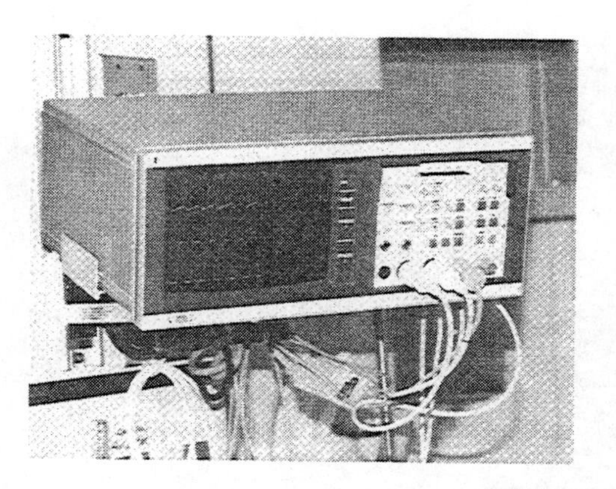

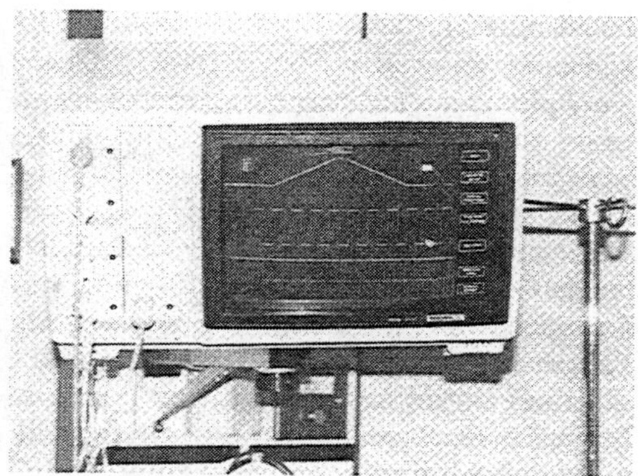

FIGURE 8-3

that became popular in the 1970s and continues to be popular today (even though models have changed and improved over the years).

The traces on both monitors shown in Figure 8-3 reveal a built-in self-test mode. Modern microprocessor electronic monitors can conduct self-tests and display the results. Thus, the unit will self-test whenever it is first turned on, and also whenever a self-test is initiated by the medical, nursing or biomedical equipment staffs. With proper design, self-test results can be reported over the data lines to the central computer and be used there for record-keeping purposes. Some self-test capability is able to locate the problems in the system at the printed circuit board level, and therefore tell the repair technician which subassembly to replace.

The concept of replaceable modules is shown more clearly in Figure 8-4. In this case (Figure 8-4A), the mainframe contains a plug-in oscilloscope module along

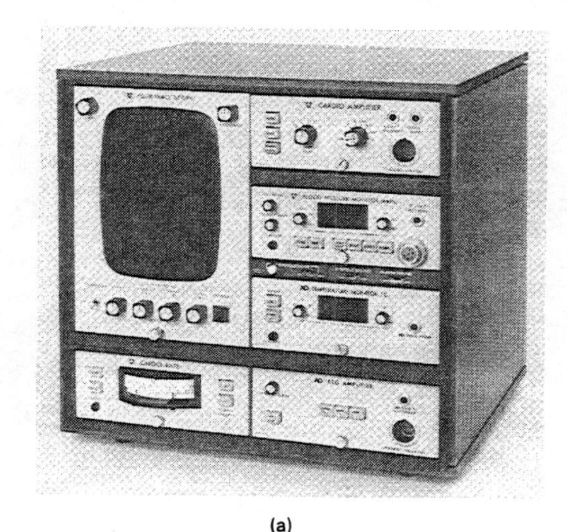

(a)

FIGURE 8-4

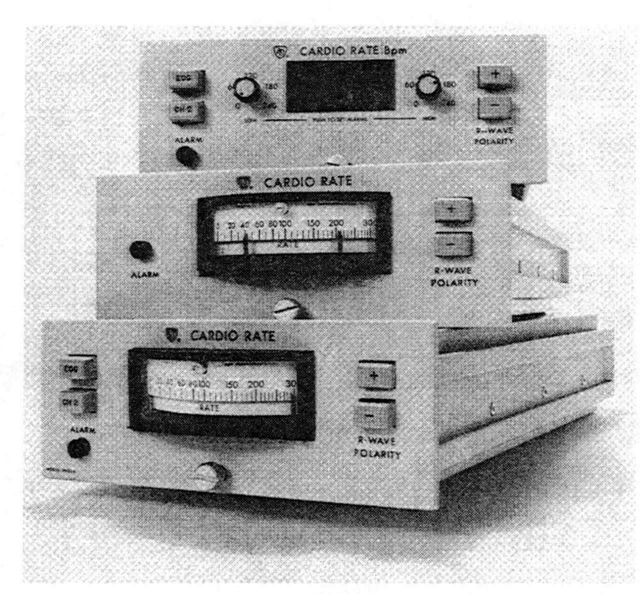

(b)

FIGURE 8-4 (continued)

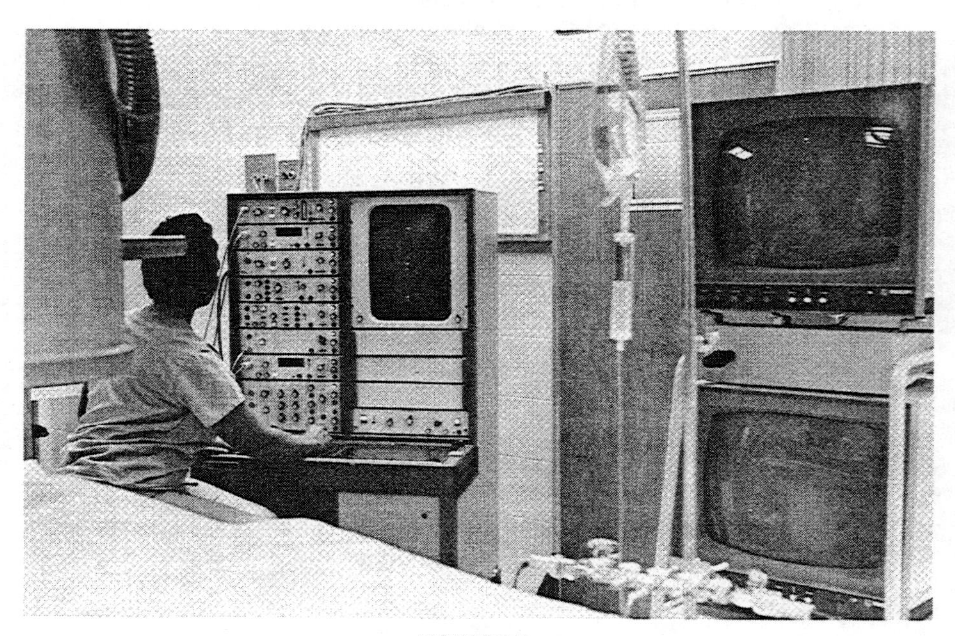

FIGURE 8-5

with five separate functional modules (in this particular configuration a cardiorate meter, ECG amplifier, EEG amplifier, blood pressure monitor, and temperature monitor are provided). Examples of the plug-in modules are shown in Figure 8-4B. A connector on the real panel of these units will interface with a mating connector in the mainframe. To install the module, it is only necessary to slide the unit into the mainframe, make sure that it is properly seated in the connector (as indicated by fitting flush with the front panel of the mainframe), and then tighten the fastener.

Bedside monitors are not limited to intensive care units. They are also found in operating rooms, postanesthesia care units, emergency rooms, and in special procedures rooms such as the catheterization laboratory. Figure 8-5 shows a typical unit from a cath lab. This type of unit is usually more extensive than the simple ICU bedside monitor because the physicians must be aware of additional parameters simultaneously.

The unit shown in Figure 8-5 is also equipped with a hard-copy printer to output the waveforms. Because some of the waveforms contain high-frequency components that would be distorted by the usual mechanical recorder, it uses a photographic process to produce renditions of the oscilloscope display on paper. Other, more modern, units digitize the analog waveform, store the data in a computer, and then output the results on a printer that uses the same dot matrix or laser technology as certain office printers. The mechanical problems that limit the frequency response of traditional printers are thus overcome.

CENTRAL STATIONS

The central station serves several functions in the intensive care environment. One thing that is immediately apparent is that it amplifies the abilities of the staff to keep track of the situation, and so reduces the number of nurses and doctors needed to staff a unit. All of the analog signals, plus numerical data and the alarm status signals, are routed from each bedside monitor to the central nurses' station unit (Figure 8-6). The console will provide an array of multichannel oscilloscopes, heart rate meters (plus occasionally blood pressure meters), a computer terminal, an alarm status annunciator panel, and a communications system. With this information a single operator can keep track of the condition of several patients at once, obviating the need to station a nurse in each patient room all of the time.

Figure 8-7 shows the block diagram of a typical central monitoring system. Electrodes and transducers (sensors) attached to the patient provide signals through an array of input amplifiers to the local bedside monitor. These signals are locally displayed on a monitor oscilloscope, various numerical (digital) readouts, and sometimes a local strip-chart (paper) recorder. Local alarms are also provided to alert the staff if any parameter (for example, heart rate) goes outside of set limits.

There will be a transmission path between the bedside monitors and the central station. The transmission path might be analog or digital, or a mixture of both. We will discuss these options.

The signals from the bedside units are routed to the central nurses' station con-

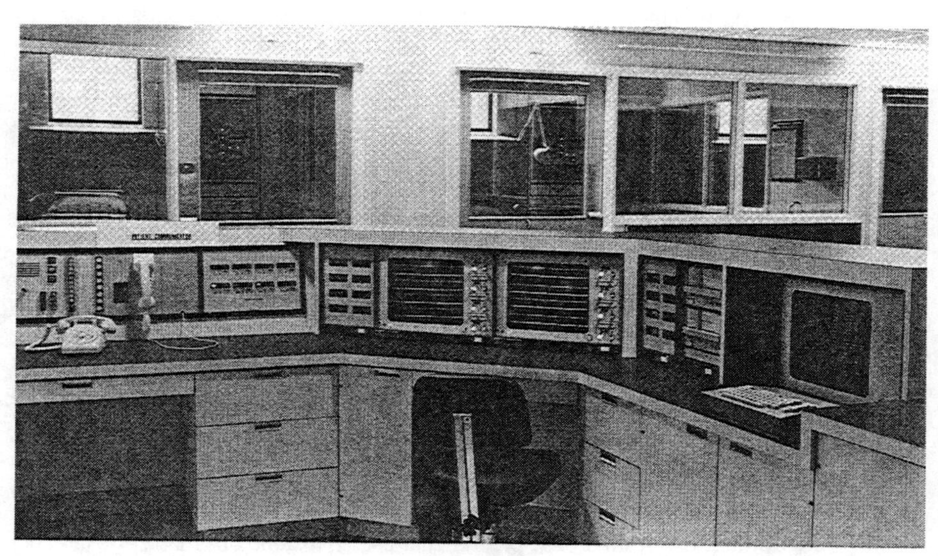

FIGURE 8-6

sole where they are displayed on slave units of the bedside monitors. Shown in this particular system are the following units: oscilloscope (usually multichannel), digital readouts for numerical data, alarms, and a strip-chart recorder. In many modern designs the numerical data and analog data are all displayed simultaneously on the screen of a video terminal.

Although older central station units (some of which are still in use) were simple analog instruments that were slaved to the bedside monitors, modern design uses a microcomputer to keep track of things and record data. The typical system will contain a computer (often an IBM-XT or AT-class machine), a manual data entry keyboard, a video/CRT display, and an interface device (not always used). The *architecture* of the central monitoring system determines how the various units relate to one another, and how the system is interconnected. Figure 8-7 shows one example of system architecture.

Older systems were strictly analog, so they used the type of system shown in Figure 8-8. The bedside monitor is equipped with an output interface that consists of a large multiconductor cable that carries two types of signals: analog waveforms and alarm/control *discretes*. A "discrete" is a single wire or wire pair that is either open circuited or closed circuited when a certain condition exists. The ECG alarm discrete, for example, is "open" when there is no alarm present and is shorted to ground when the alarm occurs. These conditions signal the central station circuits as to the alarm condition. This type of architecture required a large number of wires to implement. A 24-bed ICU system, for example, has as many as 20 discrete and analog signal lines per bed, for a total of 480 analog lines.

Note in Figure 8-8 that the output of the ECG amplifier (labeled "analog ECG signal") is not fed directly to the multiconductor cable, but rather is directed to a

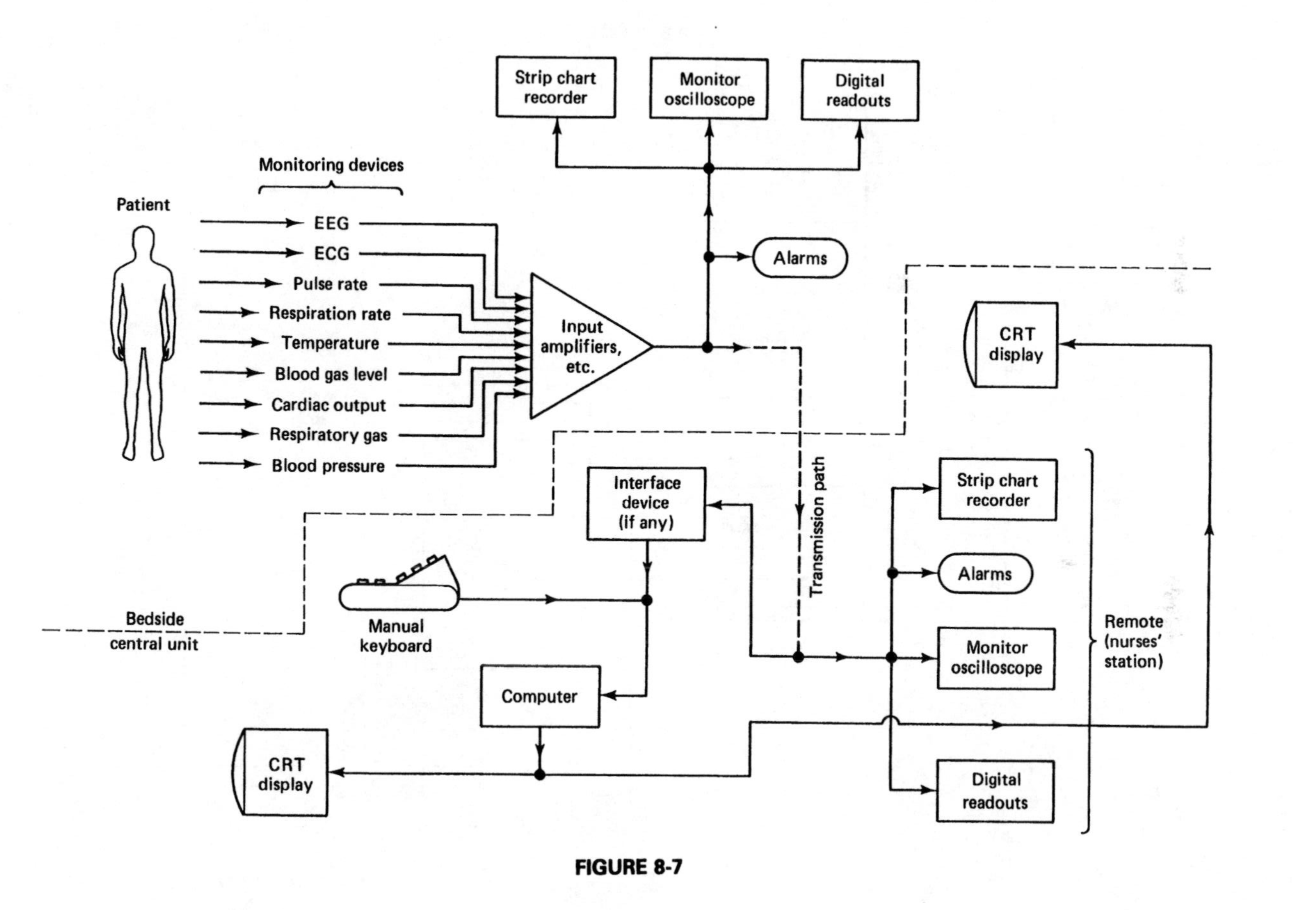
Monitoring devices
Patient
EEG
ECG
Pulse rate
Respiration rate
Temperature
Blood gas level
Cardiac output
Respiratory gas
Blood pressure
Input amplifiers, etc.
Strip chart recorder
Monitor oscilloscope
Digital readouts
Alarms
CRT display
Transmission path
Interface device (if any)
Manual keyboard
Computer
Bedside
central unit
CRT display
Strip chart recorder
Alarms
Monitor oscilloscope
Digital readouts
Remote (nurses' station)

FIGURE 8-7

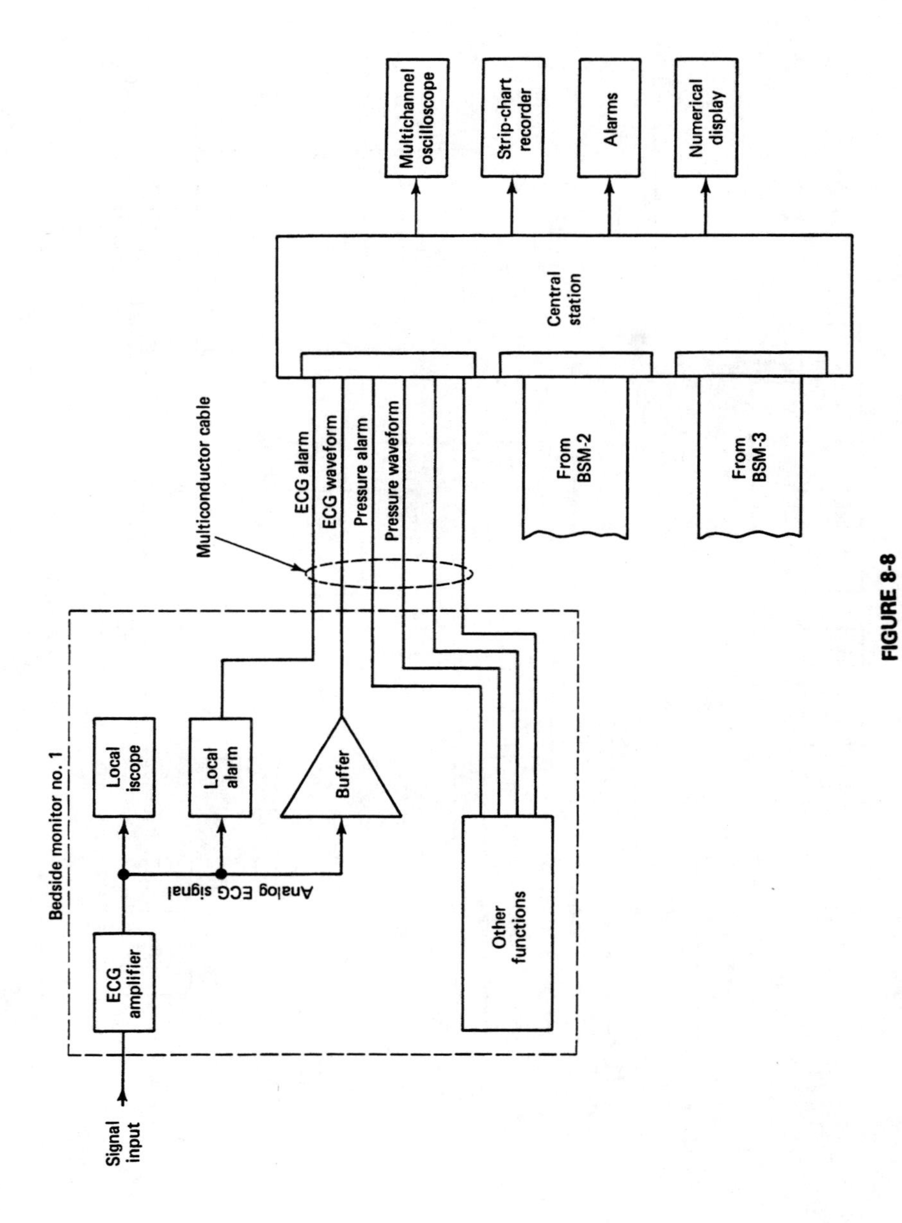

Multichannel oscilloscope
Strip-chart recorder
Alarms
Numerical display
Central station
Multiconductor cable
ECG alarm
ECG waveform
Pressure alarm
Pressure waveform
From BSM-2
From BSM-3
Bedside monitor no. 1
Local iscope
Local alarm
Buffer
Analog ECG signal
ECG amplifier
Other functions
Signal input

FIGURE 8-8

buffer amplifier ("BUFF"). This stage is used to isolate the bedside monitor from faults in either the multiconductor cable, the interconnections, or the central station itself. If, for example, a short circuit occurs in the transmission path, the output of the buffer will be shorted to ground. But, because of the buffer amplifier stage, the local oscilloscope and alarm system remains working—protecting the patient. If the external fault does not affect the alarm discrete, then even the central station alarm function will remain (even though the analog signal disappears).

Buffering in analog signals has its parallel in digital systems and represents a feature that should be required in specifying any new systems or modifications to existing systems. Some things to include in the purchase order and/or request for quotation are

1. No single-point fault will remove more than one single patient unit from service (that is, a fault on, say, bedside monitor number 2 only affects that unit and does not affect all other units).
2. No single-point fault, such as an output short, on a bedside monitor unit shall remove all functions of that unit either locally or at the nurses' station.
3. It shall be possible to disconnect any bedside monitor unit from the system without adversely affecting any other unit or function either in the local rooms or at the central station.

Most modern bedside monitor (BSM) units are digitized to allow their use with a computer. Early computerized monitoring systems were configured like any analog system, with the exception that digitization took place at the central nurses' station computer. In modern systems, however, the BSM itself may include a microprocessor to perform many of the chores once performed elsewhere (in addition to chores not offered before).

Figure 8-9 shows the block diagram for a simple digitized ECG monitor or BSM. The ECG amplifier, local alarm, and local oscilloscope are similar (often identical) to those of the strictly analog system. The difference is that no analog signals are passed to the central station. An *analog-to-digital converter* (A/D) is used to convert the analog voltage that represents the ECG signal into binary "words" that are transmitted to the central computer over a data bus. Because the voltage lev-

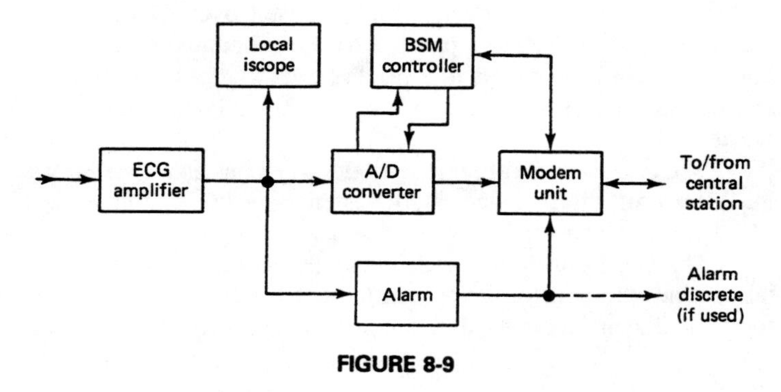

FIGURE 8-9

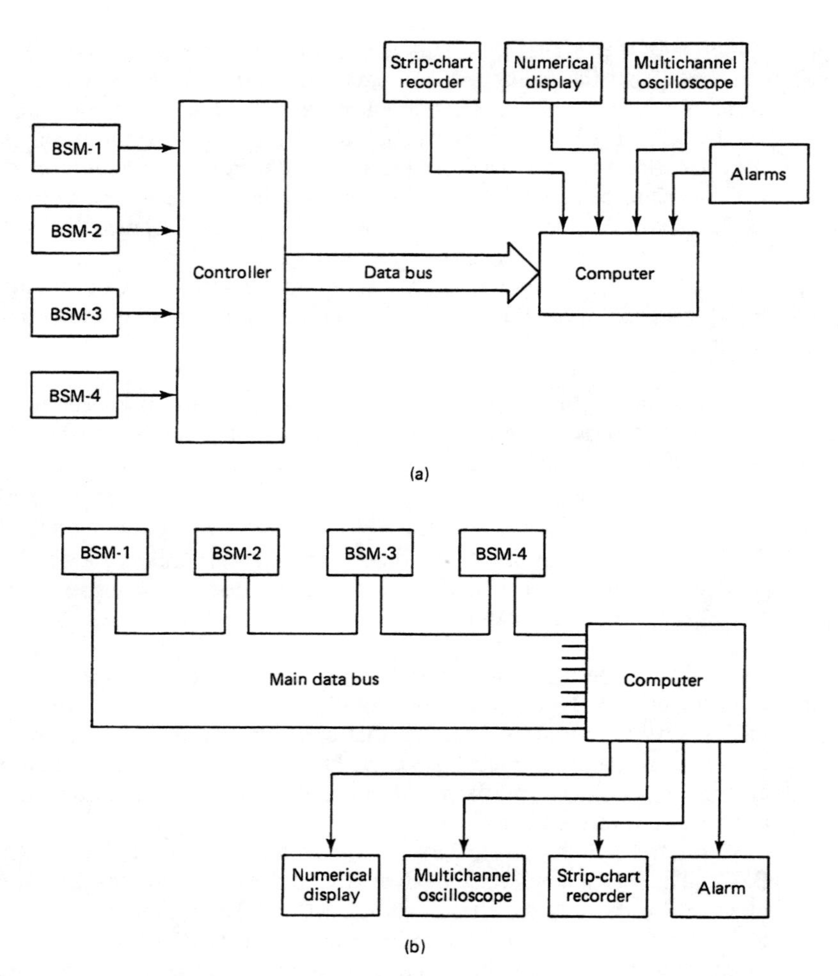

FIGURE 8-10

els of the binary word do not transmit well over distances greater than about 20 yards, or so, it is often the practice to use a modulator/demodulator (modem) unit to convert the binary signals to a series of audio tones. These tones are transmitted to the central station computer where another modem unit reconverts them to data words.

The alarms can either be sent along the bus as a tone by way of the modem, or via a separate discrete line. Both systems are known. In some cases, both modem and discrete alarms might be used as a safety feature.

The BSM controller module usually contains a microprocessor or simple digital computer to control the operation of the bedside monitor, run self-tests, and perform the alarm functions. It can communicate with the main computer unit in order to synchronize operations. In some systems "handshaking" between the central computer and BSMs indicates when data is ready or may be transmitted.

A function of the controller is to respond to the central computer when it is being polled for data. Each BSM is given a unique *address*. The BSM will not respond to traffic on the bus unless it "hears" either its own address or an "all units listen" broadcast address.

Although there are many variations on the following themes, and variations also exist in the specifics of implementation, the systems shown here represent a large number of data connection schemes between BSMs and central stations. In Figure 8-10A we see the system in which a local area controller receives the data lines from each BSM, prioritizes the signals, and then transmits the data to the central station computer. In some implementations this system is called a "star" connection.

A parallel connection is shown in Figure 8-10B. In this case, a common main data bus connects all the BSMs and the central station computer. In this case, the controller is located inside the computer. Be sure to avoid connections that are truly "daisy chained." These modules should be paralleled (and isolated to prevent a single failure from taking out the whole system). In a daisy chain system, data are passed from BSM-1 to BSM-2 to BSM-3 to BSM-4 and then to the computer. In that type of system, which is analogous to series strung Christmas tree lights, a single failure in BSM-4 blocks all data from the other three units. In other words, the entire ICU monitoring system goes down because of a single failure.

The actual data bus between the bedside units might be one of the following: twisted pair wires, multiconductor wires, coaxial cables (like TV antenna cables), or special wires.

9

X Rays and Radiation

X rays are a means of taking either photographs or video pictures of organs, bones, and foreign object that invade the inside of the body. Doctors use X rays to peer into the body without cutting. Although X rays are commonplace today, they were once viewed as somehow magical. X rays were first discovered on the evening of November 8, 1895, by physicist Wilhelm Roentgen. Using a modified Crooks' tube, Roentgen passed X rays through his wife's hand to a photographic plate. When the plate was developed, the plate showed her bones and wedding ring. Although Roentgen proposed the term "X ray" because they were of unknown origin, some of his contemporaries insisted on using the term "Roentgen rays" in honor of the discoverer. Both terms are used, but in the United States X ray is the accepted term.

THE NATURE OF X RAYS

X rays are a form of *electromagnetic radiation* similar to radio waves and light waves. To understand X rays, therefore, one should understand the terminology of waves, of which electromagnetic waves are but one form. Figure 9-1 shows a simple wave, which has a sinusoidal form. One complete *cycle* of the wave is measured between adjacent points where a feature is repeated, for example, the distance between peaks (as shown in Figure 9-1), between valleys, or between zero crossing points in the same direction.

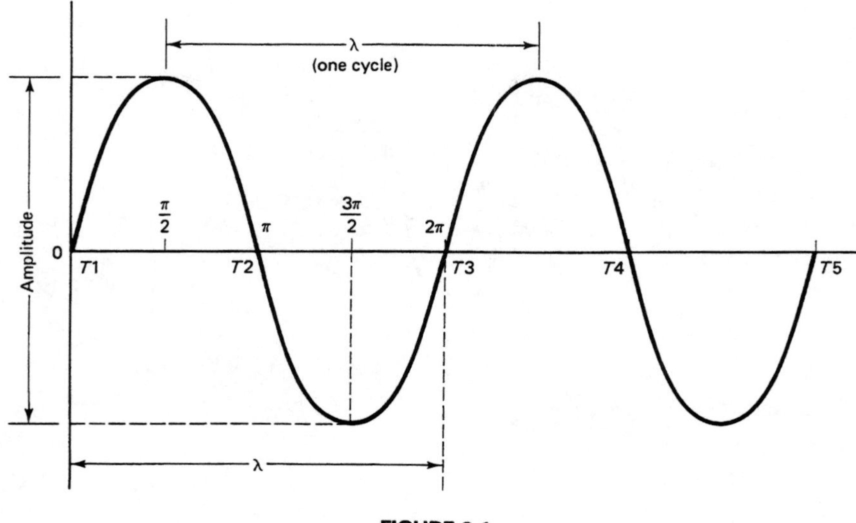

FIGURE 9-1

The wavelength of the wave is the distance that the wave travels in one cycle when it radiates out from the source. Wavelength is usually denoted by the lowercase Greek letter lambda (λ) and is measured in meters or the subunits of the meter (centimeters or millimeters).

The radiating wave does not consist of a single cycle, however, but rather a train of cycles proceeding one after another (two cycles are shown in Figure 9-1). The *frequency* of the wave is the number of cycles that occur in a unit of time (the second). The unit of frequency is *cycles per second,* also designated the hertz (Hz). Wavelength and frequency of an electromagnetic wave are related by the expression

$$c = \lambda f \tag{9-1}$$

where

c = the speed of propagation (3×10^{10} m/s)
λ = the wavelength in meters
f = the frequency in hertz (Hz)

The electromagnetic wave that propagates into space is actually a combination of two waves: an *electric field* and a *magnetic field*. These waves propagate along the same axis, but are at right angles to each other (i.e., they are said to be "orthogonal" to each other). Figure 9-2A represents a propagating electromagnetic wave. The arrows indicate the direction and magnitude of the electrical (E) and magnetic (B) field vectors at any given time in the wave's history. If the radiation emanates from a point source, and then radiates outward in a spherical field shape, we can look at the advancing wavefront at a very large distance from the source and will find that the electric and magnetic field vectors appear to be at right angles to each other in a flat (or nearly flat) plane.

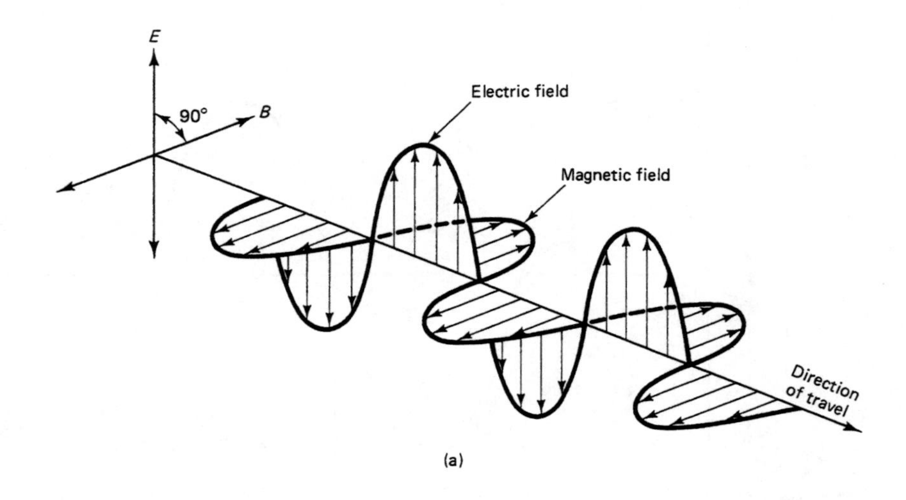

(a)

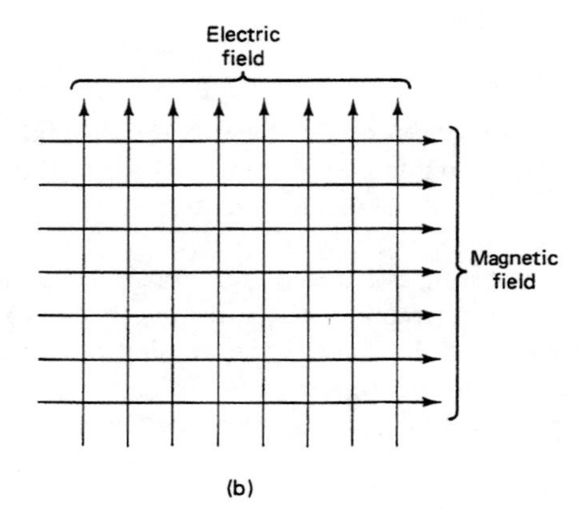

(b)

FIGURE 9-2

X rays are similar to light waves and radio in that they are electromagnetic waves with wavelengths shorter than either radio waves, visible light waves, or ultraviolet radiation. Figure 9-3 shows a spectrum chart that puts the various forms of electromagnetic radiation into perspective. Note that X rays have a higher frequency, and therefore shorter wavelength, than visible light, and that the X ray band overlaps the ultraviolet and gamma ray bands of the spectrum. The band of the diagnostic medical X rays is smaller than the range understood by physicists.

Like other forms of electromagnetic radiation, X rays can be viewed as both a particle and a wave. In other words, the X ray has a *complementary* nature. This theory was proposed by Neils Bohr, whose famous institute in Copenhagen more or less defined modern quantum mechanics and the field of nuclear physics. A deep truth about electromagnetic radiation was uncovered in 1900 by Max Planck. He was

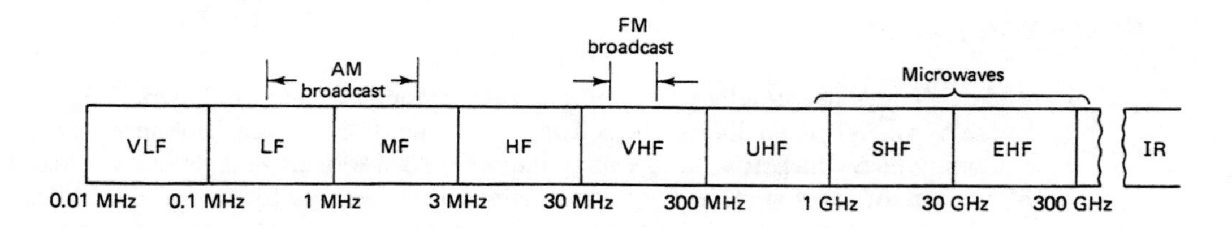

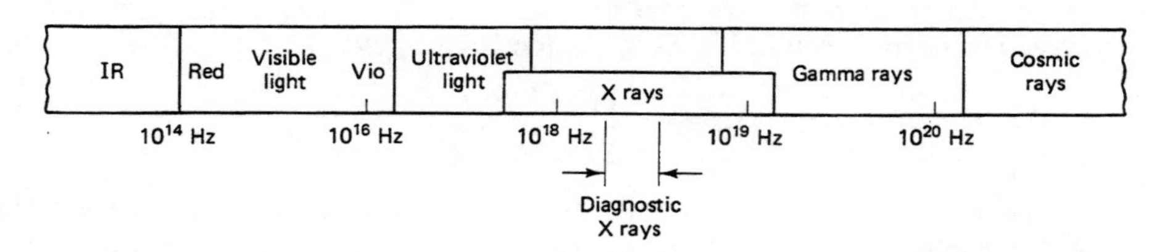

FIGURE 9-3

working on certain experimental anomalies in the thermal radiation of black bodies. The observed wavelengths did not meet the pattern that classical (Newtonian) physics had predicted. Planck proposed that electromagnetic radiation can only exist in discrete bundles, later dubbed *quanta*. Thus, the radiation can be either a wave or a photon with an energy that is proportional to the quanta by the relationship

$$E = h \times f \tag{9-2}$$

where

E = the energy level in joules
h = Planck's constant (6.624×10^{-34} J-s)
f = the frequency in hertz

As the frequency increases into the gamma ray region, it is commonplace to express energy not in joules, but rather in *electron volts* (eV), such that 1 eV = 1.602×10^{-19} joules.

As you can see, electromagnetic waves, including X rays have an energy level that is proportional to the frequency. Early in the development of X rays, it was discovered that X rays are dangerous, sadly after a number of scientists and physicians died of leukemia and other blood or lymph system disorders. The high energy of the X ray can penetrate deep organs (which is why they are medically useful), but will damage cells and turn them cancerous in some cases. The higher energy waves, such as X rays, are known as *ionizing radiation,* and are considered dangerous under the right circumstances. Lower-frequency waves are called *nonionizing radiation,* and until recently were considered safe at all intensities below that required to heat the tissue (microwave ovens cook by heating the tissue internally with very-short-wavelength radio waves). Recently, however, other mechanisms than ionization and heating were suspected of causing some forms of leukemia and non-Hodgkin's lymphomas. As a result, the responsible thing to do is to limit exposure from all sources of electromagnetic radiation.

GENERATING X RAYS

Medical X rays are usually generated using a phenomena called *bremstrahlung* (see Figure 9-4). When an incident electron, with energy E_i is smashed into a *target* containing heavy nuclei, a strange thing happens. As the electron is deflected around the nucleus, it loses some energy and assumes a new energy level, E_d. The difference between incident and deflected electron energy levels must, according to the law of conservation of energy, go somewhere, so it becomes a photon of X-ray energy. The energy level of the X-ray photon is given by

$$E_x = h \times f \tag{9-3}$$

$$E_x = E_i - E_d$$

Figure 9-5 shows an early X-ray generator tube based on the bremstrahlung phenomenon. It is a vacuum tube containing an electron-emitting cathode and a target anode. Electrons from the negative cathode are accelerated by the positive charge on the anode and antianode with a large kinetic energy (proportional to the electrical potential difference between cathode and anode). When the accelerated electrons strike the antianode ("target"), the kinetic energy is given up. Because of the conservation law, the kinetic energy of the electrons is converted to heat (infrared radiation) and X rays. The wavelength (and therefore frequency) of the wavelength is proportional to the electrical potential difference between the cathode and anode.

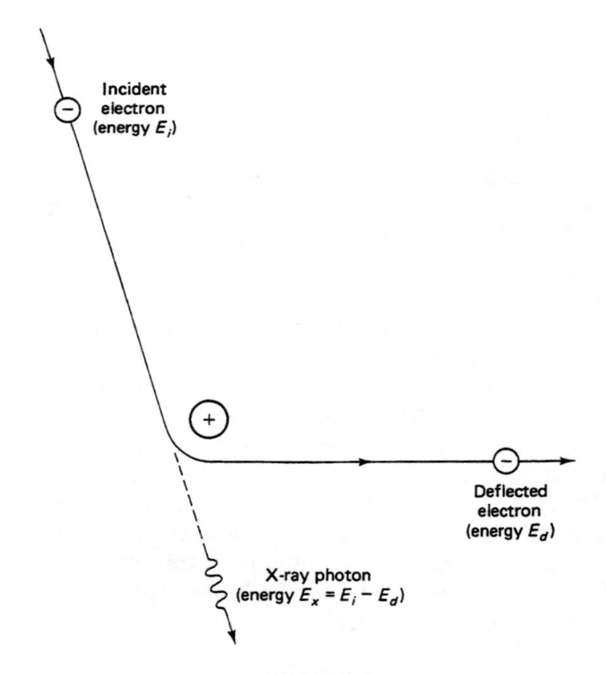

FIGURE 9-4

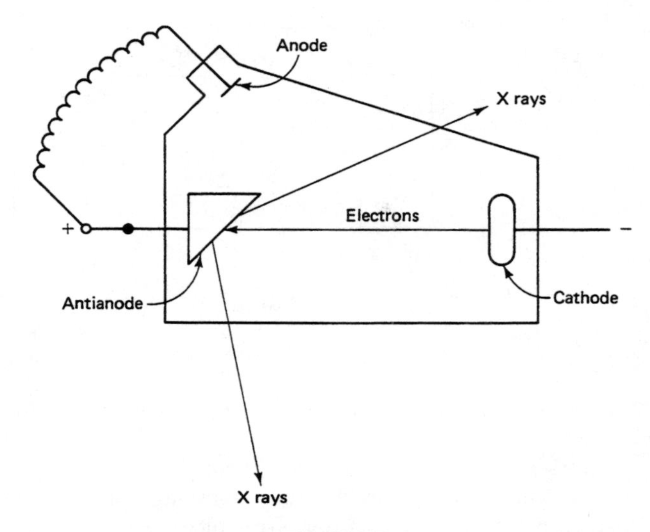

FIGURE 9-5

Where do these electrons come from? There is a phenomenon called *thermionic emission*. When a metallic surface is heated to incandescence (i.e., gives off light), a cloud of electrons are emitted from the surface. These electrons form a so-called *space charge* around the surface. In X-ray tubes (not to mention the now obsolete radio vacuum tubes), the metallic surface is in the form of a filament not dissimilar to that inside of an electric light bulb.

Thomas Edison could have kicked off the radio era 20 or 30 years earlier than he did because of an experiment he undertook to reduce the blackening of the inside the glass bulb that plagued his early commercial light bulbs. One of his early experiments used a positively charged anode inside the tube. Edison noted that an electrical current flowed between the filament and the anode, a phenomenon now called the *Edison effect*. It is the Edison effect that gives us the stream of accelerating electrons that strikes the anode target in an X-ray tube.

The materials of the target anode are selected to make X-ray generation easier. Besides the type of materials, the applied high-voltage potential ($V+$) determines the kinetic energy of the accelerated electrons, hence the frequency and wavelength of the emitted X rays. In a few very old TV sets, there was once a scare of X-ray emission caused by a new type of HV regulator tube that operated at higher than usual potentials. Medical, scientific, and industrial bremstrahlung generators are somewhat more tightly designed than TV tubes, however, so present no particular danger when used according to manufacturer's instructions.

Figure 9-6 shows the basic form of a more modern, but also very simple, X-ray tube. The anode is a beveled assembly of copper alloy inset with a tungsten alloy target region. The tungsten is better for X-ray generation, but the copper is a better heatsink. The cathode in this case is an incandescent filament. Electrons leave the surface of the filament, and then accelerate with an increasing velocity V toward the anode/target. When the electron strikes the target, its kinetic energy is given up

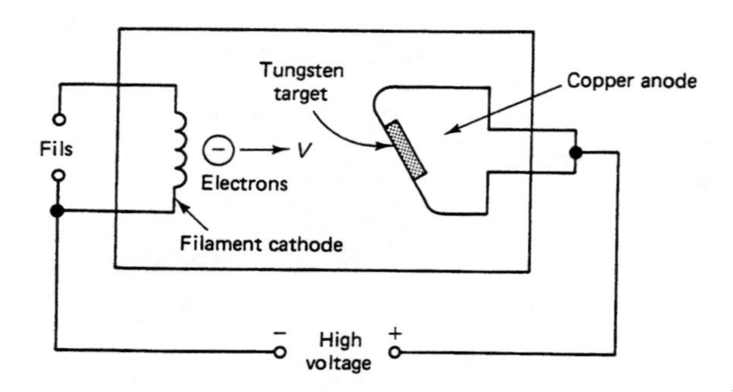

FIGURE 9-6

as heat and X radiation. The target is beveled in order to direct the X rays in a desired direction.

A variant on the basic tube uses a rotating anode (Figure 9-7). The heat created by the kinetic energy of electrons smashing into the target is tremendous, and overheating is a major cause of lost X-ray tubes. The rotating anode spreads the heat energy over a larger volume of metal, and incidentally produces a more narrowly focused beam.

Many of the sensors used in light-operated devices will also work at X-ray wavelengths. Certain phototubes, photomultipliers and photodiodes (and transistors) will also work in X-ray measurements. In this chapter we will look at certain sensors that are unique to X-ray measurements: the Geiger-Mueller tube, the scintillation cell, PN junction diode, and the photomultiplier tube.

Geiger-Mueller Tubes

The Geiger-Mueller tube (Figure 9-8) is a glass or metallic cylinder that has been evacuated of air and then refilled to a less than atmospheric pressure with an ionizing gas (usually argon with a touch of bromine, at 100-torr pressure). When radiation impinges such a gas, its energy forces the gas into ionization, thereby altering the electrical characteristics of the G-M tube. Those electrical characteristics are our transducible event.

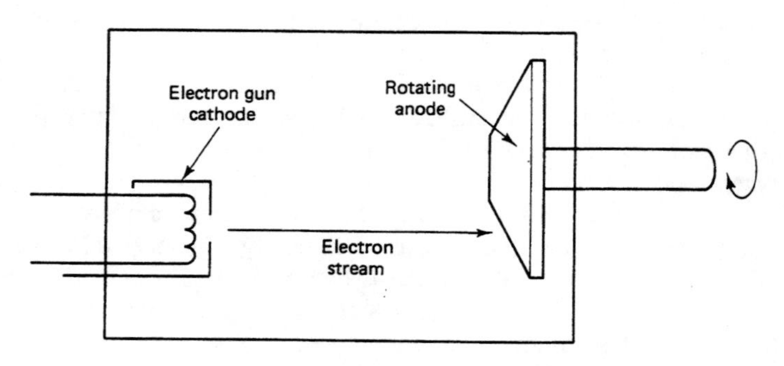

FIGURE 9-7

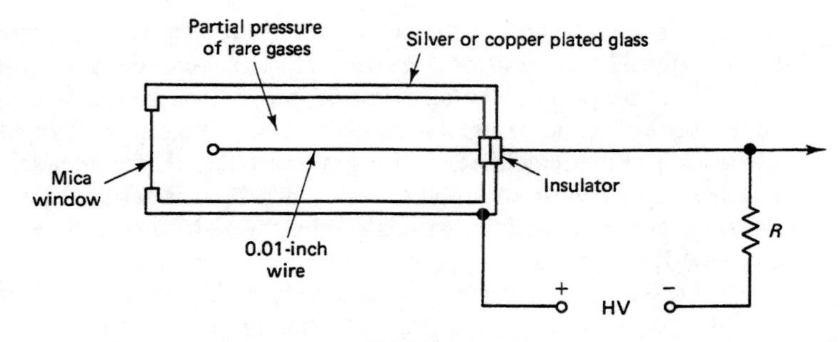

FIGURE 9-8

The general circuit for the G-M tube is shown in Figure 9-8. In most applications, the external circuitry consists of a power supply and a series current limiting or load resistor. There are three modes of operation for the G-M tube, and these modes affect both the subsequent circuitry and the voltage level required. These regions are shown in the curves in Figure 9-9 and are designated as follows: (1) ionization chamber mode, (2) proportional counter mode, and (3) geiger counter mode; these modes are reflected in the labels A, B, and C in Figure 9-9.

In the ionization chamber mode, a weak electric potential is applied across the G-M tube, so only a few electrons are generated by the radiation. Nearly all of these

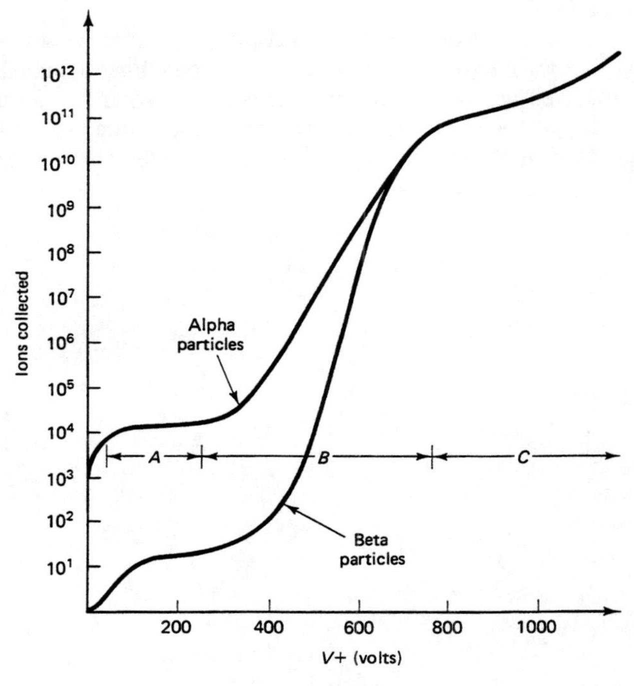

FIGURE 9-9

electrons are collected by the electrode. Therefore, we can assume that the current in the external load resistor is a measure of the amount of radiation.

In the proportional counter mode, the electric field is stronger, so the electrons generated by the ionizing gas reach sufficient kinetic energy to release additional electrons by kinetic collisions with gas molecules. The output across the load resistor will be a spike with an amplitude that is proportional to the kinetic energy of the ionizing radiation particle. In this mode, the G-M tube can count ionizing particles on a one-for-one basis.

The Geiger counter mode uses very high potentials, on the order of 800 to 2000 volts. The operation is similar to that in the proportional counter mode, except that kinetic energies are so high that a multiplication effect takes place; the tube operates in avalanche condition.

The output pulses are of approximately the same amplitude ("all or nothing" operation) every time the tube fires. An external counter circuit will tell us the number of pulses per unit of time, hence the level of radiation.

Photomultiplier Tubes

The *photomultiplier tube* (PMT), shown in Figure 9-10, is an amplifying device that uses the photoelectric effect to generate a current that is proportional to the impinging radiation. The photoelectric effect calls for the emission of electrons when a light wave (or higher-frequency radiation) strikes a metallic surface (called the "screen" in Figure 9-10).

Albert Einstein won his Nobel prize for his explanation of the photoelectric effect, not for his theory of relativity as is sometimes assumed. The problem that Einstein solved was something of an enigma to earlier physicists who studied the problem. It had been noted that the energy of the emitted electrons was not increased by increasing the intensity of the light striking the surface. The number of electrons

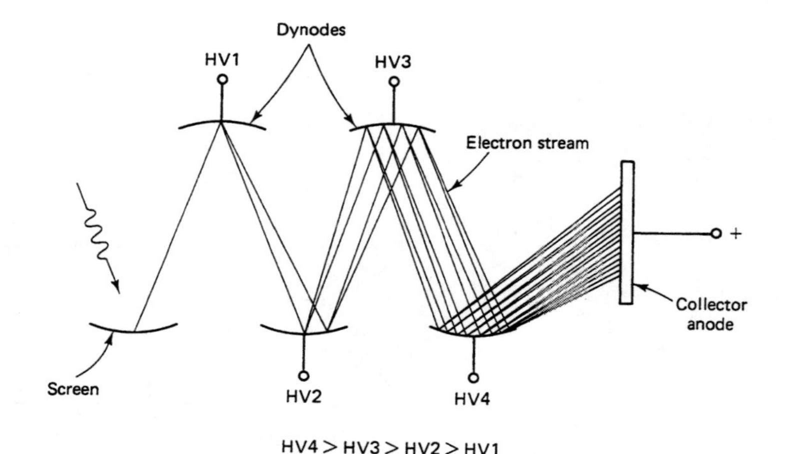

FIGURE 9-10

may increase, but their energy level was the same. But, it was noted, the energy of the electrons varied as the *color* of the light was varied. In visible light, color is a manifestation of differing frequencies and wavelengths. Einstein applied Planck's principle to the photoelectric effect, and thereby explained the observed phenomenon.

In the PMT (Figure 9-10), photons strike the screen and cause electrons to be emitted. They are attracted to a series of anodes (called *dynodes*) in succession, each of which has a slightly higher positive potential. When electrons strike each dynode, they knock loose other electrons. Each electron is therefore multiplied as the electron stream accelerates toward the final collector anode. Thus, a large current is output from the collector in response to a relatively small energy of radiation applied to the screen.

The photomultiplier (PM) tube is used in medical X rays in at least two applications. One is in fluoroscopic X-ray systems in which the output of the PM tube is applied to a video input of a television system. Thus, the X-ray picture is projected onto a TV screen. The other application is in computer-assisted tomography (CAT) scanners. The PM tube is considerably more sensitive than ordinary X-ray film, so one can take a multiple-position X ray (as needed for a CAT scan) using relatively small doses of radiation.

Scintillation Counters

An example of a scintillation cell or counter is shown in Figure 9-11. The word scintillation is a word used to denote a process similar to that which generates light on the screen of a cathode ray tube. When a radiation particle strikes an atom of certain phosphorous materials, its kinetic energy may be added to the energy of the orbital electrons. When the electrons are thus excited, they jump to a higher energy state, which is unstable. When they fall back to their ground state, the energy absorbed goes off in the form of a photon of light. Certain crystal materials possess this property.

Figure 9-11 shows a scintillation device in which a scintillation crystal window is attached to the light input window of a photomultiplier tube. Radiation causes the crystal to scintillate, and the light thus produced is picked up, and amplified, by the PM tube. The current at the output of the PM tube is proportional to the light, hence the radiation level.

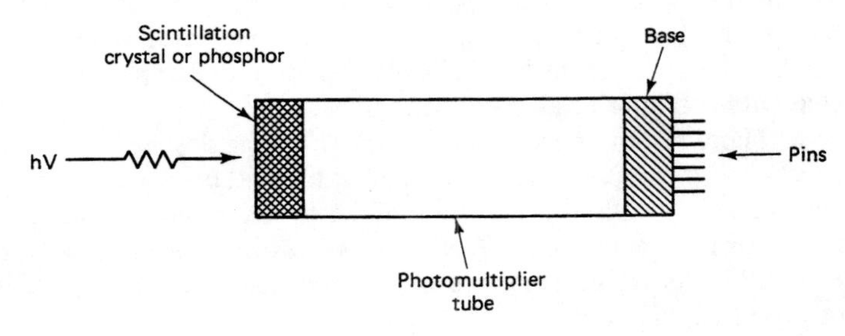

FIGURE 9-11

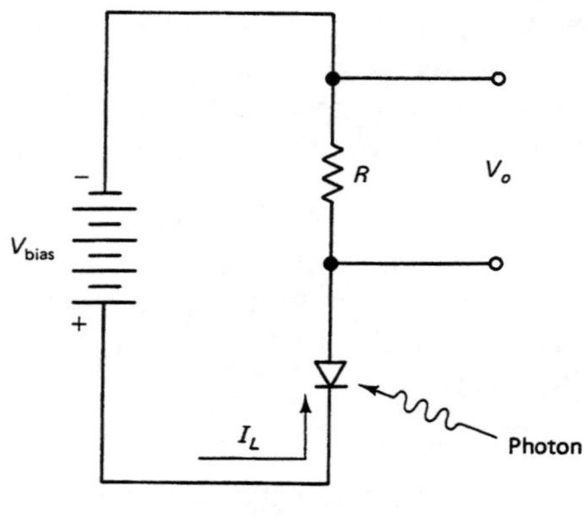

FIGURE 9-12

PN Junction Diodes

The PN junction diode is used extensively in electronics, and indeed was the first commercially available solid-state device on the market. The PN junction diode is formed by placing a region of N-type semiconductor material in contact with a region of P-type semiconductor material. When a PN junction diode is forward biased, a current will flow. But if the diode is reverse biased, no current flows—or almost no current. There will be a tiny *leakage current* (I_L) across the reverse biased PN junction. This current can be affected by impinging X rays.

Figure 9-12 shows a PN junction diode connected as a radiation detector. A reverse bias is supplied by V_{bias}, and the current is limited by a series resistor, R. The voltage drop across R is proportional to I_L. If radiation causes an increase in leakage resistance, then the voltage drop (V_o) across R will vary proportionally to the applied radiation levels.

SIMPLE X-RAY MACHINES

The field of medical X-ray apparatus is quite complex because development has kept pace with other technologies. We can, however, take a look at a simple X-ray machine in block diagram form (Figure 9-13). This sample machine contains the basic elements common to all X-ray machines.

There are three elements that make up the dosage of X rays that the patient receives: (1) the applied peak potential (kilovolts, or kV) across the X-ray tube, (2) the current level (milliamperes) emitted from the cathode, and (3) the time (seconds) the beam remains on. The unit of X-ray energy (joules) is the product $K \times$ kilovolts $\times$ milliamperes $\times$ seconds; the factor "K" is dependent on the type of power supply applied to the high-voltage circuit.

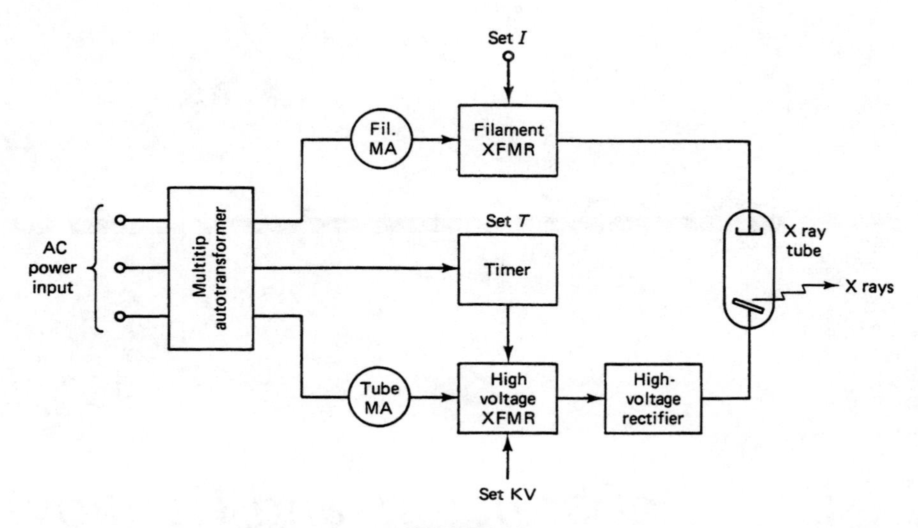
Set I
Fil. MA
Filament XFMR
AC power input
Multitip autotransformer
Set T
Timer
X ray tube
X rays
Tube MA
High voltage XFMR
High-voltage rectifier
Set KV

FIGURE 9-13

10

Defibrillators and Cardioverters

No medical device so clearly represents emergency and, in some aspects, intensive care medicine as much as the *defibrillator*. These are electric shock devices that are used to correct fatal cardiac arrhythmias such as ventricular fibrillation and ventricular tachycardia. Although usually characterized as a "random" shallow beating of the heart, the process is known by more modern research to be actually "chaotic" (which has very specific mathematical meaning in science). Prior to 1960, all defibrillators were AC models, although that form of machine is now obsolete. They applied a 60-Hz alternating current (AC) of 5 to 6 amperes for a period of 250 to 1000 milliseconds. AC defibrillators had a rather poor success rate. In addition, the technique was totally ineffectual for correcting atrial fibrillation and in fact could often induce fatal ventricular fibrillation when the attempt was made.

Since the early 1960s a series of direct current (DC) defibrillators have been created. These machines store a DC charge that can be delivered across the patient's heart. The job of the defibrillator is to cause all muscle fibers in the heart to contract simultaneously and deeply. If the attempt is successful, the heart will become resynchronized on its own. The most common forms of DC defibrillator are classified by their output waveforms: the *Lown, monopulse, tapered DC delay,* and *trapezoidal.*

The most common waveform today was introduced at Harvard in 1962 by Doctor Bernard Lown. That waveform now bears his name and is shown in Figure 10-1. During its charging period the capacitor is isolated from the patient. But when the emergency medical person initiates the electrical shock, the capacitor is connected across the patient. The applied voltage is a little less than 3000 volts, and the cur-

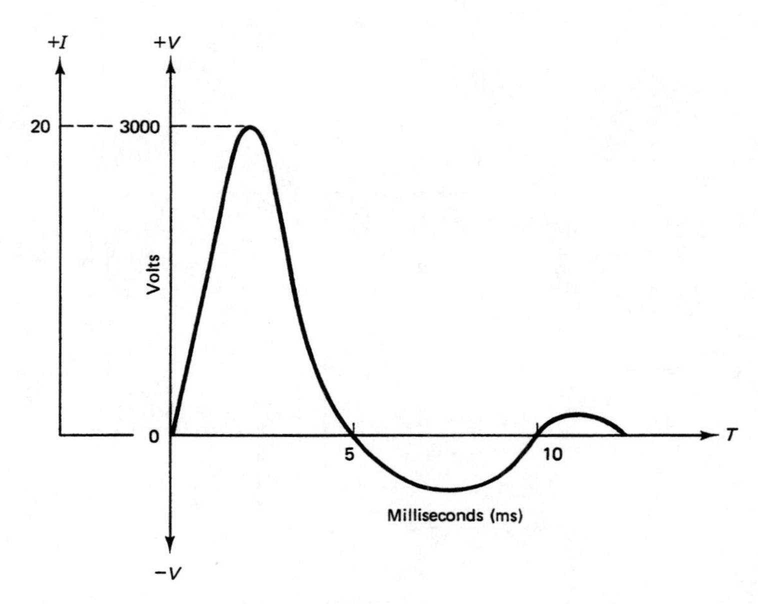

FIGURE 10-1

rent rises to approximately 20 amperes for a brief period. The waveform rises to a peak, and then drops back to zero in a period of approximately 5 milliseconds. Because some energy is stored in an inductor as well, there is a small counter current lasting about 5 milliseconds following the main burst.

Figure 10-2 shows the schematic diagram of the simplest form of defibrillator. The main charge storage element is a capacitor (C1), which in the classical Lown machines was 16 μF. Capacitor C1 must be rated at a high voltage because a typical maximum charge will be 7000 volts or so. The energy stored in a capacitor is given by

$$U = \frac{CV^2}{2} \tag{10-1}$$

where

U = the energy in joules (i.e., watt-seconds)
C = the capacitance in farads
V = the fully charged voltage

To see how the high-voltage and charge level are closely related, look at the rearranged version of Equation 10-1:

$$V = \left(\frac{2U}{C}\right)^{1/2} \tag{10-2}$$

Example

Calculate the voltage across a 16 μF defibrillator capacitor when the stored energy is 400 watt-seconds.

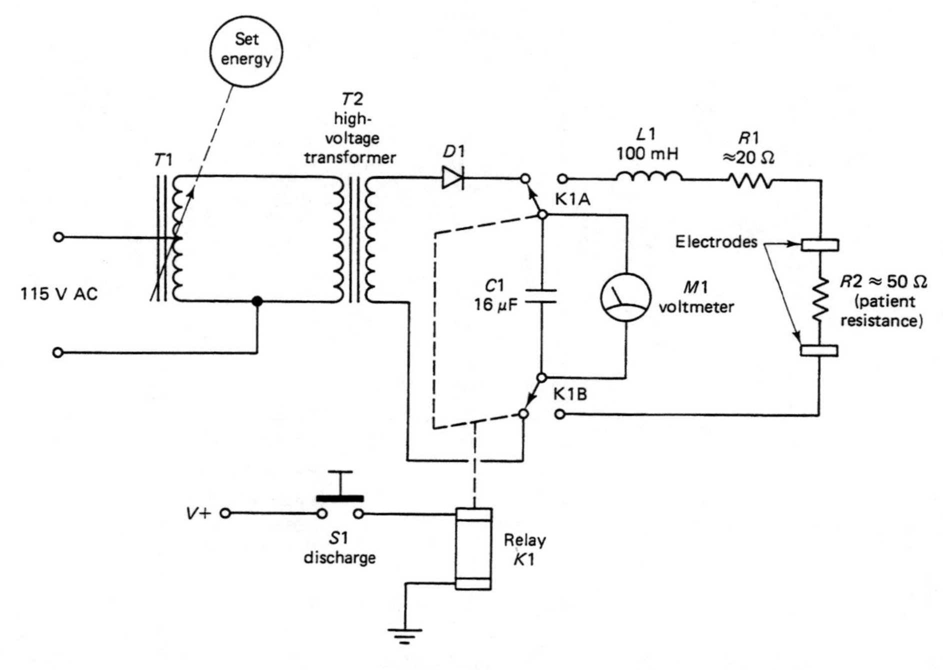

FIGURE 10-2

Solution:

$$V = \left(\frac{2U}{C}\right)^{1/2}$$

$$= \left[\frac{(2)(400 \text{ watt-second})}{1.6 \times 10^{-5} \text{ farads}}\right]^{1/2}$$

$$= \left[\frac{800}{1.6 \times 10^{-5}}\right]^{1/2}$$

$$= (5 \times 10^{7})^{1/2} = 7072 \text{ volts}$$

As can be seen from the example, the most common defibrillator energy set point (400 w-s) yields a voltage of >7000 volts. As a result, these capacitors are rated at more than 8500 volts, although some of the better quality units are rated at 10,000 volts as a safety margin. At least one model was rated at 7500 volts, but it is no longer on the market—and its reliability was poor.

Warning! Some older defibrillators used oil-filled capacitors in which the oil was PCB—a known severe carcinogen. These capacitors should be replaced if still in service. Consult the manufacturer to determine if a PCB capacitor was used, and then get expert advice from local authorities regarding disposal of the old unit. If one of these capacitors leaks, or explodes, then it is possible that a major cleanup effort is required.

A double-pole, double-throw (DPDT) high-voltage relay (K1) is used to control the capacitor in the circuit. During the charge period, the relay connects the capacitor across a high-voltage DC power supply consisting of rectifier D1, transformers T1 and T2, and the 115-volt AC power lines. The charge across the capacitor is monitored by a high-voltage voltmeter (M1), which is calibrated in watt-seconds (by virtue of Equations 10-1 and 10-2). The units *watt-seconds* are used, even though the more modern unit is the *joule*. However, because 1 J = 1 w-s, little harm is done. The charge level is set by the applied voltage, which in the case of the simplified machine is set by an autotransformer (T1).

Another note about obsolete older defibrillators is in order. Although these units are largely out of service, they are still found occasionally in veterinary offices, research facilities, and overseas. Some early machines used a single-pole double-throw relay for K1. A consequence of this type of circuit is the so-called "live ground" problem. If the operator is touching the patient, even indirectly (as in touching the bed with his or her knees), then a nasty shock will be felt. When the operator indicates that he or she is about to discharge the defibrillator, then stand back—that's a nasty jolt.

The output network of the defibrillator consists of the alternate set of relay contacts, a 100-mH inductance, and a pair of resistances (R1 is the lumped resistance of the inductor, the relay contacts, electrode contacts, and conductors, while R2 is an equivalent patient resistance). The inductor is responsible for the heavily damped Lown waveform, as well as the recharge loop between 5 and 10 mS. When the operator presses the discharge button (switch S1), the relay is transferred from the charge position to the discharge position. This action connects the capacitor across the output network. The current and voltage at the output terminals rises dramatically, but because of the retarding action of the inductor, it rapidly becomes heavily damped. The voltage and current drop off exponentially until it reaches zero at approximately 5 milliseconds. At this point the energy stored in the magnetic field of the inductor (L1) is then reintroduced into the circuit as a counter electromotive force (CEMF). Because the CEMF is of the opposite polarity as the main pulse, the polarity of the minor pulse from 5 to 10 mS is opposite.

The *monopulse DC* waveform is shown in Figure 10-3. It is a modified Lown waveform, and is commonly found in portable defibrillators. It is created by the same form of DC capacitor charging system as the Lown, but lacks the inductor in the output waveform. As a result, the waveform drops exponentially to zero after passing the peak, and does not have the minor negative swing characteristic of the Lown. The tapered DC waveform is merely the standard resistor-capacitor (R-C) discharge waveform.

The *tapered DC delay* waveform is shown in Figure 10-4. This waveform is able to achieve the same energy level using lower voltages across the storage capacitor. This fact makes it more useful for portable machines. Energy is characterized in the graphs of this chapter as the area under the voltage versus time curve. Thus, in order to have the same energy at a lower amplitude, the waveform must last longer.

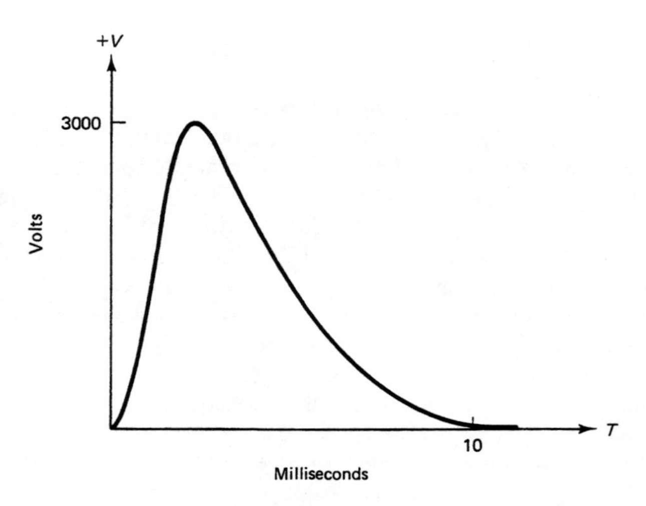

FIGURE 10-3

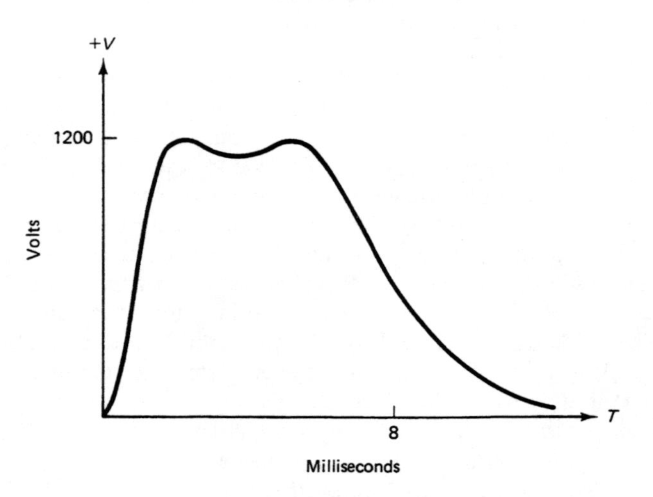

FIGURE 10-4

The basic circuit is similar to a Lown machine in which two capacitor-inductor networks are connected in cascade. The dual nature of the circuit results in the double-humped waveform as shown in Figure 10-4.

The trapezoidal DC waveform is shown in Figure 10-5. It is another of the low-voltage waveforms, and in fact uses somewhat lower voltage levels than the tapered form. The initial output voltage rises to 800 or 900 volts, and then drops linearly to about 500 or 600 volts. A dump circuit then drops the voltage to zero in a short period of time.

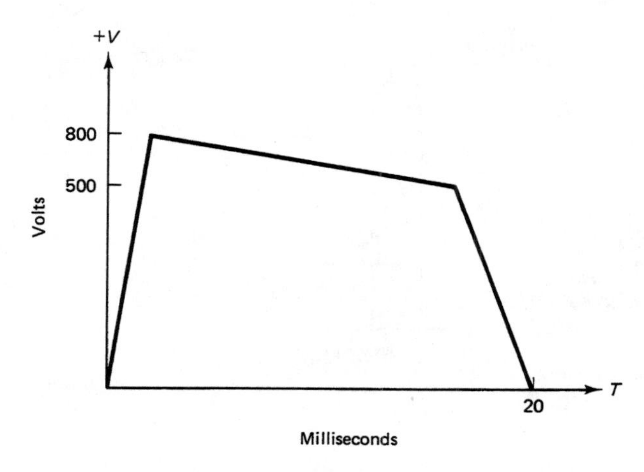

FIGURE 10-5

PADDLES

Energy is transferred from the defibrillator to the patient through a pair of electrodes called *paddles*. While the shape of current models is less "paddlelike," the name persists. Several common types of defibrillator paddles are shown in Figure 10-6. The form shown in Figure 10-6A is the standard (if older design) *anterior* paddle. This type of paddle is designed to be applied directly to the chest. The *posterior* paddle is shown in Figure 10-6B. This form of paddle is used on the patient's back. In typical applications, the posterior paddle is smeared with an electrolytic cream to make better electrical contact, and is then inserted under the patient. The patient's weight makes electrical contact possible. Some defibrillators are equipped with an anterior/anterior pair, while others are equipped with anterior/posterior electrodes. None to my knowledge is equipped with a posterior/posterior pair.

The electrode shown in Figure 10-6C is a D-ring anterior electrode. This form is probably the most common form used today, especially on portable models. The D-ring shape is superior for most applications because it is easier and more natural to hold in the strained position under which defibrillators are usually used.

A final form of paddle is the *interior* paddle. The defibrillator used for direct application of electrical charge to the open heart (which is used during open heart surgery) will have a pair of these electrodes. *Pediatric* paddles are similar, except for a minor difference in shape and a size.

The push-button discharge switch is sometimes mounted on the front panel of the defibrillator, but in most cases, it is mounted on one or both paddles. On most modern machines there are two discharge switches wired together in an AND-gate manner as shown in Figure 10-7. Both switches must be pressed before the defibrillator will fire, and this is a significant safety device. A prematurely fired

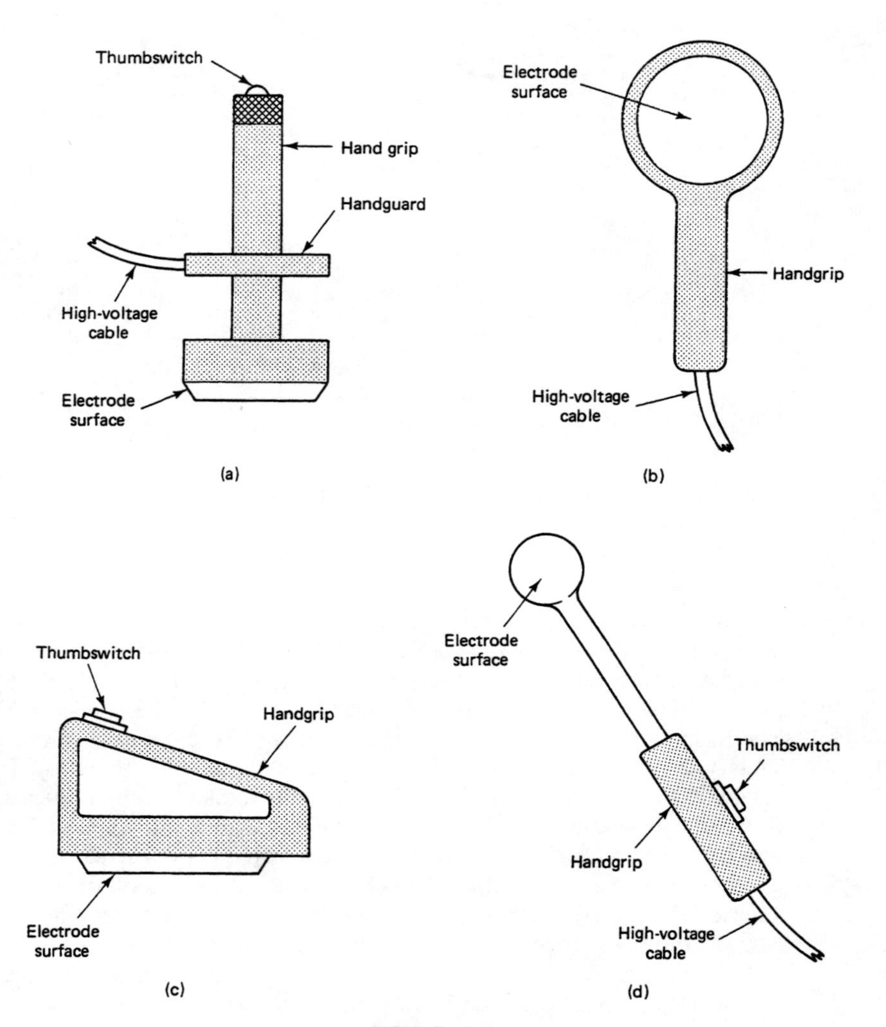

FIGURE 10-6

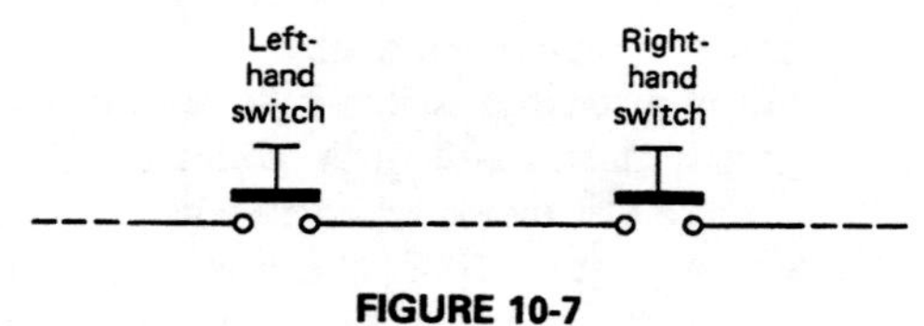

FIGURE 10-7

defibrillator is a hazard to both the patient being resuscitated and the medical staff attending the patient.

ADDITIONAL DEFIBRILLATOR CIRCUITS

The simple defibrillator shown in Figure 10-2 was once widely available, but is now obsolete. It was shown here because it reduces the defibrillator to its barest essentials. Figure 10-8 shows a somewhat more complex version than is representative of the type of machine available today. The high-voltage DC power supply is electronically controlled.

During the charge cycle the voltage across the capacitor is monitored by a resistor voltage divider (R1/R2) and a differential amplifier, A1. The differential amplifier is used as a voltage comparator in which the desired output level is set by a potentiometer (R3) and a reference voltage source, V_{ref}. When the operator selects an output level, the potentiometer output voltage V_{set} is applied to the noninverting input of A1. At this point, the voltage across the capacitor (V_c) is zero, so the output of A1 is high positive. As the capacitor charges, V_c rises so the voltage divider output (V_a) also rises. When $V_a = V_{set}$, the output of the comparator drops to zero, causing the electronic DC power supply to cease supplying current to the capacitor. This circuit makes a lighter and more reliable charge method than the autotransformer version.

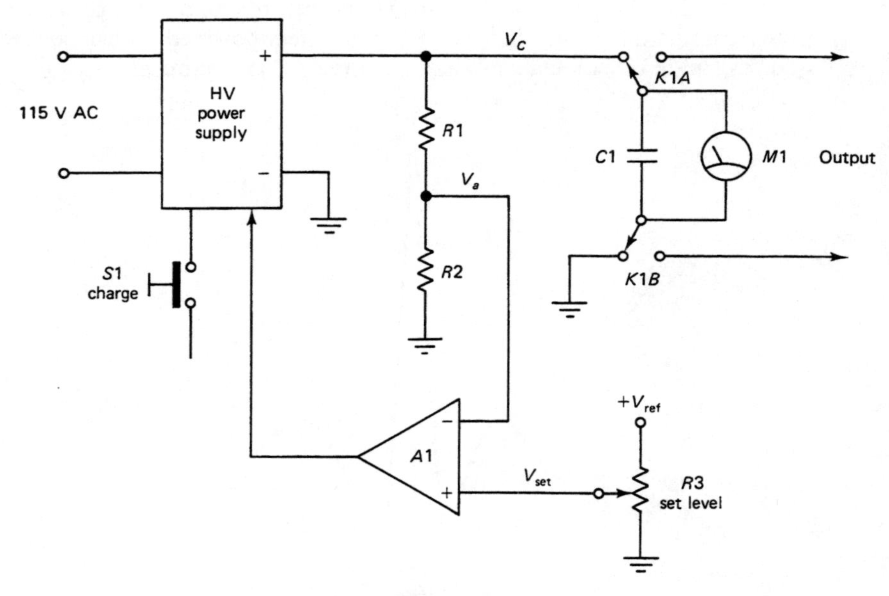

FIGURE 10-8

CARDIOVERSION

Certain types of cardiac arrhythmia, for example, atrial fibrillation, are treated with a defibrillator (usually) set to a low energy level. But the defibrillator is an asynchronous device, so cannot be used for such *cardioversion* cases. It must be redesigned to make the machine *synchronous*. The problem is that the electrical charge can induce fatal ventricular fibrillation if it occurs on the T-wave portion of the ECG waveform. The cardioverter is a special form of defibrillator that causes synchronous discharge of the capacitor. The usual standard is to detect the QRS complex on the upswing (see Figure 10-9), and then cause the discharge on the downswing.

A sample (if simplified) cardioverter synchronizer circuit is shown in Figure 10-10. A silicon-controlled rectifier (SCR) is a special rectifier that remains open circuited (no current flows) until a current pulse is applied to the gate (*G*). At that point the anode (*A*) cathode (*K*) path becomes a low resistance. In the circuit of Figure 10-10 the SCR is in series with the discharge switch, so *both* must be turned on for the defibrillator to fire.

The gate control signal is derived from the ECG waveform. Two criteria are used to detect the QRS complex: amplitude or level detection and the rate of change. If the rate of change circuit is not used, and only level detection is used, then an unusually elevated P-wave or (more likely) T-wave could fire the circuit.

An example of a modern portable defibrillator is shown in Figure 10-11. This instrument uses D-ring paddles as shown earlier. The defibrillator also includes an ECG monitor 'scope and a paper strip-chart recorder to make a permanent record of the resuscitation event. This instrument is battery powered, so can be used on ambulances and in other situations away from the AC power mains.

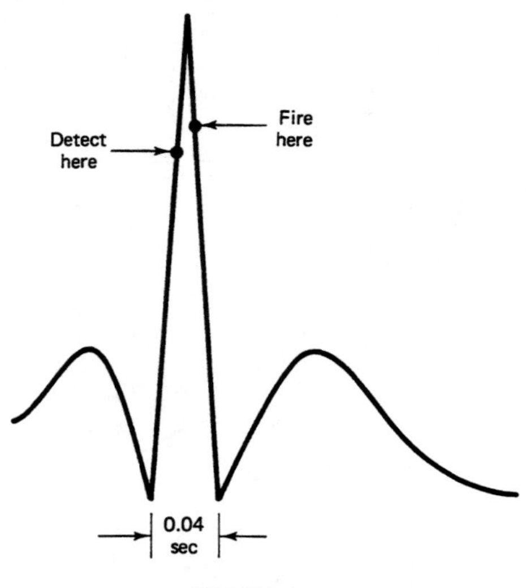

FIGURE 10-9

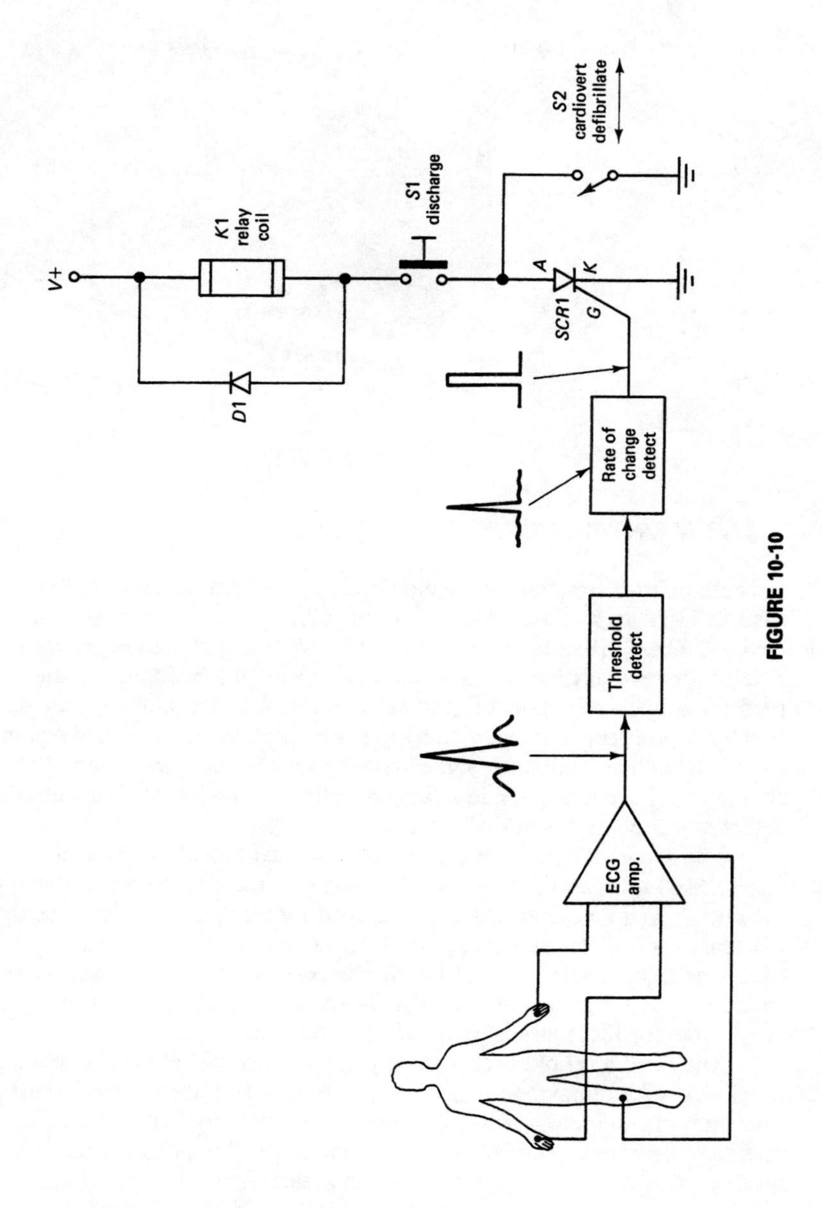
V+
K1
relay
coil
D1
S1
discharge
A
K
G
SCR1
S2
cardiovert
defibrillate
Rate of
change
detect
Threshold
detect
ECG
amp.

FIGURE 10-10

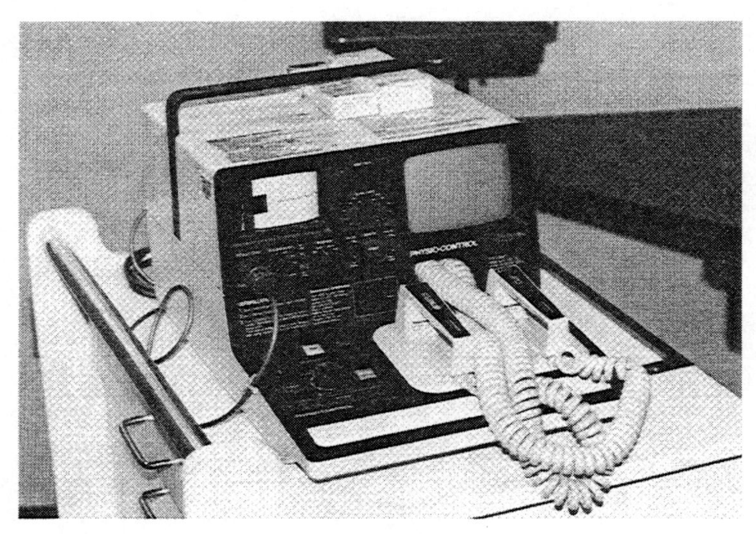

FIGURE 10-11

TESTING AND MAINTAINING DEFIBRILLATORS

Because defibrillators are high-voltage, high-powered devices, and because they are used in high-stress situations, a constant diligence is required in maintaining these devices. There are at least three levels of testing that should be performed. First, on a daily (or several times weekly) basis, or more, the operators of the device should perform a quick operational test to see that it is functioning as expected. The time to find out a problem exists is *not* during a resuscitation. A simplified test instrument or fixture (which is built into some models) makes this job easier. The daily check should also include a quick look at connections and wires visible from the outside to detect any fraying or signs of wear.

The second level of testing should be a qualified biomedical equipment technician (BMET), or similarly qualified person (not medical or nursing staff) examining the output on a special instrument designed for that purpose. It is the author's opinion that an oscilloscope photograph be made of the output waveform at this time. I have seen cases where a defibrillator tester passed the unit as good, but the waveform check revealed a defective relay that would have failed in the near term. Perhaps a good cycle for these checks is monthly or quarterly.

The third level of check, which perhaps could be called a "depot maintenance" check, calls for removing the defibrillator from active service for a short period. The instrument is taken to a laboratory where it is provided with an annual preventative maintenance check. The lab will make the same checks as are made by the BMET on a monthly basis. Controls and circuits are checked for signs of wear. In addition, the battery (if used) is checked and/or replaced as directed by the defibrillator manufacturer. At this time also, the manufacturer's recommended maintenance replacements are performed. A reasonable cycle for these checks is usually recommended by the maker and should be followed.

SAFETY NOTE

Defibrillators are high-voltage devices that are quite capable of inflicting serious injury, up to and including death. Extreme care must be used in operating and maintaining these units. If common sense and the manufacturer's directions are followed religiously, then the danger is substantially reduced. But don't fool around with these machines! I have seen medical students (they are the ones in the short lab coats) and interns (the ones in the dirty lab coats, and with a brain-dead, exhausted look on their faces) play with defibrillators. One neat trick was to hold the electrodes close together while firing the discharge button. The resultant spark between the close proximity electrodes was, I suppose, exciting to a juvenile. But it also harmed the machine and pitted the paddles (which could cause burns on the patient).

There have been other foul-ups over the years. One experienced anesthesiologist was handed the two anterior paddles (Figure 10-6A) by a cardiologist. The cardiologist had both discharge buttons pressed (mindlessly), and the anesthesia doctor grapped the paddles by the electrode surfaces—taking the full 400 watt-seconds across his arms. Fortunately, he was not killed.

In another incident, a young intern on his first resuscitation event was holding the paddles. The patient was stabilized, but the young man did not return the paddles to their holders. He instead had the bare metal electrode surfaces pressed against his hips. While watching more senior physicians evaluate the patient, he fiddled with the buttons—first the recharge button, which rearmed the machine, and then both discharge buttons. The machine discharged 400 watt-seconds across his hips. The ol' sphincter gave way and he, er, well, he "filled his pants" with the content of his large descending colon.

Be careful.

11

Temperature Sensors

Temperature is a key measurement in medicine, biological science, biomedical engineering, and, indeed, daily life. There are a number of different types of temperature sensors available to the medical instrument designer. In this chapter we will take a look at some of the more popular types. But, first, let's review the different measurement scales used to define temperature.

DIFFERENT MEASUREMENT SYSTEMS

There are three different scales used in the measurement of temperature. The familiar *Fahrenheit* and *Celsius* (aka *centigrade*) scales, along with the less familiar *Kelvin* scale, are frequently used in medical, scientific, and industrial measurements. The Celsius and Fahrenheit scales are arranged such that 0°C is the same temperature as 32°F. Both points can be defined by the freezing point of water at standard temperature and pressure. On the Fahrenheit scale, water freezes at +32°F, while on the Celsius scale water freezes at 0°C. The two scales can therefore be converted to each other by the equation

$$F - 32 = 1.8C \tag{11-1}$$

where

F = degrees Fahrenheit (°F)
C = degrees Celsius (°C)

The Kelvin scale uses the same size degree steps as the Celsius scale. That is, a 1°K change of temperature is the same as a 1°C change of temperature. However, the two scales define the zero degree point differently. In the Celsius scale, 0°C is the freezing point of water, while in the Kelvin scale it is *absolute zero* (the point where molecular activity ceases). Thus, 0°K = −276.16°C. The Celsius and Kelvin scales are converted by

$$°K = °C - 273.16 \tag{11-2}$$

$$°C = °K + 273.16 \tag{11-3}$$

Before temperature can be measured by an electronic instrument there has to be a *sensor,* so it is to temperature transducers that we now turn our attention.

TEMPERATURE TRANSDUCERS

Several different temperature sensors are commonly used in medical and other life sciences applications: *thermistors, thermocouples,* and *PN semiconductor junctions*. There are also cases where a *bimetallic strip* sensor is used. Although applications (clinical, research, control) for these different forms of transducer overlap, there are key parameters and other factors that often favor one or the other in specific situations. Let's examine each of these in turn.

THERMISTORS

Thermistors (i.e., *therm*al res*istors*) are resistors that are designed to change resistance value in a predictable manner with changes in applied temperature. The amount of change is designated by the *temperature coefficient* (*a*) of the material, which is measured in ohms of resistance change per ohm of resistance per degree Celcius. A *positive temperature coefficient* (PTC) device (see Figure 11-1) increases resistance with increases in temperature. Alternatively, *negative temperature coefficient* (NTC) devices decrease resistance with increases in temperature. The usual circuit symbols for thermistors are shown in Figure 11-2. The indirectly heated variety uses an internal heating element. Several popular packaging styles are shown in Figure 11-3.

Most thermistors have a nonlinear curve when it is plotted over a wide temperature range, but when limited to narrow temperature ranges, the linearity is considerably better. When such thermistors are used, however, it is necessary to ensure that the temperature will not go on excursions outside of the permissable linear range. There are methods for linearizing the thermistor, and these will be discussed in a later section.

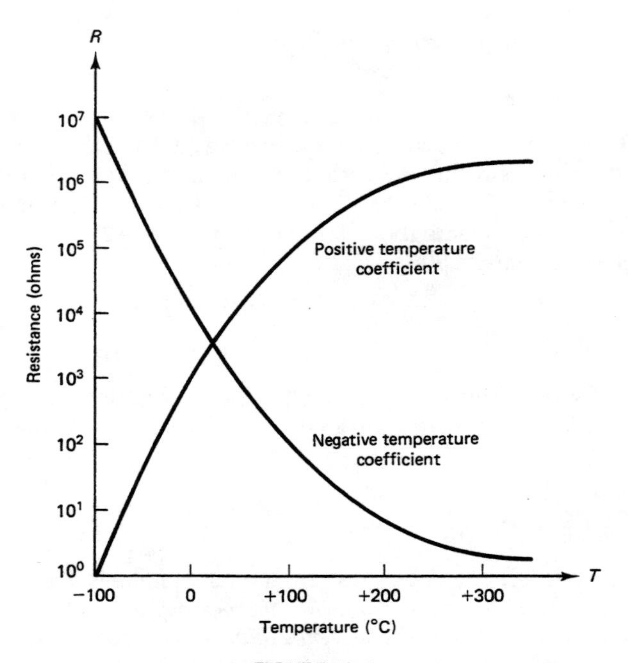

FIGURE 11-1

Thermistors are among the oldest temperature sensors available. The temperature sensitivity of electrical resistance in silver sulphide was noted by physicist Michael Faraday in 1833. There are several different types of thermistor, but the simplest is the wire element. Simple wire thermistor elements are based on two physical phenomena. First, materials tend to change physical dimensions with changes in temperature. Metals, for example, tend to expand when heated. Second, the resistance of a material is directly proportional to the length of the sample. Thus, when a metal is heated, it tends to expand so its electrical resistance increases.

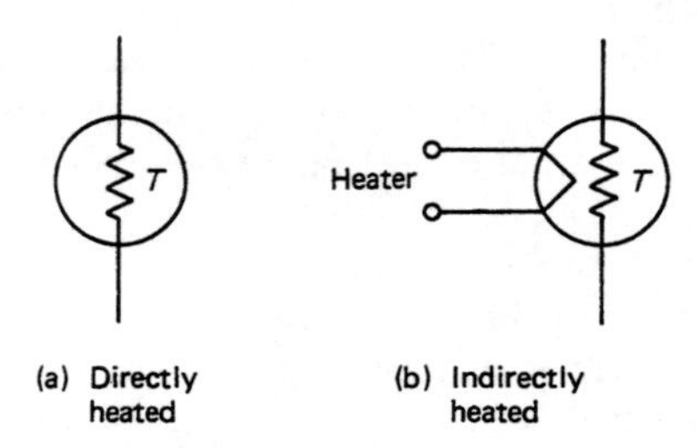

FIGURE 11-2

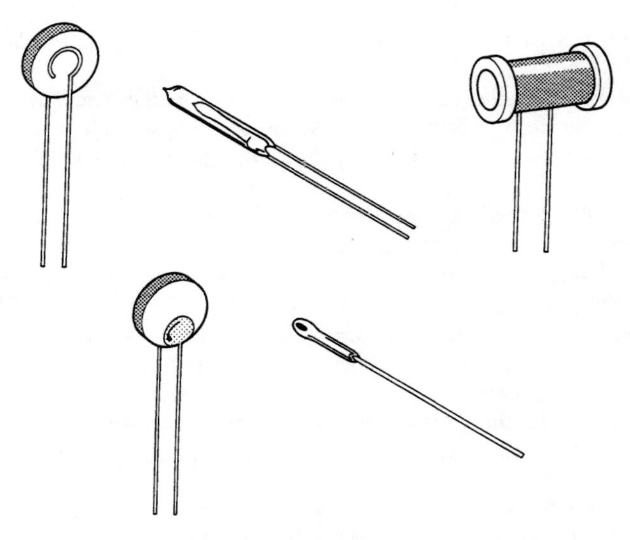

FIGURE 11-3

Most metals have a positive temperature coefficient ($a > 0$). Copper, for example, has a temperature coefficient of +0.004 ohm/ohm/°C.

Not all materials have positive temperature coefficients, however. Some materials, like carbon and some ceramics, have a negative temperature coefficient ($a = -0.0003$ ohm/ohm/°C). Other materials, including certain metal alloys, have temperature coefficients that are nearly zero. For example, in *manganin* and *constantan* the temperature coefficient is approximately +0.00002 ohm/ohm/°C, and for *nichrome* it is +0.00017 ohm/ohm/°C.

The change in resistance caused by changes in temperature is a function of a and the value of temperature change. For a wire element, the new resistance is found from

$$R_{T2} = R_{T1}[1 + a(T2 - T1)] \tag{11-4}$$

where

R_{T1} = the starting temperature resistance
R_{T2} = the final temperature resistance
a = the temperature coefficient
$T1$ = the starting temperature
$T2$ = the final temperature

Wire elements are sometimes used as thermistors in medical applications. Taut platinum wire elements, for example, are sometimes used in respiration sensors. Other thermistors are made of evaporated films; carbon or carbon compositions; or oxides of cobalt, manganese, magnesium, nickel, or uranium.

Thermistor Parameters

Before one can successfully apply thermistors it is necessary to first understand some of the basic properties of the thermistor. These are expressed in the form of certain standard parameters. Among the most commonly needed are

Cold (zero-power) resistance This parameter is the resistance of the thermistor at a standard reference temperature (usually either room temperature—25°C—or the ice point of water—0°C), under conditions of no self-heating power dissipation. This parameter is the cold resistance that is listed in the specifications sheet as the *nominal resistance*. For example, a device listed as a "1000-Ω thermistor" has a resistance of 1000 Ω at the standard reference temperature (25°C unless otherwise specified). The conditions under which the thermistor is operated for measurement of the cold resistance include a requirement that the current through the device be sufficiently low to avoid self-heating.

Hot resistance The hot resistance of the thermistor is measured when the device is operated at a higher temperature than the cold resistance temperature. The higher temperature is due to ambient temperature, the current flow through the thermistor, the applied heater current (indirectly heated types only), or a combination of all these factors. Equation 11-4 can be modified to find the hot resistance of wire elements:

$$R_T = R_o[1 + a(T - T_o)] \tag{11-5}$$

For other forms of thermistor the expression is

$$R_T = R_o e^{B[(1/T)-(1/T_o)]} \tag{11.6}$$

where

T_o = the reference temperature (25°C)
T = the new temperature
R_o = the thermistor resistance at the reference temperature
R_T = the resistance at temperature T
a = the coefficient of resistance
B = a factor with units of temperature (usually between 1500°K and 7000°K)

Example

A thermistor has a positive temperature coefficient of +0.002 ohm/ohm/°C at 25°C. What is its resistance at 98.6°F (37°C) if the nominal resistance is 12.1 kΩ?

Solution:

$$\begin{aligned} R_T &= R_o e^{B[(1/T)-(1/T_o)]} \\ &= (12{,}100\ \Omega)[1 + (0.002)(37 - 25)] \\ &= (12{,}100\ \Omega)[1 + (0.002)(12)] \\ &= (12{,}100\ \Omega)(1 + 0.024) = 12{,}390\ \Omega \end{aligned}$$

Resistance versus temperature This parameter is an expression of the characteristic shown in Figure 11-1. The exact shape of the curve is a function of the thermistor in question, but it will be of the form shown in Figure 11-1 and is nonlinear.

Resistance ratio (R_T/R_o) The resistance ratio is essentially a simplified expression of the *R*-versus-*T* curve. It states the ratio of the thermistor resistance at a specified resistance (50°C, 100°C, or 125°C) to the cold temperature (25°C) resistance.

Voltage versus current (V versus I) Directly heated thermistors have an unusual voltage-versus-current curve (Figure 11-4) that includes both ohmic and negative resistance regions. Assuming a constant ambient temperature, an increase in current through the thermistor will cause a linear increase in voltage drop across the thermistor. Because this behavior is in accordance with Ohm's law, $V = IR$, that portion of the curve is called the *ohmic region*. At a certain current, however, internal self-heating becomes dominant over ambient temperature and begins to alter the resistance of the thermistor. At this point the voltage drop begins to *decrease with increasing current flow*. In other words, in this region the thermistor is a *negative resistance* device.

Current versus time A typical thermistor current-versus-time curve is shown in Figure 11-5. The thermistor current would ideally snap to the level V/R_T when a step-function voltage is applied (or the applied level is changed). However,

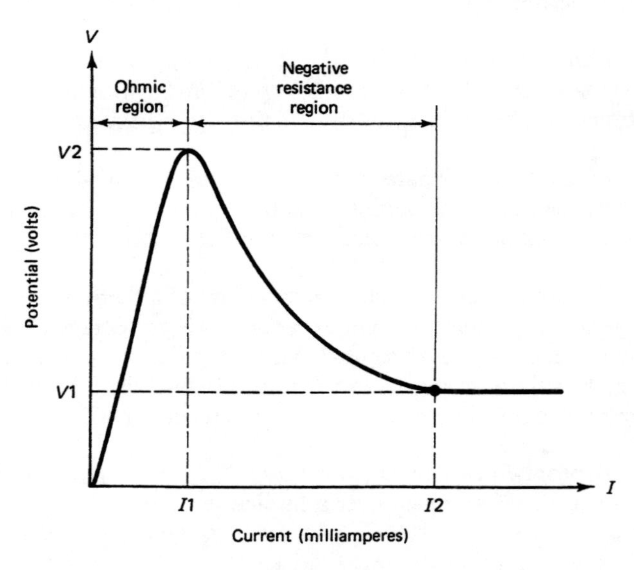

FIGURE 11-4

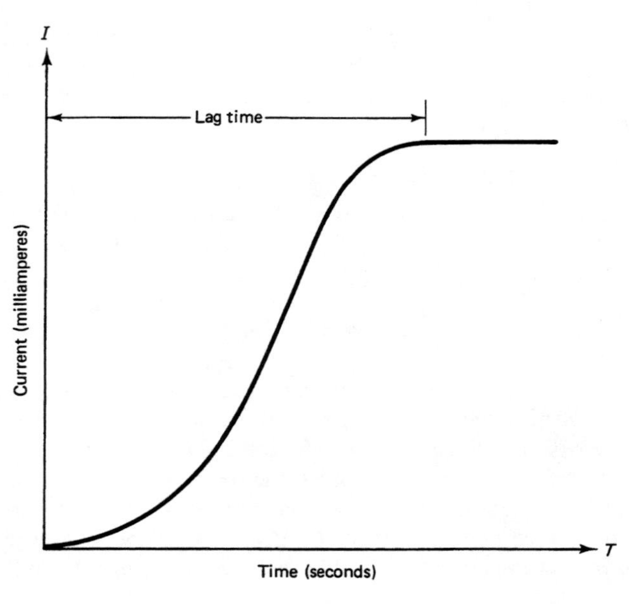

FIGURE 11-5

because there is always a small amount of self-heating involved in any thermistor, this response is not linear. There is always a time lag between a change in applied voltage and the current in the thermistor reaching the level mandated by that voltage for the thermistor resistance.

Maximum power (P_{max}) This parameter is the maximum allowable constant power level that the thermistor will handle without destruction, permanent alteration of characteristics, or degradation of its performance.

Dissipation constant (Δ) This factor, symbolized in the specifications sheet by capital Greek *delta* (Δ), is the ratio of the change in power dissipation for small changes in the body temperature of the thermistor.

Sensitivity (Φ) The sensitivity (σ) of a thermistor is the ratio of resistance change to temperature change, expressed as a percentage change per degree of temperature. Because the *R*-versus-*T* curve (Figure 11-1) is nonlinear over most of its range, sensitivity factor numbers are valid only over a limited range. Typical values for σ run from 0.5 percent per °C to 4 percent per °C.

Temperature range (Including T_{min} and T_{max}) The thermistor's characteristics are only specified over a limited temperature range, T_{min} to T_{max}. The value of T_{min} is typically −200°C, while T_{max} is typically +650°C (although there are devices with a narrower range).

Thermal time constant (t) The body temperature of a thermistor does not change instantaneously in response to a step-function change in ambient temperature. If T_i is the initial temperature, and T_f is the final temperature, then the thermal time constant is the time required for the body temperature of the thermistor to change 63.2 percent of the range between these two temperatures.

LINEARIZING THERMISTORS

The resistance-versus-time curve seen earlier in Figure 11-1 is nonlinear over most of its range. For some measurements, therefore, it is necessary to either restrict the use of the device to a limited range of temperatures, or to actually linearize the *R*-versus-*T* curve. There are several ways to linearize the curve. Some of them involve electronic circuits. There are, however, two methods that only involve simple resistors or other thermistors. Figure 11-6A shows a linearization network used by a thermistor manufacturer. Although the network functions (to an outside observer) like a single, two-terminal thermistor, it actually consists of a network of resistors and thermistors.

A relatively easy method for linearizing a thermistor is shown in Figure 11-6B. This method involves shunting a low-temperature coefficient resistor, R_s across the thermistor, R_t. The total value of the network is the parallel resistance of the two elements

$$R_{\text{total}} = \frac{R_s R_t}{R_s + R_t} \tag{11-7}$$

The value of R_s is the mean value (R_m) of R_t over the temperature range of interest. Suppose, for example, that you want to linearize a thermistor over the physiological temperature range (e.g., 30°C to 45°C). The value of R_m in this case, hence the value of R_s, is the thermistor resistance at a temperature of [30 + (45 − 30)/

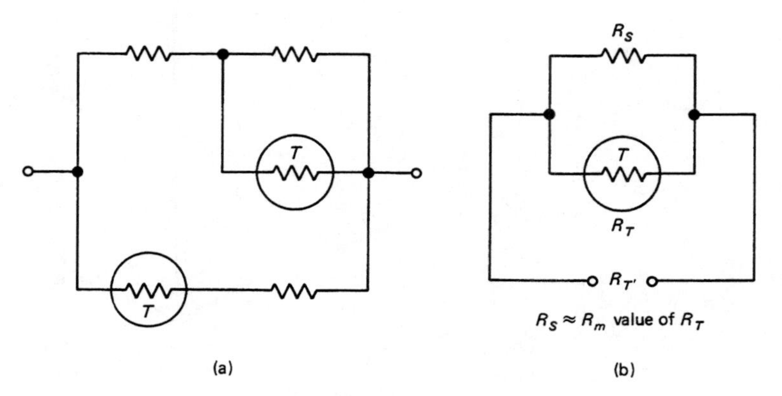

FIGURE 11-6

2]°C, or 37.5°C. Modifying Equation 11-4 gives us the expression for the value of the total resistance $R_{t'}$:

$$R_{t'} = \frac{R_m}{2}\left[1 + \frac{a}{2}(T - T_m)\right] \tag{11-8}$$

The thermistor is easy to use, and is reasonably well behaved within the temperature range for which it is rated. But when a wider temperature range is needed, especially when the temperature measurement is in a very hot environment, then the sensor of choice may well be the *thermocouple*.

THERMOCOUPLES

An example of a thermocouple is shown in Figure 11-7. This type of transducer consists of two dissimilar metals or other materials (some ceramics and semiconductors are used) that are fused together at one end. Because the *work functions* of the two materials differ, there will be a potential difference generated across the open ends whenever the junction is heated. The potential is approximately linear with changes of temperature over relatively large ranges, although over very large ranges of temperature (for any given pair of materials) nonlinearity increases markedly.

Thermocouples are typically used in twos (Figure 11-8) or even in threes. One junction will be used as the measurement thermocouple, while the other is the *cold junction*. Its name derives from the fact that some early systems required this junction to be bathed in an ice-water bath. In modern systems, a synthetic cold junction, or just room temperature, may be used for the cold junction.

There is also a third junction in the circuit, even though some texts fail to rec-

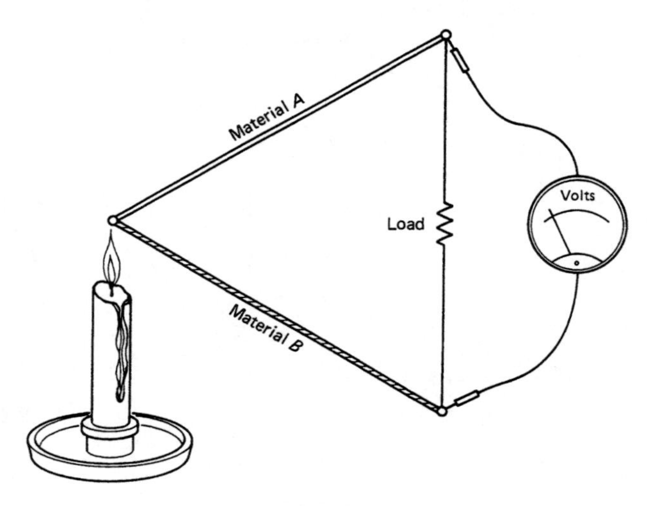

FIGURE 11-7

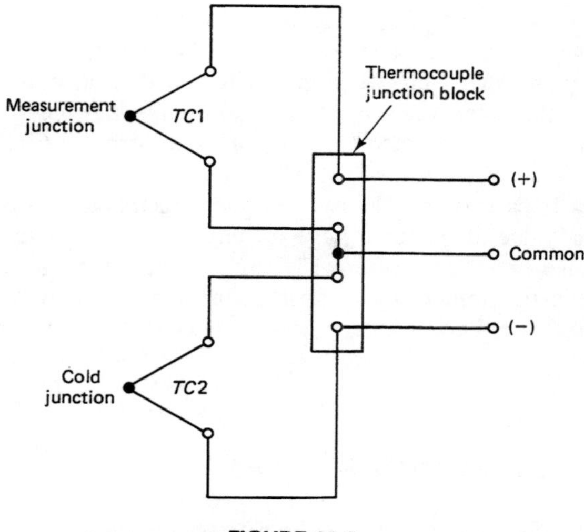

FIGURE 11-8

ognize it: the connection of the thermocouple wires to the brass or copper junction block also forms a thermocouple. These junctions should be located at a distance from the cold junction and measurement junction in order to prevent heating from the same source.

The differential voltage between the two thermocouple junctions is proportional to the temperature difference and is used as the output voltage. This potential is found from the cubic equation

$$E = a + bT + cT^2 + dT^3 \tag{11-9}$$

where

E = the output potential in volts
T = the temperature of the measurement junction
a, b, c, d = constants that are a function of the materials used in the thermocouple

Linearizing a Thermocouple

The equation governing the thermocouple demonstrates a strong nonlinear characteristic, and is, in fact, a cubic dependence of the output voltage on temperature. In some cases, an approximation of the temperature is made using just the quadratic version of the equation (cubic term deleted or approximated with an additional constant). This practice was only reasonable in days when better linearization methods were not easily available. Analog circuits to solve the quadratic equation are, after all, somewhat easier than circuits for the cubic equation. But today there is no reason to opt for the lesser of the two linearization methods.

As with other systems, there is more than one way to linearize the thermocouple. One could, for example, design a diode breakpoint generator with a cubic response, and then sum its output with the thermocouple signal. But that system is both cumbersome and subject to, of all things, thermal drift in the breakpoint generator diode circuits (this same phenomenon forms the basis for our next category of sensors—*semiconductors*.) It is also possible to use a computer or computerlike circuit for linearization. The two computer methods involve (1) a lookup table to correct the value of output voltage for any given temperature and (2) an algorithm that will solve Equation 11-9 for T given an output voltage. In both cases, the computer can be programmed with information on the specific type of thermocouple being used so that either the correct lookup table or the correct values of the coefficients of Equation 11-9 are selected.

SOLID-STATE TEMPERATURE SENSORS

The last class of temperature sensor which we will consider is the *solid-state PN junction*. If you take an ordinary solid-state rectifier diode (Figure 11-9) and connect it across an ohmmeter, then you can see the temperature effect on diodes. Note the forward-biased diode resistance at room temperature. Next, heat the diode temporarily with a lamp or soldering iron. The diode resistance drops dramatically as temperature increases.

Most temperature transducers, however, use the diode-connected bipolar transistor such as shown in Figure 11-10. We know from semiconductor theory that the

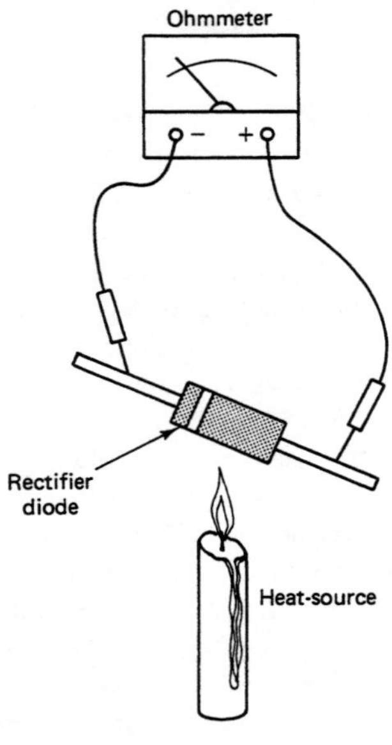

FIGURE 11-9

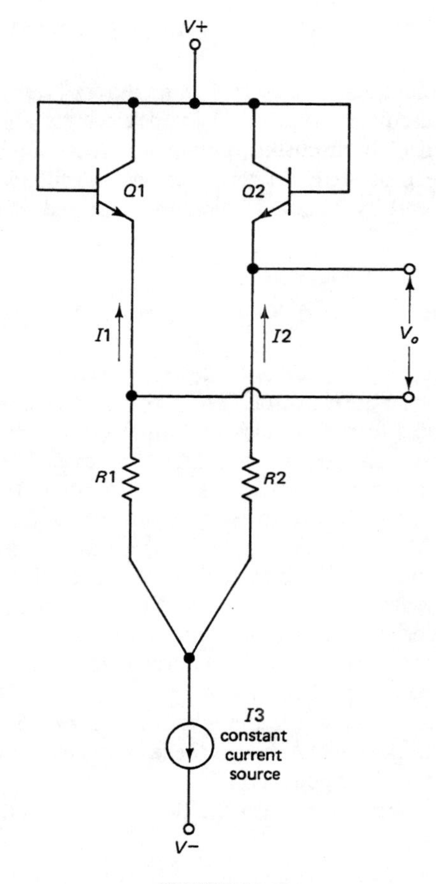

FIGURE 11-10

base-emitter voltage (V_{be}) of a bipolar transistor is proportional to temperature. For a differential pair, as in Figure 11-10, the transducer output voltage is given by

$$\Delta V_{be} = \frac{KT \ln (I_{C1}/I_{C2})}{q} \tag{11-10}$$

where

K = Boltzman's constant (1.38×10^{-23} joules/K)
T = the temperature in degrees Kelvin
q = the electronic charge (1.6×10^{-19} coulombs per electron)

The K/q ratio is constant under all circumstances and the ratio I_{C1}/I_{C2} can be held artificially constant by making I_3 a constant current source. The only variable in the equation, therefore, is temperature. In the sections following we are going to take a look at some commercial integrated circuit temperature devices based on this physical principle.

COMMERCIAL IC TEMPERATURE MEASUREMENT DEVICES

Several semiconductor device manufacturers offer temperature measurement/control integrated circuits (TMCIC). These devices are almost all based on the PN junction properties already discussed, although at least one by Analog Devices, Inc., uses an external thermocouple. In this section we will look at the semiconductor TMCIC devices offered by National Semiconductor and Analog Devices, Inc.

THE LM-335 DEVICE

The National Semiconductor LM-335 device shown in Figure 11-11 is a three-terminal temperature sensor. The two main terminals are for power (and output), while the third terminal, shown coming out the body of the "diode" symbol, is for adjustment and calibration. The LM-335 device is basically a special zener diode in which the breakdown voltage is directly proportional to the temperature, with a transfer function of close to 10 millivolts per degree Kelvin (10 mV/°K).

The LM-335 device, and its wider-range cousins, the LM-135 and LM-235 devices, operates with a bias current set by the designer. This current is not critical, but must be within the range 0.4 to 5 milliamperes. For most applications, designers seem to prefer currents in the 1-mA range.

Accuracy of the device is relatively good even without adjustment, and is more than sufficient for most control applications. The LM-135 version offers uncalibrated errors of 0.5 to 1°C, while the less costly LM-335 device offers errors of <3°C. Of course, clever design can reduce these errors even further if they are out of tolerance for some particular application.

One difference between the three devices is the operating temperature ranges, which are as follows:

DEVICE TYPE NUMBER	TEMPERATURE RANGE (CENTIGRADE)
LM-135	−55 to +150
LM-235	−40 to +125
LM-335	−10 to +100

There are two packages used for the LM-135 through LM-335 family of devices. The TO-92 is a small plastic transistor case "Z" suffix to part number, e.g., LM-335Z), while the TO-46 is the small metal can transistor package (smaller than

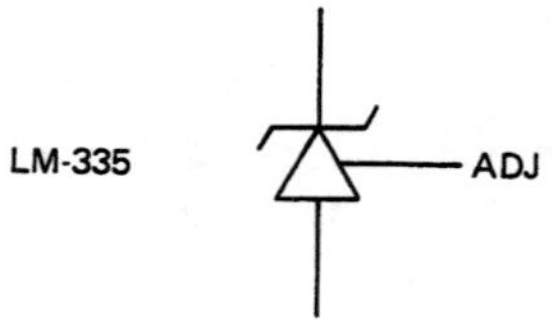

LM-335 ADJ

FIGURE 11-11

the familiar TO-5 case). This case is identified with the suffix "H" or "AH" (for example, LM-335H or LM-335AH).

The simplest, although least accurate, method of using the LM-335 device is shown in Figure 11-12A. The LM-335 is treated essentially like a temperature sensitive zener diode. The series current-limiting resistor limits the current to around 1 mA. This value of R1 (4700 ohms) is appropriate for +5-volt power supplies as might be found in digital electronic instruments. The resistor value can be scaled upward for higher values of DC potential according to Ohm's law (keeping $I = 0.001$ amperes):

$$R_{ohms} = (V+) \times 1000 \qquad (11\text{-}11)$$

For example, when the power supply voltage is +12 volts DC, the value of the resistor in series with the LM-335 is

$$R_{ohms} = (V+) \times 1000$$

$$R_{ohms} = (12 \text{ volts}) \times 1000 = 12{,}000 \text{ ohms}$$

The output signal in the circuit in Figure 11-12A is taken across the LM-335 device. This voltage has an approximate rate of 10 mV/°K. Recall from earlier that degrees Kelvin is similar to degrees Celsius, except that the zero point is at absolute zero (close to −273.16°C) rather than the freezing point of water. Using ordinary arithmetic shows us how much voltage to expect at any given temperature. For example, suppose we want to know the output voltage at 78°C. The first thing to do is convert the temperature degrees Kelvin. This neat little trick is done by adding 273.16 to the centigrade temperature:

$$°K = °C + 273.16$$

$$°K = 78°C + 273.16 = 351.16$$

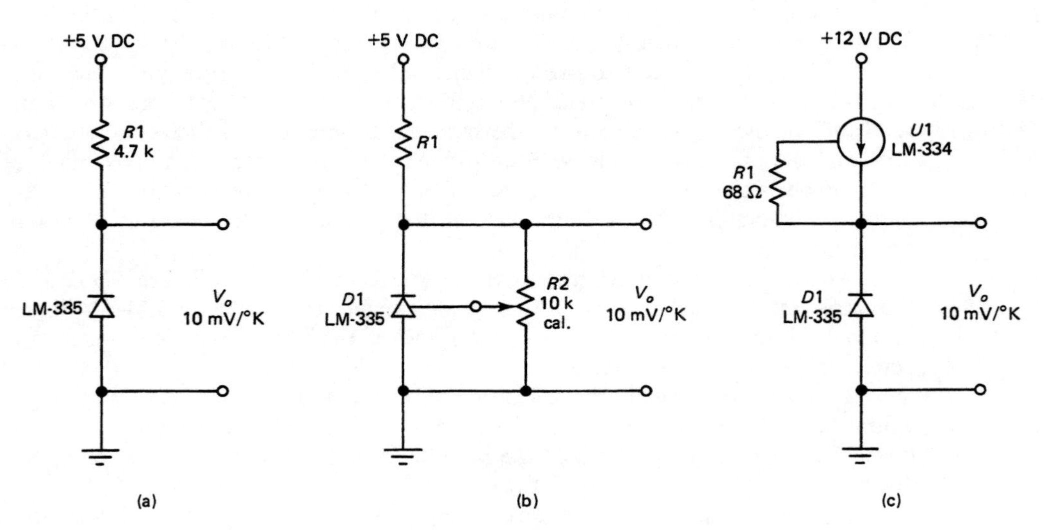

FIGURE 11-12

Next, we convert the temperature to the equivalent voltage:

$$V = \frac{10 \text{ mV}}{K} \times 351 \text{ K}$$

$$= (10 \text{ mV})(351)$$

$$= 3510 \text{ mV} = 3.51 \text{ volts}$$

One problem with the circuit of Figure 11-12A is that it is not calibrated. While that circuit works well for many applications, especially those where precision is not needed, for other cases it might be better to consider the circuit of Figure 11-12B. This circuit allows single-point calibration of the temperature. The calibration control is obtained from the 10 KΩ potentiometer in parallel with the sensor. The wiper of the potentiometer is applied to the adjustment input of the LM-335 device.

Calibration of the device is relatively simple. One only needs to know the output voltage (a DC voltmeter will suffice) and the environmental temperature in which the LM-335 exists. In some less than critical cases, one might take a regular glass mercury thermometer and measure the air temperature. Wait long enough after turning on the equipment for both the mercury thermometer and the LM-335 device to come to equilibrium. After that, adjust the potentiometer (R2) for the correct output voltage. For example, if the room temperature is 25°C (i.e., 298°K), then the output voltage will be 2.98 volts. Adjust the potentiometer for 2.98 volts under these conditions.

Another tactic is to use an ice-water bath as the calibrating source. The temperature 0°C (273.16°K) is defined as the point where water freezes, and is recognized by the fact that ice and water coexist (the ice neither melts nor freezes, it is in equilibrium). A mercury thermometer will show the actual temperature of the bath. The potentiometer is adjusted until the output voltage is 2.7316 volts.

Still another tactic is to use a warmed oil bath for the calibration. The oil is heated to a temperature somewhat above room temperature (for example, 40°C) and is stirred slowly. Again, a mercury thermometer is used to read the actual temperature, and the potentiometer is adjusted to read the correct value. The advantage of this method is that the oil bath can be a constant temperature situation. There are numerous laboratory vessels on the market that will keep water or oil at a constant preset temperature.

Another connection scheme for the LM-335 is shown in Figure 11-12C. In this variation on the theme we are using a National Semiconductor LM-334 three-terminal adjustable current source for the bias of the LM-335 device. Again, the output voltage will be 10 mV/°K.

All applications where the sensor is operated directly into its load suffers a potential problem or two, especially if the load impedance either changes or if it is lower than some limit. As a result, the buffered circuit of Figure 11-13 is sometimes justified.

A buffer amplifier is one that is used for one or both of two purposes:

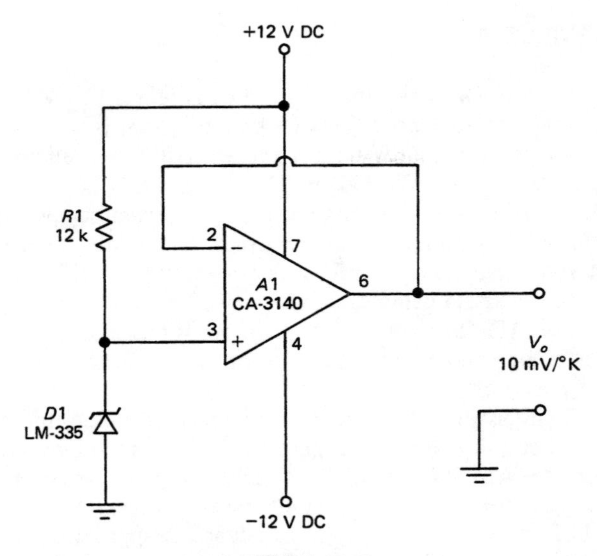

FIGURE 11-13

(1) impedance transformation or (2) isolation of the circuit from its load. The impedance transformation factor is used when the source impedance is high (not true of the LM-335). The isolation factor is somewhat more concern to us here. The operational amplifier in Figure 11-13 places an amplifier between the sensor and its load. The gain of the amplifier in this case is unity, but a higher gain could be used if desired. In that case, simply substitute one of the gain amplifier circuits shown later in this book.

The operational amplifier shown here is a GE/RCA CA-3140 device. The reason for this is simply the freedom from bias currents exhibited by the BiMOS GE/RCA operational amplifiers. The bias currents found on many other (notably BiFET) operational amplifiers could conceivably introduce error. The CA-3140 is not the only operational amplifier that will work, however. Any low-input bias current model will work nicely.

The noninverting input of the operational amplifier is connected across the LM-335. In this respect, this circuit looks somewhat like the voltage reference circuits using zener diodes seen elsewhere. The bias for the LM-335 is derived from a 12 KΩ resistor. Because there is no voltage gain in this circuit, the output voltage factor is the same as in previous designs, 10 mV/°K.

A circuit like Figure 11-13 sometimes proves useful in monitoring remote temperatures. If the operational amplifier is powered, a four-wire line is needed ($V-$, $V+$, ground, and temperature). The advantage is that the line losses are overcome by the higher output power of the operational amplifier. The LM-335 is a rugged little low-impedance device, however, and in many cases such measures would not be needed.

ANALOG DEVICES AD-590 DEVICES

The Analog Devices, Inc., AD-590 (Figure 11-14) is another form of solid-state temperature sensor. This particular device is a two-electrode sensor that operates as a current source with a characteristic of 1 microampere per degree Kelvin (1 μA/°K). The AD-590 will operate over the temperature range −55°C to +150°C. It is capable of a wide range of power supply voltages, being happy with anything in the range +4 to +30 volts DC. (This range is more than sufficient for most solid-state circuit applications.) Selected versions are available with linearity of ± 0.3°C and a calibration accuracy of ± 0.5°C.

The AD-590 comes in two different packages. There is a metal can (TO-52) that is recognized as the small-size transistor package (smaller than TO-5). There is also a plastic flat pack.

Being essentially a two-terminal current source, the AD-590 is simplicity itself in actual circuit operation. Figure 11-14 shows the most elementary calibratable circuit for the AD-590. Since it is a current source that produces a current proportional to temperature, we can convert the output to a voltage by passing it through a resistor. In Figure 11-14, the total resistance is approximately 1000 Ω, and consists of the resistance of R2 (950 Ω) and R1 (a 100-Ω potentiometer). From Ohm's law we know that 1 μA/°K converts to 1 mV/°K when passed through a 1000-Ω resistance. We can calculate the voltage output at any given temperature from this simple relationship:

$$V_o = \frac{1 \text{ mV}}{°\text{K}} \times T \qquad (11\text{-}12)$$

Thus, if we have a temperature of 37°C, which is (37 + 273) or 310°K, then the output voltage will be

$$V_o = \frac{1 \text{ mV}}{°\text{K}} \times T$$

$$= \frac{1 \text{ mV}}{°\text{K}} \times 310°\text{K} = 310 \text{ mV}$$

Potentiometer R1 is used to calibrate this system. You can make a "quick and dirty" calibration with an accurate mercury thermometer (laboratory-grade recommended) at room temperature. Connect a digital voltmeter across the output, and allow the system to come to equilibrium (should take about 10 minutes). Once the system is stable, adjust the potentiometer for the correct output voltage. For example, assume that the room temperature is 25°C, which is 77°F. This temperature converts to (273 + 25), or 298°K. The output voltage will be (1 mV × 298), or 298 millivolts (0.298 volts). Using a $3\frac{1}{2}$-digit voltmeter is sufficient to make this measurement.

In some cases it might be wise to delete the potentiometer and use a single 1000-Ω resistor in place of the network shown. There might be several reasons for this action. First, the calibration accuracy is not critical for the application at hand.

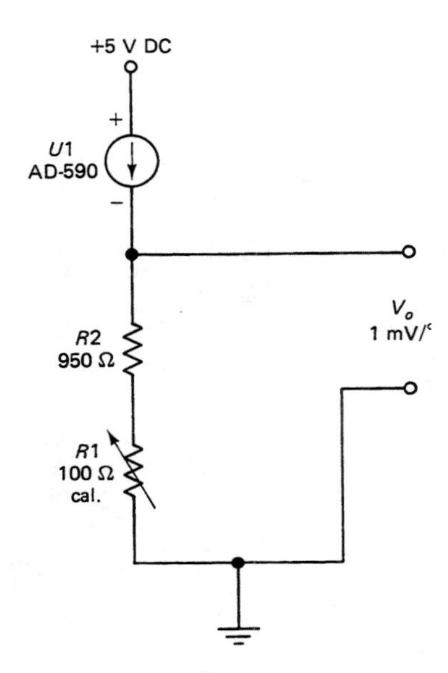

FIGURE 11-14

Second, potentiometers are points of weakness in any circuit. Being mechanical devices they are subject to stress under vibration conditions and may fail prematurely. If the temperature accuracy is not crucial, and reliability is, then consider the use of a single fixed 1 percent tolerance resistor in place of the network shown in Figure 11-14.

The circuit of Figure 11-14 is used sometimes to make a temperature alarm. By using a voltage comparator to follow the network, and biasing the comparator to the voltage that corresponds to the alarm temperature, we can create a TTL level that indicates when the temperature is over the limit. A "window comparator" will allow us to have an alarm of either under or over temperature conditions. Some electronic equipment designers use this tactic to provide an overtemperature alarm. In one application, a commercial minicomputer generated a large amount of heat (it used a 65-ampere +5-volt DC power supply!). The specification called for an air-conditioned room for housing the computer. An AD-590 device was placed inside at a critical point. If the temperature reached a certain level (45°C), then the comparator output snapped low and created an interrupt request to the computer. The computer would then sound an alarm and display an *overtemperature warning* message on the operator's CRT screen.

The circuit of Figure 11-14 suffers from a problem: it allows calibration at only one temperature, which does not allow for optimization of the circuit. We can, however, improve the situation using the two-point calibration circuit of Figure 11-15. In this case, we see an operational amplifier in the inverting follower configuration.

The *summing junction* of the amplifier (inverting input) receives two different currents. One current is the output of the AD-590 (that is, 1 μA/°K), while the

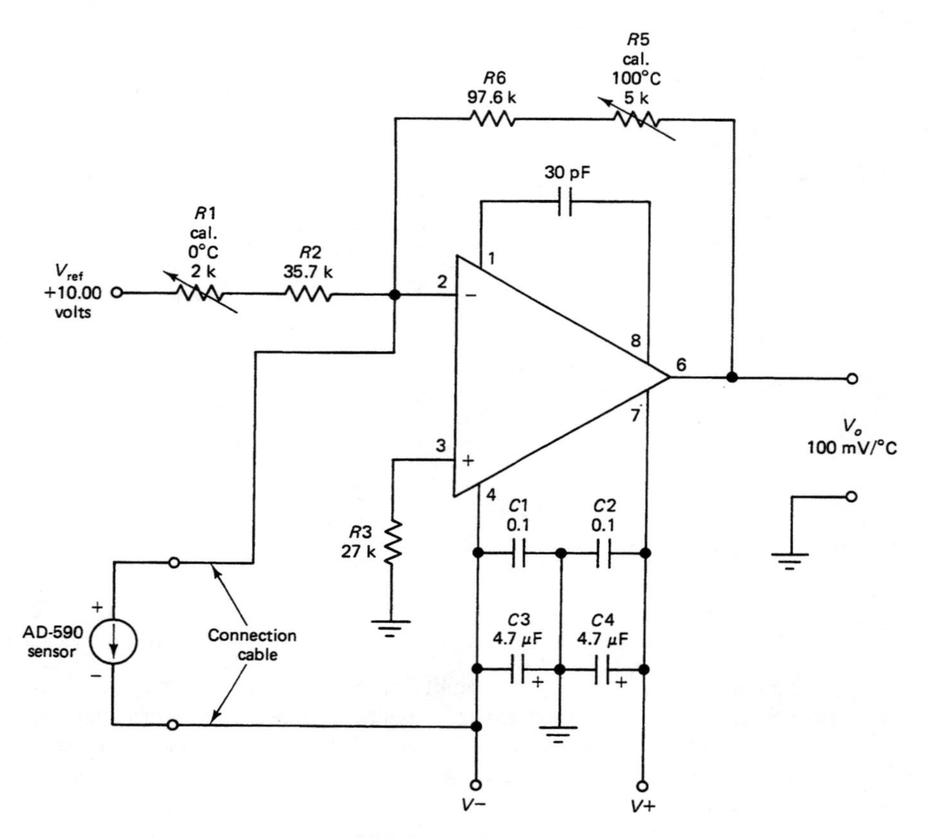

FIGURE 11-15

other current is derived from the reference voltage V_{ref} (10.000 volts). Adjustment of this current provides our zero reference adjustment, while the overall gain of the amplifier provides the full-scale adjustment.

The operational amplifier selected is the LM-301 device, although almost any premium operational amplifier will suffice. The RCA CA-3140 BiMOS device, or some of those by either Analog Devices or National Semiconductor will also work nicely. If the LM-301 or similar device is used, then be sure to use the 30-pF frequency compensation capacitor.

The $V-$ and $V+$ power supply lines are bypassed with 0.1-μF and 4.7-μF capacitor. The 0.1-μF capacitors are used for high-frequency decoupling and must be mounted as close as possible to the body of the operational amplifier. The values of these capacitors are approximate, and they may be anything from 0.1 μF to 1 μF.

Calibration of the device is simple, although two different temperature environments are required. The 0°C adjustment (R1) can be made with the sensor in an ice-water bath (as described). The upper temperature can be room temperature, provided that some means is available to measure the actual room temperature for comparison.

BIMETALLIC STRIPS

The *bimetallic strip* is an on-off temperature sensor that will allow the construction of a temperature-sensitive switch. An example of this form of temperature sensor is the water temperature sensor that plugs into the engine block of an automobile. When the water temperature reaches a certain level, the bimetallic strip closes a switch that lights up the "temp" or "hot" alarm lamp on the dashboard.

Figure 11-16A shows the construction of a bimetallic strip thermoswitch. The two metals are selected to have radically different thermal coefficients of expansion and are bonded together. When they are heated, the two pieces of metal try to expand at differing rates, so the strip is forced into a radius of curvature, R. The value of this deflection radius is

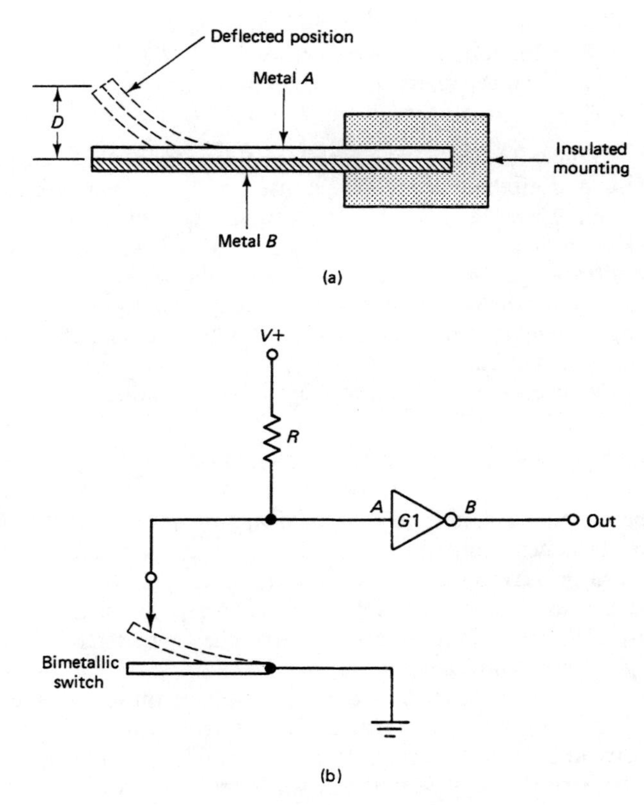

FIGURE 11-16

$$R = \frac{(t_1 + t_2)^3}{6\delta(T_2 - T_1)t_1 t_2} \tag{11-13}$$

where

R = the radius of curvature
t_1, t_2 = the thicknesses of the two metal elements in the thermal strip
$T1$ = the resting temperature before curvature begins
$T2$ = the final temperature (both $T1$ and $T2$ in degrees celsius)
δ = the difference in the thermal coefficients of expansion for the two metals

The deflection of the end, D, is found from

$$D = \frac{KTL^2}{t} \tag{11-14}$$

where

D = the deflection in inches
L = the length of the strip in inches
T = the temperature difference $T2 - T1$
t = the thickness of the strip in inches
K = a constant, typically 3×10^{-6} to 7×10^{-5}

Figure 11-16B shows a typical electronic alarm circuit based on the bimetallic strip. A digital inverter, G1, is used as the sensor electronics. The rules of this device are simple: when the input (point A) is high (near $V+$), the output (point B) is low (near ground), and when the input is low, the output is high. Under normal conditions, below the alarm threshold, the bimetallic switch is open so the input of the gate is held high by resistor R connected to the $V+$ source. Under this condition, the output of the gate is low. But when the temperature passes a critical threshold, the bimetallic switch closes, the gate input is shorted to ground so is forced to the low level—and the output snaps HIGH to indicate an overtemperature condition.

Medical Device Uses of Bimetallic Strips

The bimetallic strip is used in medicine to control temperatures and to sound alarms over or under temperature conditions, especially where the application is either non-critical or backed up by other sensors. One common application, for example, is the warmer used in certain infant incubators. The main temperature controller is a bimetallic strip thermostat not unlike the thermostat in your home, except that it might not be adjustable by the staff.

The backup in this case is a fail-safe circuit using a mercury thermometer such as Figure 11-17. The thermometer has two embedded metal electrodes that are in electrical contact with the mercury column inside the thermometer. One electrode is at the base of the glass column, while the other is at the critical temperature. If the

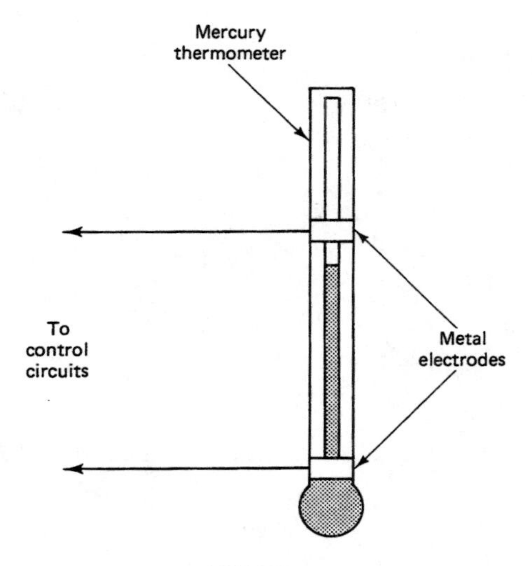

FIGURE 11-17

mercury column rises to that height, indicating a dangerous temperature situation, then the circuit between the two electrodes is closed, and this condition is sensed by external circuitry. The circuit will turn off the temperature and sound an alarm.

There was once an incubator that was designed such that the fail-safe mercury thermometer could be inadvertently damaged when the unit was cleaned or serviced. The damage was hidden from view, so the staff had no means of telling whether or not the fail-safe feature worked. At least one infant was killed because of this situation. It is, therefore, critical to test for this problem. The only way to test reasonably for the effect is to overtemperature the unit in the workshop or laboratory (*not* with a patient on board), and see if the fail-safe actually works. On the engineering level, the correct solution would have been to shield the thermometer, and to design its installation so that it was both less hazardous and more inspectable.

PREDICTIVE TEMPERATURE MEASUREMENTS

One of the disadvantages of both physical thermometers, such as the mercury variety, and some electronic thermometers is the length of time that it takes to make the measurement. The temperature inside the thermometer must come into equilibrium with the "external world" temperature being measured before the measurement is valid.

This situation is shown in Figure 11-18. Consider case 1. In this situation the patient's temperature is not very high, so the difference between room temperature (at which the thermometer was previously stabilized) and the patient temperature is small. The indicated temperature read from the thermometer rises slowly until it

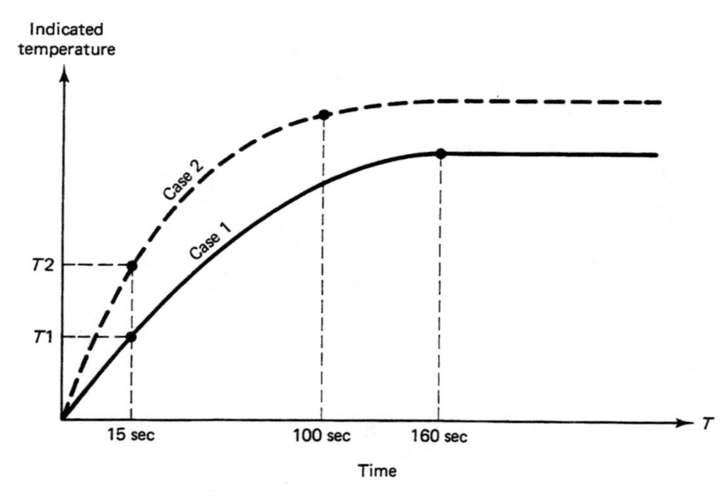

FIGURE 11-18

reaches equilibrium at about 160 seconds. Now consider case 2. There the difference temperature is much greater, so the rate of change of the indicated temperature is faster, that is, the curve rises more sharply than previously. But it still requires about 100 seconds to reach an accurate reading.

The predictive thermometer measures the rate of change of the indicated temperature over the first 15 seconds or so of the curve, and then extrapolates where the temperature will end up when it equilibrates. The method is accurate within the limits required for clinical applications if the nature of the temperature sensors is known. For this reason, one must not mix sensors and instruments from different manufacturers unless authorized to do so by the terms of the unit's warranty or other authority.

12

Medical Equipment Maintenance: Some Thoughts on Management, Facilities, and Equipment

Several alternative options exist for maintaining medical equipment. An organization such as a hospital, local government emergency medical service, or medical practice can look to several forms of maintenance repair organization (MRO) to take care of their equipment service problems. The general ground rules in this chapter assume either a commercial MRO, an in-house hospital-based MRO, or a shared service MRO. Each of these organizations has several clients (or departments served in the case of an in-house shop), served by more than two technicians. With either too few clients, or such a light work load that only one or two technicians are needed, a somewhat more ad hoc work plan insinuates itself into the picture.

Similarly, with regard to city EMS and medical practices, options are somewhat more limited because the total work load is relatively light. For them, service à la carte, or a service contract with each manufacturer, may prove both sufficient and cost effective. Alternatively, a local commercial MRO may well serve your needs. While an argument can be made that hospital in-house service can be cheaper, it is rare that a small medical organization needs such staff. However, it is not unprecedented for medical practices to use either the same outside shared services MRO as the local hospital where they have staff privileges or even the hospital's own in-house department.

TYPES OF MROS

Although the complexion of MROs varies considerably there are several important categories: manufacturer's service shops, commercial MROs, in-house hospital-based MROs, shared services MROs, in-house contractors, part-time shops, and single-employee shops. In addition, there are various levels of capability. Borrowing shamelessly from the military logistics world, we will call these levels organizational (O level), intermediate (I level), and depot (D level). The type of service program employed by any given organization should be tailored from these alternatives and may well be a blend of several. It is important for managers and administrators to understand these distinctions in order to make solid decisions on the types of organizations employed.

Levels of Capability

The concept of levels of capability is not intended to reflect on either the competence or integrity of the people involved, but rather on the design and mission of the repair organization. For example, an organization may find it worthwhile to employ a single highly skilled electronics technician in a partially management and partially technical role. Although the technician could easily perform higher-level tasks (and indeed does on some systems), logistics considerations (e.g., test equipment, spare parts) may preclude higher than O-level repairs despite the personal ability of the technician(s). The main tasks of that person would be to manage service contracts and be the decision point as to what is either beyond capability of maintenance (BCM) or beyond economic in-house repair. The person selected for this type of billet must be capable of making such decisions unemotionally. Many highly competent technical people are self-confident (and properly so), capable and action oriented. If the logistic infrastructure is not in place, however, then such enthusiasm quickly results in an overextended employee.

Consider the various levels of capability:

O level This level of capability is the most local, least expensive; it requires the smallest amount of training and support, but is also the least capable. The O-level shop, however, is not to be disdained, for it offers a "first line of defense" that can

1. Determine whether or not a fault actually exists or whether an operator error was the cause of an anomaly. One of the most common findings in medical equipment shops is no fault found (NFF). An O-level worker can reduce this finding and therefore the lost time of equipment sent for repair when none is needed.
2. Perform module or equipment substitution to bring the medical capability back on line rapidly, while the defective equipment is taken back to the shop for repair. The result is rapid return to service of the medical function involved.
3. Perform such minor technical tasks as can be trusted to on-the-job trained non-

technical personnel. For example, on most equipment nursing and paraprofessionals can perform many "repair" tasks such as stylus replacement, battery replacement, and so forth.

4. Serve as an inventory control point for management to monitor equipment that was referred to higher-level maintenance groups.
5. Keep records pertaining to equipment maintenance histories. Such records are useful in analyzing future procurement options and for defending malpractice actions based on supposedly improperly maintained equipment. In addition, the organization may find the records useful for prosecuting product liability lawsuits or regulatory actions against the manufacturers of defective equipment.

The O-level maintenance activity is almost always in-house. Higher capability levels, however, may be either in-house or out-of-house.

I level This level MRO is more highly skilled than the O-level MRO. Electronics and mechanical technicians, biomedical equipment technicians (BMETs), or even professional engineers with graduate school degrees may be employed, depending upon the scope of the MRO's mission. The I-level MRO can handle any task that can be done at O level, and more. An I-level shop is one that can

1. Test medical equipment to verify performance and adherence to specifications and safety standards.
2. Diagnose and troubleshoot equipment at least to the subassembly level. These subassemblies are sometimes called shop replaceable assemblies (SRA) and are those that can be stocked as spare parts. For example, an I-level shop should be competent (and equipped) to replace printed circuit boards, front or rear panel components or controls, DC power supplies, and bolt-on mechanical parts (motors, pumps, etc).
3. Adjust, align, or "harmonize" internal controls that are not normally available to the operator. This type of operation assumes that the I-level shop has the test equipment required to verify performance and the validity of those settings.

The I-level shop requires sufficient spare parts inventory, or a blanket purchase authority with the vendor, to assure relatively quick repair action turnaround time. It is often the case that the hospital cannot afford to have the technician go through the usual purchasing department in order to obtain parts. At least some limited trust must be placed in the person, outside the system—or be willing to accept less than rapid repairs. A component I-level technician who lacks a replacement internal assembly is not able to perform up to the level of expected capabilities. Most locally situated MROs are basically I-level shops (although a few are depot capable).

D level The depot is the highest level of repair activity. For many systems, only a major local or regional MRO will qualify. In these cases, the manufacturer's plant may be the only available depot. The D-level shop is capable of troubleshooting to the piece-part level. While the I-level shop works to a subassembly level (for example, printed circuit boards), the D-level shop can find and replace the faulty component on the subassembly (for example, the blown transistor or "microchip" that caused the problem).

It is frequently the case that D-level shops work not on equipment as a whole, but rather on the subassemblies that are sent in from I-level shops. In a typical scenario, an I-level technician will replace a printed circuit board (PCB) to bring a piece of equipment back in service. The faulty PCB is then sent to a D-level shop for detailed troubleshooting to the piece-part level.

Which Level to Employ?

A large organization that must grapple with managing a large medical technology base faces the decision as to level of shop capability required. Although there is a strong temptation to seek easy solutions, that approach is not always the best for any given organization. For example, a commercial MRO may propose taking over all equipment maintenance within the hospital. Such claims are rarely supportable by the facts.

Similarly, in-house staff, perhaps feeling threatened by the prospect of being replaced by a contractor, may also claim capability that is not supportable by facts. Rarely are the technical abilities of the employee an issue, but rather whether it is economically feasible logistically to support such a facility.

A proper management approach is to inventory the equipment that requires support, and then study the staffing and support requirements for each level of support. The decision of whether in-house support is D level, I level, O level, or none at all rests on costs versus the speed with which repairs must be performed.

TYPES OF ORGANIZATION

Earlier in this chapter several different broad categories of MRO were identified. Although that list was not intended to be exhaustive, it does serve as a guide to generic types of MRO. Let's discuss each class in turn.

Manufacturer's service department This class of MRO are those owned and operated by the manufacturer of the equipment. It may be located at the factory (usually D level) or locally (usually I level). As a general rule, the manufacturer can provide among the best and most competent service on their particular equipment. They have better information, deeper experience, and more rapid access to spare parts. However, because of certain problems the manufacturer MRO may not be the best suited for your situation.

First, there is a potential "Better is the enemy of good enough" situation—Is the "better" (if it truly exists) worth the higher cost? Manufacturer's service is usually more expensive than either in-house or commercial MRO service because the manufacturer's overhead is typically higher.

Second, the actual proximity of "local" service may make a sham out of any claims of rapid service. If the shop serves a region rather than a small locale, then response time may suffer.

Third, the promise of "local service" is sometimes met by placing a single technician in either a "desk space–only" office or the basement of his or her own home. Whether this arrangement works out depends on the size of the service area covered and the number of clients served. One company that used that form of service also used the same people to install equipment when new installations were done. As a result, the single technician in the area may be tied up on an installation and therefore unable to assist you (with your "down" coronary care unit) for several days.

Finally, the manufacturer may not have a total commitment to service. To most manufacturers the money is in sales of new systems and support products (electrodes, gel, supplies)—service is a loss center that is viewed as a "necessary evil" by the company management. In those cases the service department receives little support or resources in an effort to minimize losses. Make sure the manufacturer views service in a kindly light before committing to its service department. An indicator of the future is your experience during the warranty period when you have no choice. If it seems unwilling to meet warranty obligations, then do not trust the firm to make a sudden recovery postwarranty.

Commercial MROs These shops are commercial firms that provide service on medical equipment. Some commercial MROs provide the best solution for cost-effective management of the maintenance problem. As with any type of contractor, the desirability of entrusting work to them depends on their technical abilities, the depth of their spares inventory, and their ability to respond to customer demands. Each MRO must be evaluated on its own merits. There are, however, a few guidelines for look out for.

First, it is often the case that the marketing claims belie the actual capability of the company. Contract performance is at risk when the technical staff is not actually in place at the time of proposal. Too often commercial managers shrug off their lack of staff with the promise that staff will be hired as needed. While that flexibility may exist for low-skill–level billets, it is a pipe dream at the higher-level billets needed for many types of medical equipment service.

Second, the financial condition of the company may not be adequate to support the level of service expected. Even world-class technical staff is unable to perform well if adequate spart parts, service literature, and test equipment are not available. Both the level of technology and the prospect of product liability tend to drive up the cost of medical equipment and the supporting spares. Some electronics components companies are so fearful of product liability suits that they publish a disclaimer against use of their products in medical equipment. In most cases, the price charged for simple components destined for medical equipment, even at the original equipment manufacturer level, is huge compared with the price of the same component for general industrial products. The same problem afflicts the local service company, and increases both their own liability and the costs of the spares they sell.

Third, there is frequently an imprudent "can-do" attitude on the part of commercial MROs. Although such an attitude is often admired by action-oriented managers, it often conceals a lack of real ability to perform. The "can-do" attitude that isn't backed up with real or potential capability is a dangerous illusion.

Fourth, the smaller MRO may be insufficiently covered by liability insurance. The author has seen repairs done by inexperienced commercial MRO personnel that could have been called "malpractice." In one case, a defibrillator failed during a routine test. The fault was traced to inexcusably poor workmanship practices by the commercial MRO—and may have resulted in a death if the hospital inspector had not found it first. If that MRO lacked coverage, or the resources to self-insure, then the hospital might have had a severe liability problem.

Hospital and EMS managers are rarely equipped to evaluate the technical capability or the depth of spares inventory of any commercial MRO. However, their armamentarium is not empty if the company has a track record. Demand a list of present and past customers who can be contacted for references. Unless other peer group managers are hopeless liars, a manager should be able to elicit good information about the company's past service record. A string of lost customers, service contract nonrenewals, or dissatisfied clients is not a good indication that they can do a good job.

In-house MROs This category of MRO is owned and operated by the organization or hospital that it serves. A properly staffed and equipped department can provide competent service in an extremely short response time. Experience has shown that equipment emergencies that would otherwise affect patient care can be dealt with promptly by an in-house MRO. The author has repaired equipment in an operating room during open-heart surgery procedures. Although repair during a case is bad practice under most situations, there were several cases where the surgeon ordered it done because he believed it critical to have the instruments to bring the patient back off the heart-lung pump—and because the hospital lacked the spare equipment to back up the main system. Neither commercial MROs nor manufacturer service departments can provide that level of service.

The in-house shop can also supply "around the clock" service through the simple expedient of issuing a beeper to the on-call technician. Although other forms of MRO can also offer that service, the reality is often a bit different from the salesman's claims. For one thing, odd-hours service may be at a higher cost than normal hours service. Also, it may be a matter of dispute as to the definition of "24-hour service." In one contract, we understood "24-hour service" to mean "around the clock at any hour of the day or night." However, the company responded to our complaints of noncompliance with the suggestion that "24-hour service" meant that they had to provide the service sometime within the next 24 hours after logging in the call from the customer. Ambiguity in a contract can be devastating.

Although cost and convenience advantages are considerable, there are also some disadvantages to in-house service. A big one is the availability of properly trained I-level and D-level technical staff. It is difficult to balance the kind of salaries and benefits required to attract and hold good people with the need to contain costs. In addition, in-house shops often lack the room for career growth for the technician. As a result, the better person leaves within a short time—often disgruntled. Alternatively, the person settles down into a long term of gray mediocrity that leads to a rut that requires occasional management "attitude adjustment" actions.

Shared service MROs Equipment maintenance is an expensive proposition, especially if full I level is required on all systems (plus D level on selected systems). There are many institutions that simply cannot afford their own repair facility beyond the most basic. Even large institutions with adequate resources may find it economically desirable to share the cost of such facilities with other institutions.

A shared service is an MRO that is owned and operated by two or more cooperating institutions that are also the users of the service. In some cases, the shared service is owned by one of the institutions, but serves the others on contract. In still other cases, the shared service is a separate entity on its own, but is owned and managed by the member institutions. The shared service is a separate corporation in which the chief officers and/or directors are also officers or directors of the member institutions.

Some shared service MROs are actually more like consortiums. Each institution has its own service facility, but each group is highly specialized in the type of work it handles. For example, one group might be heavy on electronics patient monitoring equipment, while another is expert on anesthesia machines and respirators, while still another is an expert on dialysis machines. The overall capability of the consortium is greater because of nonduplicated efforts.

Shared services can be an effective and low-cost solution to the overall maintenance problem of several institutions. However, as with the other options there are some problems to solve. Perhaps one of the most difficult problems is the tendency of one institution to dominate the resources of the shared service. Usually, the majority (or most senior) member siphons off service capability that is rightfully due other members.

Another problem with shared services is the tendency to build empires. This problem especially afflicts consortiums because each hospital may want to develop local capability that would ordinarily be allocated to another shop. Perhaps most guilty of this practice are the service shop managers who see their career potential enhanced by accretion of duties, capability, and power.

If the problems can be solved, and peace maintained, then a shared service MRO can be a well-managed, low-cost solution to the equipment maintenance problem. However, the track record of shared services is spotty in this regard because of the aforementioned problems.

In-house contractor MRO This category represents a cross between the in-house concept and the commercial MRO concept. In this arrangement, a contractor will place either an entire technical and management team, or a manager who oversees hospital personnel, in the hospital to manage the in-house repair facility. Only a few of these groups exist, so little can be said about them. However, the concept has worked with housekeeping management, so should work well with medical equipment maintenance.

Part-time shop In this case, a small repair organization does medical equipment maintenance for the local hospital on a part-time or ad hoc basis. In general, it is a bad idea unless the owner of the shop (or key personnel) is familiar with the repair of biomedical equipment. In that case, it might be a good "first line of defense" for a rural or remote hospital. I recall one shop that normally repaired commercial video equipment and two-way radios and also repaired the equipment in the coronary and intensive care units of the local hospital. The nearest commercial MRO or manufacturer service shop was a six-hour drive through the Nevada desert. The manufacturer of the patient monitoring system sold the hospital a stock of spare printed wiring boards and mechanical parts and trained the local shop owner to provide a minimal I-level capability. It worked in that case, but is otherwise fraught with difficulty.

Single-technician department In some smaller hospitals a single repair technician is employed in plant operations (erroneously called "engineering" in most hospitals—even when there are no college graduate engineers employed there). If adequately supported with test equipment and spares, the properly trained technician can provide O-level or even I-level service for a limited number of in-house client departments. However, be careful to ensure the employment of an adequate technician. Many hospitals have been known to employ an electrician who thinks he knows something of electronics or some kid with an amateur radio license as the electronics technician. Insist on credentials for such an employee (a further discussion follows).

TECHNICAL PERSONNEL

One of the mysteries of medical equipment maintenance for managers and administrators is the types of technical personnel involved and their level of training. Unfortunately, too many titles are less than descriptive to the uninitiated. In addition, there are titles that are shared by different people. For example, consider the title "engineer." If you asked most medical people to define an "engineer," you would elicit images of a fellow with little education, a blue-collar plant operations uniform, and a leather tool pouch on his belt. The use of the term "engineer" by those people is illegal in some states, and only tolerated by the law in others because of long history. The title derives from the use of the word "engineer" to describe steam and boiler technicians, whose city licenses are often referred to as first-class, second-class, or third-class steam engineer. We will discuss true engineers shortly. Various levels and categories of technician are found in medical equipment maintainance. Some of them are highly specialized, while others are generalized. Several levels of education are common:

1. On-the-job or self-trained This type of person is trained as an apprentice to others and is generally capable of limited tasking. Although there are exceptions, these workers are not generally capable of more than the simplest tasks. However, certain factors are indicators of higher than elementary achievement. Included are status as a certified electronic technician (CET), certification as a biomedical equipment technician (BMET), certain other industrywide certifications, a diploma from a recognized home study school. Although often the butt of jokes, the home study route is an old, established tradition in electronics. There are a number of programs that are well regarded in the electronics industry because they turn out knowledgeable graduates.

2. Vocational technical school graduate The vocational-technical school is one in which subcollege but post–high school training is offered. Some of them offer the last year or two of high school, plus additional work that is normally beyond the high school level. These schools may be local or state government operated or commercial in nature. Unfortunately, some commercial schools are little more than mills to rip off guaranteed loan payments offered to immigrants or disadvantaged people to upgrade their economic prospects (check the reputation of the school).

The emphasis in vocational-technical training is on the practical aspects of electronics theory and differs from the higher levels in the amount and type of mathematics employed in the curriculum. These technicians can perform O-level maintenance and many I-level tasks depending upon the quality of the school.

3. Associates degree technicians The Associates degree requires two years of academic training in a community college or technical institute. The level of training is more theoretical and mathematically oriented than the vocational-technical. These graduates can handle O-level, I-level, and some D-level tasks. It is common to find bright, highly talented people in this category who prefer the technical "hands-on" type of work that requires an Associates degree, but who disdain the more paper-oriented tasks of the engineer.

4. Bachelors degree technicians At one time the Bachelor of Science degree differentiated the technician from the engineer. Today, however, there are many four-year, accredited degree programs that offer a Bachelor of Science degree in electronics technology (BSET) degree. It is perhaps fitting to refer to these people as "technologists" or something similar rather than "technicians." They can handle all tasks and indeed can often manage the shop on a professional level.

5. Biomedical equipment technicians (BMET) The title "BMET" is an indicator of certification in medical equipment maintenance. Some applicants may have earned a degree or diploma in medical equipment technology and thereon base a claim to the title. However, to avoid confusion, it is perhaps best to reserve the title BMET for those who have passed the appropriate certification examinations.

6. Engineers The true engineer is a graduate of a college or university engineering program, or a program in a related science that leads one to the same body of knowledge as engineers. The general rule is simple: no Bachelor of Science degree, no title of "engineer," unless the state government has seen fit to issue the person a professional engineer certificate. (Note: Very few "nondegree" PE certificates still exist, although a few states still allow the old method of qualification.)

It annoys engineers to be compared with, or thought of, in terms of the plant operations "engineers" because the true engineer holds one of the hardest to earn degrees the university has to offer. Indeed, a physician told the author that he switched from engineering to premed because he was not smart enough to survive the freshman year in engineering school. A common experience for engineers working in hospitals is to be looked down on or disdained by nurses with BSN degrees (or even other nurses) as somehow intellectually inferior. There is no nursing degree, even at the graduate school level, that compares in difficulty or intellectual level to even the Bachelor of Science level in engineering. Anyone who doubts that claim would do well to enroll in the first semester of engineering school to find out the truth—a typical engineering school has a 45 to 55 percent flunk-out or quit rate at the end of the freshman year. It is not uncommon for deans of engineering schools to address the incoming freshman and say: "Look at the person next to you—in June one of you will not be here—half flunk out or wisely change their major by the end of the first year."

The Bachelor of Engineering degree is the usual qualification for an engineer. Some applicants will list their degrees as BSEE (electrical engineering), BSME (mechanical engineering), BSCE (civil engineering), or BSChE (chemical engineering). In addition to these categories, there are also materials engineers, engineering mechanics degrees (which is a cross-disciplinary degree), and biomedical engineering degrees. In the latter case there is some doubt as to what curriculum was followed. It is not unusual to find that these graduates are really one of the traditional types of engineers with a little biology and a few medical instrumentation courses. For example, one friend of mine has a Bachelor of Science degree in biomedical engineering, but took only six credit hours fewer chemical engineering courses than a BSChE graduate. There are other examples of specialty engineering Bachelor of Science degrees, but in the main specialization beyond the basic traditional engineering disciplines is done in graduate school.

In some cases, graduates with degrees in science (physics particularly) or mathematics are accepted as engineers after a certain amount of relevant training and professional experience. Examples are listed here.

1. Certified Clinical Engineer (CCE) The CCE is a professional board engineering certification. It requires a level of education (B.Sc.) plus four years of relevant experience in a hospital or similar facility. Some older clinical engineers were "grandfathered" into the program on the basis of experience, but newer certificates require full compliance with the educational requirements.

2. Registered Professional Engineer (PE or RPE) This title indicates that the applicant possesses a state license to practice engineering. It is unfortunate that not all engineers are required to have a state license. In general, only those who are in private practice, who work on public projects, or who must routinely appear as an expert witness in court are required to possess an engineering license. Although some states legally limit those who may use the title "engineer" to describe themselves, there are exceptions. For example, some states exempt engineers employed in manufacturing, as junior engineers to a PE, or (in some cases) those who are employed in institutions such as academia or hospitals. There are also occupational exemptions under which railroad train drivers, crane and heavy equipment operators, and steam mechanics can call themselves "engineers." A "sanitary engineer," by the way, is not a garbage collector with a sense of humor, but rather is a speciality subset of civil engineering that designs sewage systems and water treatment plants.

The PE license is based on education, two levels of examination, plus four years of experience. The first level of examination, called the engineer in training (EIT) exam, is opened to seniors in engineering programs with 90 hours of acceptable course work completed and to all graduates of engineering programs. After four years of progressively more responsible professional experience the engineer may take the specialty examination for the type of engineering he or she is qualified to practice. While all EITs take the same exam, the PE exam is tailored to civil, electrical, mechanical, or chemical disciplines. Although not strictly required, some people feel that major hospitals ought to employ a PE, who also holds the CCE certificate, as the administrator over both biomedical engineering and plant operations.

There are a few states that allow licensing of professional engineers without a degree or with degrees other than engineering. These states call such qualification by the term "eminence." If a person demonstrates the body of knowledge required, plus a 12-year-long record of "progressively more responsible professional experience," then the board may vote to issue the license despite the lack of an engineering school degree. This method of qualification especially benefits foreign graduates whose schools are based on the European model where one "reads engineering" rather than takes specific courses. Small departments or the departments in smaller hospitals can be managed by a technician with a BSET degree or a related degree. Alternatively, with adequate training and experience less educated people will also work out well. Larger hospitals, however, should insist on filling the job of director of Biomedical Engineering Department with a graduate engineer with a certain minimum (two years) relevant experience level. While these people are hard to find, they are also professional people who are able to relate to the medical professionals they serve.

YOUR SYSTEM AFTER THE WARRANTY EXPIRES

When a system is first installed it is common practice for a warranty to be in place. If the "system" consists of a couple of modular units and a mainframe rack, then the ordinary equipment warranty is usually in effect. On the other hand, when the system is extensive the warranty may also be extensive and forms what amounts to a service contract. Regardless of the extent of either the system or the warranty (or service contract) the day may come when the owner or operator of the system must consider "going bare" and maintaining the equipment without help from vendor technical personnel. In that case, some considerations are in order.

Repair of electronic equipment is much like insurance in that many of us never consider the matter until something catastrophic happens. A little prior planning can make the difference between quick success and the discomfort (or severe impact to operations) of being off the air for weeks while the equipment makes it through the repair "pipeline."

The very first time to consider repairs is when planning the new system. Ask hard questions of the sales representative selling the system before signing the purchase contract. You want to know about the availability of a local repair shop. What "local" means varies from one situation to another, but keep in mind that a 100-mile one-way trip translates into two factors: high cost and usually slow service. Ask the representative for references of other users in your area who could testify as to the quality and responsiveness of the maintenance department (or subcontractor). These considerations form a large part of the equation in determining whether or not to do your own maintenance. If you cannot afford the cost of maintenance, or if the penalty for being down for several days while awaiting service is too large, then the matter is all but settled for you.

There may come a time when equipment must be shipped back to the manufacturer's repair shop in a distant city. The original shipping container is probably the best shipping container available to you if it has formed styrofoam inserts that take up the entire volume of the box. Take care to unpack the equipment carefully, being sure to not destroy the carton (or compromise its shipping integrity).

You think that's a bit extreme? After all, who has the room to store that large cardboard shipping crate? I called the repair shop manager for a major company. He told me that all too often improper packing results in (often hidden) shipping damage that must be repaired at the owner's expense before the warranty problem can be examined. Sometimes the shipping damage completely masks rightful warranty repairs (for example, a broken printed wiring board track).

An old cardboard carton and three inches of newspaper are not proper shipping materials! Nor is it prudent to use a single wrap of masking tape to seal the carton—equipment has been "lost in the mail" from inadequate sealing of a perfectly adequate shipping container. Use two runs of broad nylon filament tape in both directions on the carton, topped by an ample amount of plastic film tape or paper packing tape (the kind you have to dampen). Still, it is prudent to tape a card with your hospital name, the name of a person responsible for the equipment (a "point of contact"), the hospital shipping address and telephone number to the equipment—just in case. And make sure that the card is well affixed.

It is also not prudent to ship more than one item in a single container. My service manager contact told me of one unlucky owner who shipped an in-warranty radio telephone transceiver in the same substandard carton as its 26-lb, 12-volt DC, 20-ampere AC supply. That heavy power supply bounced around the newspaper-lined cardboard box like a cannonball—and smashed the transceiver to bits! Unfortunately, neither the shipper nor the manufacturer covered the repairs on grounds that the improper packing was the cause of the damage.

In general, it is wise to not ship items like external power supplies, microphones, loudspeakers, headphones, hand controller units, keyboards, and other accessories unless told to do so by the repair shop. Almost 20 years working in various repair shops left me many memories of lost customer property. If your unit is bad, then ship only the unit—keep the accessories at home; you can be assured that an authorized repair shop will have an adequate supply of accessories for testing the equipment.

Determining Whether You Really Have a Problem

In one shop where I worked our service jobs ran about 40 percent "NFF" (no fault found). That means equipment was out of service for no reason at all! The user diagnosed a fault when none existed. Eliminating the NFF takes a little common sense. Check all connections and accessories, check all switch settings, and consult the troubleshooting chart in the owner/user manual. I know it sounds dumb, but many a "probable blown fuse" complaint results from the AC power cord being disconnected from the wall socket. You might be surprised how often a "no ECG trace" complaint is traced to a broken electrode wire in the patient cable connector. In this case, try several leads.

Modern medical equipment often includes a built-in test (BIT) capability. These tests can often pinpoint a fault to the plug-in assembly level (which is great for the repair technician). In almost all cases, however, the BIT will take a more macro view and allow staff to determine whether the fault is internal or external. The decision to call the repair technician is based on the results of the BIT.

What to Fix

Although some better quality technicians loathe the very idea of not being able to repair all equipment types in every case, it is nonetheless necessary to recognize that some combination of knowledge and/or assets will put some problems "beyond capability of maintenance" (BCM). If the unit is BCM, then it needs to go to the higher-level service shop. Managers need to decide what repairs they are willing to undertake locally. Part of this decision is based on the design of the rig, while part is based on available workshop test equipment and other resources.

In general, the repair of purely mechanical problems, minor controls (for example, toggle switches or potentiometers), digital readout devices, printed wiring board (PWB), solder joint problems (ones that are visible), and DC power supply problems are well within the capability of most on-site technicians even if not well trained in the deeper aspects of electronic servicing.

If the design of your equipment is such that most assemblies are on removable PWBs, then swapping boards is also within the capability of most maintenance shops. It is common practice to keep a set of "golden cards" (i.e., known good) to aid in troubleshooting. Even in equipment covered by either internal built-in test equipment (BITE) or external automatic test equipment, there is always the possibility of ambiguity groups of PWBs that cannot be discriminated without swapping out with known good boards.

It is true that problems with electronic equipment tend to be common to a lot of individual sets within a model group. A professional repairman sees the same problems over and over, and soon develops a "sense" for the symptoms. The point in mentioning this fact is to encourage technicians to call the repair technician at the manufacturer's facility, describe the symptoms of a tough dog, and receive advice—he or she has probably seen that problem before and might be able to help you. Also ask him or her if there are any updates, retrofits, or engineering changes that he or she would normally incorporate into your unit if it were on their bench. You would probably be surprised how often manufacturers and importers update equipment returned for repair at little or no cost to the owner. Such a courtesy often eliminates future problems.

SHOP LAYOUT AND OPERATION

Efficiently maintaining or repairing medical equipment requires an efficient work environment. In this section we will examine some principles of shop layout and discuss the principles of efficient shop operation. While the main remarks apply to those readers who are in, or anticipate entering, the service business as a commercial MRO, other equipment service personnel will benefit from them also. After all, running a hospital- or fire department–based shop is essentially similar to the commercial MRO, except that remaining within budget is the driver—not the baseline profit. Service shops are sometimes very inefficient because a large amount of energy is expended, even though little real work is actually accomplished.

How is it possible that two shops in the same locality, both employing technically qualified personnel, can produce such widely different results? On the one hand, Shop A operates well, and has a healthy roster of satisfied, consistent clients. Shop B, however, barely manages to eke out a living and has unfaithful clients who rarely come back for additional work—they are too frustrated over previous work. Shop A has consistent service contract renewals, while Shop B enjoys only a few renewals. Once you reduce the problem to its bare essentials, it is often found that the difference is that Shop A is laid out and operates in a superior manner, while Shop B is laid out in a way that seems carefully planned to reduce the efficiency, work the technicians to death, and exacerbate the manager's ulcer.

A properly laid out workshop, one that reduces the steps (therefore time) needed to accomplish each job, will increase profits significantly for two reasons. One is that the physical work flow is made easier. When fewer steps are required, when it is easy to locate parts and the equipment to be serviced, then it takes less time to do each job. Less time on each job means that more jobs can be done per week, and customers receive their equipment back faster.

Second, there is a morale boost for the technicians and other workers in the shop. Efficient work flow reduces the tension and aggravation on each worker and, as a result, makes them all more productive. There is a definite psychological boost for people who work in a clean, warm, well-lighted place. Some industries in the past, and probably a few today who have not learned anything since 1920, narrowly viewed some of the amenities as too expensive. Others discovered that "sweatshop" conditions produce unhappy workers, and unhappy workers are unproductive workers. As a consequence, some companies now spend considerable sums of money in efforts to fine-tune the work environment.

Let's discuss some of the factors that enter into the creation of an efficient working environment. Part of our discussion will involve the layout of the physical plant, while part will discuss the other elements of making a shop more productive. Although some of these concepts are so basic as to appear self-evident, they are often overlooked.

Reduce wasted effort The basic goal when designing a work space layout is to maximize efficiency by minimizing wasted effort. The main way to accomplish this goal is to place the facilities inside the shop in such a way that the number of steps required to get each job done is minimized. If you think that is begging a point, then go to a camping supplies store and purchase a hiker's pedometer (a device that measures how far you walk every day). When you see just how fast the miles pile up, and remember that walking technicians are not repairing sets, then perhaps you will have the impetus to reconsider shop layout and give it a higher priority.

No book can tell you exactly what is best for your shop; there are far too many variables for that. But you really only need a few pointers, some case histories as examples, and your own native intelligence to begin thinking through your own problems. In fact, all a consultant would do is come in and make some recommendations that, on reflection, are little more than applied common sense.

Any shop layout plan is a trade-off between several competing interests, so must be considered carefully in light of your own policies, operating practices, work load, and the relative profitability of each business activity (i.e., sales, service, installation, design, construction). Several factors must be weighed and balanced:

1. *Shop floor space is terribly expensive*. The $300 a month shop is a rarity. Recent quotations in larger cities of the East Coast run from $10 per square foot per year to $50 per square foot per year. A modest 1000-square-foot shop, therefore, can cost you $10,000 to $50,000 per year (or $800 to $4200 per month). Obviously, wasted space is terribly expensive.
2. *People are expensive to employ*. If your people waste time through poor practices, bad policies, or inefficient layout, then your overhead costs will be increased by the amount of waste.
3. *Time is money*. This is an admittedly hackneyed old expression, but is as true now as ever—perhaps even more so. The major thing that a service shop has to make money on is time. If there are two technicians working on the repair of equipment, and they work a 40-hour week, then you have only 80 work-hours per week in which to make a profit. Regardless of whether you charge a flat rate for each job, an hourly charge, or work on contract repairs, it is an elementary fact that more repairs means more income. In a few moments you will read how shop policies sometimes reduce the efficiency (that is, repairs per unit of time) of the workers.

Departmentalize Consider some typical shop policies for a moment. Do technicians wait on customers? Do technicians answer the telephone? Does each technician price the finished ticket, or do they go to a supervisor, dispatcher, or control desk for pricing? Do these policies affect shop layout plans any? Yes, they surely do! Some of these policies are poor practices, but are unavoidable. In order to reduce the cost of the policy to the business, one must plan the shop layout such that these jobs involve as few steps as possible (remember that pedometer).

In smaller shops, especially, it may be necessary for the service technicians to wait on customers. In general, this is a poor practice, and should be changed as soon as the shop is large enough to support a counterperson or receptionist (depending upon the type of business). Technicians are skilled labor, and belong at the workbench or in the laboratory where their skills can earn the company some profit. Most counter work can be done by less skilled persons, and even high school students can accomplish most tasks successfully.

Let's examine the cost of using technicians at the front counter, and see if there is any way that the cost can be reduced for the shop which must use this practice. Assume that a technician is paid $14.00 per hour (which is low by current standards for experienced help). Because of overhead and other considerations, this wage translates to a cost of $30.00 to $40.00 per hour. Let's use the $30 figure to make some interesting observations. Keep in mind that $30 per hour is $0.50 a minute.

One shop used technicians to work the customer counter; no matter how simple the counter job was, a skilled, certified BMET did the job. The situation was aggravated by the fact that the service benches were at the extreme rear of the shop, and it took an average of 26 seconds to walk up to the front counter and another 26 seconds to walk back to the workbench. In other words, it took 52/60th (0.867) minutes, or $0.43 per trip to the front counter. With an average of 10 minutes waiting on each customer, the technician spent nearly 11 minutes of technical time per customer, or a cost of $5.50 per customer. If we have an average of 3 customers per hour, then we waste $16.50 per hour, or $132 per day just to wait on customers. Considered on a weekly, monthly, and yearly basis, those figures add up to $660, $2640, and $132,000.

The figures just given are admittedly hypothetical, but serve nonetheless to illustrate that poor planning policies have a profound effect on service shop profitability. The same calculations also serve for telephone time, incidentally. Using the technician to answer the telephones also costs about $0.50 per minute.

Interruptions cost more money than linear lost time Recall that $0.50 per minute is the linear time cost of interrupting a working technician. But that figure is based only on transit and waiting-on time. There is a much larger hidden cost of interrupting working technicians. It is harder to estimate, less easy to recognize, but costs you more than simply adding up lost time: lost train of thought adds to service time. Servicing complex electronic equipment is a mental activity; technicians have to think through each service problem. When they are interrupted, they forget where they were more often than not; thus they are likely to have to repeat steps or tests, or may even totally miss things that would otherwise be obvious. It is simply a fact that a technician puts out fewer jobs per day, at a higher cost per job, if he or she waits on customers or answers the telephone.

Where you must use technicians in that way, then it is essential that they be given work space that is close to the counter so that delays are minimized. Similarly, if they are to answer the telephone, then it is essential that an extension phone be within arm's reach and that the service job records be handy (most calls are requests for information on the status of jobs).

Now consider some implications of pricing and the handling of tickets after the job is finished. The key question to ask is how often technicians must leave the workbench and how far they have to walk to hand in a ticket. In many shops a supervisor prices all job tickets. Typically, the tickets are brought to the pricer or placed on a dispatcher or control desk that is usually located in either a business office or at the customer walk-in counter. A technician who has to walk up to the desk after every job is wasting time! A possible solution is to keep some tickets on the bench, or if you use a multipaged ticket just give the technician one copy (a practice borrowed from automobile dealer service shops). This way, tickets are left at the bench until there are enough there to justify a trip "up front"—or there is another pressing reason to make the trip. This matter becomes exceptionally important on low-dollar benches (e.g., warranty or contract service) or where repair time is usually short.

In one shop, technicians are assigned tickets for 2–4 hours at a time. There is an office-type "in/out" file tray at each bench with slots for finished, order parts, estimate, and to-do tickets. When the "to-do" pile is exhausted, or there is another reason to go to the control desk, then the tickets are transferred. Again, the whole idea is to reduce the number of steps taken by each employee.

Space allocations It is sometimes difficult to assess how much floor space to dedicate to each activity in your shop. Of course, if you are all service, then this matter is simplified. But in shops that do several things, then the allocation of space and other resources becomes proportionately more difficult. It is important to know the relative profitability of each shop activity. If your bookkeeping system does not separately break out income and expenses for each activity, then it may be impossible to make correct decisions on this matter. But if your books are properly divided, then you can look at them and tell which activity is paying best.

Do not be tempted into thinking of sales as only the sales floor and service as only the workbench area. Also consider the space used for new equipment or parts storage. If you are located in an area where a local distributer can resupply needs in short order, then the extra savings realized by quantity buying may well be offset by the reduced cost of using less floor space. Two factors must be considered in evaluating the desirability of using floor space for storage. One is the cost per square foot (rent plus overhead) figure, but the second (often overlooked) figure is the lost income that could be realized if the same space is occupied by a working technician.

Efficient paperwork The efficiency situation in electronic service shops is enhanced by a well-designed service record ticket. Paperwork can make or break a maintenance repair organization, so some thought must be paid to the design of the form used. Large-volume printings (5000 and up) don't cost much on a per ticket basis.

In this day of computerized everything, it is reasonable to install a personal computer and database system in which the service ticket is logged in and tracked.

The computer can replace the logbook formerly kept by the more successful shops. The ticket and the database must be keyed to show the technician where the stored equipment can be located, and any other pertinent information.

Test equipment In the ideal work space, every piece of test equipment that a service technician will normally require is right at fingertip. But in the real world we have to deal with the fact that some test equipment is both very costly and not used frequently enough to allow each technician to have a complete set. But moving equipment around can also be terribly time consuming. Solutions to this problem involve making the instruments portable, but in an integrated way.

Field technicians can use briefcase toolboxes and luggage carriers to get to their work. But those boxes need to be carefully designed to the needs of the particular MRO. Rarely is a tool-manufacturer–defined selection of tools totally adequate for real service technicians (they usually have too many useless tools, and certain items are missing). In a repair organization where the technicians are stationed at the same site with the customer activity, each technician can have a folding "clutch notebook" leatherette tool case with zipper closure and a few frequently used tools. These cases are a lot easier to carry around (underarm, not on a luggage cart) and can service up to 90 percent of the jobs. Less frequently used tools can be brought from the shop when needed.

MANAGEMENT APPROACHES

Over the years the author was associated with many maintenance or repair shops, in both technician- and engineer-level positions. In addition to practical experience in the workplace, my insights have been organized by exposure to certain modern management theories that proved themselves in a wide variety of environments.

Hospitals, and often the associated commercial vendors supplying services, are among the least well-managed enterprises in the country. Indeed, one of the many reasons for the runaway costs of health care is the fact that medical enterprises often suffer from defective management. It is the responsibility of management to find and correct causes of extra or hidden costs in order to make their enterprise more economically viable.

It is not intended here to cover all the problems in health care management, for indeed the author is not qualified to do so, but rather the problems and issues related to small-unit management are discussed. Both biomedical engineering and nursing personnel would be wise to consider some of the issues raised herein.

While one is quick to recognize the inefficiencies of medical enterprise management, one must just as quickly be certain to point out that it is not necessarily the fault of present managers and supervisors. But rather, it is the fault of the system that these people inherited and learned under. Part of the problem faced by these people is that they are professionals in other fields than management. For example, head nurses and directors of nursing are drawn from the ranks of the registered nurses, just as directors of biomedical engineering are drawn from the ranks of the engineering profession. Their training, the poorly thought out claims of the proponents of the

BSN degree notwithstanding, lacks relevance to management. Yet, there is hope, for those people tend to be high-quality individuals who care about the health of the organization—and the skills situation is easily correctible with training.

The principal technique of small-unit management in most industry, including health care, is also the most incompetent and least effective. In fact, it is counterproductive and often leads to exactly the opposite effect than that intended. One might be tempted to call this method the "drill sergeant" approach. Namely, coercion and intimidation rule the unit. Wherever this method is employed, the supervisor (and usually his or her superiors as well) operates from a set of basic premises that require elements of the following worldview:

1. People are inherently no good and lazy, and want a free ride. Any quality resulting from their efforts is merely coincidental, or the result of supervisory browbeatings. It is exemplified by a cartoon of a tabby cat pulling a piano upstairs under a whip lash: "If you whip the cat hard enough, it will pull a piano upstairs."
2. There is no pride of workmanship. That is, the lazy or incompetent worker (which includes all of them) does not want to do a good job, cannot be convinced to do a good job, and will not do a good job unless coerced.
3. A proper employee is one who keeps quiet, stays in his or her place, never makes waves, never rocks the boat, and never offers any opinion or suggestion whatsoever. "Just do the job, don't comment on it" exemplifies this view.
4. All—or at least the overwhelming majority of—problems in the unit, especially production-related issues, are the fault of workers who will not do their best.

These views are fundamentally flawed. The concept that all employees are somehow lazy is often implicitly accepted by supervisors and managers, even though considerable evidence to the contrary exists. If a set of employees seems to fit the foregoing description, then it is a sure bet that some problem in management is responsible for that morale problem. Perhaps the apparent laziness or incompetence is actually due to severe demoralization brought on by irrational, inconsistent, or insensitive management.

As to the belief that the cat will pull the piano upstairs if whipped hard enough, experience suggests exactly the opposite—the "cat" will walk out. This problem is often obscured in the medical, nursing, and medical equipment industries because, in any one locality, it is often the case that other employment opportunities in the field are lacking. Perhaps that's why so many nurses claim to "burn out" so young—they are totally demoralized by the ineffective management of their supervisors.

A key factor to research when a unit has a high turnover rate is the kinds of jobs taken by those who leave. If their new jobs are predominantly career advances, then the problem is mere attrition and no action need be taken. But if the jobs tend to be laterals, dead-ends, or otherwise not career enhancing, then that is evidence that the employees are leaving for reasons of very bad management.

The only way that any organization can remain economically viable over the long haul is to be in a state of constant improvement. This process is the job of management to stimulate, but requires the best efforts of all employees. Unfortunately, there is a tendency in management (not just in health care) to assume that employees cannot make improvements. In fact, they often believe that employee suggestions are boat rocking. There is even record of a head nurse who demanded that the personnel department select interviewees for a position who are "introverted and not the least bit innovative." That prescription is a blueprint for disaster. It is a simple fact that the person who does the job is the one who knows the most about it, and is therefore one of the principal people who should be in on solving problems.

If an organization is in such serious trouble that innovative employees are shunned or beaten into demoralization, then theirs is a boat that doesn't need freedom from boat rockers, but rather needs very much to be rocked—and hard.

One of the most destructive attitudes seen among managers is the mistaken belief that problems in a unit are due to employees not pulling hard enough. Often accompanied by exhortative slogans, this attitude demonstrates a management that does not know its business—or are unwilling to think hard about the problem. According to W. Edwards Deming, writing in *Out of the Crisis* (MIT-CAES, Cambridge, MA), the truth is exactly the opposite. In Deming's view, the overwhelming majority of problems are due to the system—which is management's responsibility—not to the employee.

As an aside, let's take a quick look at Deming. He is the master of management who is, along with a very few others, responsible for the post–World War II resurgence of Japanese industry. He taught them statistical quality control techniques (variants of which can be used by all organizations), and that approach made them the economic powerhouse that we know today. Deming is practically deified by the Japanese, and their most prestigious industrial award is called the Deming prize. It is interesting to note that Deming is an American, and that many older Japanese managers called Japanese management (which is such a popular buzzword today) "American management." Many companies in the United States once practiced statistical quality control, but we largely lost it. Deming's books, and those of his competent disciples, are well worth reading by anyone with supervisory or management aspirations.

Some of the problems seen by management specialists such as Deming include the ranking of employees in an annual (or otherwise periodic) evaluation system. These systems are essentially lotteries, for they reward and punish according to criteria that are not within the span of the individual's control.

One manifestation of the problem is the habit of some supervisors in rewarding all of those who are above average and counseling (or worse) those who are below average. What is missing in this situation is the basic understanding of the meaning of "average." After all, in every system, where the average is correctly calculated, about half the employees are above average and half will be below average. A supervisor with 100 employees will, therefore, be in the unenviable position of having to work with 50 "below-average" employees.

Of more significance is a statistical determination of whether or not the unit is working in a statistically stable manner (Deming provides the methods for doing this job in his book). The method involves measuring the performance of all individuals and plotting the data on a control chart. The performance indices might be time to repair equipment, errors made in record keeping, or, in the nursing field, medication errors. From the data, upper and lower control limits are calculated (*not* set by management—the idea is to discover how the system is working). If all of the employees fall inside the control limits, then the system is in statistical control, and is therefore stable. It might not be at a desirable stability point, but that is not something that employees can help—only management can—because the employees are given all they have to give within the context of that system.

If a system is not producing the desired results, but is in a state of stability, then something must be done to find means of improving the system—not the work effort of the employees—to make the work turn out better. The system needs something that will permit the employee to work smarter, not harder. Obviously, if the system is not in a state of stability, then the causes must also be found—and once again, that's the job of management.

If an employee falls outside the control limits, then there is a possibility of a special cause that needs attention by the supervisor. If the employee exceeds the control limits in a good direction, then that person should be observed to determine what can be learned by the rest of the staff from their method of doing things. If, on the other hand, the employee is outside the limits on the poor side, then one must find the cause. Poor eyesight? Poor training? Lack of communications? Personal problems? It is the job of the supervisor to find and correct such problems.

Problems should be solved with a view toward making the system better. One of the principal errors made here is the setting of work standards or objectives. One thing that you will reap when setting standards is that you often get exactly what you measure—and no more. Often, what you measure was selected because it is easy—not because it is somehow relevant. Let's consider some examples.

1. In maintenance shops it is common to rate employees on the number of repair jobs completed per week or the average amount of time spent to repair each unit. The measured parameter that affects the technician's pay next year (and self-esteem this year) is quantity, not quality. Thus, the technician is naturally directed to turning in completed "tickets," rather than ensuring that the hospital's equipment does what it is supposed to do.
2. In many hospitals, nurses are treated severely for medication errors—and there is no doubt that medication errors are a serious issue. One hospital fires nurses who make three medication errors in 12 months. As a result, in response to a new nurse who wanted formally to report her medication error, a supervisor was heard to say: "On this unit, we don't have medication errors!" Which is more dangerous to patients—a system in which medication errors can be freely admitted, or one where it is in the nurse's best interest to hide the truth and pray no harm comes to the patient?

In both of the preceding examples, it is the superior management technique to evaluate the work performance statistically and determine if the system is stable. If the technician does not produce enough repair jobs, then perhaps training, equipment, or spare parts supplies are at fault. Similarly, if there are a lot of errors in medication, then perhaps there needs to be an evaluation of the system to determine how it can be tweaked to overcome the potential for error.

OVERCONTROL

Overcontrol is the last problem which we will address at this time. It is the habit of many supervisors to monitor closely, and frequently tweak, employee performance. An example of this is seen in word processing or data entry departments where computers automatically record the number of keystrokes made per minute. Rather than having the desired effect, which is improvement of employee performance, these data and their use actually breed resentment and poorer performance. Keystrokes up, errors up too.

Another insidious form of overcontrol is the habit of some supervisors who make rules or take general disciplinary action on the entire unit for the sins and problems of a few—or even one. Poor managers think that every special problem that arises needs a new regulation. Of course, the new regulation will seem to work for a while, but it is soon ignored. When confronted with special problems, the supervisor needs to evaluate the situation in order to discern whether the problem is systematic or is singular. It never seems to occur to some people that happenings are often not systematic (the only kind that succumb to general rules), but rather are either random happenings or single-point failures that may never happen again. In the absence of evidence of a wider cause, any generalized action taken will probably be counterproductive and is definitely little more than wheel spinning.

13

Respiration Monitors and Apnea Alarms

There are several ways to measure respiration signals on humans. Some of them are capable of rendering quantitative measures of flow volume and rate, while others only yield information about the existence of the flow and the respiration rate. The latter information occurs because the human respiration is pulsatile, and that fact can be used to form the basis of a pneumotachometer and alarm system. The simple "existence" form of respiration measurement device is used in clinical medicine to monitor patients, especially infants, under situations where it might be difficult or inconvenient to use visual techniques.

Figure 13-1A shows a schematic diagram for the *impedance pneumograph,* while an equivalent circuit is shown in Figure 13-1B. The method is based on the fact that the AC impedance across the human chest varies a small amount as the lungs inflate and deflate during breathing. The change of impedance, ΔR, is tiny but sufficient for our purposes.

A low-voltage (100-mV p-p or less) 50- to 500-KHz (200-KHz being common) excitation is applied to the chest through a pair of 100-KΩ matched precision (0.1 percent) resistors. A differential AC amplifier (drift stabilized and optimized for the excitation frequency) receives the signal from chest electrodes. In most cases, the same electrodes as used in lead I ECG recordings can do double duty as respiration monitoring sites. The output of the AC amplifier, which signal contains the respiration signal, and a sample of the 200-KHz oscillator are fed to a synchronous detector that extracts the respiration waveform. Because of the distortions in the system, no

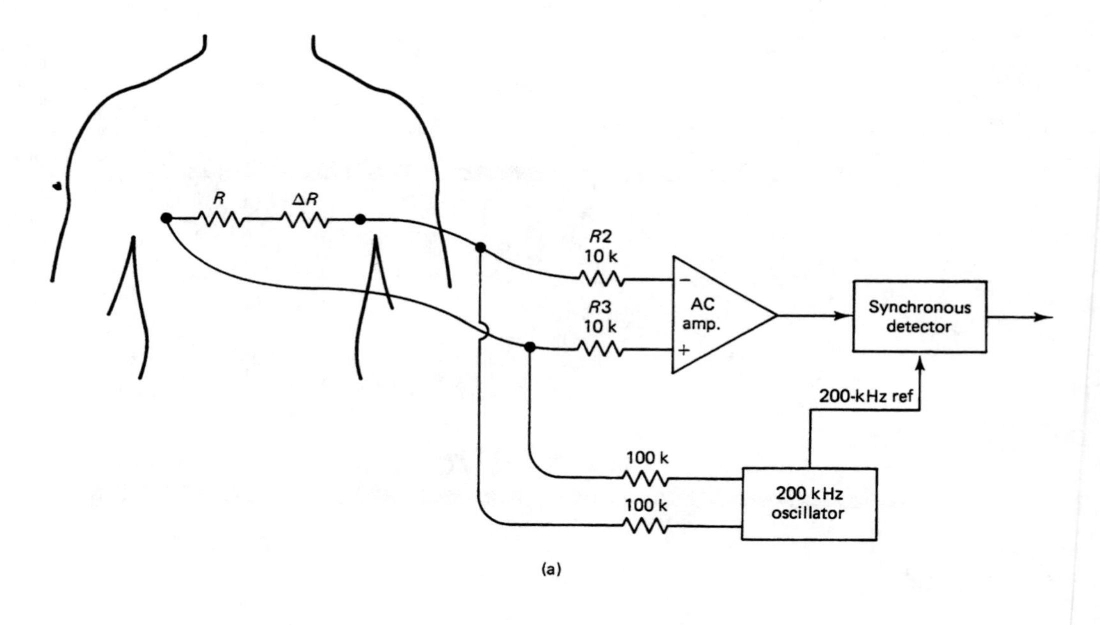

(a)

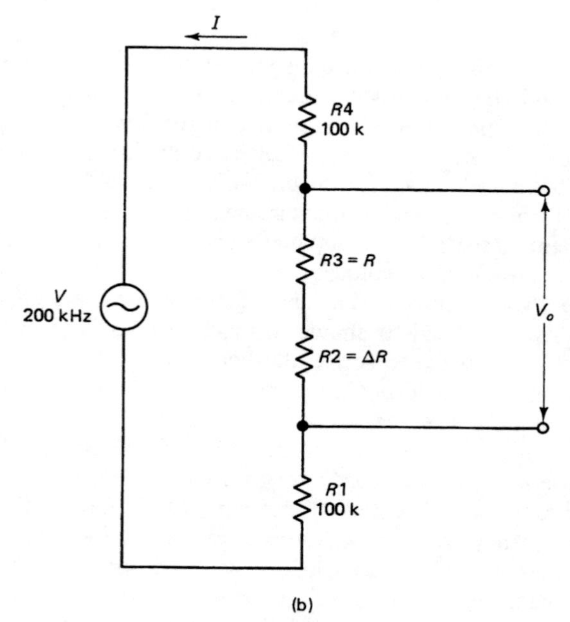

(b)

FIGURE 13-1

data other than respiration rate (breaths per second) are retrievable from this method.

You can infer from Figure 13-1B how this instrument works. R1 and R4 are the isolation resistors (each 100 KΩs); resistor R is the chest impedance at rest (lungs empty), and ΔR is the change of value of R as the patient inspires air. The output voltage, V_o, is determined by either of the following methods:

$$V_o = I(R + \Delta R)$$

or

$$V_o = \frac{(V)(R + \Delta R)}{(\mathrm{R1} + \mathrm{R4} + R + \Delta R)}$$

Assuming an amplifier input impedance high enough to make R2 and R3 too small to need consideration, either of the given expressions will yield the respiration signal. If this signal is integrated using pulse counting techniques, we have a respiration monitor, also called an *apnea monitor*. Although these instruments are commonly called "apnea" monitors, they measure chest movement, not true apnea. The FDA does not prefer the term "apnea monitor" since it conveys a sense of capability that is not actually present. Nonetheless, the respiration monitoring method shown is a valuable means for acquiring respiration rate data.

FLOW MEASUREMENTS

The measurement of flow is the art of determining how much fluid or gaseous material is passing through a given pathway. We might be measuring blood in an artery, respiratory gases into and out of a ventilator tube, the amount of water passing though a pipe, or any of a number of other similar situations.

Flow can be either turbulent or smooth. The measurement of turbulent flow is notoriously difficult, and until modern chaos theory (a new science) arose, it was even difficult to characterize theoretically. Therefore, we will concern ourselves with the measurement of clinically significant laminar-style (or nearly so) airflow situations. Fortunately, most of our transducers have inertia, so tend to integrate out small variations due to turbulence. Not so, however, with ultrasonic systems, which are covered elsewhere in this book. In those systems, the transducer should be designed to minimize introduced turbulence.

Flow Volume versus Flow Rate

Most transducers (but not all) measure *flow rate,* that is, the amount of material passing a point per unit of time. For example, a popular medical respiratory flow meter measures the patient's inspiration or expiration in *liters per minute* (l/min). Similarly, a certain fluid transducer measures fluid flow in cubic centimeters per second (cc/s). (Note: Some such transducers measure in milliliters per second—ml/s—which is the same thing. For water, at standardized temperature and pressure, 1 cc = 1 ml by definition). The definitions for gas and fluid flow rates are similar.

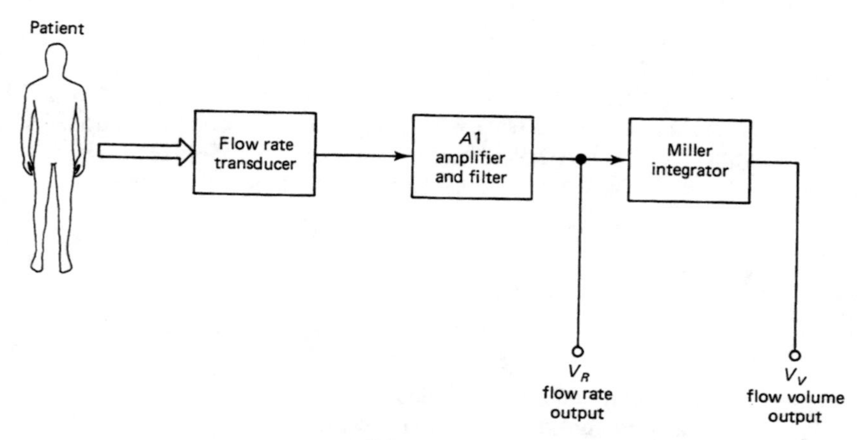

FIGURE 13-2

We can obtain the *flow volume* from flow rate data by the simple expedient of *integrating the flow signal,* as in Figure 13-2. The output of the flow transducer is amplified (and possibly further processed) in amplifier A1. The output of A1 is proportional to the flow rate. This same signal is applied to an integrator. Although an operational amplifier Miller integrator is shown here, it is likely that modern computerized systems would contain the integration as a software algorithm.

FLOW DETECTORS

A flow detector is a circuit that informs the operator of the presence of flow, but does not necessarily quantify either the flow rate or the flow volume. Two such systems are shown in Figure 13-3. In Figure 13-3A we see a *thermistor bridge* flow detector. Two thermistors, RT1 and RT2, are placed inside of the flow container. In this particular case shown, the container is a tee-connector used in a respirator pneumatic hookup. The idea here was to detect whether or not air was getting to the patient; "how much" was less important because this transducer was a simplified alarm scheme. Thermistor RT1 is placed in the airstream, while RT2 is in a dead space off the main flow; it makes the ambient measurement.

The two thermistors in Figure 13-3A are connected in an ordinary Wheatstone bridge circuit. When R1/RT2 = R2/RT1, the output voltage V_o is zero (R3 balances inequalities, and is adjusted for $V_o = 0$ when no air is flowing in the tube). The $(V+)$ voltage biases the thermistors to the point of self-heating (but not greater). At this point, the thermistor resistance is the most sensitive to small changes in airflow, which cools the surface of the device. When airflow changes the device resistance, the output voltage will be

$$V_o = (V+) \times \left(\frac{RT2}{R1 + RT2} - \frac{RT1}{R2 + RT1}\right)$$

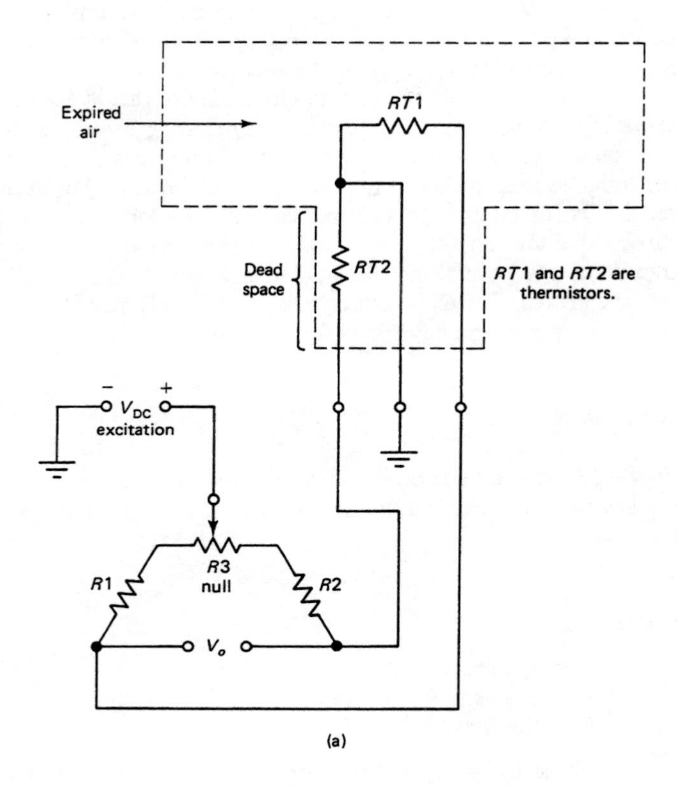

(a)

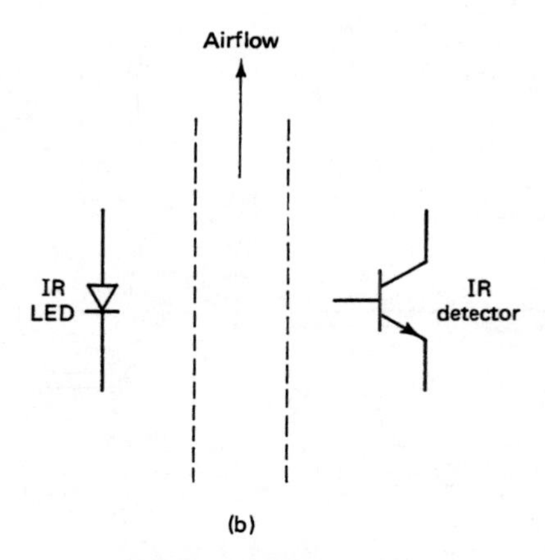

(b)

FIGURE 13-3

The output voltage is proportional to the temperature change caused by the flowing air. While it is not impossible to calibrate this temperature change over a narrow range of flow rates, it is too difficult to consider in most applications. There are better suited transducers on the market.

Figure 13-3B shows a photooptical device that is used to detect flow. Here we see a light source (an LED in this case) shining across the flow path to a detector (phototransistor in this case). Either the fluid or gas must be opaque to the light, or the light frequency chosen for maximum attenuation. For example, ordinary visable red LEDs (or other light sources) can be used for an opaque liquid. For a gas like carbon dioxide, on the other hand, we can appeal to the fact that CO_2 absorbs infrared energy. By making the light source and the detector IR sensitive, we can detect the presence of CO_2. Other gases and liquids may absorb other wavelengths, so each system must be developed for its own capabilities.

OTHER SYSTEMS

Figure 13-4 shows a common form of flow rate transducer. An obstruction placed in the gas path will create a pressure drop that is proportional to the square root of the flow rate:

$$P_d = K\sqrt{F}$$

where

P_d = the pressure drop
K = a sensitivity constant
F = the flow rate

In some transducers, the obstruction is a narrowing of the path at a point. In

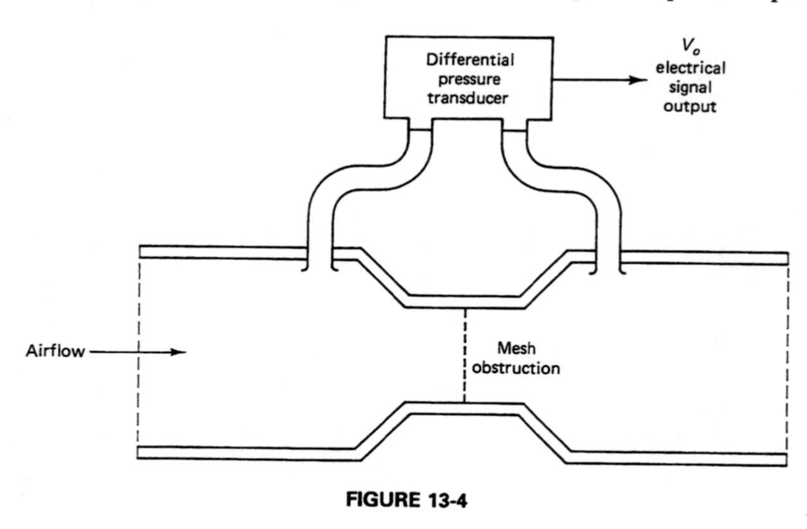

FIGURE 13-4

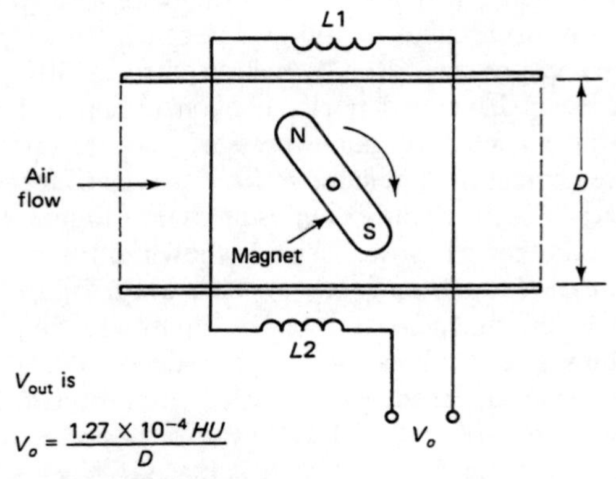

V_{out} is

$$V_o = \frac{1.27 \times 10^{-4} HU}{D}$$

V_o = Output voltage
D = Airway diameter in inches
H = Magnetic field in gauss
U = Flow in cubic antimeters per second

(a)

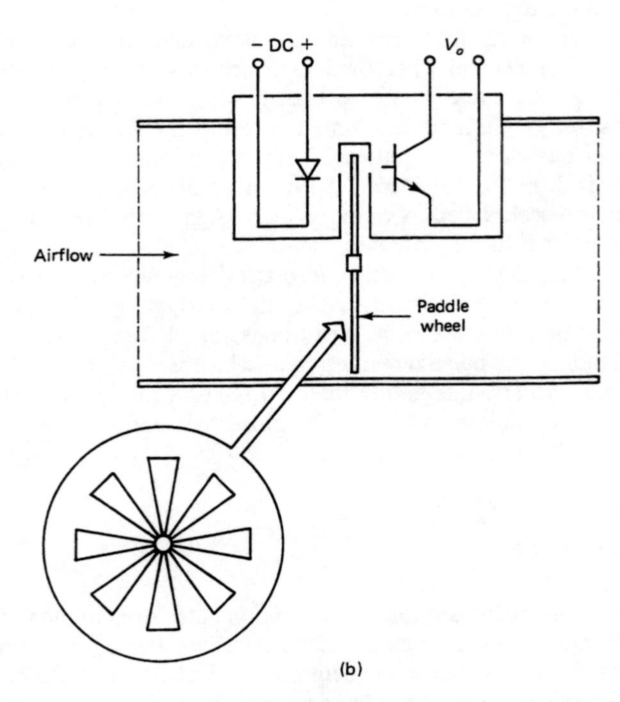

(b)

FIGURE 13-5

others, including most medical transducers, the obstruction is a wire or plastic cloth mesh stretched across a constant diameter airway. The usual mesh for medical respiratory measurements is 400 grid per inch.

The pressure drop is measured by a differential pressure transducer. These transducers have two ports, one on either side of the diaphragm. Most pressure transducers measure gauge pressure, so are open on one side to the atmosphere. Those devices are not suitable for this type of measurement. We need, instead, a differential pressure transducer as shown in Figure 13-4.

Another gas flow system is shown in Figure 13-5. Two versions are presented; Figure 13-5A is a magnetic system, while Figure 13-5B is optical.

In the magnetic transducer, Figure 13-5A, a small magnet is introduced into the flow stream. This form of transducer is used for both liquids and gases and is also usable in closed systems where it is difficult to introduce other forms of transducer. A pair of coils, L1 and L2, are placed at right angles to the flow path, at the point where the magnetic rotor is placed. When a moving magnetic field cuts across the turns of a coil, a current is introduced into the coil. Thus, a voltage, V_o, is found at the output of the series-aiding connected coils. The amplitude of the voltage is proportional to the magnetic field, while its frequency is proportional to the rotational frequency of the magnet. The rotational frequency of the magnet is related to the flow rate. Transducers of this type are used in a wide variety of medical instrumentation applications.

Figure 13-5B shows an optical version. An optointerrupter is a device that places an LED and a phototransistor across an open path. When the path is blinded, then the phototransistor is darkened; when the path is not blinded, then the phototransistor is illuminated. Similar interrupters are used in applications such as the "paper out" sensor in computer printers, type sensors in recorders, and others. The light path in the transducer of Figure 13-5B is interrupted by a multibladed fan or paddle wheel placed in the flow path. Again, the frequency of the output signal is proportional to the flow rate.

With the right circuitry, a rotating flow rate transducer can also produce a flow volume signal. By using the AC signal to trigger a one-shot multivibrator, we obtain a pulse train of pulses that are of constant duration and constant amplitude; the only variation is the pulse repetition rate (which is equal to the AC signal frequency from the transducer). Integrating these pulses produces a DC voltage that is proportional to the total area under all of the pulses per unit of time—in other words the flow volume (that is, integral of rate).

ALARM CIRCUITS

One of the main uses for the respiration detector is to monitor patients in emergency medical and intensive care situations. There are several forms of alarm circuit used in these circuits. Some of them are the same sort of alarm used on other forms of monitor, so will not be discussed again here. But there is a common form of alarm circuit used in medical respiration monitors that deserves separate treatment.

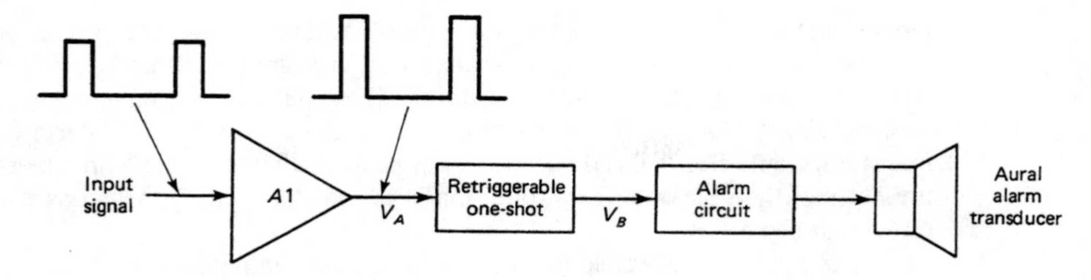

FIGURE 13-6

The transducer shown earlier in Figure 13-3A is derived from an alarm used in the expiration line of a respirator. A particular problem existed in some respirators when the patient was on intermittent mandatory ventilation (IMV). The patient might be weaned to the point of one mandatory breath per minute. If he or she stopped breathing immediately after the last IMV, then it would be one full minute before being ventilated again. The McCullough alarm was placed in the expiration line because all expirations—mandatory or voluntary—caused pulsatile flow in that line. Therefore, regardless of whether the patient breathed or the respirator breathed for him or her, a pulsatile flow existed in the line. The problem was to alert the staff to a cessation of breathing between IMV pulses.

Figure 13-6 shows a simplified version of the circuit used in this alarm. The three main stages are a *voltage comparator* (A1), a *retriggerable one-shot* (i.e.,

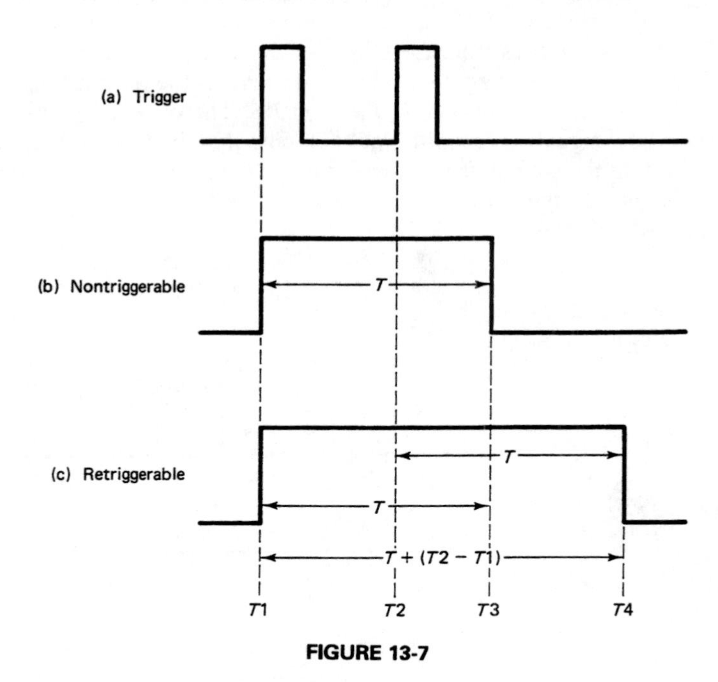

FIGURE 13-7

monostable multivibrator), and an *alarm circuit*. The voltage comparator is used to produce nice, square output signals when triggered by the rather sloppy respiration signal that one expects from the transducer. These pulses are used to trigger the one-shot circuit. As long as the one-shot circuit remains "in time" the alarm circuit remains dormant. But if the duration of the pause between expired breaths exceeds a preset time, then the one-shot "times out" and the alarm circuit responds with an audio output alarm.

The operation of retriggerable and nonretriggerable one-shots can be seen in Figure 13-7. By definition, a one-shot will produce an output pulse of fixed duration T when a trigger input signal (Figure 13-7A) is received. In the nonretriggerable circuit (which is the usual type seen), the one-shot will not accept further input pulses until the period is completed. Figure 13-7B is the output response of the nonretriggerable one-shot circuit. At time $T1$ a trigger pulse is received, so the output of the non-retriggerable one-shot snaps high. It will remain high until time $T3$ when period T has expired. But note that a second trigger pulse is received at time $T2$. The nonretriggerable one-shot ignores this pulses—it cannot be retriggered again until after T expires at time $T3$.

Now note the response of the retriggerable one-shot in Figure 13-7C. In this case, the first trigger pulse is received at time $T1$, so the output snaps high with the intention of remaining high from $T1$ to $T3$, that is, for the period T. Again, a second trigger pulse is received at $T2$. In the retriggerable version, the circuit fires again for a second period T. Thus, the circuit output will remain high from $T1$ to $T4$, or a total of T plus the expired term of the first period $(T2 - T1)$.

The application of the retriggerable one-shot to the alarm circuit is shown in Figure 13-8. Pulses from the output of the voltage comparator (refer back to Figure 13-6) become the trigger signal, V_A. As long as the patient breathes regularly, there will be a series of pulses $T1$, $T2$, and $T3$. The one-shot continues to retrigger, so the output signal V_B remains high. But note that the pulse expected at $T4$ is missing, indicating the patient ceased breathing. The one-shot now "times out," so the output drops low. In the alarm circuit this action will trigger an aural alarm signal to alert the medical staff.

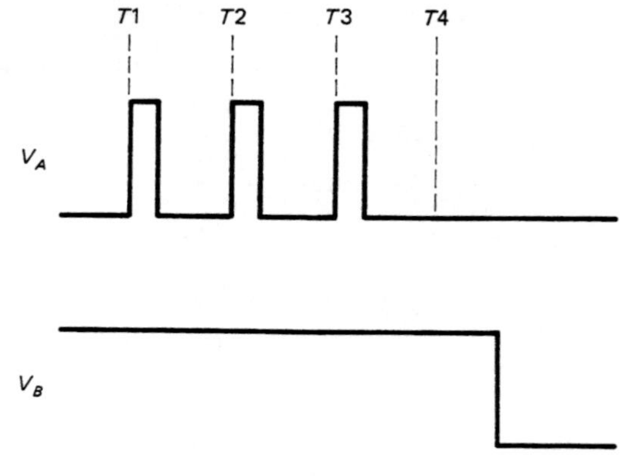

FIGURE 13-8

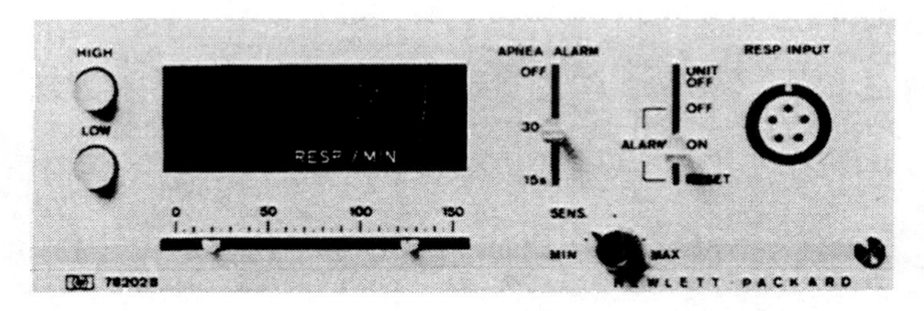

FIGURE 13-9

Figure 13-9 shows a typical medical respiration monitor. This particular model is a Hewlett-Packard 78202B and is a plug-in for a mainframe. It contains a digital output reading in respirations per minute, high and low settable alarms, and a series of controls that allow the operator to custom-tailor the alarm situation.

NEONATAL APNEA ALARMS

Sudden infant death syndrome (SIDS) is a terrifying possibility for many young families. Some newborn infants for some reason seem to stop breathing, and will die unless someone revives them. In some cases, merely being aware of the problem and picking the infant up and handling it will cause the breathing to restart. At one time, the parents of the potential SIDS child were unable to monitor breathing without being physically present all of the time throughout sleep periods. But a new form of instrument was designed about a decade ago, and it will monitor the infant's breathing.

Some infant apnea alarms were based on the impedance pneumograph described earlier in this chapter. But a new design (Figure 13-10) used an inflatable cuff around the infant's body. The pressure inside the cuff will vary slightly as the baby breathes, and these variations can be used to excite an electronic alarm.

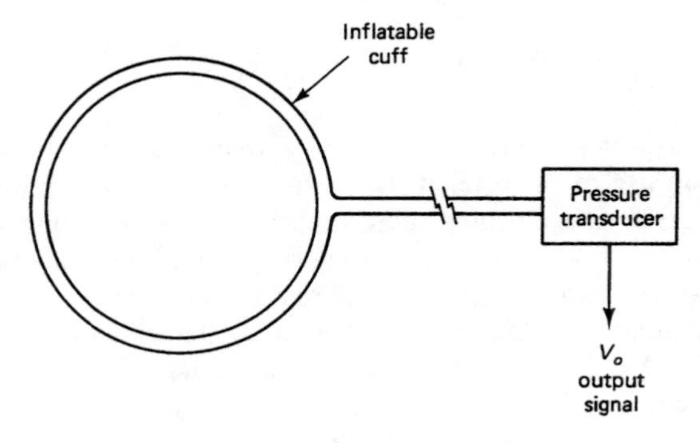

FIGURE 13-10

14

Patient Telemetry Systems

Telemetry systems are special cases of patient monitor systems (see Chapter 8) in which the monitoring is done from a remote location. There are two basic forms of telemetry system: *radio telemetry* and *landline telemetry*. The radio form uses a small radio transmitter attached to the patient that picks up electrocardiograph (ECG), or some other electrophysical parameter, and transmits it via radio waves to a central monitoring point. The landline form of telemetry uses an audio tone to represent the analog ECG or other signal and then transmits over telephone lines. In this chapter we will take a look at both forms and discuss some of the problems and parameters that pertain to designing and troubleshooting such systems.

RADIO TELEMETRY SYSTEMS

Many hospitals used radio telemetry systems to monitor certain patients. The most common use of radio telemetry is to keep track of improving cardiac patients while at the same time keeping them ambulatory. These units are sometimes called *post-coronary care units* (PCCU), *step-down CCU,* or some other name that indicates a less rigorous monitoring and care regime than the full coronary care unit where new heart patients are treated. The telemetry unit is sort of a "halfway house" between the full-up CCU and either the general medical floor patient population or discharge to home care.

The telemetry unit uses a tiny cigarette pack–sized VHF or UHF radio transmitter that is attached to the patient either by a belt clip or in a small sack hung around the patient's neck. The transmitter contains an analog ECG section that acquires the signal and uses it to frequency modulate (FM) the radio transmitter. The nurse's station is equipped with a bank of radio receivers tuned to the same frequencies as the various transmitters. The receiver demodulates the FM signal to recover the analog ECG waveform. The waveform is then displayed on an oscilloscope and/or strip-chart recorder as in any other patient monitoring system. The signal may also be input to a computerized monitoring system (indeed, today it probably will be so processed).

It is common practice to use either specialized frequencies set aside by the Federal Communications Commission (FCC) for medical telemetry use or television channel frequencies. It is not unusual for a telemetry transmitter to operate in the quietest "guard band" between the video carrier and sound carrier on TV channels. These VHF and UHF frequency selections allow the telemetry system designer to use hardware that was originally designed for the master antenna TV (MATV) or cable TV industries to process signals for the medical system.

Figure 14-1 shows the block diagram of a typical analog patient telemetry system. Several patients (A, B, and C) are wearing the miniature transmitters that pick up and then transmit the ECG waveform over a VHF or UHF frequency. In each case, a radio receiver picks up and demodulates the signal, recovering the analog waveform. This waveform is output to an oscilloscope display and a pulse rate meter. The pulse rate meter will also have a high rate ("tachycardia") alarm and a low rate ("bradycardia") alarm built in. In addition, the analog signal is also sent through a patient selector switch to a strip-chart recorder that can provide a "hard copy" of the waveform for the nurses and doctors who care for the patient.

Some telemetry systems are now using an analog-to-digital (A/D) converter inside the transmitter to digitize the analog ECG waveform prior to transmission. The transmitter then sends out a series of tones that represents the ones and zeros of the binary numbers system recognized by the computer.

A practical analog telemetry system is shown in Figure 14-2A. The corridors around the nurses' station is set aside for use of ambulatory patients. However, there are defined limits of the patient's permitted zone of travel. Some hospitals paint the walls of the permissible area a different color than the walls beyond the zone. Alternatively, some hospitals paint a stripe on the wall of the permissible area. Still other hospitals make no modifications of the paint scheme at all, but rather depend on telling the patient where to stop walking, or rely on a prominent landmark such as a fire door or elevator area. The nurses' station is located so that the entire area can be kept under surveillance all of the time in case a patient gets into trouble.

The transmitters carried by the patient are very low power, on the order of a few milliwatts at best. Therefore, it is possible for the signal levels to be too low for the receiver, even though the permissible area of travel is not extensive. As a result, a series of small whip antennas are placed at strategic locations throughout the unit. These antennas usually hang from the false ceiling (Figure 14-2B) in a manner that does not interfere with pedestrian traffic in the corridor.

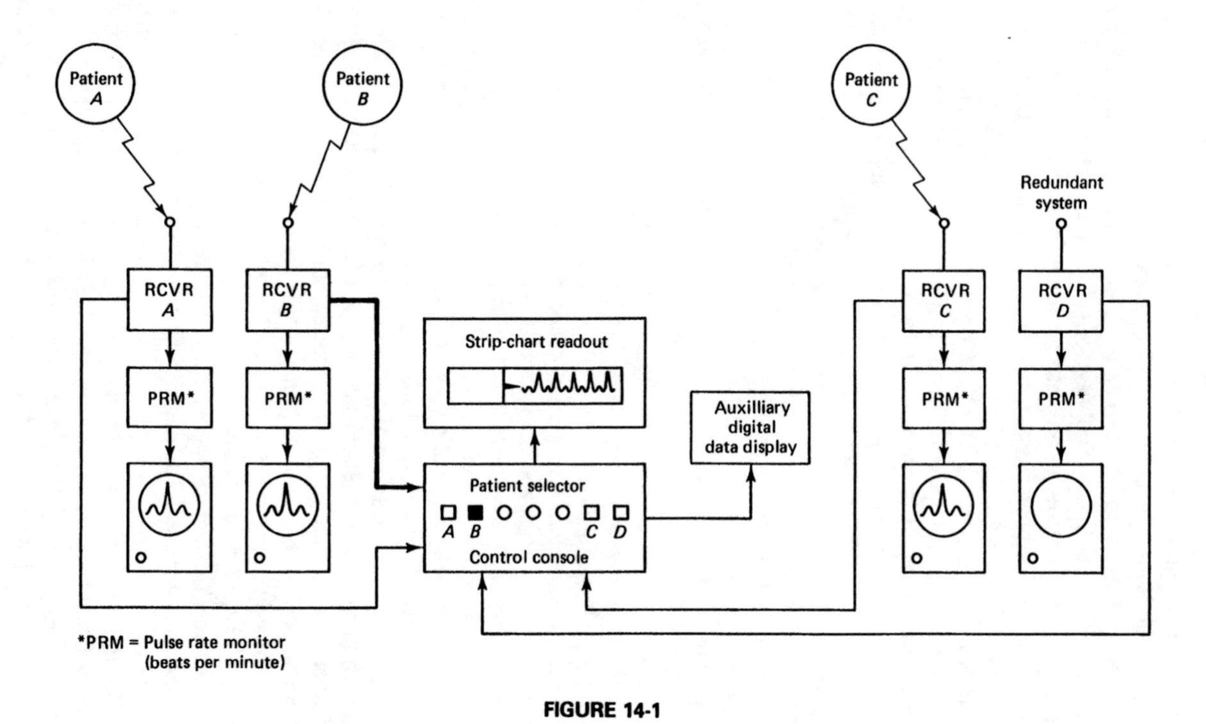
Patient A
Patient B
Patient C
Redundant system
RCVR A
RCVR B
RCVR C
RCVR D
PRM*
PRM*
PRM*
PRM*
Strip-chart readout
Auxilliary digital data display
Patient selector
A B C D
Control console
*PRM = Pulse rate monitor (beats per minute)

FIGURE 14-1

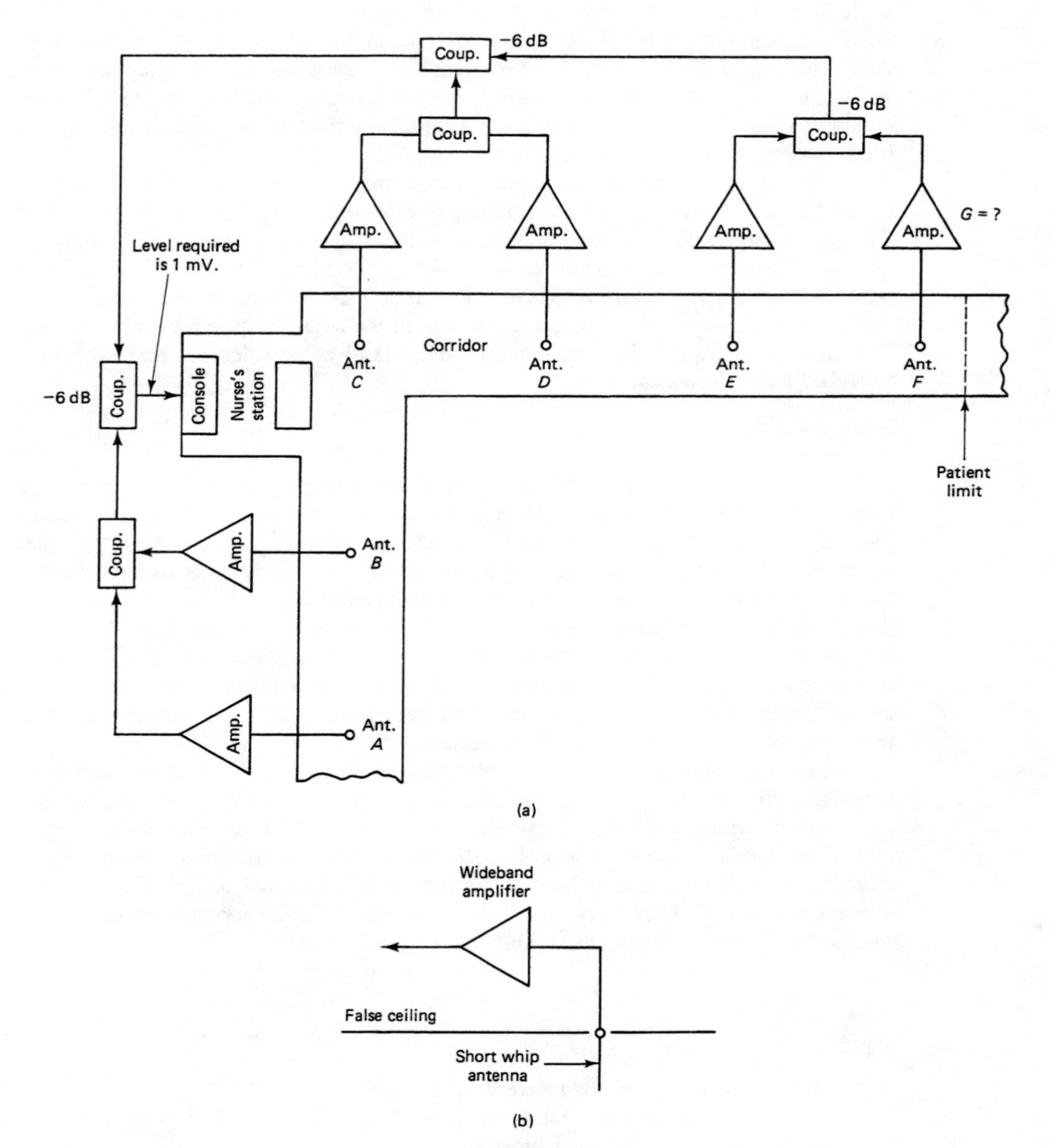

Coup.
−6 dB
Coup.
−6 dB
Coup.
Amp.
Amp.
Amp.
Amp.
G = ?
Level required
is 1 mV.
Corridor
Ant.
C
Ant.
D
Ant.
E
Ant.
F
−6 dB
Coup.
Console
Nurse's
station
Patient
limit
Coup.
Amp.
Ant.
B
Amp.
Ant.
A
(a)
Wideband
amplifier
False ceiling
Short whip
antenna
(b)

FIGURE 14-2

Even with several antennas in place, however, the losses in the system added to the low power of the original signal conspire to prevent adequate reception. As a result, booster amplifiers (labeled "Amp." in Figure 14-2A) are placed at each antenna site. Gains up to 60 dB are required. The amplifiers are usually selected from MATV and cable TV equipment. These amplifiers are wideband, so therefore cover the entire VHF, UHF, or VHF/UHF television spectrums. Some models offer selectable voltage gain, so are able to accommodate tailoring the gains to account for differing signal levels and loss situations.

The outputs of the various amplifiers are mixed together linearly in standard VHF/UHF two-set or multiset TV couplers (designated "Coup." in Figure 14-2A). It is commonplace to find ordinary television receiver system couplers used in this application. These devices are passive, and so will offer a loss of −2 to −9 dB. System losses consist of the radiation loss between the transmitter and the nearest antenna, the losses of the various coupler, and the loss in the coaxial cable transmission line. The cable loss is dependent on the type of coaxial cable selected, and can reach 6 dB/100 feet in low-cost types.

System Design

System design requires the signal levels to be anticipated, and the losses overcome by either the sensitivity of the receiver or the gain of the wideband amplifier used to boost signals from the antennas. One can assume certain levels and design to that standard. Alternatively, one can also make practical measurements using a sample transmitter supplied by the manufacturer. The signal levels at various points in the permitted ambulatory area are measured using a television antenna or cable field strength meter (FSM). These instruments are now relatively common in TV and cable service organizations, so can easily be obtained. The continuously tunable types are preferable over the strictly channelized models because the telemetry channels might not fall exactly on the standard television channel.

Once the signal level in microvolts or millivolts is determined, it should be converted to decibel notation. In master antenna or cable work the system impedance is typically 75 Ω, as opposed to the standard 50 Ω used in other RF systems. The standard reference level is designed 0 dBmv. In this system of measurement, the zero decibel voltage level is taken to be 1 millivolt (1 mV or 1000 μV) developed across a 75 Ω resistive load. All other signal levels are referenced to this standard using the following equation:

$$\text{dBmv} = 20 \log \left(\frac{V}{1 \text{ mV}}\right) \tag{14-1}$$

where

dBmv = voltage decibels referenced to 1 mV
V = the signal level being measured
log = the base 10 logarithms

Example

A VHF signal on a frequency of 174.125 MHz measures 50 μV across a 75-Ω resistive load. Calculate the level in dBmv.

Solution:

a. Convert to millivolts:

$$50\ \mu V \times \frac{1\ mV}{1000\ \mu V} = 0.05\ mV$$

b. Calculate dBmv:

$$\text{dBmv} = 20 \log \left(\frac{V}{1\ mV}\right)$$

$$= 20 \log \left(\frac{0.05\ mV}{1\ mV}\right)$$

$$= (20)(-1.3) = -26.02\ \text{dBmv}$$

Design of the system at the hospital level is a matter of adding up the losses and gains in order to present the required signal level to the input of the receiver. Let's assume that the receiver in Figure 14-2A needs to see 0 dBmv (which is 1 mV or 1000 μV) to produce proper, full quieting, analog demodulation. Antenna F is located near the end of the corridor where patients are permitted, and normally receives a signal level of 50 μV or −26.02 dBmv. There are three lossy two-set couplers ($L_c = -6$ dB) in the system. There is also a total of 100 feet of coaxial cable in the system ($L_a = 4.5$ dB). Calculate the gain (G) required of the amplifier (Amp.) in order to input 1000 μV to the receiver antenna connector reliably. The operant equation is

$$S_{req} = S_{ant} + G - L_c - L_a \tag{14-2}$$

Or plugging in the values,

$$0\ \text{dBmv} = -26.02\ \text{dB} + G - (3 \times 6\ \text{dB}) - 4.5\ \text{dB}$$

Solving for G,

$$G = (0 + 26.02 + 18.0 + 4.5)\ \text{dB}$$

$$= 48.52\ \text{dB}$$

In the system discussed here the normal losses and signal levels required in excess of 48 dB of gain in the amplifier (Amp.) colocated with the whip antenna.

Normally, the gain of the amplifier will be set higher than this figure in order to account for aging losses and failures in the system. For example, one of the failure modes of antenna couplers is to increase the signal loss while not completely eliminating the signal. Such losses might be accommodated by a well-designed system.

Another consideration in designing a system is the selection of operating frequencies. In some cases, the manufacturer will not allow selection of operating frequencies, but in others there are enough options to custom-tailor the selection of frequencies for a given unit. There are two basic considerations in this matter: *interference* and *intermodulation problems*.

Interference is an obvious problem. If there is a strong local transmitter operating on a proposed frequency, then it is unlikely that the weak ECG transmitter will "break through" the noise even when the transmission distance is short. For example, when the telemetry transmitter frequencies are in the guard bands of the television channels, it may be prudent to select frequencies of channels that are inactive in your local area. In other cases, the transmitter frequencies are not on TV channels, but rather on designated spots used for telemetry. Unfortunately, some of these channels are multiuse, so there might be another form of transmitter on the same frequency.

These comments are for cochannel interference, that is, interference from other transmitters operating on the same frequency. But there is also a problem with adjacent channel interference. A radio receiver, such as used in telemetry systems, does not accept only single frequencies. Rather, it picks up a small band of frequencies surrounding the designated frequency. The width of that band is called, appropriately enough, the *bandwidth* of the receiver. If a signal on an adjacent channel is strong enough, then it will also be accepted by the receiver if it is within the passband of the receiver.

Intermodulation is a form of interference that can be quite perplexing because it is generated by frequencies that seemingly bear little or no relationship to the receiver frequency. The intermodulation occurs when a nonlinear mixing element heterodynes two or more frequencies together to produce one or more additional frequencies. The frequencies produced follow the rule

$$F_{out} = mF1 \pm nF2 \tag{14-3}$$

where

F_{out} = the product frequency
$F1$ = the frequency of the first signal
$F2$ = the frequency of the second signal
m, n = integers representing harmonics of $F1$ and $F2$.

The typical system will produce at least the sum and difference of $F1$ and $F2$. In some systems, however, there may be multiple harmonics (that is, several values of m and n) or several frequencies present in the system. Those systems become very complex.

Example

Calculate the output frequencies of a nonlinear system in which a 174.15-MHz signal is mixed with the third harmonic of an 88.5-MHz FM broadcast signal.

Solution:

a. First frequency (sum):

$$\begin{aligned} F_{out1} &= mF1 + nF2 \\ &= (174.15 \text{ MHz}) + [(3)(88.5 \text{ MHz})] \\ &= (174.15 \text{ MHz}) + (265.5 \text{ MHz}) = 439.65 \text{ MHz} \end{aligned}$$

b. Second frequency (difference):

$$F_{out2} = (265.5 \text{ MHz}) - (174.15 \text{ MHz}) = 91.35 \text{ MHz}$$

In this case, a pair of frequencies (174.15 MHz and 265.5 MHz) are heterodyned together to produce a sum frequency (439.65 MHz) and a difference frequency (91.35 MHz). If either of these frequencies is your telemetry channel, then the modulation of the interfering FM broadcast station will override the weak ECG signal.

And how is this possible? After all, all we have to do is design the system to be linear, isn't it? That's a good start, but it is not sufficient. An amplifier or receiver can be overloaded by the outside signal, even if the signal is supposedly outside the passband of the receiver. This situation is especially likely to affect the wideband amplifiers used in the antenna system. If a strong external signal is present, then it may overload the amplifier and drive it into a nonlinear region of operation—creating multitudinous harmonics.

Interfering signals that generate intermodulation problems can come from surprising sources. Once, when the author was working as a bioelectronics technician at a major university medical center, a particularly annoying intermodulation problem was found. It turned out the the local oscillator inside of an FM radio receiver was causing interference that resulted in an intermodulation problem. The result was that a patient's ECG waveform was appearing on the wrong channel on the oscilloscope and in the computer. The radio had been placed on the receiver cabinet by a night nurse who wanted some easy listening entertainment while she worked the "graveyard shift" (bad choice of words). The antenna of the FM receiver was only inches from one of the whip antennas for the telemetry system. Because the radio is both unshielded and lacks a totally unilateral RF amplifier in the front end, the local oscillator signal inside the radio was radiated directly into the telemetry receiver antenna! As a result, the hospital director of bioelectronics engineering banned FM receivers in the nursing unit where telemetry was used.

Another potential source of "extra" signals is amateur "ham" radio operators, citizens band enthusiasts, and others who own and use portable radio transmitters. Some of these operate on frequencies that can "intermod" into the telemetry channel.

In some locations the only hope for solving severe intermodulation problems is to use a spectrum analyzer to locate potentially offending frequencies. Special computer programs, which are actually quite simple, will predict the effect of these signals on the proposed telemetry frequencies. Some consultants can perform a site survey and make recommendations on the most desirable frequencies from those that are available.

TRANSMITTER/RECEIVER DESIGNS

Two major design philosophies are found in standard, single-channel medical telemetry links. These approaches can be classified according to the modulation type and are usually designated *direct FM* (or simply *FM*) and *FM/FM* (frequency modulation, or FM, is used almost exclusively—only a few low-cost research systems use AM).

Direct-FM Systems Figure 14-3 shows the block diagrams for the transmitter (Figure 14-3A) and receiver (Figure 14-3B) used in typical direct-FM telemetry sys-

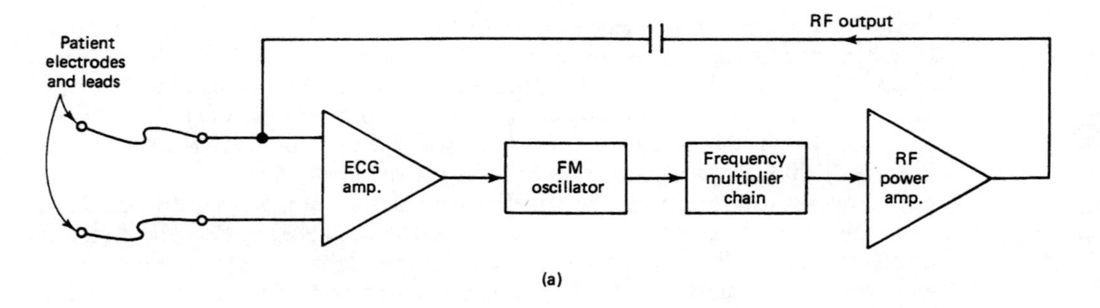

(a)

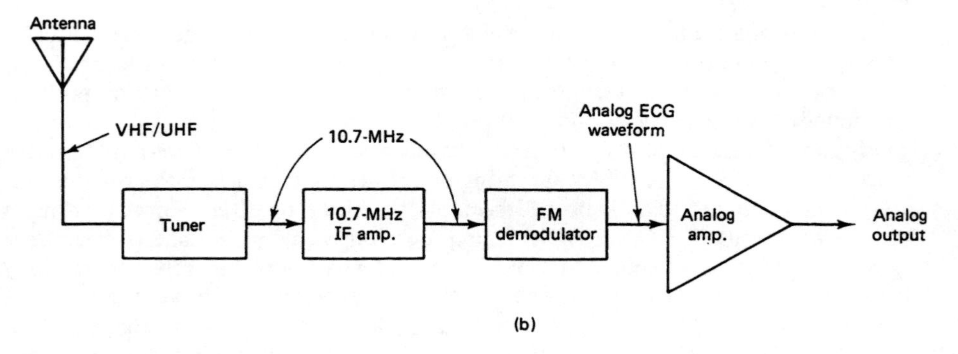

(b)

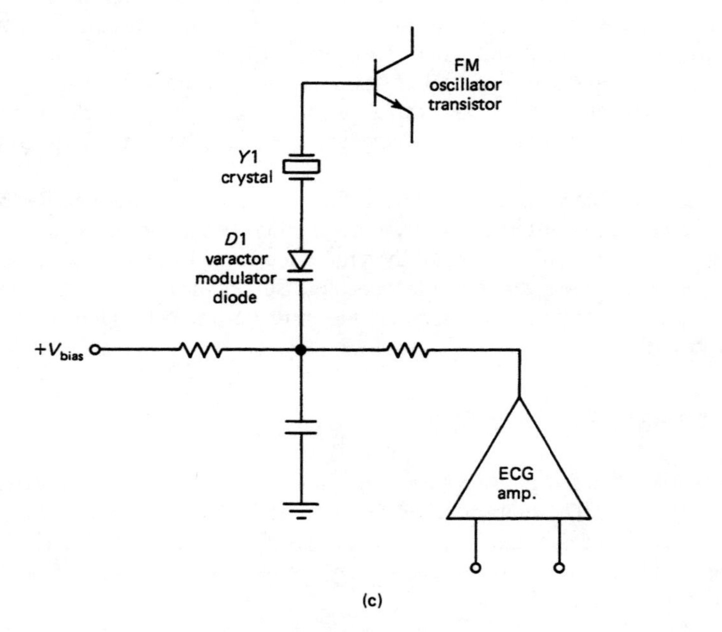

(c)

FIGURE 14-3

tems. The stages shown here are *ECG amplifier, FM oscillator, frequency multiplier chain,* and *RF power amplifier*.

The patient's ECG signal is a 1-mV or less analog signal with a bandwidth of 0.05 Hz to 100 Hz for diagnostic purposes and 0.05 Hz to 40 Hz or so for monitoring systems (the reduced bandwidth reduces muscle artifact, but increases the probability that important features will be missed). In telemetry systems, the monitoring standard is typically used.

The ECG amplifier boosts the 1-mV, or so, signal to a level between 0.5 volts and 3 volts for application to the FM oscillator stage. As a result, this amplifier will have a gain of 500 to 3000 depending upon the design of the system. It has differential inputs in order to accommodate the standard ECG lead I or lead II configuration.

An FM transmitter does not transmit on a strictly fixed frequency, but rather the frequency of the transmitter varies as a function of the amplitude and frequency of the modulating signal (in this case, the ECG waveform). When no modulating signal is present, the frequency of the FM oscillator remains constant at a center value F_o, also called the *unmodulated carrier frequency*. But when the modulating signal is applied, the RF signal deviates from this value. The amplitude of the modulating signal determines how far the signal deviates from the carrier frequency, while the frequency of the modulating signal determines the rate at which the signal deviates.

On positive excursions of the modulating signal, the carrier frequency will shift upband an amount ΔF (read "delta F") to a new frequency $F_h = F_o + \Delta F$. The term ΔF is proportional to the amplitude of the applied modulating signal. Similarly, on negative excursions of the modulating signal, the carrier deviates to a new frequency $F_L = F_o - \Delta F'$. In a perfectly symmetrical direct-FM transmitter, the two ΔF terms have an equal magnitude for equal amplitude but opposite polarity signal voltage levels:

$$|\Delta F| = |\Delta F'| \tag{14.4}$$

The *deviation* rating of the transmitter is the magnitude of either ΔF term (assuming symmetry), while the total *frequency swing* is the maximum excursion from F_L to F_h, or $2\Delta F$.

In Figure 14-3A the carrier frequency and deviation is determined by the *FM oscillator* stage. This oscillator usually operates on a frequency that is a subharmonic of the actual assigned output carrier frequency. The *frequency multiplier* stage (or stages) increase the operating frequency and deviation in integer ratios. For example, if the oscillator frequency is 30 MHz, and the multiplier is a tripler stage, then the output frequency is 3×30 MHz, or 90 MHz. The deviation is similarly multiplied. If the original deviation is 6 KHz, then the output signal deviation from the tripler will be 3×6 KHz, or 18 KHz.

In most modern telemetry transmitters, the FM oscillator is a crystal-controlled stage. The crystal frequency is a subharmonic of the operating frequency (determined by the ratio of the frequency multiplier stages) and sets the channel that the transmitter operates on. Figure 14-3C shows the basic scheme used in some transmitters for modulating the normally fixed crystal frequency. The operating frequency of most crystals is set by the physical dimensions, the location on the original quartz crystal from which the resonator was obtained, and the *circuit capacitance*. It is this last feature that makes it easy to produce a small FM transmitter with a stable crystal oscillator.

The modulating element in Figure 14-3C is *varactor diode* D1. This form of diode is also called a *voltage variable capacitance diode* because, when reverse biased, acts like a capacitor in which the capacitance is a function of the applied reverse bias voltage. If the ECG signal from the ECG amplifier stage causes this reverse bias to vary, then the effect is to change the diode capacitance as a function of the ECG signal amplitude. The result is therefore to change the frequency of oscillation of the crystal proportionally to the ECG signal amplitude.

Another form of FM transmitter that is essentially interchangeable with the direct-FM type shown in Figure 14-3A is the *phase modulation* type. In those transmitters, the crystal oscillator frequency remains fixed. The output of the oscillator is applied to a stage called a *reactance modulator* that alters the phase of the carrier signal an amount that is proportional to the modulating signal amplitude. For all practical purposes, the FM and PM types of transmitter are interchangeable, and the same receiver will process both. Both FM and PM are forms of *angular modulation*.

The RF power amplifier stage is used to boost the output power to the operating level. Because of the very low power levels involved, this stage actually functions as a final frequency multiplier (usually a doubler) and a *buffer amplifier* that isolates the circuitry from the external world.

Because the RF power amplifier uses a tuned output circuit, which is often a frequency multiplier condition, care must be used on tuning the stage. Unfortunately, this task is not like the related task of "tuning up" a regular radio transmitter because of the low RF power level involved. The RF wattmeter instruments normally used for that application are insufficient for the job. As a result, the standard method for tuning these transmitters is to view the output signal on either a tunable field strength meter (similar to that used in making site surveys for new installations) or (preferably) a spectrum analyzer. The analyzer should be set to show the second and third harmonics of the operating frequency, especially if the final RF amplifier is a frequency multiplier stage. The effect of tuning is to maximize the RF output on the correct channel, while also minimizing the output on harmonics (of which the second and third are the most important).

The output signal is capacitively coupled back to the analog patient electrode input leads, which now serve double duty as an antenna as well as for analog signal acquisition. This form of antenna is not very efficient, and is almost never resonant. For that reason, the design of the output amplifier stage must be such as to be able to handle load impedances that are both nonresistive and variable.

Frequency-modulated systems are generally divided into *narrowband* and *wideband* classifications. A narrowband system is one in which the deviation is small for a given amplitude of modulating signal. In most cases, narrowband systems have a deviation of 20 KHz or less, with 5 to 10 KHz being very common. Wideband FM systems use a wider deviation, that is, in the 20- to 100-KHz range. FM broadcasters, TV broadcasters, and most cardiac radio telemetry systems use this form of modulation. For example, the television sound signal is an FM carrier with 25-KHz deviation, while the standard FM broadcast band (88 to 108 MHz) uses 75-KHz deviation.

The concept "100 percent modulation" has physical meaning in amplitude modulation (AM) systems, but in FM systems the definition of 100 percent modulation is set by convention. In general, for telemetry purposes, the standard wisdom is that wideband FM tends to give a more faithful reproduction of the modulating waveform using low-cost components.

One reason for the popularity of FM in telemetry systems is the same nearly noise-free operation that makes FM ideal for high-fidelity broadcasting. Contrary to the claims and lies of some hi-fi and car radio salespersons, FM reception is not always totally free of noise interference, but under similar conditions of signal strength, the FM is superior to AM. The reason for this situation is that most of the types of natural and artificial electrical noises that interfere with the transmitted signal tend to amplitude modulate the carrier. As a result, an FM receiver can clip off the peaks of the signal—eliminating the noise—while at the same time no information is lost to the modulating signal. If the signal is strong enough to force this clipping action, then the reception is essentially noise free. But, if the signal level drops, then the noise signal can affect the quality of the recovered ECG waveform.

The receiver for a direct-FM system is shown in Figure 14-3B. This form of receiver is essentially the same as an FM broadcast radio receiver, and indeed, many early telemetry systems used components that were originally designed for use in the consumer electronics industry. The telemetry signal is a VHF or UHF signal and is captured by the antenna. The tuner section of the receiver consists of an RF amplifier operating at the VHF/UHF telemetry channel frequency and a converter (or oscillator-mixer) that down-converts the VHF/UHF signal to an *intermediate frequency* (IF), usually 10.7 Mz. This form of down-conversion is called a *superheterodyne* process. The main signal processing, including bandwidth tailoring and gain functions, are handled at 10.7 MHz in the IF amplifier section. The FM demodulator stage recovers the modulating signal, and presents it to the analog output amplifier.

FM/FM Systems The FM/FM system is very much like the direct FM, except there is an intermediate step in the process. Figure 14-4A shows a typical FM/FM transmitter. Most of the stages are the same as in the direct-FM transmitter, but there is an added stage: *audio VCO*. This stage is a *voltage-controlled oscillator* (VCO) operating at an audio frequency. It is permissible to call the VCO an audio band "FM" transmitter because it shifts audio frequency proportional to the applied modulating signal. The output of the VCO is usually called the *subcarrier signal* in FM/FM telemetry systems.

In most cases, the VCO operates at a center frequency that will allow the entire deviation to take place inside the passband of a standard communications channel (300 Hz to 3000 Hz). Typical unmodulated "carrier" frequencies are in the 1000-Hz to 2000-Hz region so that deviation above and below the carrier frequency will not cause the signal to go outside of the passband of the communications medium.

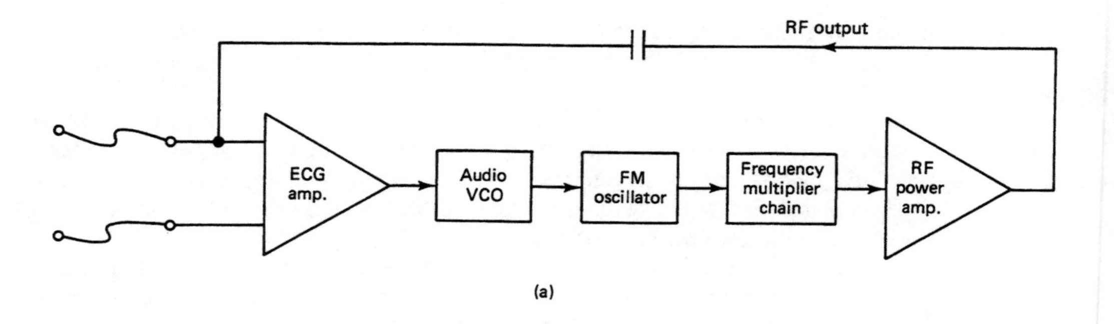

(a)

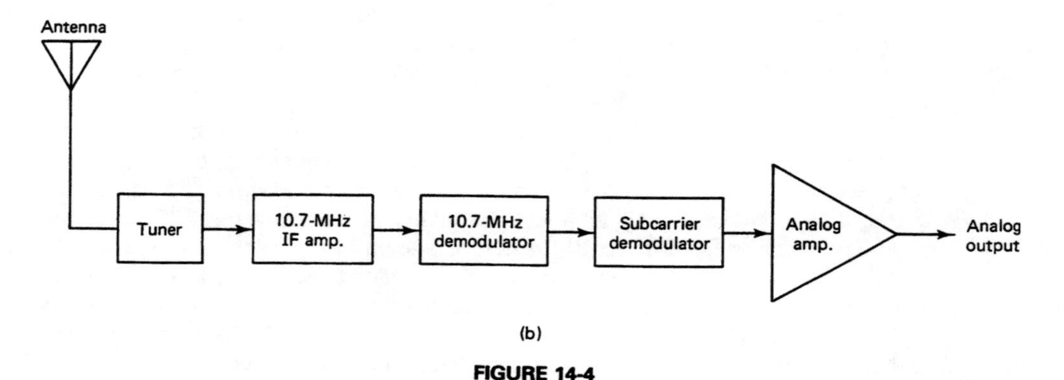

(b)

FIGURE 14-4

The output of the VCO is essentially an audio-FM carrier that contains the analog ECG waveform within the variations of the audio signal. This signal is then used to direct-FM modulate the FM oscillator in a manner exactly like the transmitter in Figure 14-3A.

The receiver in an FM/FM telemetry (Figure 14-4B) system uses a similar layout to the direct-FM receiver. The difference is that there must be a *subcarrier demodulator* stage following the normal 10.7-MHz demodulator. This stage can be a pulse counting detector, a phase locked loop, or other circuit. The output of the subcarrier demodulator is the recovered ECG waveform and is applied to the input of the analog amplifier.

TROUBLESHOOTING TELEMETRY SYSTEMS

ECG telemetry systems are like all other hardware, so from time to time they will malfunction. Some of the faults can be handled directly by the user, while others must be referred to various grades or levels of service shop.

Nurses, EMTs, and other medical personnel can perform several minor troubleshooting tests. First, the patient electrodes and the wires that connect them to the transmitter are usually replaceable by the user, so can be checked before taking a unit out of service. Second, the battery (which is the usual fault) can be replaced on most units by the user. Finally, it is permissible for users to swap telemetry transmitters and receivers on most systems, and therefore restore operation (if on a different channel) by a simple process of elimination. The problem on single-channel systems is that this process does not reveal whether it is the receiver or transmitter that is at fault.

For routine troubleshooting of the telemetry system by a service technician, much can be said for owning either a television field strength meter (which can also be used in making site surveys) or a continuously tunable VHF/UHF receiver that covers all the operating frequencies that might normally be expected to be covered. The receiver or FSM can be used to monitor the output of the transmitter to determine whether or not the transmitter is putting out a signal.

Receiver troubleshooting requires a signal generator that covers the frequency of operation. The selected instrument should be an FM generator that is capable of external modulation so that a low-frequency square wave, simulated ECG from a "chicken heart" generator, or other source can be used to modulate the FM output of the signal generator. The FM signal generator should be capable of deviating at least 25 KHz and preferably the entire range of the deviation expected in the system.

If no FM generator is available, then a common CW (i.e., unmodulated) signal generator can also be used by the technician who knows what she is doing. The telemetry transmitter can also sometimes be used as a signal source, but this approach is fraught with difficulty when there is an ambiguity over whether the receiver or the transmitter is at fault.

Also useful in this type of servicing are the usual collection of DC multimeters and oscilloscopes needed for all forms of complex electronic service work. However, be aware that most of the faults are "trauma" items like broken battery connectors, open switches, and other components that are subject to abuse in normal use. Then there is always the unit that got drenched in saline IV solution!

PORTABLE TELEMETRY UNITS

The rise of emergency medical technicians in the rescue services of local communities gives us an immensely useful tool in dealing with trauma and coronary victims outside of the hospital. Although very highly trained, the EMT is not a physician, so some means is often required to communicate physiological data to the local hospital where they are interpreted by a physician. In addition, two-way voice communications must be established for the EMT team to converse with and receive instructions from the physician at the hospital. Specialized communications equipment is often used to meet these requirements.

Figure 14-5 shows a portable telemetry system that has the range and power needed for the EMT/ambulance crew to establish a data link to the hospital. The transmitter might be a special unit, or, most often, it is a modified version of the standard walkie-talkie that is commonly used by police, fire, and rescue units. The modulating signal, however, is an analog signal such as the ECG, the output of a blood pressure transducer, or other physiological source. The signal is transmitted

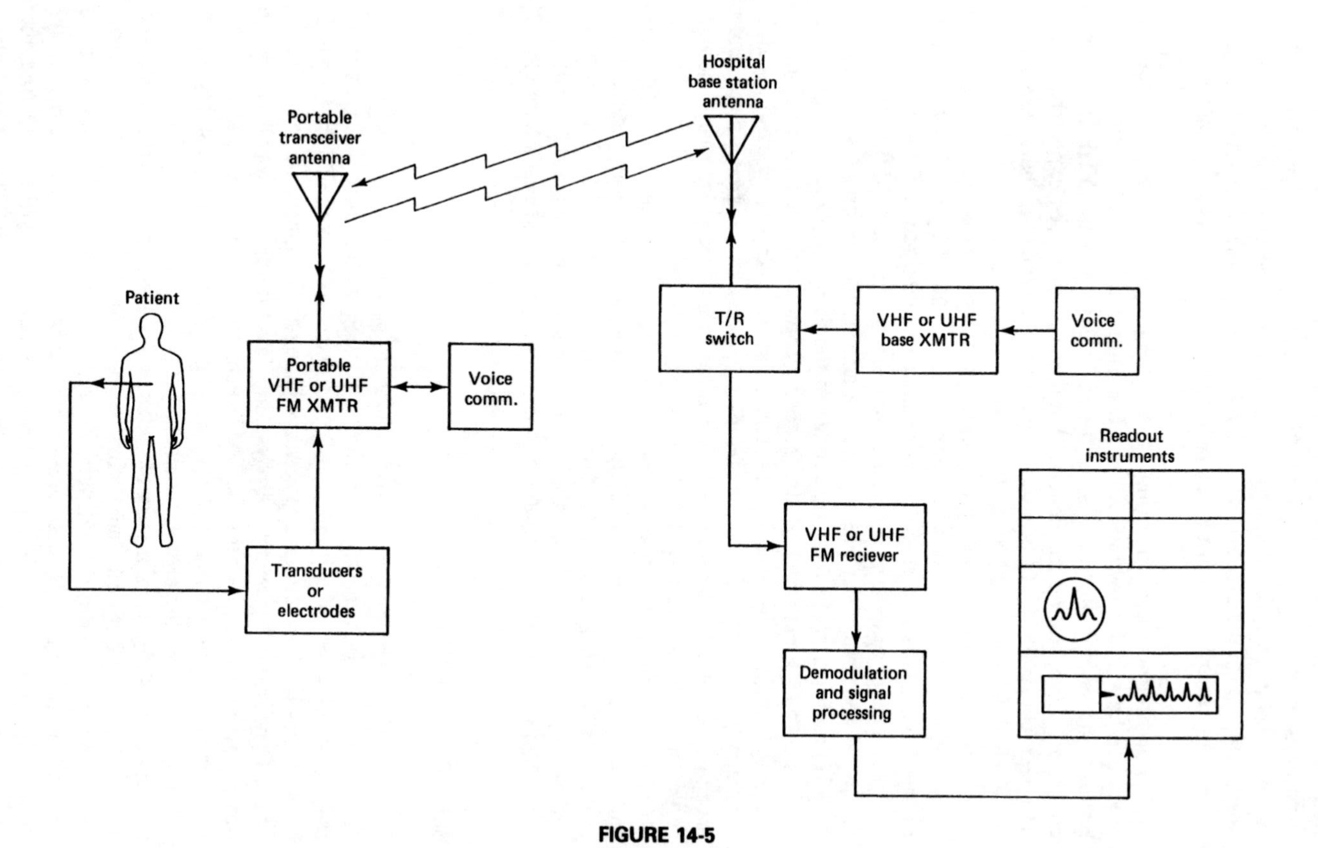
Patient
Portable transceiver antenna
Hospital base station antenna
Portable VHF or UHF FM XMTR
Voice comm.
Transducers or electrodes
T/R switch
VHF or UHF base XMTR
Voice comm.
Readout instruments
VHF or UHF FM reciever
Demodulation and signal processing

FIGURE 14-5

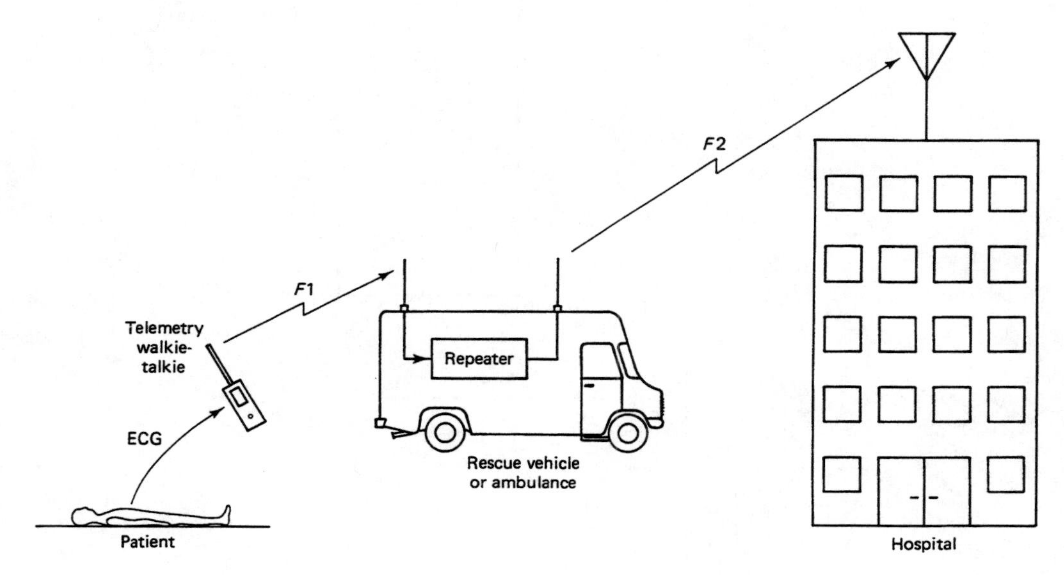

FIGURE 14-6

over the airwaves to a base station transceiver (transmitter and receiver in the same cabinet) at the hospital. From there, the demodulation and display is similar to that of other telemetry systems.

Because the size of handheld transceivers used for telemetry and voice communications is necessarily small, the available power output is low. As a result, the range is short for these units. Where the required range is greater, however, a *repeater system* can be used. At critical locations around the city receiver sites can pick up the small signal from the handheld units. Another method, shown in Figure 14-6, is to install the repeater on the ambulance itself. The handheld unit only has to transmit on frequency $F1$ as far as the vehicle, where the signal is picked up and reradiated at higher power on a different frequency ($F2$) to the hospital site.

LANDLINE TELEMETRY

Telephone lines are sometimes called "landlines" in the trade, so one can expect landline telemetry to send the ECG or other physiological parameter to a remote location via the telephone system. This form of telemetry is used for several purposes. For example, the converted ECG waveforms can be transmitted to a distant location for interpretation either by a computer or a specialist physician.

In other cases, some patients are asked to send in their ECG waveform on a periodic basis. For example, some cardiac pacemaker clinics ask the patient to start sending in the waveform after so many months because it is known that an imminent failure of the battery is usually preceded by a shift of the heart rate. Because the ap-

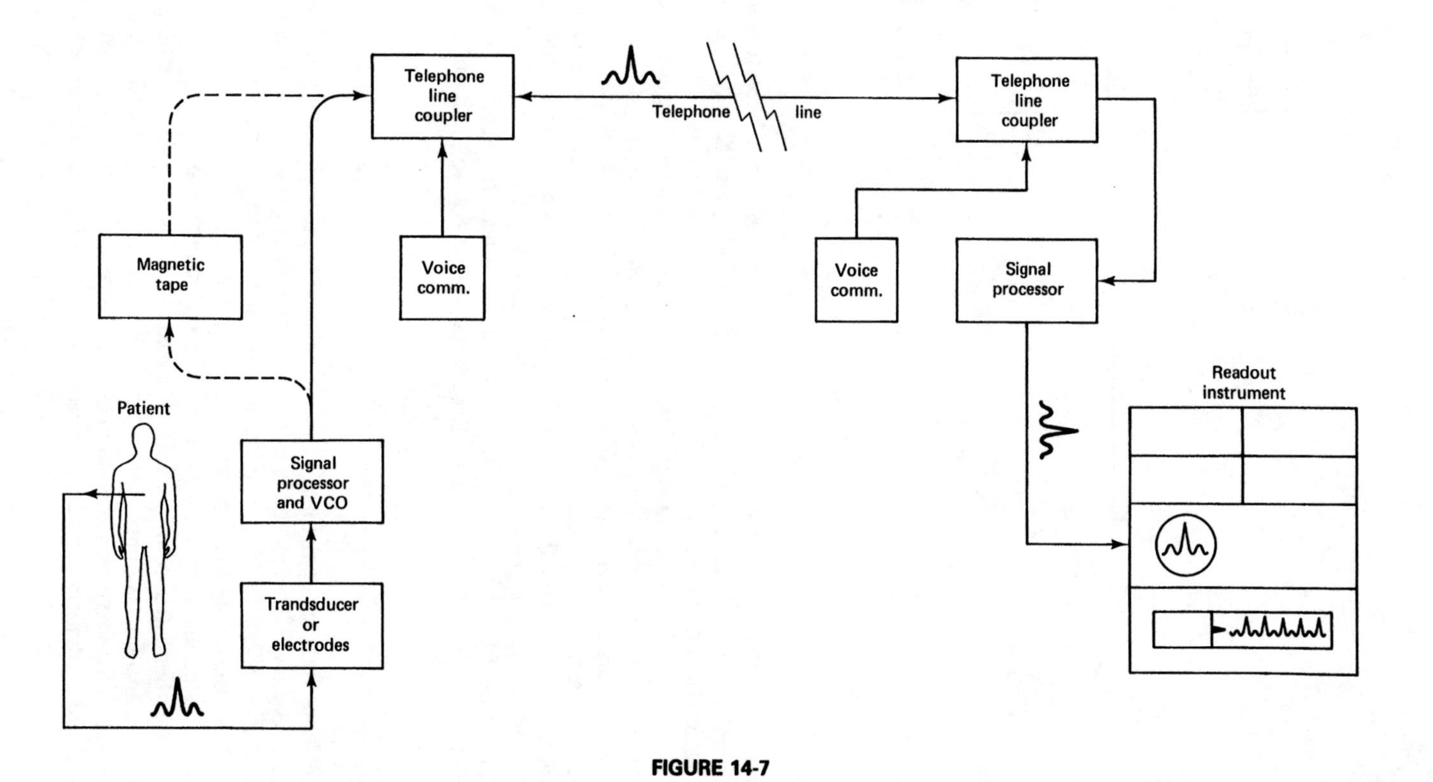
Telephone line coupler
Telephone
line
Telephone line coupler
Magnetic tape
Voice comm.
Voice comm.
Signal processor
Readout instrument
Patient
Signal processor and VCO
Trandsducer or electrodes

FIGURE 14-7

proximate life expectancy of the battery is known statistically, the monitoring can commence when the patient is in the dangerous period between the onset of premature failures and the routine replacement cycle time.

Figure 14-7 shows the block diagram for a landline telemetry unit. The basis for this system is the same voltage-controlled oscillator as was used in the FM/FM radio telemetry. The signal will be acquired from electrodes (ECG), a blood pressure transducer, or a photoplethysmograph (PPG). The waveform is applied to the input of a signal processor (usually filtering) and the VCO, where it is converted to an audio-FM signal. This signal can be recorded on an ordinary tape recorder or can be coupled to the telephone lines and transmitted over the landlines.

At the clinic or hospital where the signal is received, the signal processor demodulates and further processes the signal in order to determine either the waveshape or the interpulse interval. Because frequency (e.g., heart rate) is the reciprocal of time, the interpulse interval is an indirect measure of heart rate. An analog recording can also be made for the convenience of the medical staff or record-keeping purposes.

15

Ultrasonic Systems

A significant number of medical diagnostic and testing instruments use ultrasonic waves to provide the information required about the patient's condition. When the author entered the hospital through the emergency room with upper-right abdomen pain, the doctors arranged an ultrasonic scan to detect the presence of gallstones. The ultrasonic images are often superior to X rays. One physician told me that fully one-third of gallbladder patients show no stones under X-ray examination, while exhibiting stones under ultrasonic examination.

Ultrasonic waves are acoustical waves (that is, vibrations in a medium) that have a frequency above the range of human hearing. In the common understanding of the term, "ultrasound" usually means acoustical frequencies above 20 KHz, but only up to about 100 KHz. Typical ultrasonic burglar alarm transducers and the older form of consumer electronic remote controllers, for example, typically operate in the 40-KHz range. The prefix *ultra* is derived from the fact that these waves are above the range of human hearing (although some animals can hear sounds above 20 KHz, as proven by "silent" dog whistles).

In medical measurement applications, however, the word "ultrasonic" can mean anything from 20 KHz to 20 MHz. The important fact to remember is that the waves are *acoustical waves,* not electromagnetic (i.e., radio) waves despite the high frequencies.

There are several types of ultrasonic transducers available for medical use, but most of them are either dynamic or piezoelectric. The dynamic form (Figure 15-1A)

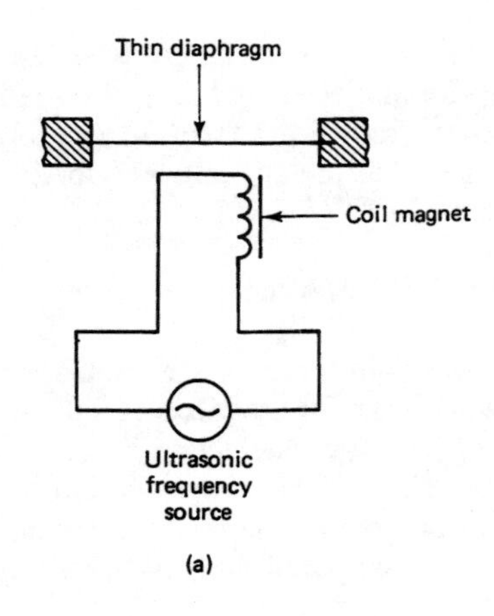

(a)

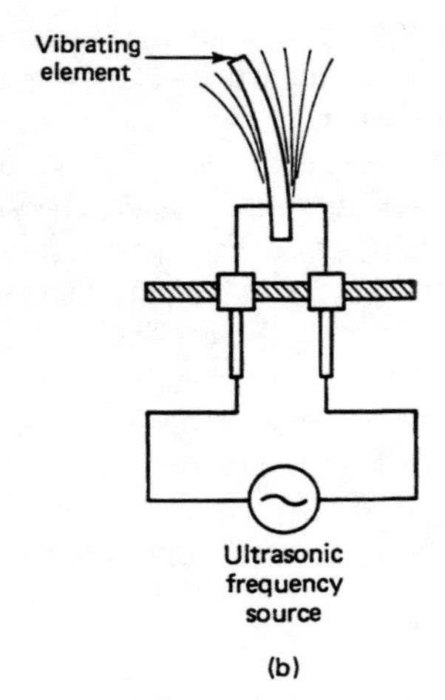

(b)

FIGURE 15-1

is analogous to dynamic microphones: a thin diaphragm stretched over an electromagnet. These transducers are used for relatively low frequencies.

The piezoelectric form of transducer (Figure 15-1B) is analogous to the crystal microphone. *Piezoresistivity* is a phenomenon in which certain crystalline structures will do two things:

1. If mechanically deformed, a slab of the crystal will generate an electrical potential.
2. If it is struck mechanically, then the crystal slab will vibrate at its resonant frequency and produce an AC electrical signal at or near that frequency.
3. If excited by an electrical signal at its resonant frequency, the crystal slab will vibrate mechanically at or near that frequency.

A piezoresistive crystal vibrates when an AC signal of its resonant frequency is applied. This vibrational energy is applied either to a diaphragm or directly to the media being measured in the form of acoustical waves. These waves are generated by the simple fact that the crystal slab vibrates in air or other media.

PHYSICS OF ULTRASONIC WAVES

We can study waves in terms of the simple sine wave, not only because the mathematics are simpler than for other forms, but also because these waves are representative of actual physical systems found in medical ultrasonic applications. Figure 15-2 shows a train of waves. This system is said to be *periodic* because the waves repeat themselves over and over. The wave train consists of peaks, where the wave reaches a maximum value compared with its at rest value, and valleys, where the value is minimum.

The *wavelength* (λ) of the wave is the distance between points where a feature repeats itself. For example, in Figure 15-2 the wavelength can be defined as the distance between either the peaks, or the distance between the valleys, or the distance between crossings of the "at-rest" line. The entire complex between wavelength measurement points is one complete *cycle*. The *frequency* (F) of the wave is the number of cycles per unit of time. For most systems, the frequency is expressed in cycles per second, or hertz (1 Hz = 1 cps). The *period* (T) of the wave is the time required to complete one cycle. Note: The period is the reciprocal of frequency ($F = 1/T$).

In human tissue, the average velocity of soundwave propagation is about the same as it is in seawater: 1500 meters per second. The actual velocity varies somewhat according to the type of tissue. Actually, it is the differences in the *density* of the material that accounts for the difference. Some common values are

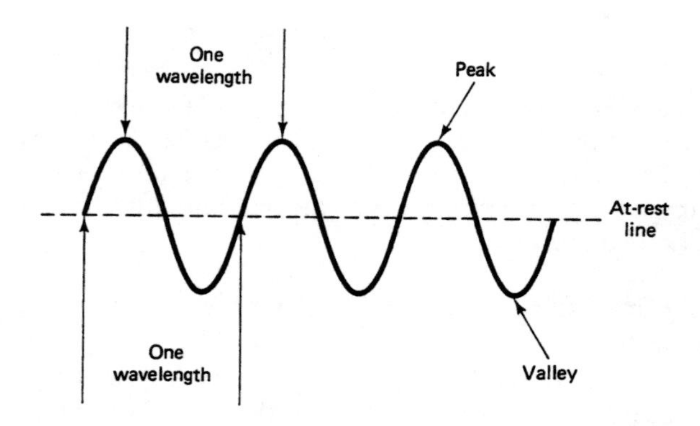

FIGURE 15-2

Bone: 3400 m/s
Muscle: 1600 m/s
Fatty tissue: 1480 m/s
Blood: 1560 m/s

All wave phenomena, whether acoustical or electromagnetic, obey a simple relationship between frequency and wavelength:

$$v = F\lambda \tag{15-1}$$

or, because $F = 1/T$

$$v = \frac{\lambda}{T} \tag{15-2}$$

where

v = the velocity of propagation of the wave through the medium in meters per second
F = the frequency in hertz
λ = the wavelength in meters
T = the period of the wave in seconds

Example

An ultrasonic wave propagating in human tissue has a frequency of 9.1 MHz. Calculate the wavelength.

Solution:

$$\lambda = \frac{v}{F}$$

$$= \frac{1500 \text{ m/s}}{9.1 \times 10^6 \text{ Hz}}$$

$$= 1.65 \times 10^{-4} \text{ meters} = 0.0165 \text{ cm}$$

There are two propagation phenomena that affect the operation of medical ultrasound devices: *reflection* and *refraction*. These phenomena also define all other forms of wave behavior, including light waves and radio waves (which are perhaps more familiar to most readers). These phenomena occur either at the boundary between materials of differing density or, in the case of refraction, in a region of varying density.

Reflection occurs at the surface boundary between two regions of different density, and is why we are able to see our images in a mirror or on the surface of still water. Refraction is a bending of the path of propagation as the wave passes between the two regions. Both of these phenomena are illustrated in Figure 15-3A. The vertical line is orthogonal (i.e., at right angles) to the the boundary and is the reference datum line for measurements involving reflection and refraction.

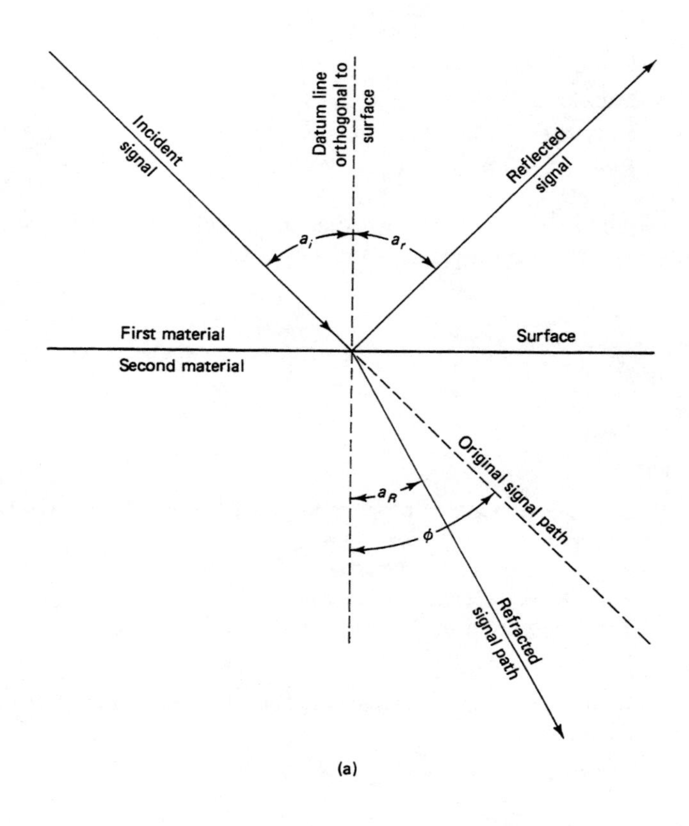

(a)

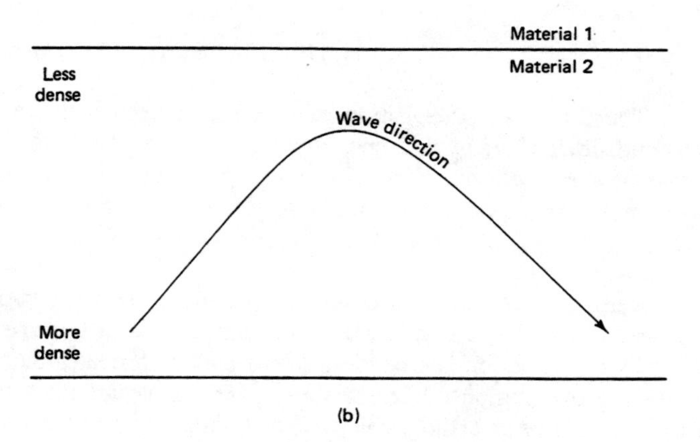

(b)

FIGURE 15-3

Reflection In reflection phenomena, the wave seems to bounce off the boundary and "reflects" back into the originating medium but at a different angle. The incident angle (a_i) is equal to the reflection angle (a_r)

$$a_r = a_i \tag{15-3}$$

where

a_i = the angle of incidence measured with respect to the datum line
a_r = the angle of reflection measured with respect to the datum line

Only at one angle, $a_i = 90$ degrees, will the incident wave be reflected exactly back on itself. At all other angles of incidence the wave will be reflected at an angle that takes it away from the source.

Refraction The phenomenon of refraction is unlike reflection (except in one case). In reflection, the wave will change direction at the interface or boundary between materials of different densities, but the wave remains in the original material. But in refraction, the wave passes from one material into the other material. If the densities are different, then the velocities of propagation are different—and the wave will change direction slightly. Note the ray segment in Figure 15-3A that is marked *refraction signal path*. It will deviate an amount that is proportional to the velocities of propagation in the two respective media. The *angle of refraction* (a_R) is a measure of the amount of deviation from the original path that takes place.

A measure of the ability of a material boundary to refract the signal is the *index of refraction* (n), which is defined as

$$n = \frac{V1}{V2} \tag{15-4}$$

where

n = the index of refraction (dimensionless)
$V1$ = the velocity of propagation in the original material
$V2$ = the velocity of propagation in the destination material

By convention, the index of refraction for light is measured against the velocity of propagation in a vacuum. The value of n for a vacuum is 1.0, while for air it is 1.003. The index of refraction for pure water is about 1.33, and for quartz it is 1.46. These indices are for light passing from a vacuum into the material listed. But for most ultrasonic applications, the important parameter is the relative index of refraction.

The *relative index of refraction* (RIR) assumes two materials of differing densities, so that Equation 15-4 holds true. Then the following equations can be written:

$$N_{2-1} = \frac{V1}{V2} = \frac{\sin a_i}{\sin a_R} \tag{15-5}$$

These equations are known as *Snell's law*.

Acoustical Impedance

Impedance in electrical circuits is a measure of opposition to the flow of current. In an acoustical system we have a similar concept: acoustical impedance (Z_a) is opposition to the propagation of the sound wave. A value for Z_a is

$$Z_a = DV \tag{15-6}$$

where

Z_a = the acoustical impedance in grams per square centimeter second
D = the density of the material in grams per cubic centimeter
V = the velocity of propagation in centimeters per second

Ultrasonic energy operates like other wave phenomena, and so can be expected to be reflected, refracted and so forth. A form of refraction that looks like reflection is *total internal refraction,* shown in Figure 15-3B. In this form of refraction, the density of the same material varies as a function of distance through the material. In this type of system, the wave path is refracted different angles at different points along the path—and is eventually bent backward into the same material.

Absorption of Energy When a wave is propagated through a medium, and then hits a medium of much denser material, some of the energy is absorbed by the denser medium (called a "load"), while some is reflected back toward the source. The total energy (E) is a combination of the reflected energy (E_r) and absorbed energy (E_a). The *coefficient of reflection* (R) is a measure of how much energy is reflected and how much is absorbed. The value of R can be determined from the acoustical impedances of the two materials:

$$R = \left(\frac{Z_{a1} - Z_{a2}}{Z_{a1} + Z_{a2}}\right)^2 \tag{15-7}$$

or, in percent notation,

$$R = \left(\frac{Z_{a1} - Z_{a2}}{Z_{a1} + Z_{a2}}\right)^2 \times 100\% \tag{15-8}$$

Note in the two equations given that the coefficient of reflection is the quotient of the difference over sum of the two acoustical impedances. In medical applications, there are transducers that must cross an air boundary into tissue. The acoustical impedance of air is on the order of 60 g/cm^2-s, while for soft human tissues (muscle, fat, etc.) it is 160,000 g/cm^s-s. The coefficient of reflection for this system is

$$R = \left(\frac{Z_{a1} - Z_{a2}}{Z_{a1} + Z_{a2}}\right)^2 \times 100\% \tag{15-8}$$

$$= \left(\frac{60 - 160,000}{60 + 160,000}\right) \times 100\%$$

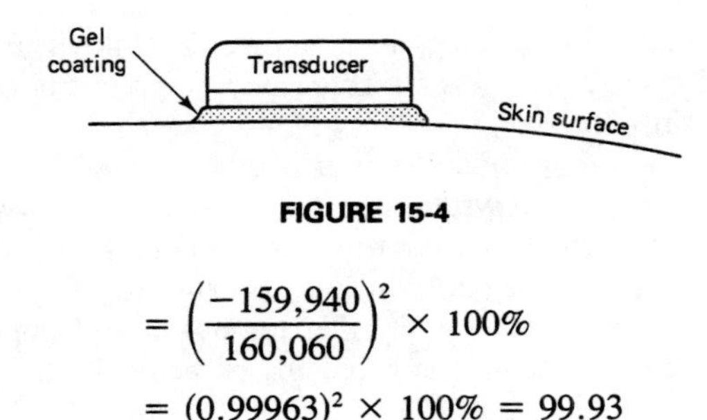

FIGURE 15-4

$$= \left(\frac{-159{,}940}{160{,}060}\right)^2 \times 100\%$$

$$= (0.99963)^2 \times 100\% = 99.93$$

Note that 99.93% of the energy is reflected back to the transducer, while only 0.074% is absorbed into the tissue. A consequence of this ratio is that a tremendous amount of power would be needed to make ultrasonic measurements. Total absorption occurs when the acoustical impedances are equal. In order to make the transducer work well when interfaced to the patient, but in an air environment, it is customary to use an acoustical gel (see Figure 15-4) between the transducer face and the skin surface.

The reflection of ultrasonic energy is not always bad, and in fact many medical ultrasound instruments use the reflection phenomenon. If structures within the path of propagation inside the body have differing densities, hence different acoustical impedances, energy will be reflected backward toward the transducer. The greater the difference in density, the greater the reflection.

ULTRASONIC BLOOD FLOW DETECTORS

Blood flow can be measured using ultrasonic flow monitors. Figure 15-5 shows a medical blood flow detector based on piezoelectric crystals. Two crystals are used, one for transmit (*TT*) and one for receive (*RT*). The frequency of the incident signal

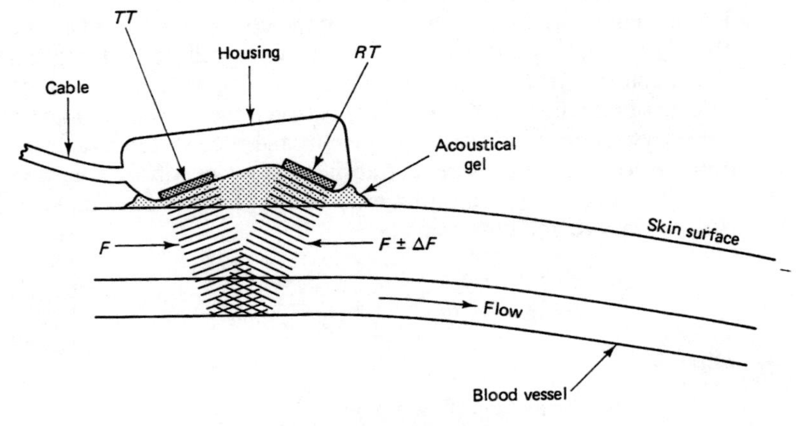

FIGURE 15-5

(F) is changed by the *Doppler effect* as blood flows underneath the transducer. The reflected energy will contain frequency components of $F \pm \Delta F$, where ΔF is the Doppler shift.

In blood flow monitors it is nearly impossible to calibrate this transducer for blood flow rate. The system is used to check for vessel patency, that is, whether or not blood is flowing, but not to measure blood flow rate. In other systems, the calibration might be possible, however, because the Doppler frequency shift is proportional to the fluid velocity. By filtering out those Doppler cells, we ought to be able to calibrate the system. The problems in medical ultrasonic systems are that

1. blood vessels are distensible, that is, they flex at blood flows.
2. blood flow is pulsatile.
3. blood vessels are not located at a constant distance beneath the surface.

The system shown in Figure 15-5 is used in emergency medicine and in surgery to determine the patency of blood vessels. The Doppler components of frequency can be compared to the transmitted frequency, demodulated in a simple product detector, and then used to drive either a meter or a loudspeaker. When blood is properly flowing through an underlying artery, the output will sound like "swish, swish." The lack of such sound tells the physician that the vessel is not passing blood and that action is required.

At one time, it was believed that using two receive transducers, one distal to TT and one proximal to TT, would allow the instrument to discern the direction of flow. One well-known instrument manufacturer gave in to the demand of its customers for the "stereo flow meter," but averred that the only real advantage was that the surgeon could tell her colleagues that ". . . *mine* is in stereo!"

The simple Doppler flow meter will not yield reliable information about the magnitude of blood flow. The flow rate can be quantified by using a *transit time flow transducer*. An example of a transit time flow transducer is shown in Figure 15-6. This system depends upon the fact that the upstream and downstream transit times of acoustical pulses are different (a phenomenon related to Doppler effect). A pair of piezoelectric crystal transducers (TA and TB) are aimed at each other in an oblique path across the flow path. The angle between the crystal path and the flow path is θ. Both crystals are used for both transmit and receive functions. We first fire a pulse from TA to TB and measure its transit time; we next fire an upstream pulse from TB to TA and measure its transit time (in reality, both measurements are made continuously). The average flow velocity is

$$V = \frac{C^2 \times \Delta T}{2D \cos \theta} \tag{15-9}$$

where

V = the average flow velocity
C = the speed of the signal in the media

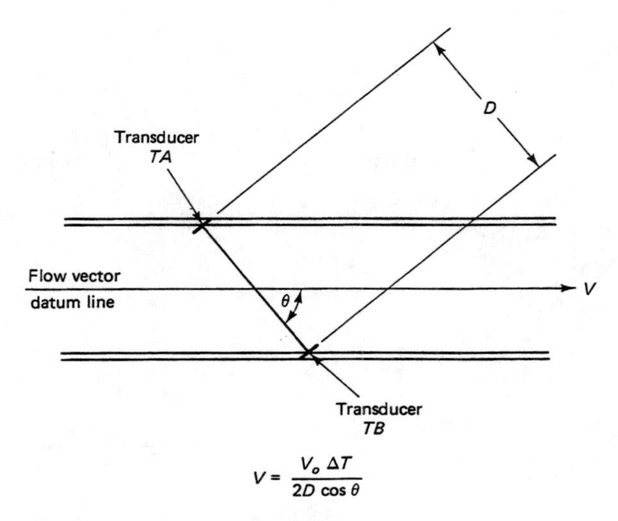

FIGURE 15-6

ΔT = the difference between downstream and upstream transit times
D, θ = as defined in Figure 9-8

A Doppler system is shown in Figure 15-7. This system uses the frequency change of a wave *scattered* from particulate matter flowing in the fluid path and is particularly useful in blood flow meters. It has been shown that the change in frequency ΔF, is given by

$$\Delta F = \frac{VFs\,(\cos\theta_1 + \cos\theta_2)}{c} \tag{15-10}$$

where

ΔF = the Doppler shift frequency
Fs = the source frequency
V = the fluid velocity
c = the velocity of sound in the media
θ_1 = the angle of the receive crystal to the flow axis
θ_2 = the angle of the transmit crystal to the flow axis

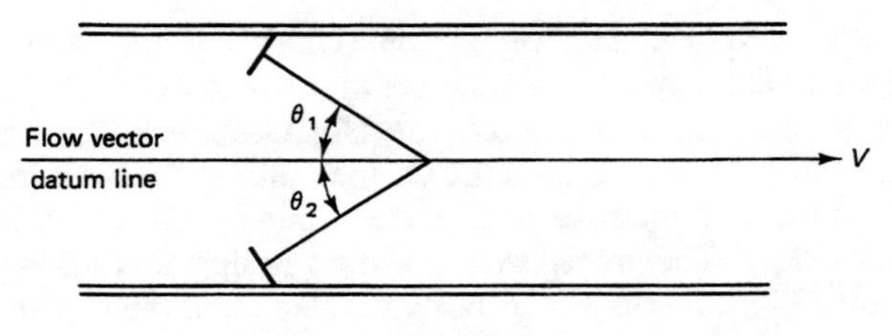

FIGURE 15-7

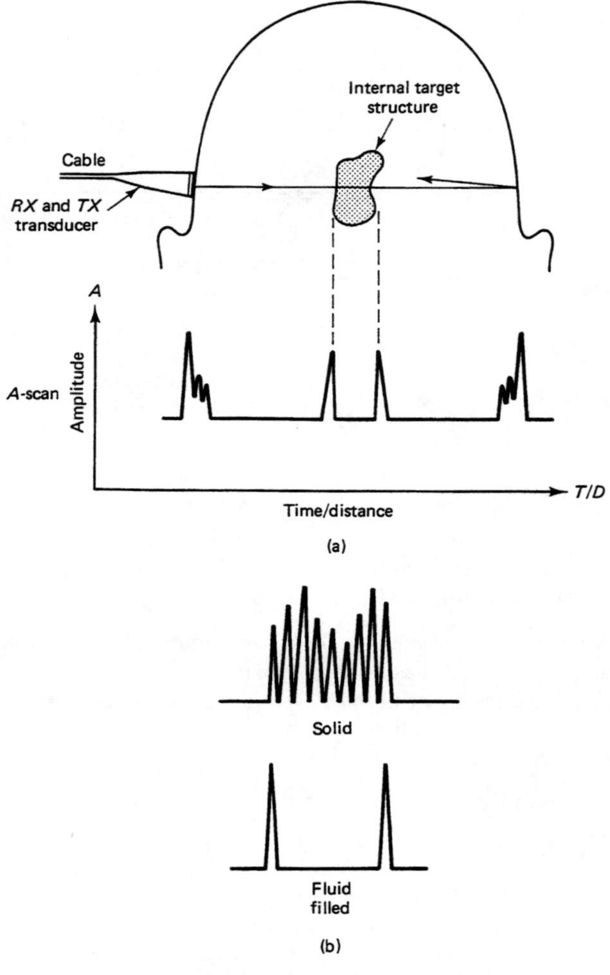

FIGURE 15-8

ECHOENCEPHALOGRAPHS

An *ultrasound echoencephalograph* (UECG) is an ultrasonic instrument that acts somewhat analogously to a radar set in order to make simple images of structures inside the brain. Like the radar, the UECG emits a short pulse of energy and then looks for reflections. In the UECG, the pulse will have a frequency of 2 to 3 MHz, a pulse width of 1 microsecond (1 μS), and a pulse repetition rate of 500 pulses per second (PPS). The transducer is a dual design that allows both receive (RX) and transmit (TX) functions. On pulsed systems the dual-mode transducer only needs a single piezoelectrical element because there is a difference in time between the transmitted and received pulses. This is the same *monostatic aperture* concept as found in most radar sets. If two transducers are used, one *RX* and one *TX*, then the configuration is said to be *bistatic aperture* (to use radar terminology).

Figure 15-8 shows schematically how the UECG works. A piezoelectric transducer is placed against the skull, using ultrasound gel to match the impedances. At the instant that the pulse is fired, an oscilloscope display is triggered. The 'scope displays the signal output from the transducer element in the *A-scan* format, that is, amplitude versus time. Because the speed of propagation is approximately constant, the time base also describes the distance traveled.

In the A-scan presentation of Figure 15-8 the large, noisy pulse on the left side is due to reflections off the two surfaces of the skull immediately beneath the transducer. The two pulses shown in the center are the leading and trailing edge reflections from an internal brain structure. The large, noisy pulse on the right side is the reflection off the far side of the skull. If the internal structures are fluid filled, then the A-scan will look like that shown, but if it is solid, the A-scan representation will more likely resemble the upper trace in Figure 15-8B.

ECHOCARDIOGRAMS

The *echocardiogram* is also similar to radar, but it is used to image the moving heart as it beats. The echocardiogram display is a *time-motion* (T-M) plot (Figure 15-9). The recorder is either an optical oscillograph, or a computer plotter/printer with

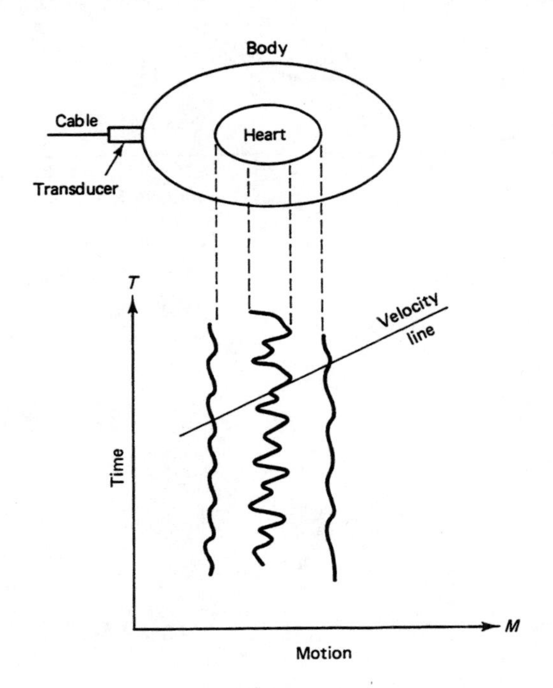

FIGURE 15-9

graphics capability. The CRO beam is typically raster scanned at 0.5 s/cm vertically and 20 us/cm horizontally. The reflections received by the transducer intensity modulate the CRO beam. Thus, when there are no reflections, the CRO beam is turned off, even though the sweeping action continues in a synchronized manner. But when a reflection is received, the CRO beam is unblanked an amount proportional to the received signal strength.

A common problem in all imaging systems is that the signal is attenuated as it traverses the path. These *path losses* can be tremendous at the acoustical frequencies used for echocardiography. As a result, it is necessary to create a receiver gain control that sets sensitivity of the receiver element as a function of distance traveled, which is the same as time elapsed since the pulse was fired. In some models, a gain curve occurs, such as shown in Figure 15-10. This concept is called *time compensated gain* (TCG). If the gain curve is set correctly, then the amplitude of the signal will remain constant from reflections from similar objects regardless of the distance. As a result, differences in reflected amplitude indicate differences in the material.

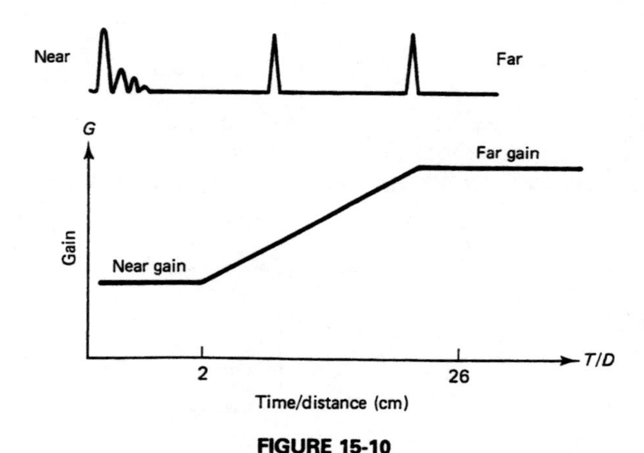

FIGURE 15-10

16

Electrosurgery Machines

The *electrosurgery machine* (ESM) is a radio frequency power generator that operates at frequencies similar to those used by AM band broadcasters (typically, 300 to 3000 KHz). Surgeons use ESMs to cut tissue and cauterize blood vessels severed during the cutting process. The use of the ESM minimizes bleeding and other problems.

The basis for the operation of the ESM is shown in Figure 16-1. The patient's body, shown in cross section, is placed on a large electrode "patient plate," also

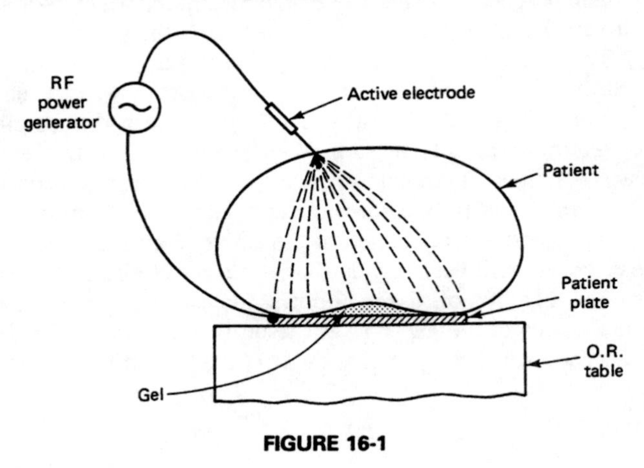

FIGURE 16-1

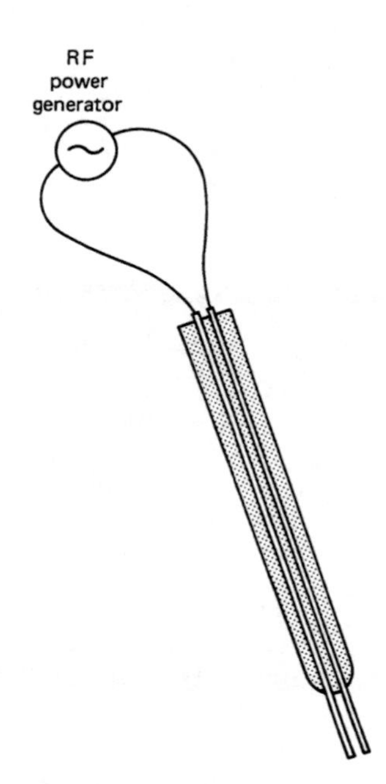

FIGURE 16-2

called the *passive electrode*. The passive electrode shown in Figure 16-1 is the classic form, that is, a metallic plate on which the patient is laid. The contact area and impedance difference between the patient and the plate are optimized by smearing a conductive gel on the plate. More modern patient plates are disposible, gel-filled cuffs wrapped around the patient's upper leg and secured with an adhesive. In either case, the surface area of the plate in contact with the patient must be 100 cubic centimeters or more.

The surgeon's tool is the *active electrode*, which is a small RF electrode that has a very small surface area in contact with the patient's skin.

The operating principle of the electrosurgery machine is quite simple. The RF current paths, lines of force, if you please, flow between the active and passive electrodes. These current paths are shown as dashed lines in Figure 16-1. The passive electrode has a large surface area, where the active electrode is a very small surface—almost a pinpoint. As a result, the current is dispersed at the patient plate, but is highly concentrated at the active electrode. Cutting action occurs because of the high current concentration at the active electrode site. The tissue under the passive electrode will heat slightly, but at the active electrode it is heated to destruction.

The heating of tissue follows the same rules as the heating of any RF-permeable material. The relevant issue is how much RF power is dissipated in the tissue. The expression in Equation 16-1 describes the RF power dissipated in the tissue:

$$p_d = pV(I_d)^2$$

where

P_d = the power dissipated in watts
p = the resistivity of the tissue in ohm-meters
V = the volume of the tissue in cubic meters
I_d = the current density in amperes per square meter

Some surgeons, especially Ob-Gyn, may elect to use a so-called *bipolar electrode* (Figure 16-2). The name "bipolar" is actually incorrect, because all RF ESM electrodes are bipolar (or the machine would not work). The unipolar electrode gets its name from the fact that the surgeon holds only one pole of the RF output, while the other pole is connected to the passive electrode. The bipolar electrode places both poles of the RF generator's output circuit into a single handpiece operated by the surgeon.

RF POWER GENERATORS FOR ELECTROSURGERY

Currently used electrosurgery machines span the range of technology from pre–World War I spark gaps to modern solid-state complex waveform circuits. The first electrosurgery machines were *spark-gap* models. These circuits (Figure 16-3) are nearly identical to the crude radio transmitters used aboard ships and by amateur radio operators in the pre–World War I era. The spark-gap transmitter was outlawed by the Federal Communication Commission in 1938. For many years, assorted vacuum tube models were prevalent. Although solid-state ESMs started to appear about

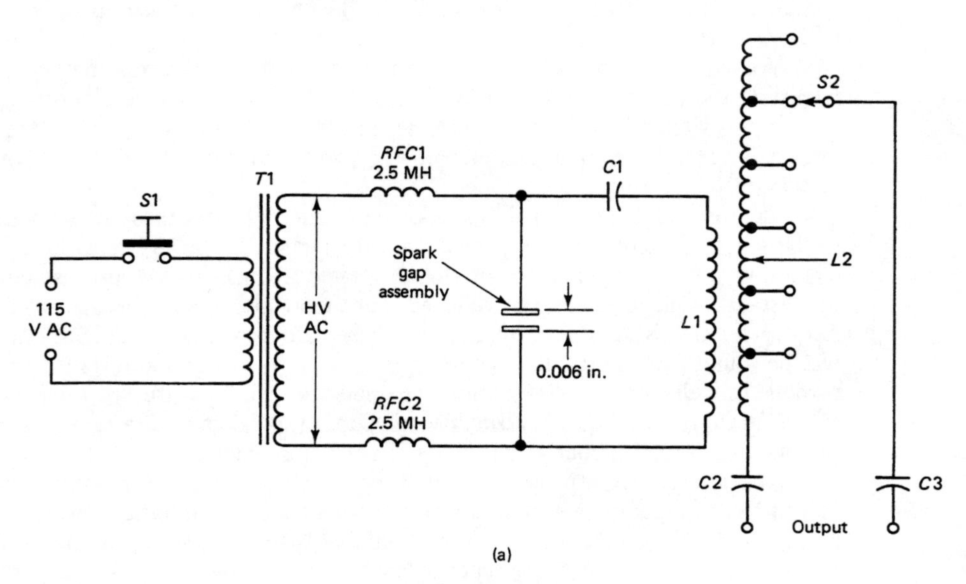

FIGURE 16-3

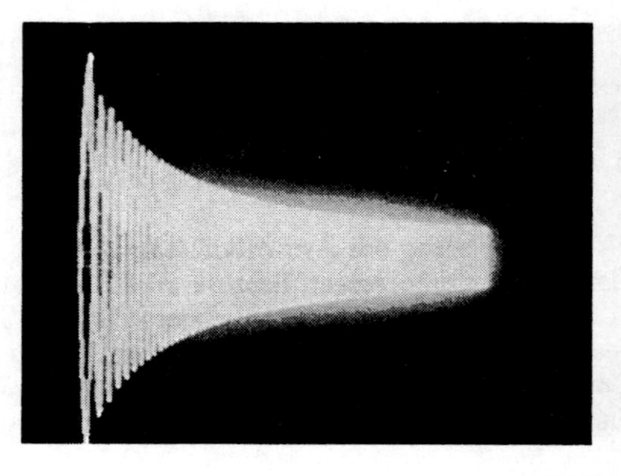

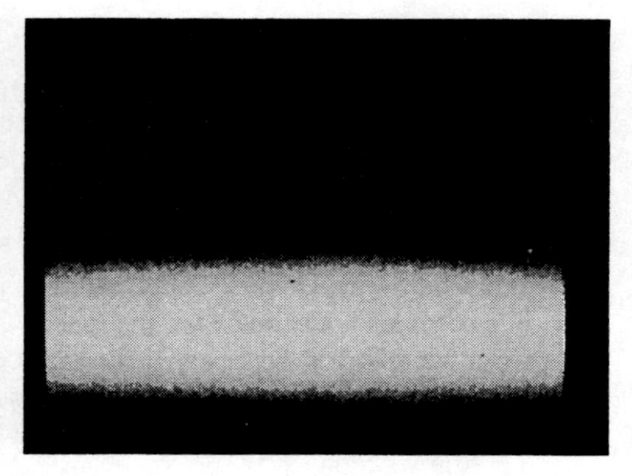

FIGURE 16-3 (continued)

15 years ago, there was a long period when the cheapest and most reliable method for generating large amounts of RF power was the vacuum tube (heresy!). Interestingly, all forms of ESM (including spark-gap models) are found in clinical medical and veterinary settings today.

Figure 16-3A shows the basic circuit for an actual spark-gap ESM, while Figure 16-3B shows the basic spark-gap RF output waveform. The spark-gap assembly is a series-parallel combination of points, each with a diameter of about quarter inch, spaced 6 mils (0.006 inches) apart. The 60-Hz, high-voltage secondary of a power transformer is applied across the spark gap, and is the source of the electrical spark. A pair of RF chokes (RFC1 and RFC2) are used to prevent RF created by the sparking from entering the AC power lines. The high voltage used is typically 2000 to 3000 volts.

Air-core inductors L1 and L2 are used to form a transformer that couples RF energy to the output. The output level, selected by the surgeon, is a function of the setting of switch S2. This switch selects the tap on L2 that is applied to the output terminals. Typical spark-gap output power levels vary from 25 watts to more than 500 watts.

Because C1/L1 form a series resonant LC circuit, only those frequencies close to the resonant frequency are passed onto the output. However, because the circuit has a low "Q," a large number of closely related frequencies are also passed. Also, the distant frequencies are only reduced, not suppressed totally. Because of the high frequencies involved, the harmonics and intermod products from ESM equipment will be found from 1/100 the operating frequency (typically 500 KHz for spark-gap models) to well into the VHF region. The noiselike nature of the spark-gap output is shown in Figure 16-3C. This oscilloscope photo was taken with a sampling link inside a dummy load (about which you will read more later).

The spark waveform is best suited for cauterization of cut blood vessels, and indeed some surgeons still maintain that it works better than other waveforms from purely electronic generators. The waveform that is best suited to cauterization, however, is also inefficient as a cutting tool. As a result, most ESMs have dual footswitch controls, one each for cut and cauterize. The best cut waveform is a sine wave, shown in Figure 16-4A and in expanded form in Figure 16-4B. If the machine does not use smooth filter circuits in the DC power supply, then the waveform will be amplitude modulated by the 120-Hz ripple. Alternatively, if (as did many earlier machines) the circuitry is power directly from the AC power lines the waveform is modulated by the 60-Hz AC power line waveform (Figure 16-4C).

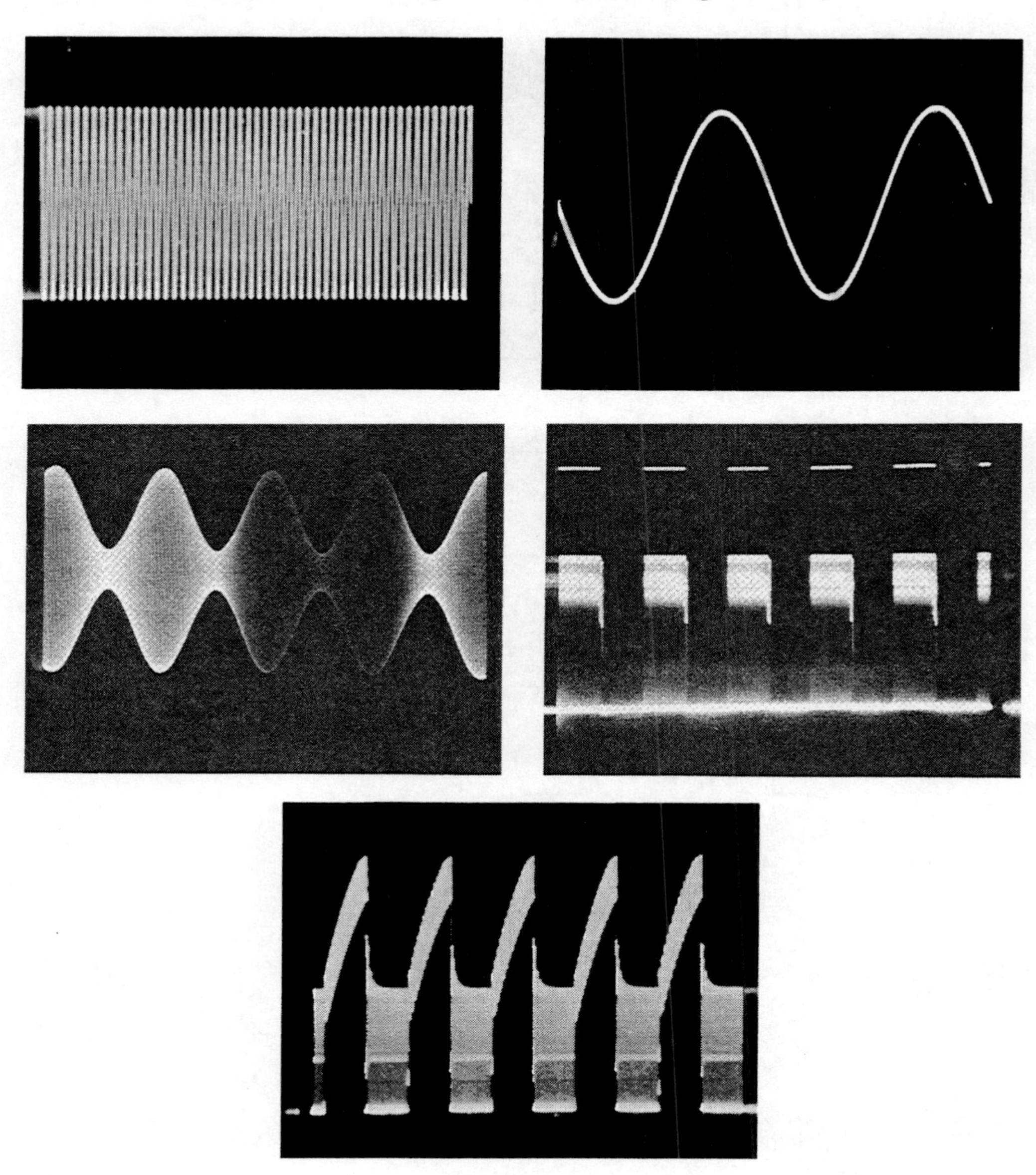

FIGURE 16-4

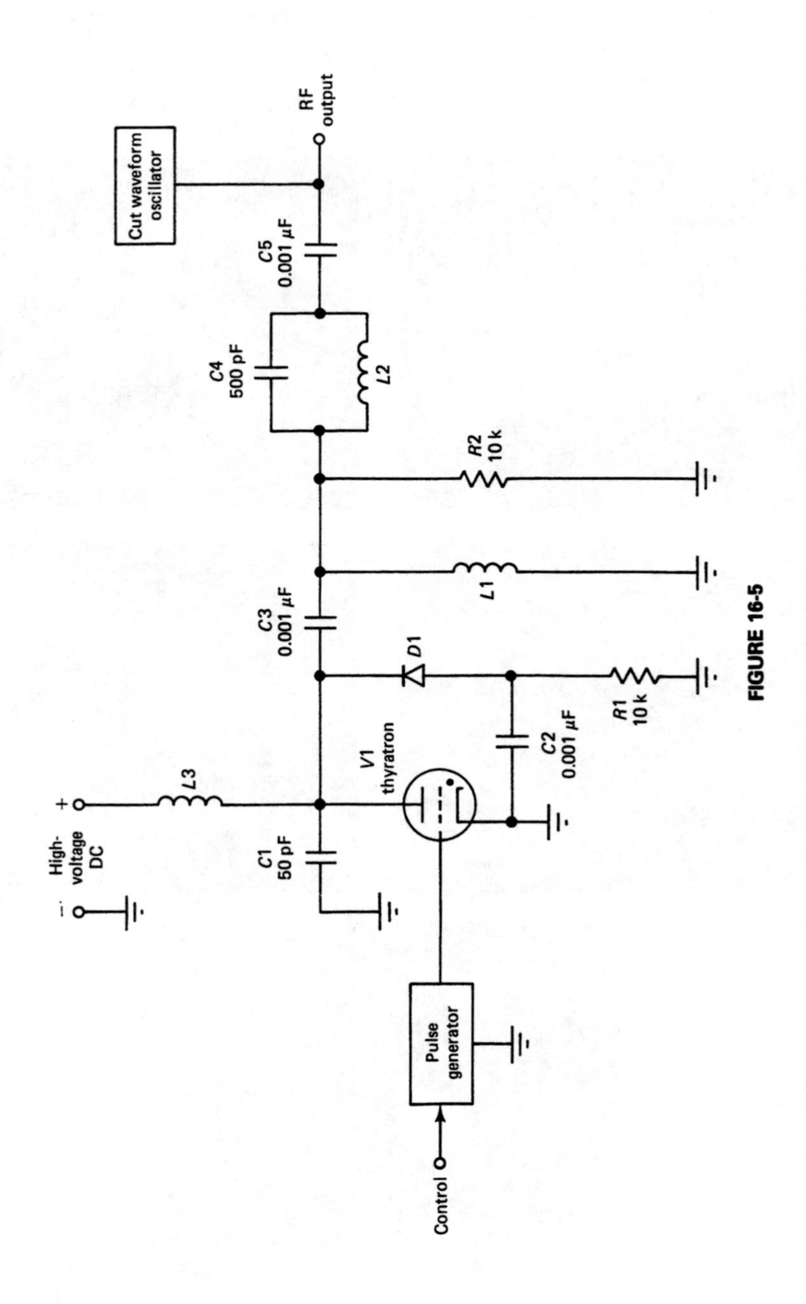
Cut waveform
oscillator
RF
output
C5
0.001 μF
C4
500 pF
L2
R2
10 k
L1
C3
0.001 μF
D1
V1
thyratron
L3
High-
voltage
DC
C1
50 pF
C2
0.001 μF
R1
10 k
Pulse
generator
Control

FIGURE 16-5

Modern solid-state ESMs attempt to mimic by the cauterization effect of the spark gap by chopping the sinusoidal cut waveform with either a square wave (Figure 16-4D) or a sawtooth wave (Figure 16-4E).

A vacuum tube circuit still used in some machines for generating the cauterization or coagulation waveform is shown in Figure 16-5. The basis for this circuit is a special gas-filled vacuum tube called a *power thyratron* (VI). The thyratron will not pass current until the grid voltage reaches a certain level. At grid voltages less than the critical threshold point, the tube acts like a high impedance. But when the voltage reaches a certain point, the gas inside the tube ionizes and the tube becomes a very low impedance.

The purpose of the thyratron in Figure 16-5 is to *ring* the LC resonant tank circuit (L1/C3). Normally, when the thyratron is turned off, capacitor C3 charges up to the level of the applied high-voltage DC. But when the grid of the thyratron is excited by a pulse waveform, the thyratron impedances are too close to zero and that causes C3 to discharge. Part of the discharge path is inductor L1, so there is an exponentially decaying RF oscillation at the resonant frequency of L1/C3.

The other LC resonant tank circuit in Figure 16-5 (L2/C4) is a parallel resonant wavetrap. It presents a high impedance to the resonant frequency, so will block energy from the *cut waveform oscillator* from interfering with the cauterization oscillator circuitry.

Figure 16-6 shows the circuit for a twin-triode cut waveform oscillator that was used in a number of popular machines for many years. The older machines used the

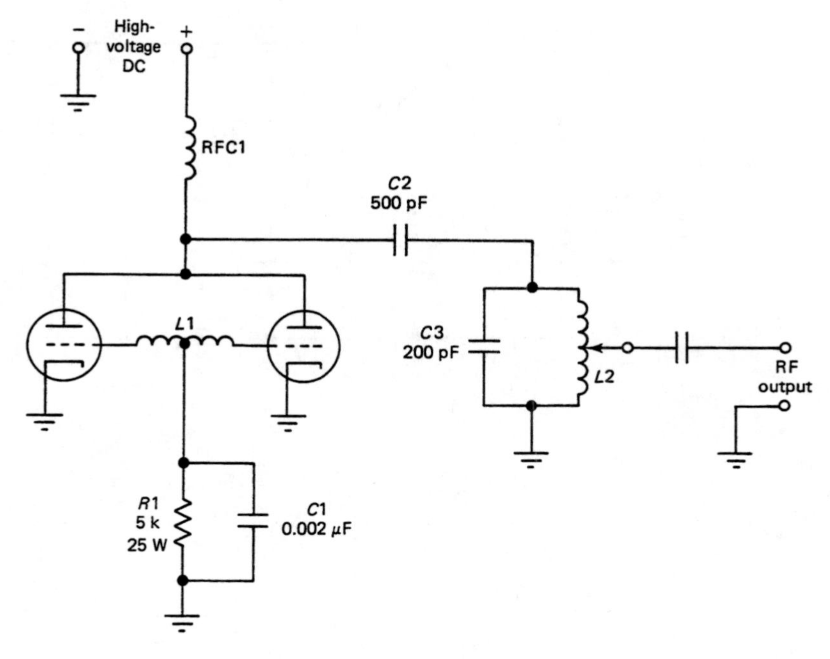

FIGURE 16-6

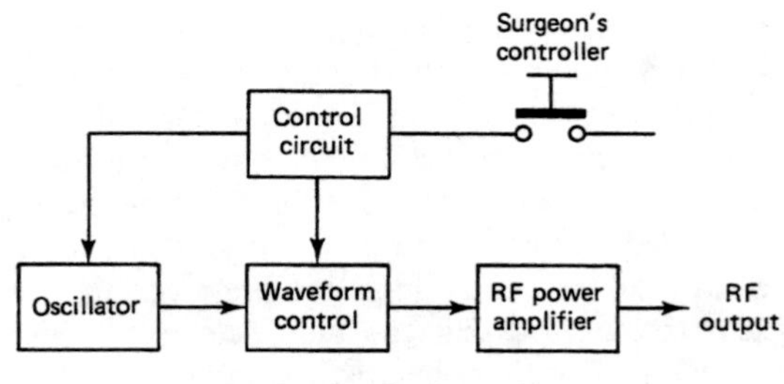

FIGURE 16-7

elderly UXCV-11 triodes, and newer types used the 7986. These tubes are somewhat hard to find, although they are still used in medical ESM machines.

About 15 years ago the manufacturers of electrosurgery machines began to use solid-state (transistor) circuits. This design approach allows the use of different kinds of circuits. Figure 16-7 shows the block diagram of a modern solid-state ESM. The signal is originated in an oscillator circuit that operates on a frequency between 300 KHz and 3000 KHz. If only a cut waveform is needed, then the oscillator signal is applied directly to the RF power amplifier. But if one of the chopped waveforms is needed, then a waveform control or modulator is needed. This circuit will superimpose the square wave or sawtooth wave onto the sinusoidal RF waveform.

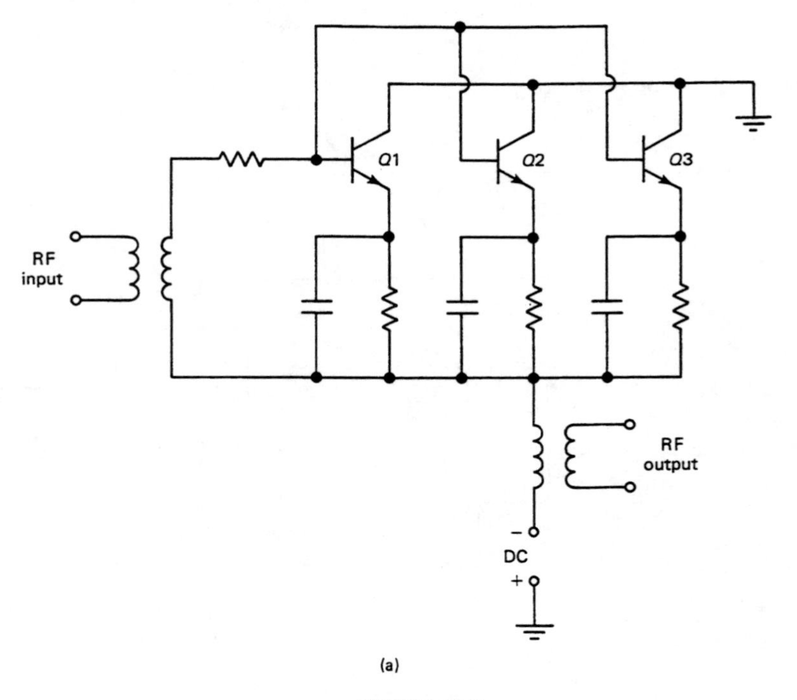

FIGURE 16-8

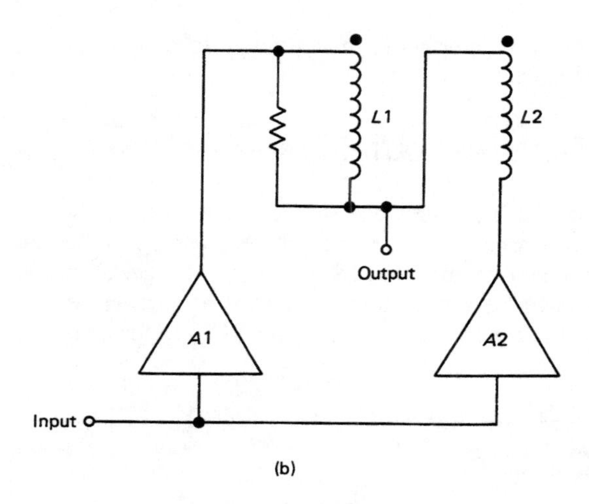

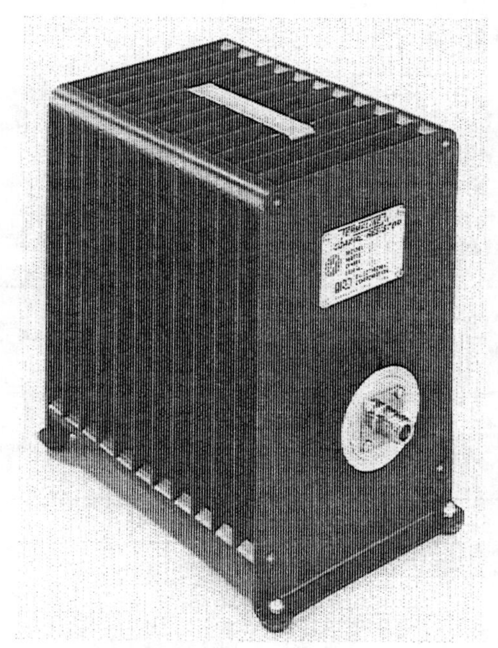

FIGURE 16-8 (continued)

Generating a large amount of RF power in a solid-state circuit is still not as easy as it is in vacuum tube circuits. Designers typically combine amplifiers in either of two ways to produce the amounts of power needed. In Figure 16-8A three RF power transistors are connected in parallel to produce a larger power level than any one alone could produce. The method shown in Figure 16-8B combines the outputs of two power amplifiers into a single load by using a broadband hybrid combiner transformer.

MEASURING RF POWER OUTPUT FROM THE ESM

The standard, perhaps one should say typical, RF wattmeter (see Chapter 26) typically measures either the RMS power, which is a measure of the power heating ability (hence is somewhat averaged), or the peak power. The relationship between RMS and peak and average powers is a function of the *waveform* and certain other factors. Table 16-1 shows different RF waveforms that are output patterns of differ-

TABLE 16-1

Transmission type and scope pattern	Frequency spectrum (C = carrier)	PEV_{rms} (arbitrary)	PEP = PEV^2_{rms}/Z_o	Average (heating) power	4311 in peak mode	4311 in CW mode (1)
Table *A* CW (100 V)	C	$\frac{100}{\sqrt{2}}$ V	100 W	100 W	100 W	100 W
Table *B* AM 100% mod. (200 V)	C	$\frac{200}{\sqrt{2}}$ V	400 W	150 W	400 W	100 W
Table *C* AM 73% mod. (173 V)	C	$\frac{173}{\sqrt{2}}$ V	300 W	127 W	300 W	100 W
Table *D* SSB 1 tone (100 V)	(C)	$\frac{100}{\sqrt{2}}$ V	100 W	100 W	100 W	100 W
Table *E* SSB 2 tone (100 V)	(C)	$\frac{100}{\sqrt{2}}$ V	100 W	50 W	100 W	40.5 W
Table *F* SSB 3 tone (100 V)	(C)	$\frac{100}{\sqrt{2}}$ V	100 W	33.3 W	100 W	–
Table *G* SSB Voice (100 V)	(C)	$\frac{100}{\sqrt{2}}$ V	100 W	–	100 W	–
Table *H* Pulse (100 V; 10%, 90%)	C	$\frac{100}{\sqrt{2}}$ V	100 W	10 W	100 W	–

Z_o = 50 ohms
(1) or model 43

ent styles of radio transmitters (which are similar enough to ESMs to be considered here). This chart is provided courtesy of Bird Electronics, Inc., a supplier of professional-grade RF wattmeters including the "industry standard" Model 43.

The waveform in illustration A of Table 16-1 is the ordinary unmodulated CW waveform. It has a single frequency spectrum and is easily measured. Suppose, as shown in the example, the peak voltage of the waveform is 100 volts (i.e., peak to peak, 200 volts). Given that the CW waveform is sinusoidal, we know that the RMS voltage is 0.707 times the peak voltage, or 70.7 volts. The output power is related to the RMS voltage across the load by

$$P = \frac{(V_{rms})^2}{Z_o}$$

where

P = the power in watts
V_{rms} = the RMS potential in volts
Z_o = the load impedance in ohms.

If we assume a load impedance of 50 ohms, then we can state that the power in our hypothetical illustration A waveform (Table 16-1) is 100 watts.

We can measure power on unmodulated sinusoidal waveforms, by measuring either the RMS or peak values of either voltage or current, assuming that a constant value resistance load is present. But the problem becomes more complex on modulated signals. Several different forms of modulation are shown in illustrations B through H of Table 16-1. As you can see from comparing the various power readings on a Bird Model 4311 peak power meter, the peak (PEP) and average powers vary markedly with modulation type.

Notice the relationship between the power levels and the waveforms in the other illustrations in Table 16-1. The RMS power varies markedly with waveform, and that fact has a direct bearing on measurements of the ESM output in the hemostasis modes (the cut modes are essentially sinusoidal, although some are AM modulated with 60 Hz).

DUMMY LOADS

Testing electrosurgery machines in the laboratory has a high potential for creating electromagnetic interference—and even damage—to nearby electronic equipment. The EMI can affect instruments at relatively far distances from the site where the machine is being examined, because ESMs are really little more than moderately high-powered radio transmitters. In testing the ESM, a *dummy load* (that is, nonradiating artificial "antenna") is required. There are also certain measurements that don't make sense when made in a live antenna because of imperfections in the load impedance (usually reactance). In those cases, the nearly ideal dummy load is a better indicator of isolated transmitter performance.

A dummy load (Figure 16-8C) is a shielded noninductive resistor that absorbs the RF power from an RF power source. Although the model shown is for radio transmitters, it is similar to models used for ESM machine measurements. The resistor *must be noninductive* and have a resistance equal to the output impedance of the transmitter being tested. Because most commercial antennas today are designed to present a 50-ohm resistive load, most commercial dummy loads are 50 ohms. Other resistance values are available on special order, or can be shop constructed locally. Electrosurgery machines typically require odd-value load resistors in their "dummy" antenna because the RF impedance of patients is not the nice, standard 50 ohms. Rather, it is more like 200 to 300 ohms.

Few dummy loads are able to withstand the full rated power for an indefinite period. Most of them have a specified duty cycle that must be observed. Determine the specified duty factor before applying RF power to the load. The typical dummy load duty factor will read something on the order of "2 minutes at full-rated power, 5 minutes off." Alternatively, there might be a derating curve in the manual (or on an affixed label) that relates applied power to permissible time at that power level.

An instrument seen in some service shops called an *absorption wattmeter* is a dummy load and RF wattmeter in a single housing. For the service bench the absorption wattmeter is often the best selection because of the convenience and the fact that less wiring is needed on the workbench. But for more general purposes, the dummy load and RF wattmeter should be separate instruments. An example is the instrument used to test mobile and marine transmitters on-site.

Dummy loads for ESM service Dummy loads for electrosurgery machines require a resistance of 200 to 300 ohms in order to match the output impedance of the ESM. There are several ways to make the load. The simplest

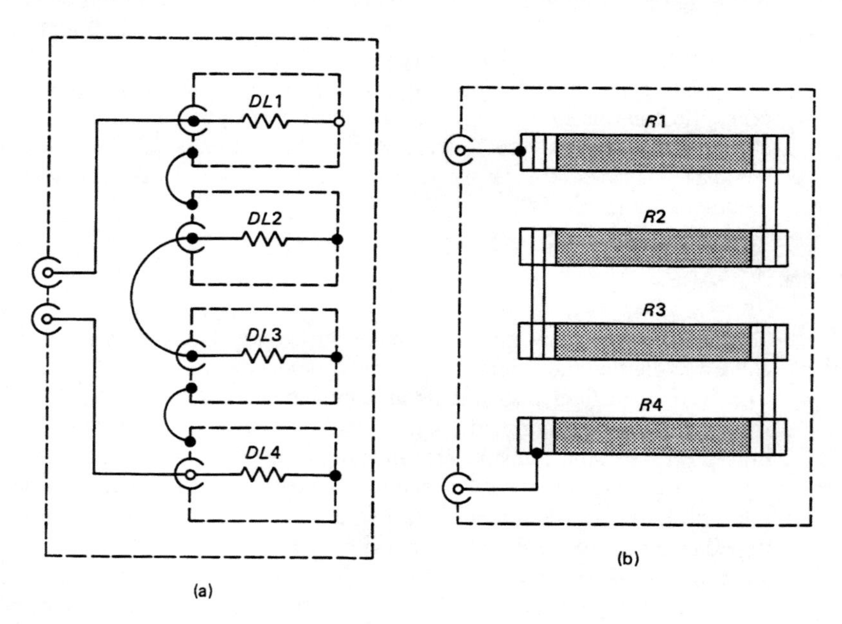

FIGURE 16-9

method is to purchase a 250-ohm, noninductive resistor. These are usually made with carbon or metalized film over a ceramic cylinder. Unfortunately, these resistors are hard to find. There is, however, a solution to the problem that is not too expensive. Amateur radio operators use 50-ohm dummy loads rated at power levels from 300 watts to 1500 watts. These can be combined in series to form a dummy load for ESM service technicians.

Figure 16-9A shows a method for combining four or five 50-ohm dummy loads into a single 200- or 250-ohm load. The four dummy loads (DL1–DL4) are 50-ohm, 300-watt, amateur loads with metal shield cases. These are connected in series in the manner shown, and then mounted inside of, and insulated from, an outer shield. The other method, shown in Figure 16-9B, is to salvage the resistor elements inside the amateur loads, and then connect them in series inside of a shielded enclosure.

It is also possible to use a high-power amateur or commercial dummy load, rated for use in the HF band, on the ESM. Recall that the output impedance of the ESM is on the order of 200 to 300 ohms. If a transformer is used between the load and the ESM, then the impedance can be transformed to the correct value. Figure 16-10 shows a commercially available amateur radio BALUN (balanced–unbalanced) transformer coupled to the dummy load. These transformers are avail-

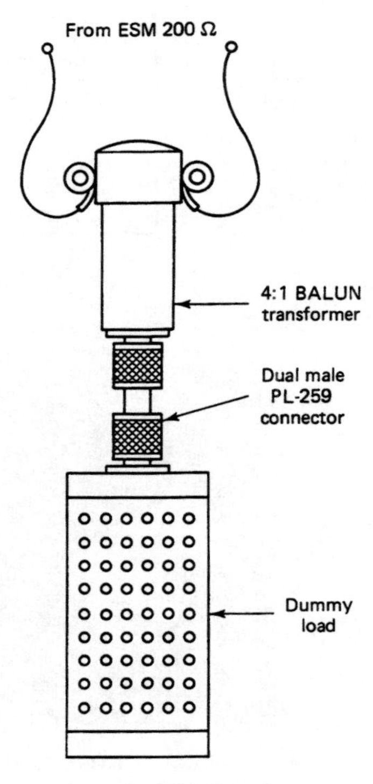

FIGURE 16-10

able in two types: one offers a 1:1 impedance transformation and the other a 4:1 ratio. It is the latter that is used for this application.

"Home-brew" impedance transformers can be made using a high-power toroidal core, such as those sold by Amidon Associates. The circuit for a 4:1 transformer is shown in Figure 16-11A, while the connection diagram is shown in Figure 16-11B. A practical implementation is shown in Figure 16-11C. These transformers will work up to several hundred watts. Because of the high voltages present in these circuits, make sure that the load and the transformer are isolated from ground. A commercially available transformer used by amateur radio enthusiasts is shown in Figure 16-12. Although intended for matching 50 ohms to other (lower) impedances, it could just as easily be used for matching 200 ohms to 50 ohms, especially on the cut waveform where high voltages are limited.

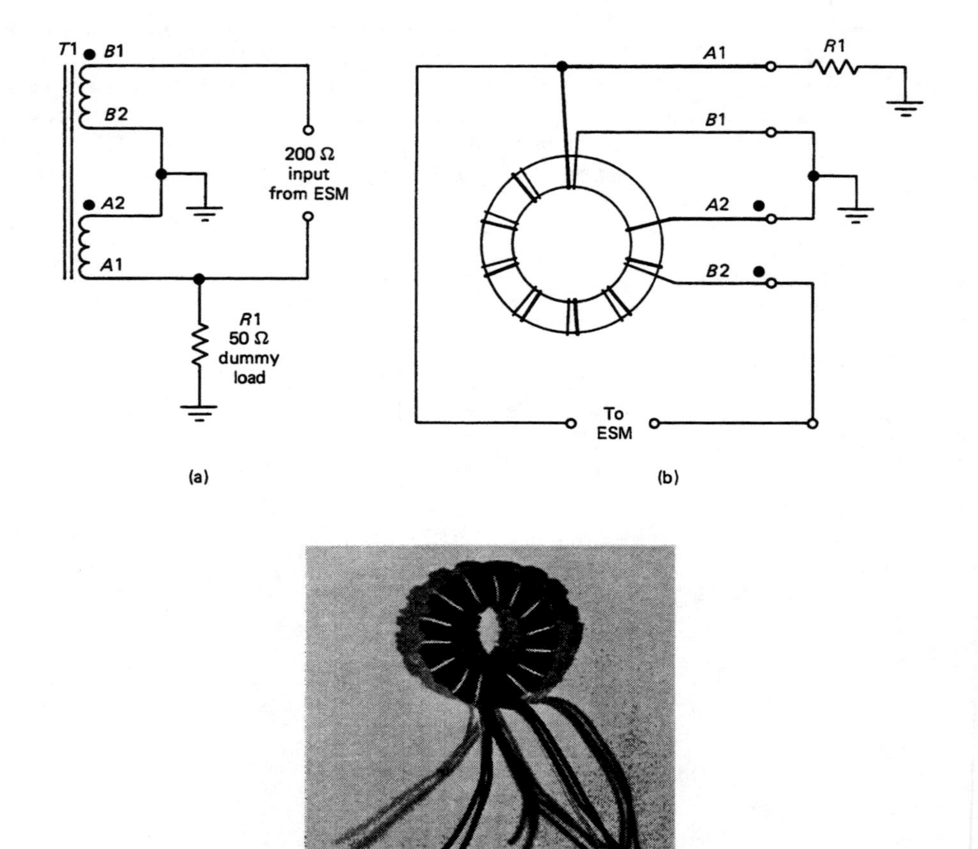

FIGURE 16-11

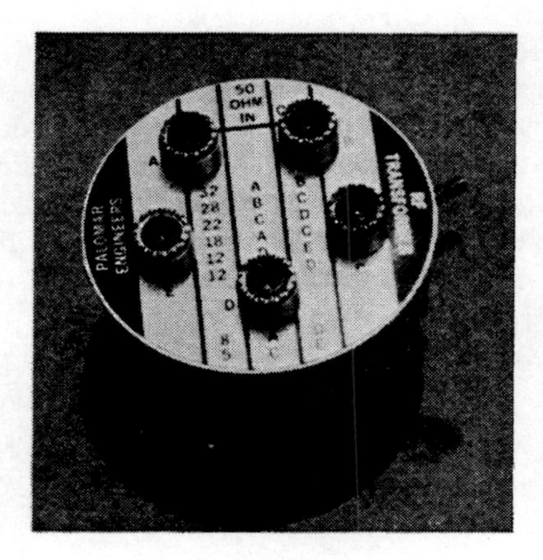

FIGURE 16-12

Displaying the ESM Waveform on an Oscilloscope

The ESM waveform is sometimes displayed on an oscilloscope so that the service technician can evaluate it, and arrive at a good understanding of how well it is working. The 'scope cannot be connected directly across the load, even with a voltage divider, because some machines (being ground referenced) will cause RF to shoot all over the work area—a potentially dangerous situation. There are, however, at least two ways to make a sampling loop from a dummy load.

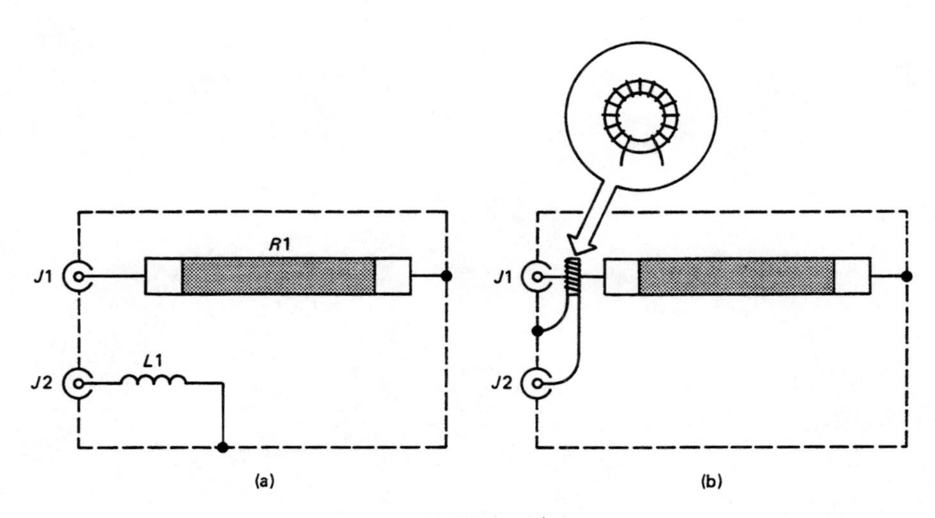

FIGURE 16-13

Figure 16-13A shows a method that depends on a small (3 to 10 turns) coil of wire placed inside the case of a dummy load. The coil is about 1 in. diameter and is made of ordinary hookup wire. One side of the coil is grounded, while the other is connected to a BNC connector (J2). The alternate method (Figure 16-13B) is to place a small toroidal pickup transformer around the wire leading to the load resistor from the connector. The small-diameter toroidal core is wound with 20 to 30 turns of #26 wire and is connected in a manner similar to Figure 16-13B.

17

Decibels

The subject of "decibels" almost always confuses the newcomer to electronics, and even many an old-timer seems to have occasional memory lapses regarding the subject. For the benefit of both groups, and because the subject is so vitally important to understanding electronics systems, we will examine the decibel.

The decibel measurement originated with the telephone industry, and was named after telephone inventer Alexander Graham Bell. The original unit was the *bel*. The prefix *deci* means 1/10, so the *decibel* is one-tenth of a bel. The bel is too large for most common applications, so it is rarely if ever used. Thus, we will concentrate on only the more familiar decibel (dB).

The decibel is nothing more than a means of expressing a ratio between two signal levels, for example, the "output-over-input" ratio of an amplifier. Because the decibel is a ratio, it is also dimensionless—despite the fact that "dB" looks like a dimension. Consider the voltage amplifier as an example of dimensionless gain; its gain is expressed as the output voltage over the input voltage (V_o/V_{in}).

Example

A voltage amplifier outputs 6 volts when the input signal has a potential of 0.5 volts. Find the gain (A_v).

$$A_v = \frac{V_o}{V_{in}}$$

$$= \frac{6 \text{ volts}}{0.5 \text{ volts}}$$

$$= 12$$

Note that the "volts" units appeared in both numerator and denominator, so "canceled out" leaving only a dimensionless "12" behind.

To analyze systems using simple addition and subtraction, rather than multiplication and division, a little math trick is used on the ratio. We take the base-10 logarithm of the ratio and then multiply it by a scaling factor (either 10 or 20). For voltage systems, such as our voltage amplifier, the expression becomes

$$\text{dB} = 20 \log \left(\frac{V1}{V2}\right)$$

In the example given earlier we had a voltage amplifier with a gain of 12 because 0.5 volts input produced a 6-volt output. How is this same gain (i.e., V_o/V_{in} ratio) expressed in decibels?

$$\text{dB} = 20 \log \left(\frac{V_o}{V_{in}}\right)$$

$$= 20 \log \left(\frac{6}{0.5}\right)$$

$$= 20 \log (12)$$

$$= 21.6$$

Despite the fact that we have massaged the ratio by converting it to a logarithm, the decibel is nonetheless nothing more than a means for expressing a ratio. Thus, a voltage gain of 12 can also be expressed as a gain of 21.6 dB.

A similar expression can be used for current amplifiers, where the gain ratio is I_o/I_{in}:

$$\text{dB} = 20 \log \left(\frac{I_o}{I_{in}}\right)$$

For power measurements we need a modified expression to account for the fact that power is proportional to the square of the voltage or current:

$$\text{dB} = 10 \log \left(\frac{P1}{P2}\right)$$

We now have three basic equations for calculating decibels, which are summarized in Figure 17-1.

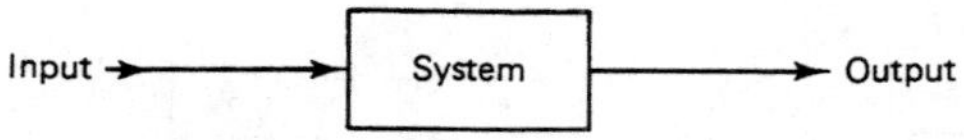

Input → System → Output

Generic: $dB = k \log\left(\frac{\text{output}}{\text{input}}\right)$

1. $dB = 20 \log\left(\frac{V_o}{V_{in}}\right)$

2. $dB = 20 \log\left(\frac{I_o}{I_{in}}\right)$

3. $dB = 10 \log\left(\frac{P_o}{P_{in}}\right)$

FIGURE 17-1

ADDING IT ALL UP

So why bother converting seemingly easy to handle, dimensionless numbers like voltage or power gains to a logarithmic number like decibels? Fair question. The answer is that it makes calculating signal strengths in a system easier. To see this effect, let's consider the multistage system in Figure 17-2. Here we have a hypothetical electronic circuit in which there are three amplifier stages and an attenuator pad. The stage gains are as follows:

$$A1 = \frac{V1}{V_{in}} = \frac{0.2}{0.010} = 20$$

$$\text{Atten} = \frac{V2}{V1} = \frac{0.1}{0.2} = 0.5$$

$$A2 = \frac{V3}{V2} = \frac{1.5}{0.1} = 15$$

$$A3 = \frac{V_o}{V3} = \frac{6}{1.5} = 4$$

The overall gain is the product of the stage gains in the system:

$$\begin{aligned} A_v &= A1 \times \text{Atten} \times A2 \times A3 \\ &= (20) \times (0.5) \times (15) \times (4) \\ &= 600 \end{aligned}$$

When converted to decibels, the gains are expressed as

$$\begin{aligned} A1 &= 26.02 \\ \text{Atten} &= -6.02 \\ A2 &= 23.52 \\ A3 &= 12.04 \end{aligned}$$

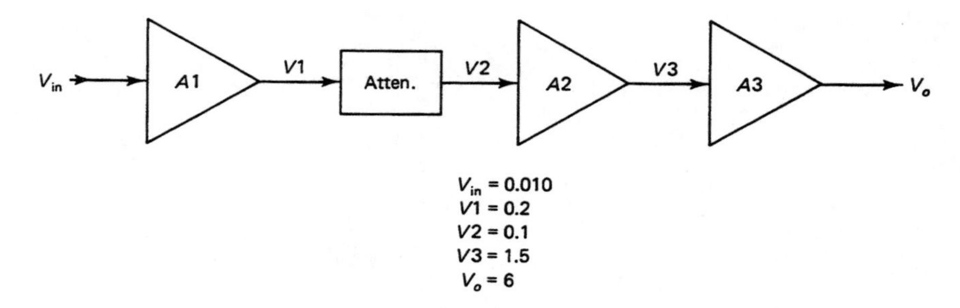

FIGURE 17-2

The overall gain of the system (in dB) is the sum of these numbers:

$$\begin{aligned} A_{v(\text{dB})} &= A1 + \text{Attn} + A2 + A3 \\ &= (26.02) + (-6.02) + (23.52) + (12.04) \\ &= 55.56 \text{ dB} \end{aligned}$$

The system gain calculated earlier was 600, and this number should be the same as that given:

$$\begin{aligned} A_{\text{dB}} &= 20 \log (600) \\ &= 55.56 \text{ dB} \end{aligned}$$

They're the same.

One convenience of the decibel scheme is that gains are expressed as positive numbers, and losses are negative numbers. Conceptually, it seems easier to understand a loss of "−6.02 dB" than a loss represented as a "gain" +0.50.

CONVERTING BETWEEN dB NOTATION AND GAIN NOTATION

We sometimes face situations where gain is expressed in dB, and we want to calculate the gain in terms of the output/input ratio. For example, suppose we have a +20 dB amplifier with a 1-mV input signal, as shown in Figure 17-3. What is the expected output voltage? It's 20 dB higher than 0.001 volt, right? Yes, that's true, but your meter or oscilloscope is probably not calibrated in decibels but rather in volts. By using a little algebra we can rearrange the expression—dB = 20 log (V_o/V_{in})—to solve for output voltage, V_o. The new expression is

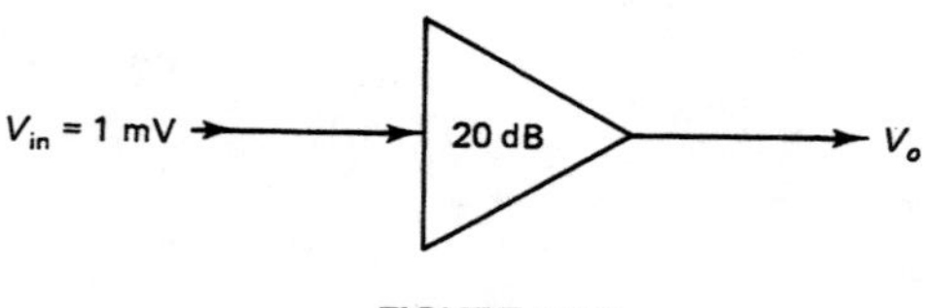

FIGURE 17-3

$$V_o = V_{in}10^{(db/20)}$$

which is also sometimes written in the alternate form

$$V_o = V_{in}e^{(dB/20)}$$

In this example we want to calculate V_o if the gain in dB and the input signal voltage are known. We can calculate it from the preceeding equations. Using the values given (20 dB and 1 mV):

$$\begin{aligned} V_o &= V_{in}e^{(dB/20)} \\ &= (0.001) \exp (20/20) \\ &= (0.001) \exp (1) \\ &= (0.001)(100) \\ &= 0.01 \text{ volts} \end{aligned}$$

For those who don't want to make the calculation, Table 17-1 shows common voltage and power gains and losses expressed both ways.

Again we see the convenience of decibel scales over gain ratios. If we want to calculate system gain of a circuit that has a gain of 10,000, and an attenuation of 1/1000 in series, then we can do it either way:

$$\begin{aligned} A_v &= 10{,}000 \times 0.001 \\ &= 10 \end{aligned}$$

or

$$\begin{aligned} A_v &= (+80 \text{ dB}) + (-60 \text{ dB}) \\ &= +20 \text{ dB} \end{aligned}$$

TABLE 17-1 COMMON GAINS/LOSSES EXPRESSED IN DECIBELS

Ratio (out/in) gain (dB)	Voltage gain (dB)	Power
1/1000	−60	−30
1/100	−40	−20
1/10	−20	−10
1/2	−6.02	
−3.01		
1	0	0
2	+6.02	
+3.01		
5	+14	+7
10	+20	+10
100	+40	+20
1,000	+60	+30
10,000	+80	+40
100,000	+100.02	+50
1,000,000	+120.00	+60

SPECIAL dB SCALES

Various user groups have defined special dB-based scales that meet their own needs. They make a special scale by defining a certain signal level as "0 dB" and referencing all other signal levels to the defined 0 dB point. In the dimensionless dB scale, 0 dB corresponds to a gain of unity (see Table 17-1). But if we define "0 dB" as a particular signal level, then we obtain one of the special scales. Consider the following scales commonly used in electronics:

1. dBm. Used in RF measurements, defines 0 dBm as 1 milliwatt of RF dissipated in a 50-ohm resistive load.
2. Volume Units (VU). The VU scale is used in audio work and defines 0 VU as 1 milliwatt of 1000-Hz audio signal dissipated in a 600-ohm resistive load.
3. dB (now obsolete). Defined 0 dB as 6 milliwatts of 1000-Hz audio signal dissipated in a 500-ohm load (once used in telephone work).
4. dBmv. Used in television antenna coaxial cable systems with a 75-ohm resistive impedance, the dBmV system uses 1000 microvolts across a 75-ohm resistive load as the 0-dBmv reference point.

Consider the case of the RF signal generator. In RF systems using standard 50-ohm input and output impedances, all power levels are referenced to 0 dBm being 1 mW (i.e., 0.001 watt). To write signal levels in dBm, we used the modified power dB expression

$$\text{dBm} = 10 \log (P/1 \text{ mW})$$

Example

What is the signal level 9 milliwatts as expressed in dBm?

$$\text{dBm} = 10 \log (P/1 \text{ mW})$$
$$= 10 \log (9/1)$$
$$= 9.54 \text{ dBm}$$

Thus, when we refer to a signal level of 9.54 dBm, we mean an RF power of 9 mW dissipated in a 50-ohm load. Signal levels less than 1-mW show up as negative dBm. For example, 0.02 mW is also written as −17 dBm.

Converting dBm to volts Signal generator output controls and level meters are frequently calibrated in microvolts or millivolts (although some are also calibrated in dBm). How do we convert dBm to volts, or volts to dBm?

1. Microvolts to dBm. Use the expression $P = V^2/R = V^2/50$ to find milliwatts, and then use the dBm expression just given.

Example

Express a signal level of 800 μV (i.e., 0.8 mV) RMS in dbm.

$$P = V^2/50$$

$$= \frac{(0.8)^2}{50}$$

$$= \frac{0.64}{50} = 0.0128 \text{ mW}$$

$$\text{dBm} = 10 \log \left(\frac{P}{1 \text{ mW}}\right)$$

$$= 10 \log \left(\frac{0.0128 \text{ mW}}{1 \text{ mW}}\right)$$

$$= -18.9$$

2. Converting dBm to microvolts or millivolts. Find the power level represented by the dBm level, and then calculate the voltage using 50 ohms as the load.

Example

What voltage exists across a 50-ohm resistive load when -6 dBm is dissipated in the load?

$$P = 1 \text{ mW} \times 10^{(\text{dBm}/10)}$$

$$= 1 \text{ mW} \times 10^{(-6 \text{ dBm}/10)}$$

$$= 1 \text{ mW} \times 10^{-0.6}$$

$$= 1 \text{ mW} \times 0.25 = 0.25 \text{ mW}$$

If $P = V^2/50$, then $V = (50P)^{1/2} = 0.707(P^{1/2})$, so

$$V = 0.707 \times P^{1/2}$$

$$= 0.707 \times 0.25^{1/2}$$

$$= 3.535 \text{ mV}$$

(Note: Because power is expressed in milliwatts, the resulting answer is in millivolts. To convert to microvolts, multiply result by 1000.)

CONCLUSION

Decibels are both easy to understand and easy to use. They make design and troubleshooting of electronic systems easier and more comprehensible.

18

The Care and Feeding of Mechanical Paper Recorders

The term "mechanical recorders" refers to a broad class of devices that make a permanent paper record of analog waveforms. To the analog data system, such as an ECG machine, the recorder serves the same function as a printer in a personal computer system. That is, it creates a permanent record ("hard copy") of the data output produced by the instrument. As you will see later in this chapter, for some modern recorders (which are actually digitally based), the analogy to a computer printer is more than merely metaphorical.

Mechanical recorders are used for a variety of reasons in a variety of applications, especially in emergency and intensive care medical equipment. First, they provide a physician with a means for evaluating the waveform in a nonreal-time situation, perhaps long after the emergency is over. The physician will not always have the time to consider carefully all the implications of a recording when he or she is tending to the emergency, but afterward may want to review the record. Alternatively, another physician may be asked to evaluate a strip. Most physicians, if they are candid, would have to admit that ECG reading is not their strongest skill and that they routinely have specialists read their patients' strips. Second, the paper recorder allows a medical record to be made of an event, and this record might be useful later. Third, the record can be sent to a specialist physician for consultation purposes (although that function is now more often handled through telecommunications). Finally, the strip can be retained for future training needs.

Also, the analog recorder permits a legal record to be made of an event as evidence in case of a lawsuit. The importance of a reliable legal record cannot be overstated. The paper recording of a heart attack episode, for example, will help establish the fact that it was correctly identified and (in some cases) that it was correctly treated.

For all these reasons, the care and feeding of mechanical recorders is a necessary topic of discussion. In this chapter you will learn how these machines operate, how they are maintained, and how they are abused.

Several different categories of analog recorders are used in medicine: *strip charts, X-Y servorecorders,* and *plotters* are among the most common. We also now have analog-digital dot matrix printing mechanisms for analog recorders. The strip-chart recorder uses paper that is continuous on either a roll (like adding machine paper) or in a Z-fold pack (like personal computer printer paper). The X-Y servorecorder uses a single sheet of paper and an analog pen. The plotter is actually a sophisticated digitally controlled version of the analog X-Y recorder. Of these, the strip-chart recorder is by far the most commonly used in medicine (especially on emergency equipment). For this reason we will begin our study with this category of recorder. But first, we must examine the principal means for writing in the strip chart recorder: the *permanent magnet moving coil* (PMMC) *galvanometer* mechanism.

PMMC GALVANOMETER MOVEMENTS

The heart of any standard strip-chart recorder is a device called a *permanent magnet moving coil* (PMMC) galvanometer, or "galvie" as it is called in the trade (see Figure 18-1). The moving coil consists of a bobbin on jeweled bearings, with a lightweight coil of wire wound over it. When an electric current is applied to the coil, a weak magnetic field is set up around the coil. The signal being recorded is applied to the coil so that it causes a current to flow in the coil. Thus, the magnetic field surrounding the coil is proportional to the amplitude of the signal applied to the coil.

The permanent magnet applies a strong magnetic field across the space occupied by the moving coil. The magnetic field of the moving coil therefore interacts with the field of the permanent magnet. Recall the standard rules for magnetic field interaction: *opposite poles attract* and *like fields repel*. The reaction of the coil will be to move when a current flows. The jeweled bearings allow rotational motion only. By attaching a pen or stylus (of which, more later) to the coil's pivot point, we produce an angular deflection proportional to the applied signal amplitude.

The pen tip is positioned over a strip of chart paper that is pulled under the pen tip at a constant speed, thereby establishing a time base. Deflection of the pen across the paper reproduces the waveshape of the signal applied to the coil.

A PMMC galvanometer with a short pen arc will write in a curvilinear manner (Figure 18-2A); the pen will scribe an arc at its tip instead of a straight line. In some

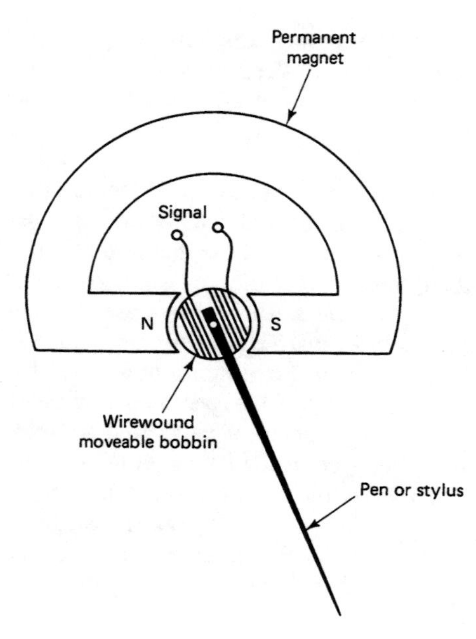

FIGURE 18-1

applications this may be tolerable, and the user merely records on a paper that has a semicircular grid marked on it. In medical applications, however, it is limited to such jobs as recording the time-varying temperature of blood lockers, incubators, and other machines that must maintain an internal temperature constant. In these cases, the amount of deflection (e.g., a temperature) is more important than the shape of the wave. Thus, this type of pen is almost useless for recording medical information and waveforms from a patient.

A solution to the problem of curvilinear recording is shown in Figure 18-2B. The PMMC mechanism is not connected directly to the pen, but through a mechanical linkage that translates the curvilinear motion of the PMMC coil bobbin to a rectilinear motion needed at the pen tip. This type of mechanism is used extensively in medical applications, although not as extensively as the knife edge method discussed next.

A pseudorectilinear technique is shown in Figure 18-2C. In this type of assembly the pen is very long compared with the arc that it must scribe (and also the chart paper width). The pen tip, therefore, travels in an arc that is very small compared with its radius, that is, the pen length. The trace, then, is nearly linear. Some curvature will exist, however, so this method is only used on some noncritical medical applications.

There are several writing methods used in strip-chart recorders, but two are amenable to a special type of pseudorectilinear writing. Both of these writing systems use a knife edge (also called "writing edge" in some service manuals), to linearize the trace effectively. The method is shown in Figure 18-2D. The pen tip still travels in a curvilinear method (which allows the simplest form of PMMC pen mechanism), but the trace is very nearly linear because the knife edge is straight. This technique works in both thermal writing and direct pressure systems (as opposed to ink) because the pen, which is actually a heated stylus, can write anywhere along its own length—not just at the tip. By keeping a straight knife edge in a fixed position

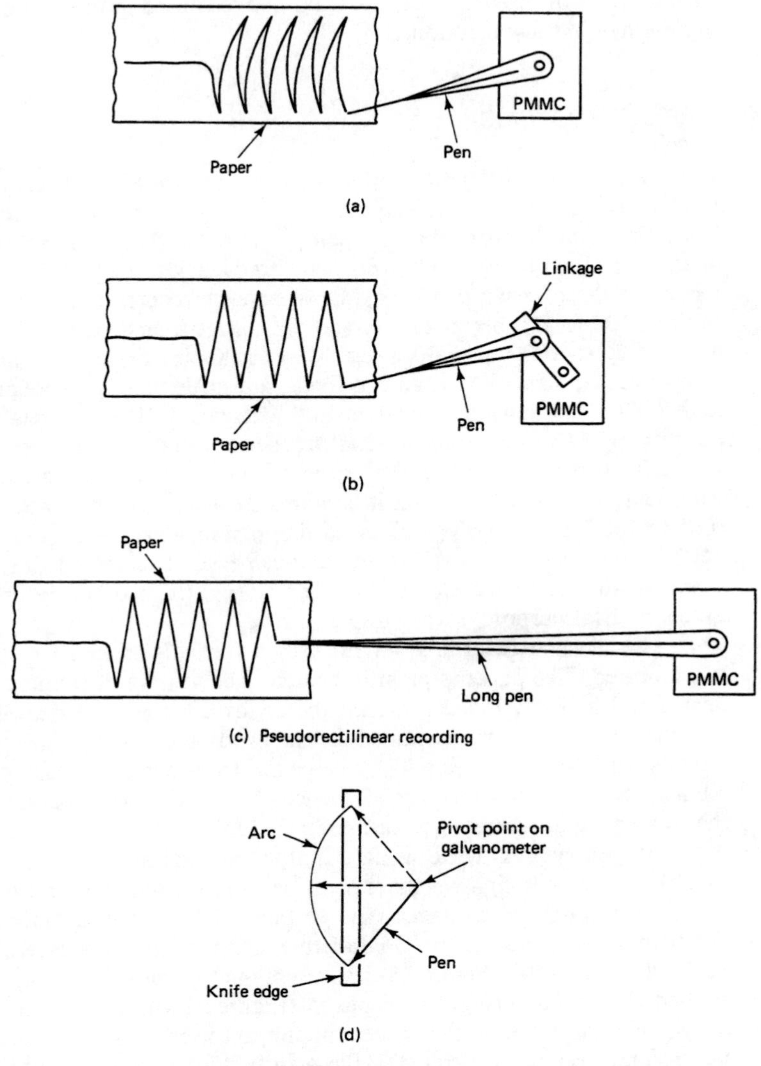

FIGURE 18-2

beneath the stylus, and allowing the stylus's point of contact with the heat or pressure-sensitive paper to vary, we obtain a rectilinear recording. It is the straightness of the knife edge that creates the rectilinear operation.

The thermal "knife-edge" recording system is used more widely than the direct contact type. The direct method uses specially treated paper similar to the "carbonless" multicopy form paper marketed by companies such as NCR for commercial purposes. The heat-sensitive paper is paraffin coated and turns black when heated. We will discuss several writing methods used in medical equipment, including the method just mentioned.

PMMC WRITING SYSTEMS

There are several different writing systems used on PMMC recorders: *direct pressure, thermal, ink pen,* and *optical.*

Those mechanisms that use pens or styluses, that is, direct pressure, thermal, or ink pen, tend to have relatively low "frequency response" due to the mechanical inertia of the massive pen or stylus. Most such recorders have an upper frequency limit of 100 to 200 hertz. Ink jet and optical recorders, on the other hand, have responses up to 1000 or 2000 hertz. Why is this important? All analog waveforms, such as ECG, EEG, EMG, and so forth, are made up of components of frequencies higher than the apparent "fundamental" frequency. For example, a 60-BPM (beat per minute) ECG has a fundamental frequency of one beat per second, or 1 Hz. But an analysis of its components in a special electronic device called a "Fourier spectrum analyzer" will show that it contains frequency components in its spectrum of 0.05 to 100 Hz. Similarly, a phonocardiogram may have spectrum components up to 1500 hertz. Therefore, a stylus recorder can easily handle an ECG waveform but not a phonocardiogram waveform. In other words, the type of recorder used for any given medical purpose is very important.

The thermal recording system uses a specially treated paper that turns black when heated. The paper is paraffin coated. The writing instrument is an electrically heated stylus. Early models formed the stylus tip from a U-shaped electrical resistance element. More modern models use a resistance element inside of a cylindrical metal stylus. In both cases a low-voltage electrical current is passed through the element, heating it almost to incandescence. The heated stylus leaves a black mark on the treated paper wherever it touches.

Ink pen systems write using a hollow pen and ink supply. In some machines, the ink is relatively lightweight (i.e., it has a low viscosity), and pressure is applied manually through an atomizer type of pump (also called a "squeeze ball" pump). Other machines, such as the Gould-Brush instruments (Figure 18-3A) and Hewlett-Packard Model 7402 (Figure 18-3B), use a thick, high viscosity ink. The pressure is applied through a spring-driven piston (Figure 18-4) inside of the ink supply cartridge. An ink manifold distributes the ink to the several pens that might be used in the system. Pressure is applied to the manifold by a solenoid that is energized when the machine power is turned on.

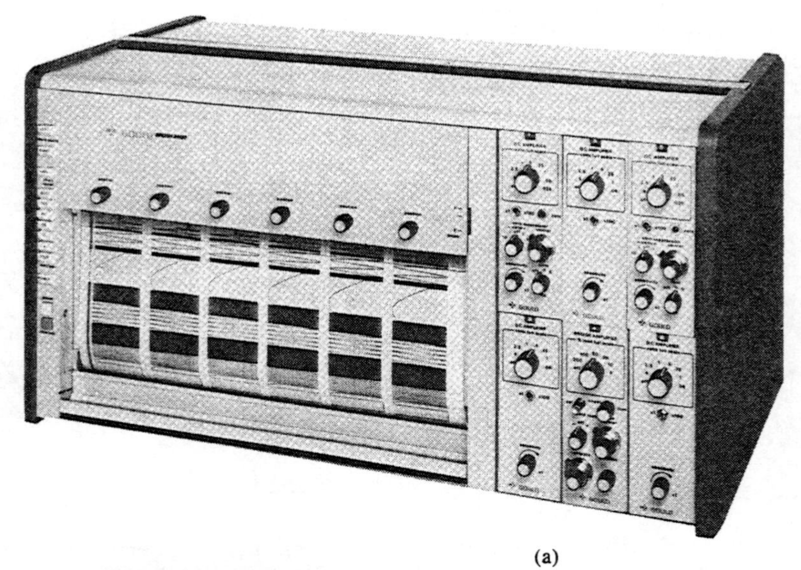

(a)

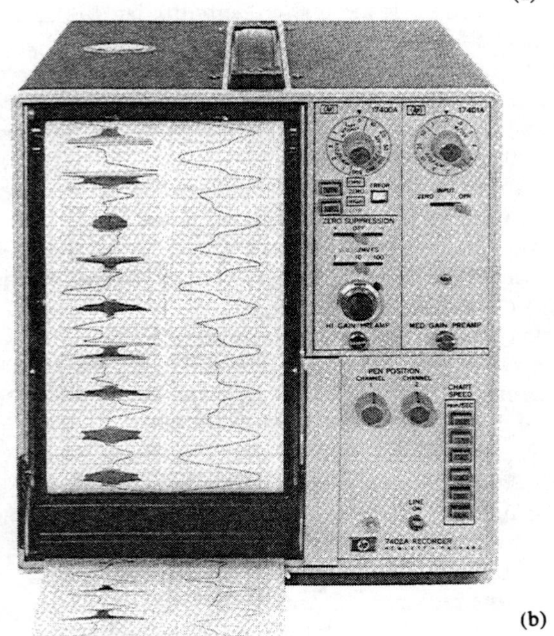

(b)

FIGURE 18-3

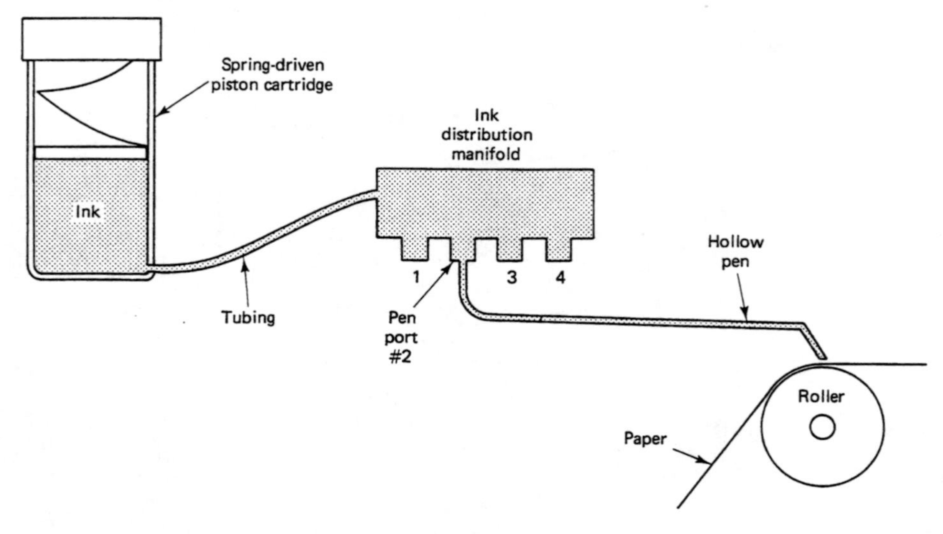

FIGURE 18-4

A related type of writing system, used in some high-frequency-response phonocardiogram machines, is the high-velocity ink jet. In that type of recorder ink under high pressure is fed to a nozzle mounted on the PMMC galvanometer in place of the pen. The ink jet is directed at the moving paper and, when the system is properly adjusted, produces a line that is almost as fine as that produced by thermal and ink pen recorders. Only a small amount of trace fuzziness is apparent, and this is due to ink splattering.

The high-velocity ink jet recorder finds use wherever a high-frequency response is needed. The low mass of the ink jet nozzle, compared with the relatively bulky mass of the ink pen and thermal stylus, gives the machine a 1000- to 2000-hertz frequency response. These recorders are sometimes used for recording phonocardiograph ("heart sound") waveforms.

An example of an optical PMMC recorder is shown in Figure 18-5A, while a cathode ray tube optical recorder is shown in Figure 18-5B. The PMMC optical writer uses a mirror mounted on the PMMC galvanometer to reflect the light beam from a collimated light source onto the photosensitive chart paper. In most such cases, the paper is at least 6 inches wide, so a greater span (or resolution) is possible. Additionally, on a multichannel recorder, the time relationships between two different traces can be more easily seen because the beams can be made to cross each other—a difficult trick to accomplish with pen or stylus recorders.

The paper is exposed to an ultraviolet light source that develops the trace as the paper comes out of the recorder. The trace will fade over a long period of time or if it is exposed to a strong light (sunlight will cause damage). Therefore, for long-term storage a light-tight box is used. Alternatively, some machines allow the paper to be wet-developed like photographic printing paper, after which process the image is stable.

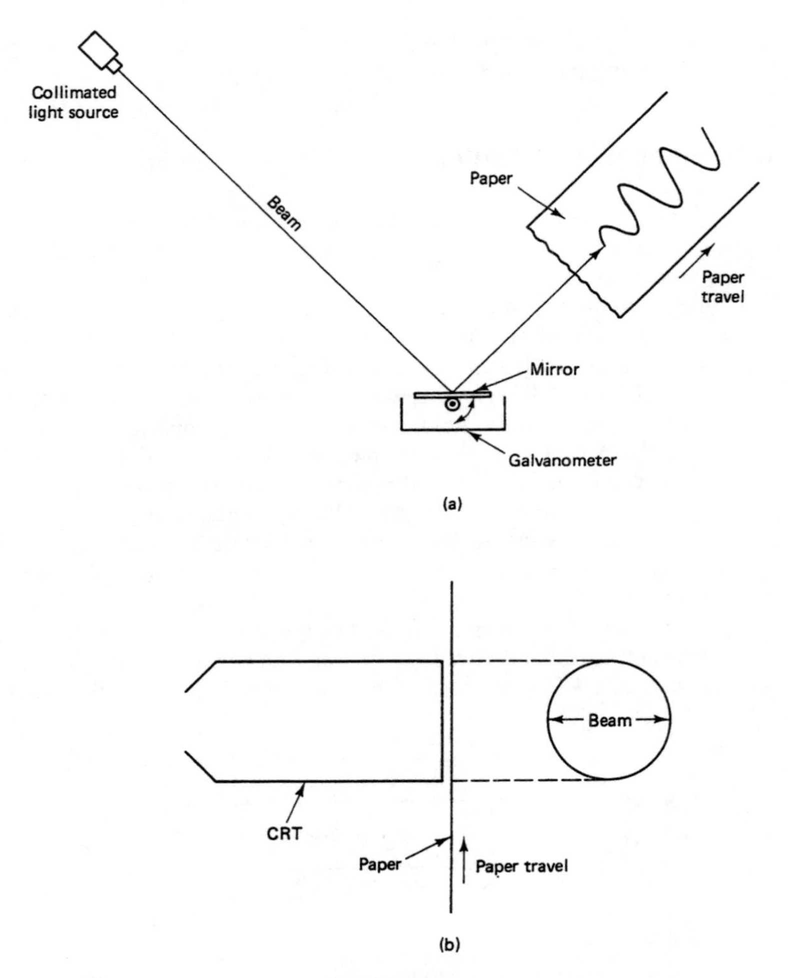

FIGURE 18-5

A few models of older recorder use a cathode ray tube (CRT) as shown in Figure 18-5B. The old VR-6 and VR-12 recorders by Electronics for Medicine are still in use. This type of chart recorder is called a *camera recorder*.

There is no time base sweep on the CRT screen. The beam sweeps back and forth along one axis in response to amplitude variations of the input signal (examine Figure 18-5B closely). A time base is provided by the constant speed at which the photosensitive paper is drawn in front of the CRT screen.

The frequency response of the PMMC optical recorder is better than that of any other PMMC system because of the low mass of the reflecting mirror. The CRT camera has an even higher-frequency response because it is limited only by the writing time of the photosensitive paper. As a result, CRT cameras often used for high-frequency medical signals such as phonocardiograph, electromyograph, and Bundle of His (and other intracardiac ECG) recordings.

RECORDING POTENTIOMETERS AND SERVORECORDERS

A *potentiometer* is a three-terminal device that acts as a variable resistor. Two ends are fixed, while the middle arm is attached to a "wiper" that selects a resistance proportional to its position. The two fixed ends are connected across a reference voltage, while the variable voltage appears at the movable wiper arm. The output voltage is proportional to the applied voltage and the relative position of the wiper on the resistance element. A galvanometer connected between the wiper and an unknown voltage will register zero deflection when the known voltage from the potentiometer is equal to the unknown voltage. This condition is called the "null" state. But if these two voltages are unequal, then the PMMC "galvie" will deflect an amount proportional to the difference between the two potentials.

It is possible to build a self-nulling potentiometer. If a pen is connected to the potentiometer's wiper drive mechanism, then the applied voltage can be recorded on paper as the mechanism constantly seeks to null out the applied voltage from the signal source.

Figure 18-6 shows the basic DC potentiometer servorecorder system. The pen is attached to a string that is wound around two idler pulleys and a drive pulley on the shaft of a DC servomotor. The pen assembly is also linked with a potentiometer

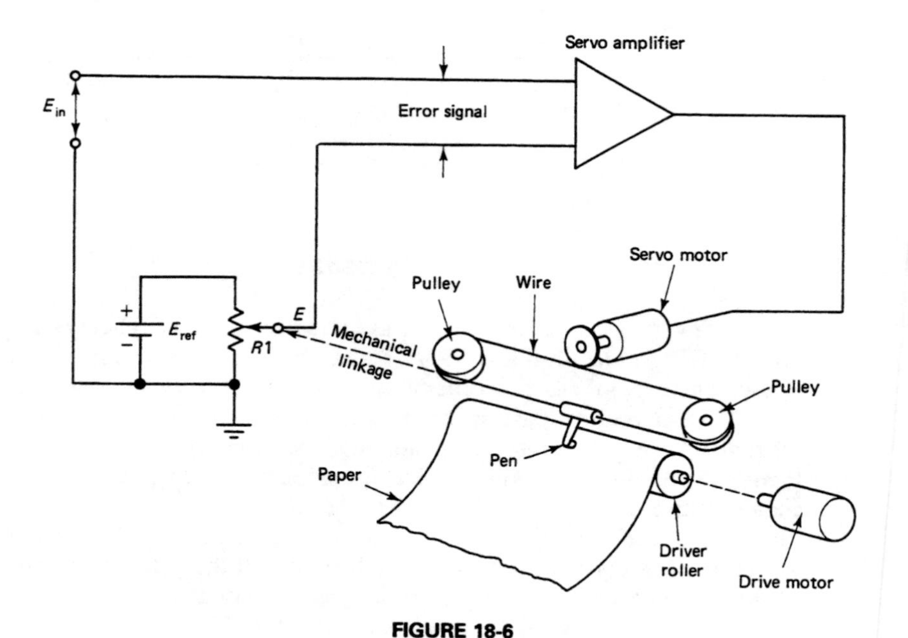

FIGURE 18-6

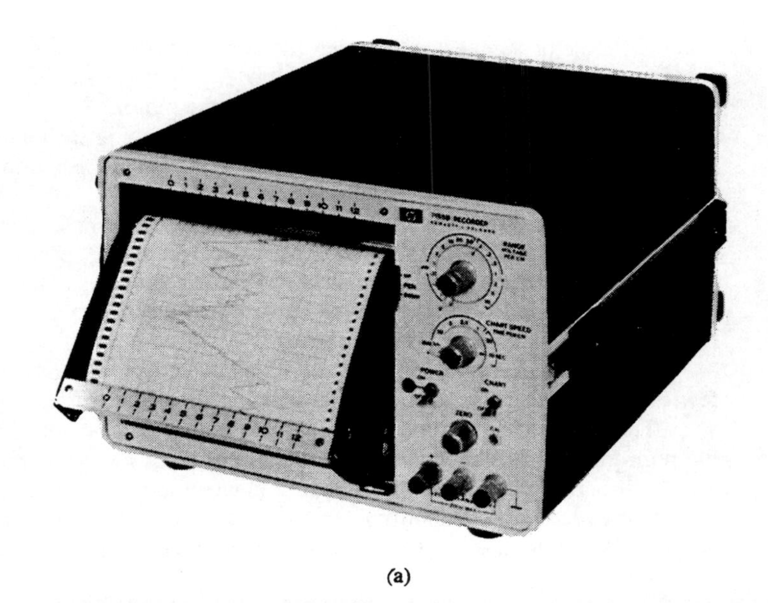

(a)

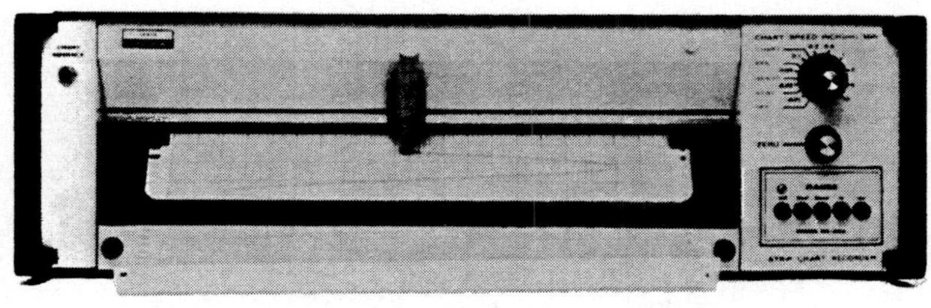

(b)

FIGURE 18-7

(R1) in such a way that the position of the wiper arm on the resistance element is proportional to the pen position.

The potentiometer element is connected across a stable, precision reference potential, E_{ref}, so potential E will represent the position of the pen. That is to say, E is the electrical *analog* of pen position. When the pen is at the left-hand side of the paper (in Figure 18-6), then E is zero, and when the pen is full scale (that is, at the right-hand side of the paper), E is equal to E_{ref}.

The pen position is controlled by the DC servomotor, which is in turn driven by the output of the servoamplifier. This amplifier has differential inputs. The input signal E_{in} is applied to one amplifier input, and the position signal E is applied to the other amplifier input. The difference signal ($E_{in} - E$) represents the error between the actual pen position and the position it should take in response to the command from E_{in}.

If the error signal is zero, then the amplifier output is also zero, so the motor remains turned off. But if E is not equal to E_{in}, then the amplifier sees an input signal and creates an output signal that turns on the motor.

The motor drives the pen potentiometer assembly in such a direction as to cancel the error signal. When the input signal and the pen position signal are equal, then the motor shuts off and the pen remains at rest.

A paper drive motor forms a time base because it pulls the paper underneath the pen at a fixed, constant rate. In most servorecorders a sprocket drive is used instead of the roller drive system popular in PMMC machines. The paper used in these machines (see Figure 18-7) has holes along each margin to accept the sprocket teeth, much like personal computer printer paper.

Most high-grade servorecorders use either a stepper motor that rotates only a few degrees for each pulse applied to its winding or a continuously running motor.

The stepper motor method is low in cost, and can be very precise when a stable reference clock oscillator is used as the source of the electronic drive pulses.

The actual potentiometer resistance element used may be any of the following: slide wire, rectilinear potentiometer, or a rotary potentiometer. The slide wire system is very common because it can be built with less friction loss and no mechanical

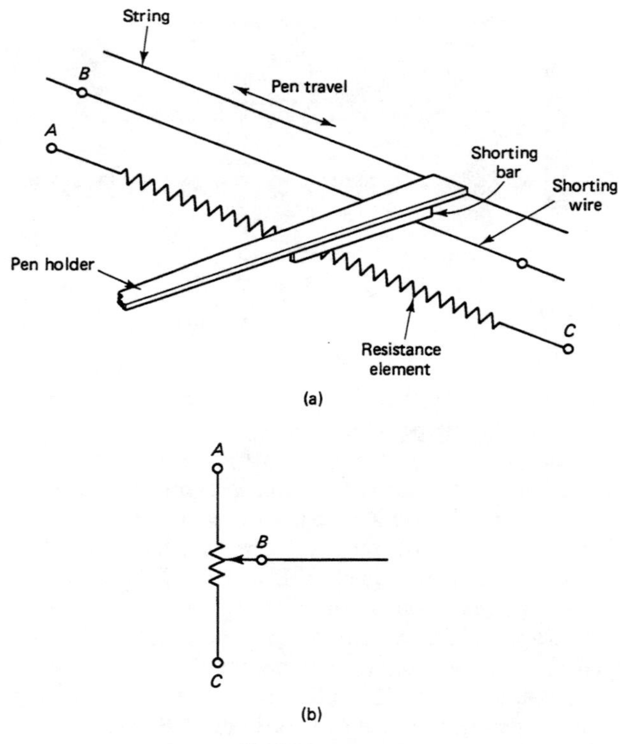

FIGURE 18-8

linkage. A shorting bar on the pen assembly serves as the wiper element on the slide wire resistance element; it also serves to connect the shorting bar to the wire. The letters A, B, and C in Figure 18-8A refer to the potentiometer terminals shown in Figure 18-8B. The shorting wire "B" serves as the terminal for the wiper.

X-Y RECORDERS AND PLOTTERS

An X-Y recorder (Figure 18-9) uses two servomechanism pen assemblies mounted at right angles to one another. The vertical (or Y-plane) amplifier moves the pen vertically along the bar, while the X-plane amplifier moves the bar back and forth across the paper.

The paper itself does not move, and is usually held in place by clamps or, in high-grade machines, a vacuum drawn by a pump connected to a hollow chamber beneath the paper platform. Holes in the paper platform create the negative pressure needed to keep the paper in place.

One advantage to the X-Y recorder over either PMMC or servorecorders is that almost any type of paper may be used. Most X-Y recorders are designed to accept the standard-size graph papers used by scientists, engineers, and physicians.

The X-Y recorder can be made to record time-varying signals by applying a linear ramp voltage to the X-plane input. The ramp is adjusted so that it traverses the horizontal width of the paper in the desired length of time.

An X-Y plotter (Figure 18-10) is an X-Y recorder that has an electrically operated pen-lift mechanism. A plotter can make patterns of complex shape, including alphanumerics. Many modern plotters are designed to do computer graphics, while others handle both analog and digital data.

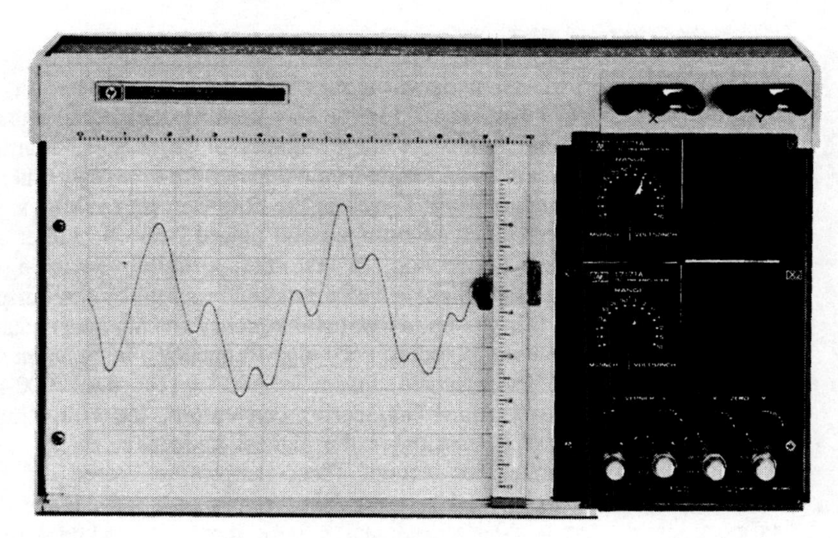

FIGURE 18-9

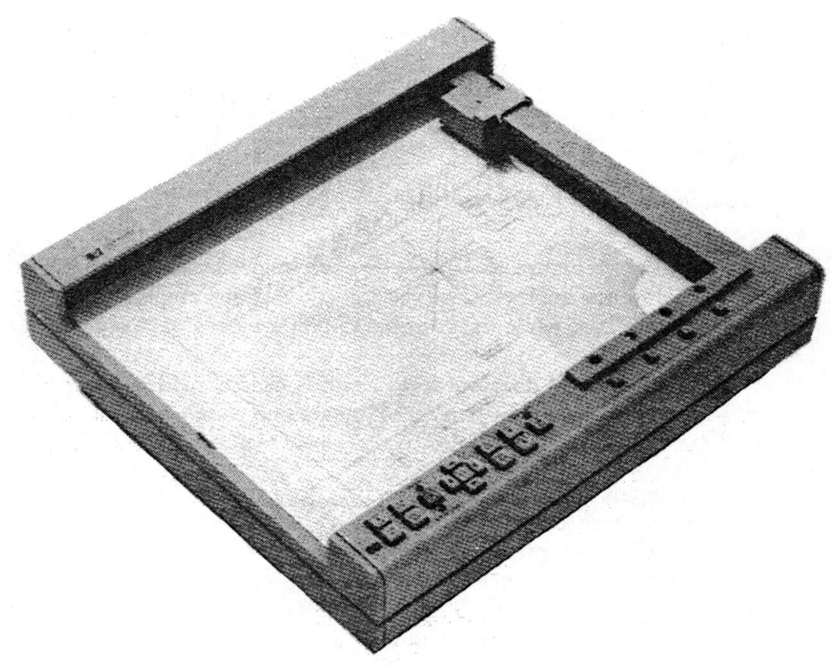

FIGURE 18-10

DIGITAL RECORDERS

A relatively new class of medical recorder is the digital type (Figure 18-11). The input signal is applied to an analog-to-digital (A/D) converter. The A/D device produces a binary output "data word" (of the sort used in computers) that is proportional to the signal amplitude. If a large number of successive "samples" of the analog waveform are taken, and stored in a computerlike memory, then the pattern of digital data in the memory will represent the time-varying analog signal.

The data in memory can be scanned and played back to either a strip-chart recorder or CRT screen for viewing. In that case, a digital-to-analog (D/A) converter is used to re-create the analog voltage signal required by the display device.

An advantage of this system is that low-frequency (which also means low-cost) paper recorders can be used to record very high-frequency analog signals simply by varying the time base. For example, suppose we want to record a 1000-hertz analog signal. According to a standard engineering convention, the sampling rate of an analog signal should be at least twice the highest frequency, so we need to take $2 \times 1000 = 2000$ samples per second. These samples are stored in the computer memory. When we want to make a recording we need only reduce the sampling rate proportionally, say, to 20/sec, and play it back through a standard low-frequency machine.

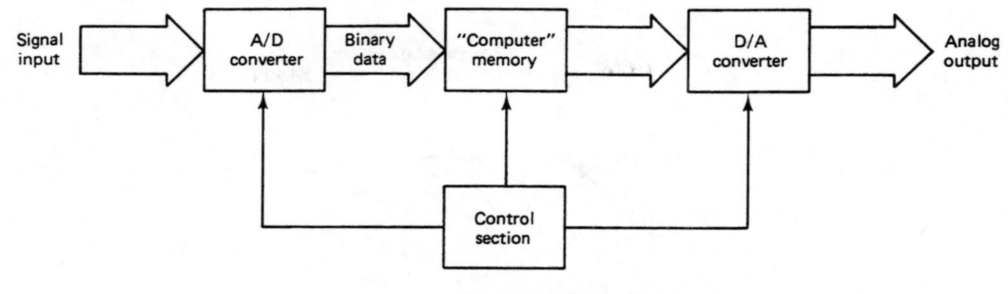

FIGURE 18-11

This method is one means for standard hospital ECG machines to be used for higher-frequency studies. The same method is also used for producing the "nonfade" oscilloscopes in ECG monitors used in emergency medicine. Normally, the ECG waveform would fade almost immediately after it occurs. But with the digital recording oscilloscope, it will remain on the screen until the memory is used up and is overwritten by newer data.

RECORDER PROBLEMS

The pen assembly always has a certain amount of inertia because of its mass, regardless of whether PMMC or servo systems are used. Because of its mass the pen assembly will not start moving until a certain minimum signal is applied. Figure 18-12 shows this so-called "deadband" phenomena. The definition of the deadband is "the largest amplitude signal to which the instrument will *not* respond." In most quality instruments the deadband is not more than 0.05 to 0.1 percent of full scale.

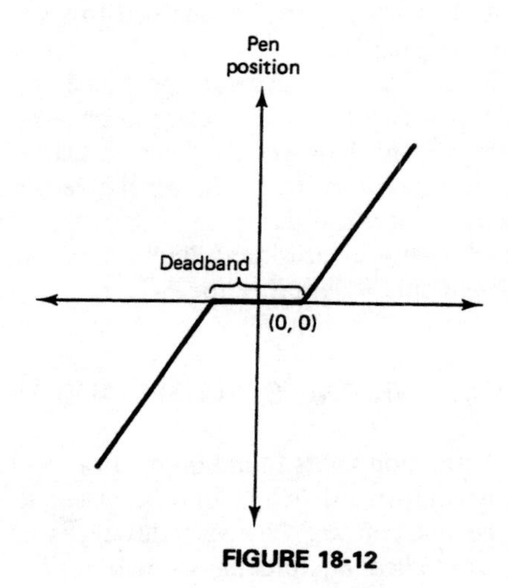

FIGURE 18-12

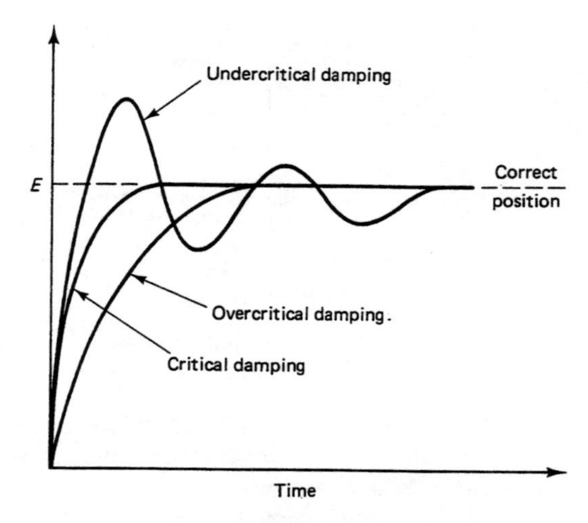

FIGURE 18-13

The deadband can cause severe distortion of the recorded trace, especially on low-amplitude signals whose level approximates the deadband itself. The solution to the problem of deadband is to slew the signal through the deadband as rapidly as possible.

Another problem is overshoot or undershoot of the pen in response to a step function (e.g., square wave). This problem also affects both forms of mechanical writer. Figure 18-13 shows three different responses. In a properly damped recorder, the pen will rise to the correct position with very little rounding of the trace. This situation is called "critical damping."

A subcritically damped signal will overshoot the correct position, and then hunt back and forth across the correct position for a few cycles before it settles on the correct point. If a square wave is applied to such a system, then the recording will appear to be "ringing."

An overcritically damped system approaches the final value very sluggishly. The pen in that type of system will appear to be very sluggish. A square wave applied to such a system will have rounded edges. Damping is an important parameter in medical recorders because it can distort the resultant traces and thereby mimic pathological traces. Subcritical damping mimics the double or "notched" QRS complex of heart block, while overcritical damping mimics the trace often found in recent heart attack patients by altering the S-T segment of the waveform.

MAINTENANCE OF PMMC WRITING STYLUSES AND PENS

There are several common faults found on medical paper recorders. These are sometimes amenable to adjustment, while in other cases repair is necessary. Let's separately consider the ink pen and heated stylus types of recorder. Because they find only limited use in medical equipment, we will not consider some of the other types (even though you need to be aware of them conceptually). In this section we will take a look at some common maintenance actions that don't always need trained engineering technicians to perform.

Figure 18-14 shows how to remove an ink blockage from an ink pen recorder that's been allowed to stand too long without being used. As a general rule, such recorders should be run for about 5 minutes or so once a week when not in regular service. Otherwise, the ink will dry up at the tip and prevent the recorder from writing. Fill a 3- to 10-cc syringe with water (or acetone if certain types of ink are used), and insert the needle end into the ink inlet on the rear end of the pen assembly. On most recorders the pen will have to be removed from the machine for this operation. The needle should be inserted up to the Luer lock hub to make a good fluid seal. Quickly, and with a single sharp motion, drive the plunger "home" so that a high-pressure jet of water or acetone is forced into the pen. The ink clot should be forced under high pressure out the other end.

This procedure usually works quite well. Some precautions are in order, however. First, always wear protective goggles over your eyes when doing this operation. Also, wear protective clothing, as ink/water will splatter everywhere. Second, make sure that the pen tip is aimed downward into a sink (there is still a laboratory at George Washington University Medical Center with a blue spot on the ceiling tiles

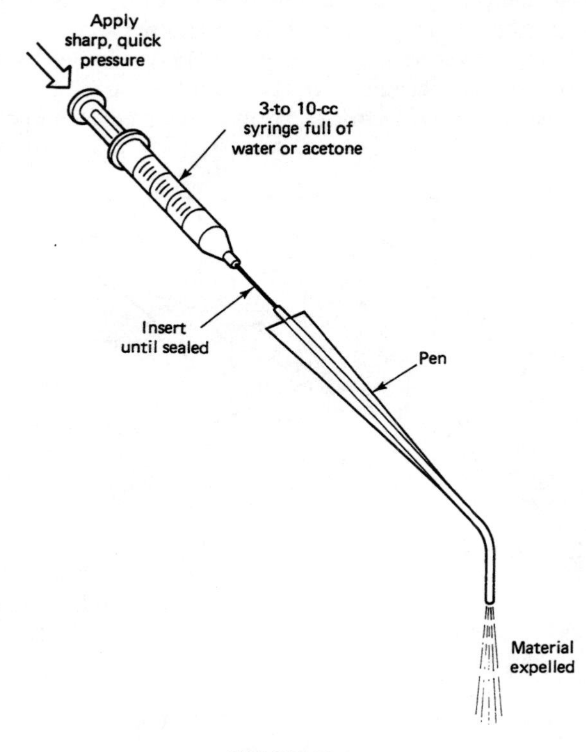

FIGURE 18-14

over the sink—where the author failed to observe this precaution). Finally, as always when dealing with needles, be careful not to stick yourself.

Also, keep in mind that the thick, high-viscosity ink used in these machines stains everything it touches and is the virtual dickens to clean.

Ink pen tips are designed to operate parallel to the paper surface (see inset in Figure 18-15). If the pen is worn, or when a new pen is installed, it is necessary to "lap" the tip in order to reestablish the parallelism. The symptom that lapping is needed will be either (or both) of the following: (1) a "blob" of ink when the machine first starts recording a waveform or (2) a too-thick trace. In most such machines the ink should be dry before the paper leaves the paper platform at the drive roller end of the surface. If it is not dry, then lapping may be needed. To lap the pen, place a piece of very fine emery cloth (a sandpaperlike material available at any hardware store) under the tip. The pen tip is worked back and forth five to ten times to "sand" the tip parallel to the paper.

The pressure of the stylus or pen is also important. If the pressure is not correct, then the waveform may be distorted. On medical equipment it is possible to make a normally healthy lead I ECG signal look like it has either a heart block or a recent myocardial infarction because of improperly adjusted stylus pressure. The manufacturer will specify a pressure in grams. These numbers vary from 1 to 10 grams depending upon the machine model (and its year of manufacture—older model machines tended to use heavier stylus pressures).

A stylus pressure gauge (see Figure 18-16) is used to lift the pen or stylus from the paper as the machine is running until the trace just disappears. The pressure reading is then made from the barrel of the gauge. Suitable stylus pressure gauges

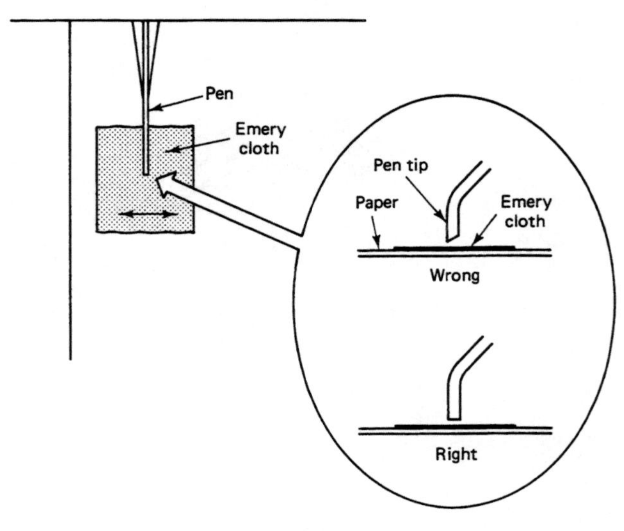

FIGURE 18-15

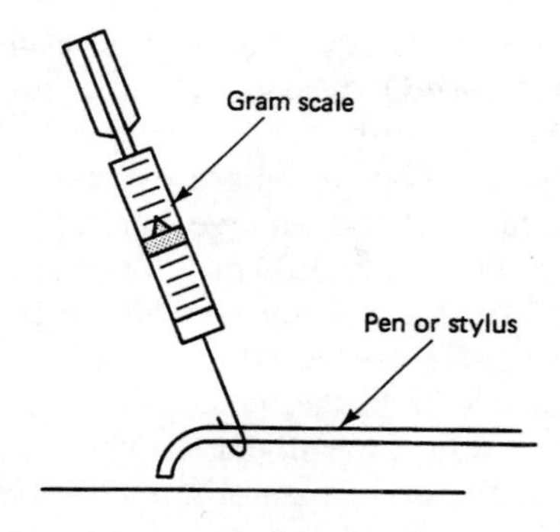

FIGURE 18-16

can be purchased from ECG machine manufacturers' service or parts departments. Alternatively, the stylus pressure gauge used for record player "tone arms" is also useful if the specified pressure is within their relatively limited range (usually 0 to 4 grams). The stylus pressure adjustment is made using a screw that is usually located on the rear of the stylus (or pen) or the assembly that holds it in place.

Figure 18-17 shows several different 1-millivolt calibration pulses from an ECG machine. These traces can be made by pressing the "1 MV" or "CAL" button on the front panel of the machine. The ideal shape is perfectly square, as shown in Figure 18-17A. But this ideal is almost never achieved in practical machines because of the inertia of the pen or stylus assembly. Usually we see the slightly rounded features of the pulse shown in Figure 18-17B. This waveform is usually acceptable. What is not acceptable, however, are the overdamped and underdamped waveforms of Figures 18-17C and 18-17D, respectively.

On all recorders there may be a damping control available for adjustment by a properly trained technician. This control is adjusted (usually internally to the machine) in order to compensate for problems. On ink pen machines the stylus pressure

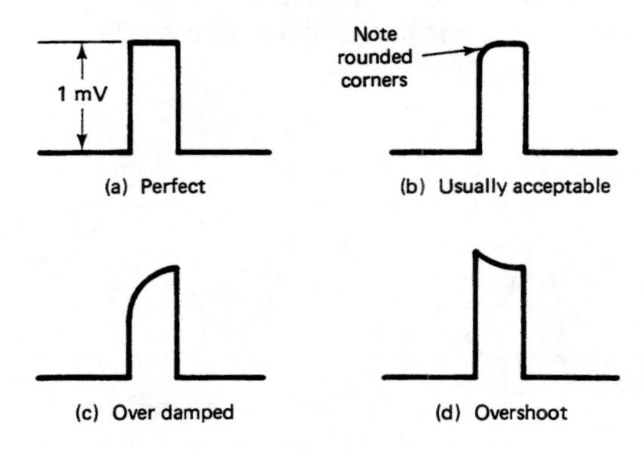

FIGURE 18-17

can affect the waveshape, especially if it is set to too high a value (it produces the overdamped waveform). On heated stylus machines, both the stylus pressure and the heat can affect the waveform.

On some heated stylus machines the standard procedure is to set the pressure to a specified value, set the voltage applied to the stylus heating element to a specified value (usually either 5.00 or 7.00 volts), and then adjust the internal damping control to produce the waveform of Figure 18-17B in response to either a square wave input or successive presses of the "1 MV CAL" button.

If the manufacturer of the machine did not provide a knob on the stylus heat control, then don't adjust it without the correct equipment (usually stylus pressure gauge and voltmeter) *and* the manufacturer's service manual! The author remembers a time when the director of the emergency room called me and snorted that he didn't really believe that the last 40 patients—only 1 of which had a cardiac complaint—all had recent myocardial infarctions. The problem was that an ambitious medical student (who also held an electrical engineering degree) *thought* he knew how to adjust the heat, but did not. He brought a small screwdriver to work and adjusted the heat to make the trace lighter "for reliability reasons." The trace was lighter, allright, but the machine would not recover from fast waveform transitions (such as an ECG QRS complex) fast enough. As a result, the extra inertia caused by insufficient melting of the paraffin on the paper of the ECG tracings all erroneously showed S-T segment anomalies.

DOT MATRIX ANALOG RECORDERS

The *dot matrix printer* is long familiar to users of computer equipment. The dot matrix printer was developed in response to the high cost of traditional computer printers. At the time that they became popular, the dot matrix printer cost about one-fifth to one-third the cost of daisy wheel, Selectric, or similar printer mechanisms. The original dot matrix printers (mid-1970s) used a 5 × 7 matrix of dots (Figure 18-18A) to form alphanumeric characters.

The dot matrix machine used a print head (Figure 18-18B) to cause the correct

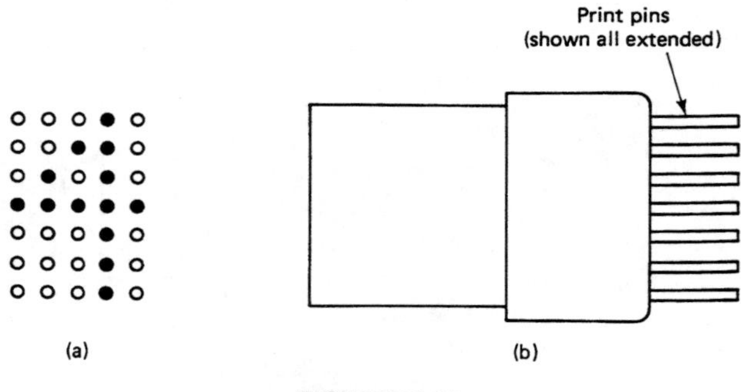

FIGURE 18-18

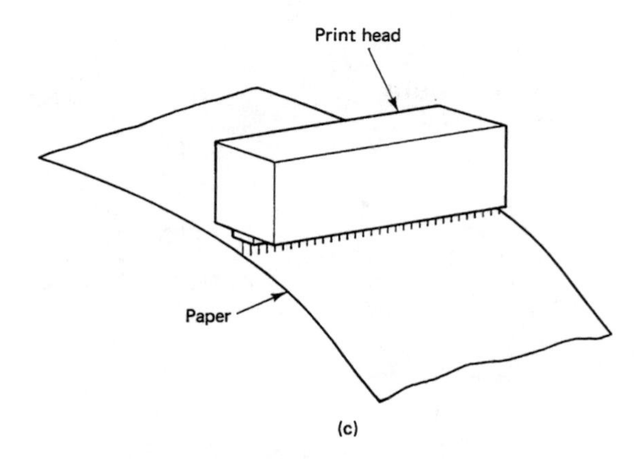

FIGURE 18-18 (continued)

dot elements to be energized to make a mark on the paper. Two different methods were once popular, although one has since faded almost to obscurity. Some of the earliest machines were thermally based. The dots were thermally connected to heating coils, and could be heated when needed. Special temperature-sensitive paper was used to receive the text. This method is no longer used widely. The second method used an array of 7 print hammers (actually pins). The pins would either extend or retract depending upon whether or not that particular dot was active for the character being printed. An advantage of the pin method is that ordinary paper can be used. The pins impact an inked ribbon to leave the impression. Although the original low-resolution printers were 7-pin models (as shown in Figure 18-18A and B), there are now available higher-resolution models with 9-, 18- and now 24-pin print heads.

It was rapidly discovered in the computer world that clever programmers could make a dot matrix print head do graphics as well as alphanumerics. The spate of newsletters, church and school bulletins, and other low-cost (but often creatively done) publications are testimony to the graphics capability of modern dot matrix technology.

Dot matrix printing can be used to make analog recorders that outperform most older mechanical analog recorders. Figure 18-18C shows the concept schematically. A dot matrix print head with a very large number of pins is arrayed over a platten. The action depends upon whether thermal, electro-arc, or plain strip-chart paper is used. Regardless of the particulars, however, the result is a strip-chart recording that mixes analog and digital data on the same chart.

Figure 18-19 shows dot matrix analog recordings. The digital computer backing up this system can print the appropriate grid (notice the difference between Figures 18-19A and 18-19B; these recordings were made sequentially on the same machine without changing paper). Printed as alphanumeric characters along the top of the strip are data including ICU bed number, time, date, ECG lead number, heart rate, and blood pressure values. Figure 18-19B is similar to Figure 18-19A, but includes an arterial blood pressure waveform along with the ECG waveform.

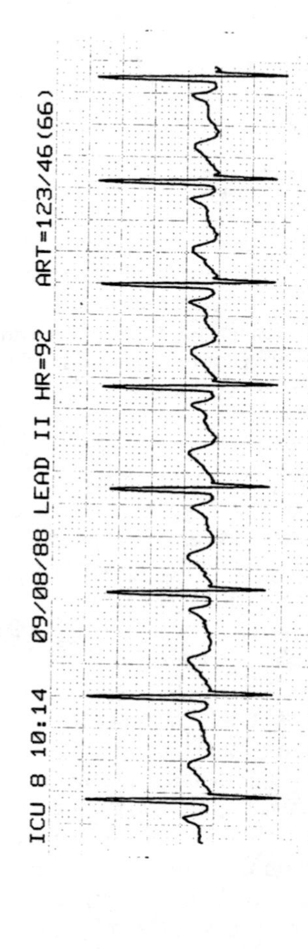
ICU 8 10:14 09/08/88 LEAD II HR=92 ART=123/46(66)

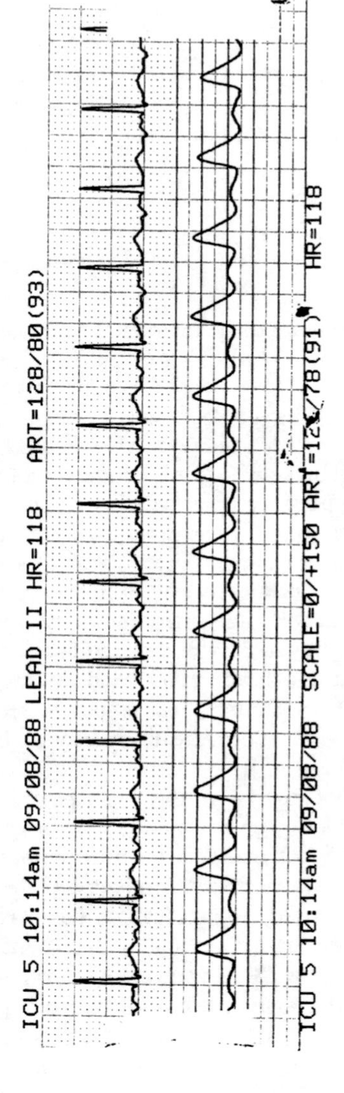
ICU 5 10:14am 09/08/88 LEAD II HR=118 ART=128/80(93)
ICU 5 10:14am 09/08/88 SCALE=0/+150 ART=12
/78(91)
HR=118

FIGURE 18-19

19

Care and Feeding of Battery-Operated Medical Equipment

Much medical equipment uses batteries of one sort or another. The "care and feeding" of batteries is a critical element in keeping the equipment ready for use and is thus especially problematical in emergency equipment.

The author worked for a long time in a biomedical electronics laboratory and was employed by a large eastern university medical center. We used batteries for a lot of different reasons. Some equipment was battery powered for reasons of portability. A defibrillator, for example, might be needed almost any place—heart attack victims didn't always have the good sense to die near an electrical outlet. Although most of our defibrillators were AC powered (or dual powered), we also had a number of purely battery-powered models. We also had patient monitors that ran on batteries. These were used to keep track of ECG and blood pressure as the patient was transferred between units, for example, from emergency room to the intensive care unit. Still other devices used batteries for reasons of patient safety. A cardiac output computer, for example, makes measurements based on a thermistor inserted into the heart. Small amounts of AC "leakage" current could be fatal, so batteries are used to isolate the instrument completely from the AC power line.

A "cell" is the most basic element, and sets the minimum voltage for that sort of device. Additional voltage is gained by connecting the cells in series, and extra current is available by connecting them in parallel. To be strict, we would refer to single entities as "cells" and multiple-cell entities as "batteries." But in common usage, it is usually acceptable to be less than rigorous, so all cells and batteries are called "batteries."

In this section we will discuss mostly the nickel-cadmium batteries (NiCd) commonly used in portable electronics equipment. These batteries have a nominal terminal voltage at full charge of 1.2 volts, except immediately prior to turn-on after a fresh charge (at which time the "open-terminal" voltage is 1.4 volts). Shortly after turn-on, however, the open-terminal voltage drops from 1.4 volts to the nominal value of 1.2 volts for the duration of the operation. As the stored energy is used up, however, the terminal voltage drops lower.

NiCd batteries are rechargeable, and will typically sustain a charge-discharge cycle lifetime of 1000 times before becoming unusable. In most cases, manufacturers rate a battery as unusable when the capacity of the battery drops below 80 percent of its original specified value.

The capacity of a battery is measured in ampere-hours. That is, the product of current load (in amperes) and time required to reach the officially designated discharge state. The NiCd battery is capable of delivering tremendous currents. For example, the size D (4 A-H) and size F (7 A-H) can deliver short-duration currents of 50 amperes, or more. That is why they are used in medical defibrillators and why certain medium power portable radio transmitters can use them. As a result of their ability to deliver huge currents, NiCd batteries should be fused in order to protect printed wiring tracks, wires, and other conductors. The author has seen copper foil-printed wiring board tracks and an on-off switch vaporized by a shorted capacitor across the DC line.

The amount of time that a battery will last is a function of the discharge time, which in turn is determined by the amount of current drawn. Figure 19-1 shows two different discharge scenarios: one for a current of one-tenth the A-H rating and one for a current equal to the A-H rate. In Figure 19-1A the battery will be fully discharged in ten hours, while in Figure 19-1B discharge occurs in one hour. This particular chart is derived from the data published for a size D cell rated at 4 A-H.

The standard cell ratings for NiCd batteries are as follows:

BATTERY SIZE	AMPERE-HOUR RATING
AA	0.4/0.5/0.7
C	2
D	4
F	7

As you can see, the "AA" cells are found in three ratings from 400 to 700 mA-H, depending upon the manufacturer and style. You will find a lot of variation from this chart, especially among consumer product NiCd batteries. Some "size C" cells are rated at both 1 and 1.2 A-H, and size D rated at 2 A-H. Suspect that these are actually lesser cells dressed in size C and size D packages. One manufacturer's representative actually admitted to me that the consumer "D cells" were actually size C cells inside of a D package.

This chicanery is of little consequence to most consumer electronics users and actually results in a lower-cost product. But if you use or service commercial, medical, or communications equipment, then make sure that you get the correct ampere-

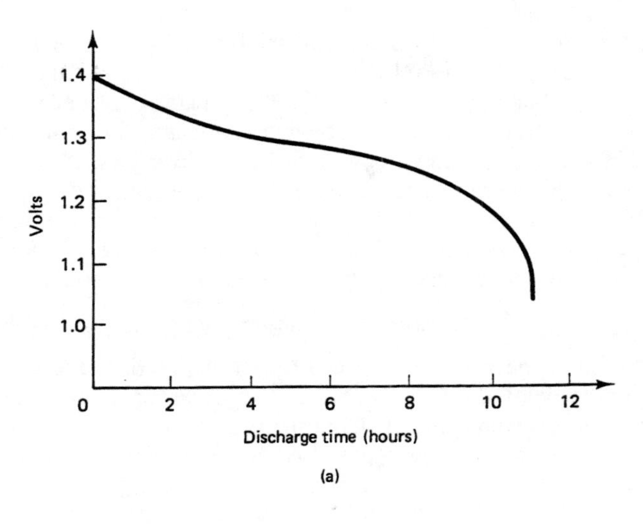

(a)

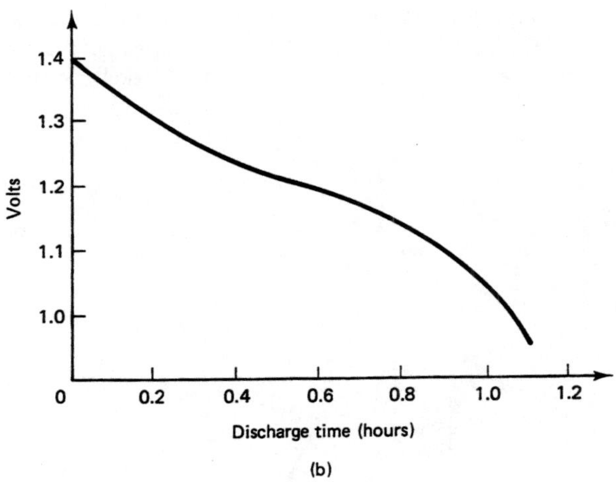

(b)

FIGURE 19-1

hour rating. It has been my experience that Gould brand cells are fully rated, while certain others require caution. I would not want to be the guy who reduces a heart patient's chance of survival by replacing 4 A-H NiCd cells in the defibrillator with a collection of 2 A-H consumer replacements intended for power toothbrushes and "blaster" radios. *Be sure of the rating of replacement batteries and cells!*

Rating games are also played by some distributors by quoting different discharge rates. One standard method of measuring A-H capacity is the current required to discharge a cell to 1.0 volts in one hour. Some makers, however, define it in terms of the 10-hour discharge rate normalized to ampere-hours. From analyzing

Figures 19-1A and 19-1B you can see how this might result in a warm, fuzzy—but false—feeling of capacity.

The charging protocol for the NiCd battery depends somewhat on application and manufacturer. In general, though, the charge current must be at least A-H/20, and in many commercial consumer battery chargers, it is often A-H/15. For most applications where you can control the charge rate, it is safe to use a charge rate of A-H/10. That is, charge the battery at a current not greater than one-tenth the ampere-hour rating. In addition, the battery must be charged to 140 percent of capacity, so a charge time of 14 hours at A-H/10 is mandated. The general rule is

charge at 1/10 ampere-hour rating for 14 hours

Some chargers are designed to fast charge the battery in as little as one hour, with most being three to four hours. Fast charging should not be done unless the battery maker recommends it. Even then, be a little cautious about fast charging (cells can explode from charging too fast). NiCd batteries can be dangerous, so don't ad-lib: follow the maker's recommendations rigorously.

NiCd batteries can also lose energy from merely sitting. Some users find that a battery charged up, and then stored, is unusable at the time when it is eventually turned on. Figure 19-2 shows a storage discharge curve for a typical NiCd battery. As you can see, the battery or cell will be of doubtful use after only a few weeks.

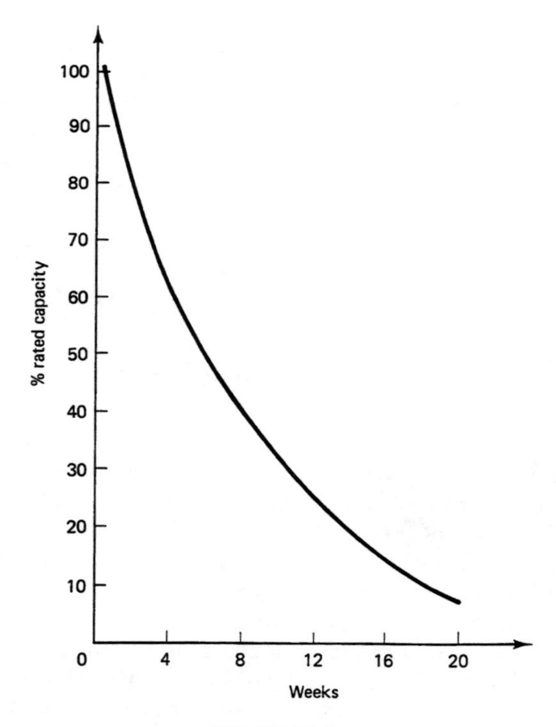

FIGURE 19-2

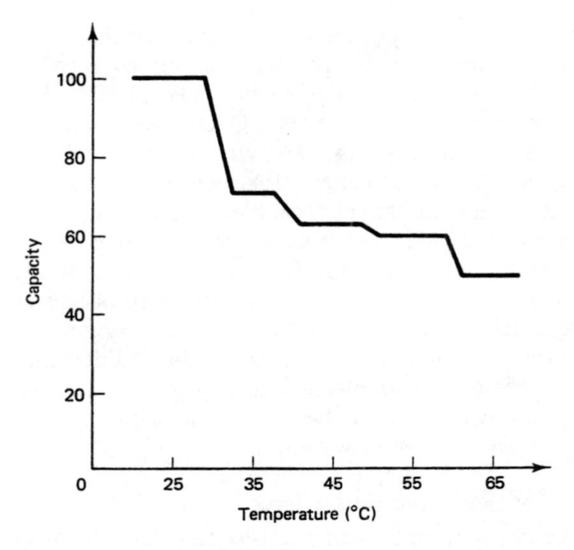

FIGURE 19-3

storage. I can recall many times when nurses in our neonatal intensive care unit complained bitterly about an instrument (and my ability to keep it fixed), when the truth was that the instrument was never plugged into the charger. The cure for this form of problem is a trickle charge at a rate between A-H/30 and A-H/50. Some commercial battery chargers have a switch that allows either an A-H/10 regular charge rate or an A-H/30 trickle charge.

Another problem with NiCds is the operating temperature and its effects on available capacity. As shown in Figure 19-3, the available current capacity is a function of temperature. As the temperature increases above room temperature (25°C), the available capacity diminishes.

NiCd "MEMORY"

You will hear a running debate that NiCds do/do not have a memory problem. "Memory" means that a battery will not allow deep discharge after repeated shallow discharges. For example, if a battery is repeatedly discharged in some particular application to only 80 percent of capacity, after a while it will "remember" the 80 percent level as the fully discharged point. The battery will then exhibit the fully-discharged potential when the charge level is only 80 percent of fully charged. That makes the battery look like a premature failure. A NiCd battery suffering memory problems can sometimes be reformed by repeatedly fully charging it and then immediately deep discharging it. After a while the memory phenomenon would work itself out.

The best "cure" for the memory phenomenon is to avoid it altogether. I have a friend who lives in constant pain and as a result uses an electronic pulse generator called a "transcutaneous electronic nerve stimulator" (TENS) to keep the pain at a manageable low level. His physician prescribed a device that runs on small internal NiCd batteries instead of replaceable cells. My friend complained that the $90 battery pack lasted only a few weeks. Questioning him, I found that he routinely placed the TENS unit in the charger every night, even though he didn't use it all the time. Hence, the TENS unit battery was routinely shallow-cycled—and developed memory. I instructed him to keep two battery packs available. One is kept in an insulated bag in his brief case, and is used when the other one goes dead; the other was installed in the unit. When the TENS unit battery was low, it didn't work as well, so my friend would swap battery packs. He used one battery pack for two years, and had been averaging at least one year on each—instead of six-weeks.

When equipment is subject to routine maintenance, it is possible to keep the batteries healthy by following a certain routine. For most equipment the manufacturer recommends that the batteries be periodically discharged and then recharged. The protocol for most is as follows

1. Fully charge the battery or cell.
2. Discharge it fully with a resistor that draws a current of A-H/10 for about 8–9 hours for multicell batteries and 10 hours for single cells.
3. Recharge the battery at the A-H/10 rate for 14–16 hours.

A phenomenon called "polarity reversal" might result if the battery is fully discharged. The cause of this problem is that not all cells have the same terminal voltage at any given time. It might occur that one cell will become charged backward by the others in the series chain. For this reason, multicell batteries are only discharged to 10–20 percent of capacity.

Do not leave the battery in a discharged condition for a lengthy period of time. The battery may then develop interelement shorts. Little whiskers called "dendrites" grow internally from plate to plate and cause a short circuit. The cell potential drops to zero or near zero, and the cell will refuse to accept a charge. In some cases we would have to regard the cell as lost and replace it. There are, however, some cells that can be salvaged from short circuits.

Figure 19-4 shows a revitalization circuit for shorted NiCd cells. It works by vaporizing the internal dendrites that short the plates together. A known good cell of the same type is placed across the shorted cell through a push-button or spring-loaded toggle switch. It is important to use this type of switch instead of a regular switch: you don't want to keep the circuit closed for too long (battery explosion could result). Press the switch several times in succession, and then measure the terminal voltage. If the current from $V1$ successfully vaporizes the dendrites inside of $V2$, then the terminal voltage will rise.

Caution. A word of caution is in order for people using this method: be sure to wear safety goggles or glasses when performing this operation. NiCd batteries have been known to explode under high current, and it could conceivably happen when deshorting a cell. Most equipment maintenance technicians have never seen it happen under this circumstance, but those who are smart wouldn't bet their eyesight on it never happening!

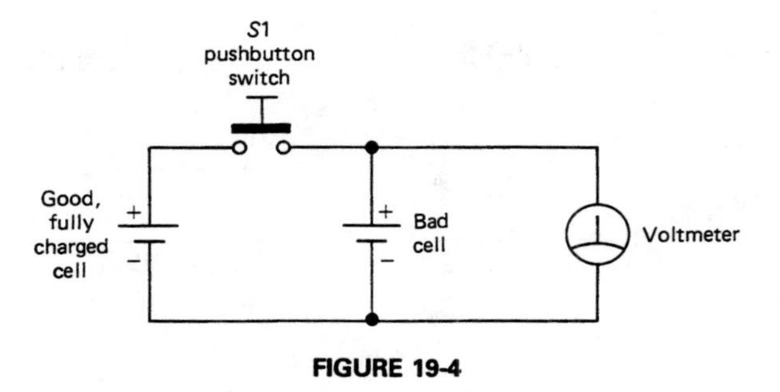

FIGURE 19-4

CHARGING NiCd BATTERIES

There are two basic forms of charger for NiCd batteries: constant current (CI) and constant voltage (CV). Regardless of the type, it is important to not use a charging current greater than A-H/10 unless specifically instructed to do so by the battery manufacturer (not the equipment maker, by the way). The A-H/10 rate is one-tenth of the ampere-hour rating. For a 500-mAH "AA" cell, for example, a charging current of 50 mA is used. Similarly, for a 2 A-H size C cell use 200 mA, and for the 4 A-H size D cell use 400 mA. Be cautious to not overcharge batteries using other A-H ratings, incidentally.

Figure 19-5 shows the basic circuit for a constant current charger of simple design. The transformer secondary voltage should be 2.5 times (or more) the cell or battery voltage. A resistor in series with the rectifier has a value that limits the output current under short-circuit conditions to the official A-H/10 charging rate. This circuit is the basic circuit for most low-cost chargers.

Figure 19-6 shows two electronic constant current chargers based on three-terminal IC voltage regulators. A variable circuit is shown in Figure 19-6A, and it is based on the LM-317 (up to 1 ampere) or LM-338 (up to 5 amperes). Both circuits require a filtered DC input voltage several volts higher than the battery or cell potential. The actual value is not critical so long as it is sufficiently high enough to turn on the circuit (in general, V_{in} must be equal to or greater than V_{batt} + 3 volts). We can set the charge current by setting the value of resistor R. For example, for a 400-mA charger for 4 A-H size D cells, we would use a resistor value of $1.2/I = 1.2/0.4 =$ 3 ohms. Charging currents down to 10 mA can be accommodated by the circuit of Figure 19-6A, so both regular and trickle chargers can be designed.

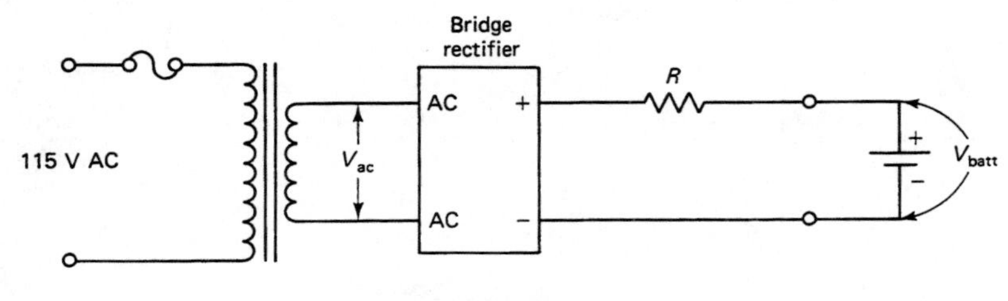

FIGURE 19-5

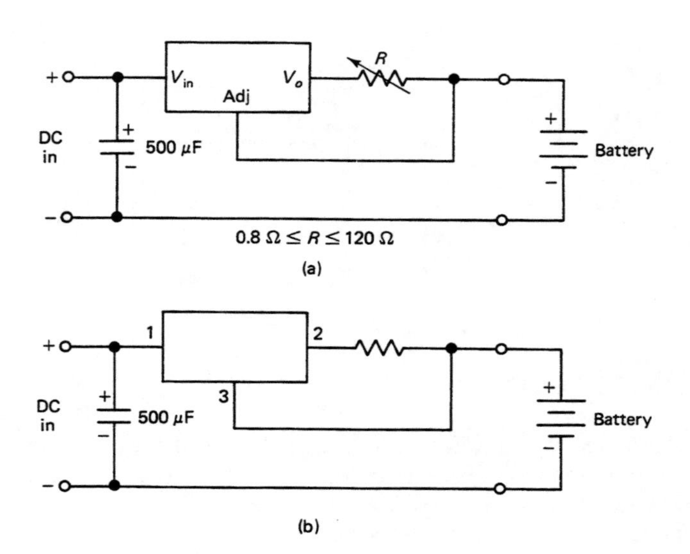

FIGURE 19-6

The circuit of Figure 19-6B will charge batteries up to 4 A-H with terminal voltages up to 12 V DC. It is similar to the circuit of Figure 19-6A, but is based on the 5-volt fixed regulator such as the LM-309, LM-340-05, or 7805 devices.

A constant voltage charger is shown in Figure 19-7. The output voltage of the charger is set by the ratio of R1 and R2, and is determined by the equation

$$V_o = 1.25 \times \left(\frac{\text{R2}}{\text{R1}} + 1\right)$$

A series resistor, R3, prevents the current from exceeding the A-H/10 value and is set to allow the short-circuit current to that value. The required charger output impedance must be the resistance V_o/I_{max}, where V_o is the open-terminal battery voltage and I_{max} is the maximum permissible charging current. For a 12-volt, 4 A-H

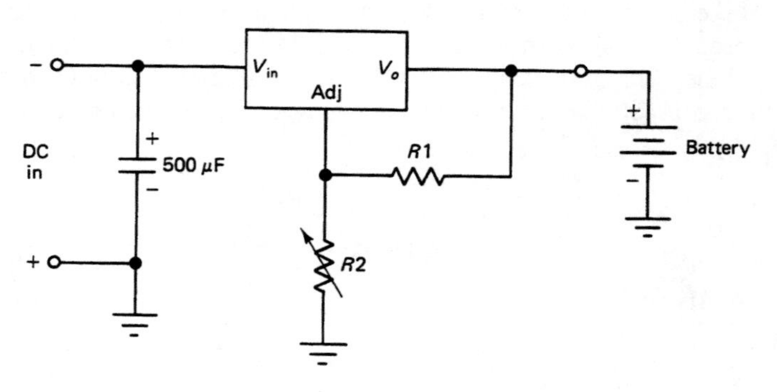

FIGURE 19-7

battery, for example, the required impedance is 12/(4/10) = 12/0.4 = 30 ohms. We can solve the equation in the figure for R3, and place that resistor value in series with the output of the regulator. The power rating of the resistor must be $V_o \times I_{max}$.

USING BENCH POWER SUPPLIES

A bench power supply should not be used to charge NiCd batteries unless it has both a variable output voltage control and a current limiting control. Set the output voltage to exactly the full terminal voltage of the NiCd battery, and adjust the current-limiter for a short-circuit current equal to the A-H/10 value. Disconnect the output short from the power supply and connect it across the battery.

MULTIPLE-CELL BATTERIES

A large number of multiple-cell batteries are used in electronic equipment. Most are typically 6-volt, 12-volt, or 24-volt models. In most cases, these batteries are made up of individual AA, C, D, or F cells. It is possible to take apart the original battery packs and replace individual cells to restore the battery to normal operation. Some battery packs are put together with screws or snaps, while others are glued together.

The pain sufferer (mentioned earlier) who uses a TENS unit paid $90 apiece for the battery packs. One afternoon we took apart one of the "bad" packs using a utility knife and a lot of care. We found that the pack consisted of three "AA" cells connected in series. We went to a supplier that sold commercial solder-tab AA cells and returned with $18 worth of cells to make a "new" battery. I showed him how to solder them in, and then used superglue to reclose the plastic package; that pack lasted nearly 18 months.

When selecting cells for replacement, keep several factors in mind. First, of course, is the right size (AA, C, D, F) and the right A-H rating (not all C and D cells are created equal). Also keep in mind whether regular cells or solder-tab cells are needed. Some consumer NiCd cells are in nonstandard packages. One brand of "AA" cells is a millimeter or so shorter than standard "AA" cells. As a result, intermittent operation is sometimes experienced when these replacement cells are used. To avoid the necessity of shimming these cells, or retensioning the contact spring, avoid buying them and use the standards instead. Medical equipment is simply too critical for those batteries.

OTHER BATTERIES

There are several other types of batteries used in medical equipment. For mobile (e.g., ambulance) and portable applications, for example, there is the lead-acid automobile battery. These are the familiar batteries used to start automobile engines. Very heavy, and dangerous because of the wet-cell acid content, they are nonetheless popular because they are generally well behaved and easily available. In addition, many radio communications sets are designed to operate from the nominal 13.6 volts DC produced by the typical automobile battery.

In addition to the 13.6-volt (aka "12-volt") battery, there are also available 6-volt, 24-volt, 28-volt, and 32-volt lead-acid batteries on the market. Some of these are marine (boat) batteries, others are military batteries (28 V DC) and still others are truck batteries. The terminal voltage can be increased by connecting batteries in series, while current availability is increased by connecting batteries in parallel.

Mobile operation is usually carried out with the vehicle battery. But in certain cases, it is wise to have a separate battery for the equipment in order to have battery power in the event of main vehicle power supply failure. Some users might want to consider the type of system shown in Figure 19-8. This system is common in recreational vehicles to power the creature comforts separately from the vehicle battery. The point is to keep your capability, even if you accidently discharge the vehicle battery by leaving the lights on or suffer some other problem. The backup battery could then be used to start the vehicle or summon help (depending upon the situation).

The charger will be a generator or alternator installed on the vehicle. Although the ideal system would be to have separate charging and regulating systems, that ideal is not always achievable for certain practical reasons. Thus, we have a single charger and voltage regulator for two (or more) batteries. Isolation between the batteries is provided by a pair of large-current silicon diodes (D1 and D2). The rating of these diodes should be at least 1.5 times the maximum charge rate of the charger. In most cases, large stud-mounted diodes are used for D1 and D2, and they are mounted on a finned heat sink. Keep in mind on vehicular installations that ambient temperature is high in some locations, and that will affect diode reliability.

For portable operations some means must be provided to charge the lead-acid battery. In most cases, a small gasoline or kerosene engine–powered generator (called a "light plant" in some catalogs) is used to provide battery power. In some cases, an "auto parts store" type of battery charger is needed to convert the AC output from the generator to DC for the battery. It is increasingly common, however, to find small 500- to 2000-watt generators that include a "12-volt" output that provides from 6 to 35 amperes for purposes of powering radio equipment or charging batteries.

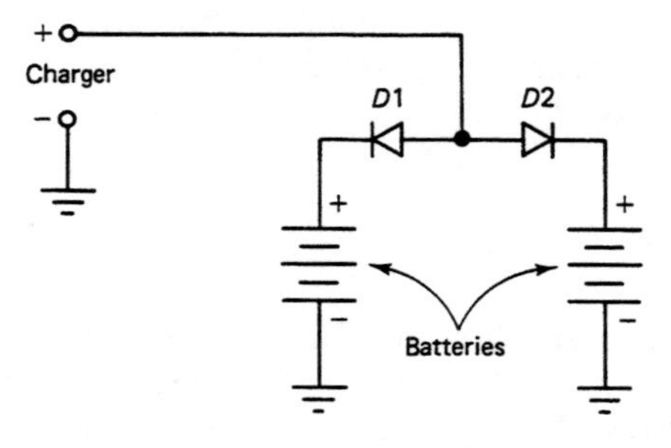

FIGURE 19-8

Other forms of charger are also used. Some people use wind power, while others use falling water (somewhat easier in isolated locations than you might think possible), and still others use sunlight. A Swedish medical missonary works in the deserts of Sudan. In the area of Africa where he was sent, the "roads" are littered with dead animals (including camel) corpses, an indication of how dreadful the place is. His organization does not allow him to set up camp without taking a 6-MHz band Stoner Communications transceiver and an amateur radio transceiver. One thing that they have lots of in those latitudes is sunshine, so a set of solar panels (intended originally for boaters) was procured to charge the lead-acid batteries. A 6-ampere charging system cost him about $2300 at the time it was purchased several years ago (probably cheaper now).

Maintenance of lead-acid batteries is relatively easy but is needed. The water level in each of the cells must be checked periodically. For people with a critical need for the battery, the level should be checked weekly. Although distilled water works best (because of the lack of additional chemicals), ordinary tap water will work in the cells. There are vents in the caps that cover the cells, and these holes must not be blocked. If dirt jams up the opening, then either replace the cap or clean it.

Warning! Lead-acid batteries produce hydrogen as a normal by-product. If you fail to observe proper procedure, then this hydrogen may blow up the battery and cause *serious* injury to people and damage to equipment. First, never allow the battery to become overcharged. Second, turn off all circuits connected to the battery (*especially* the charger) before disconnecting the wires to the battery. If current is flowing in those circuits, then a spark will occur—and that spark can create an explosion. This is not a hypothetical possibility, but a *real danger*.

Gel-cell batteries Another form of battery that is popular in portable equipment is the gel-cell. I have seen these batteries in commercial, medical, and radio communications equipment. Several years ago I worked with a piece of medical equipment used to transport cadaver kidneys to sites where a transplant was performed on a dialysis patient. If you have ever known end-stage renal disease (dialysis) patients, then you know the tragedy of the loss of a donor kidney. We kept losing kidneys because of battery failure in the transport unit. The manufacturer sent us a new design internal battery charger, but it too was deficient. All of the battery chargers found were high-tech models that depended upon sensing small variations in terminal voltage to determine charge or discharge state. Unfortunately, the analog sensing circuitry drifted enough to give bad results. In desperation, the engineer in our laboratory called the battery maker, instead of the device maker, and asked him. The applications engineer asked if we'd ever heard of Kirchoff's voltage law. Allowing that we'd heard that one before, we let the applications engineer guide us to a solution (see Figure 19-9).

The circuit in Figure 19-9 will allow charging of a gel-cell (and other forms of battery) without resorting to a lot of unreliable high-tech circuitry. The charger power supply must have two features: a precisely controlled output voltage and a current limit control. With switch S1 open, set the output voltage to exactly the value of

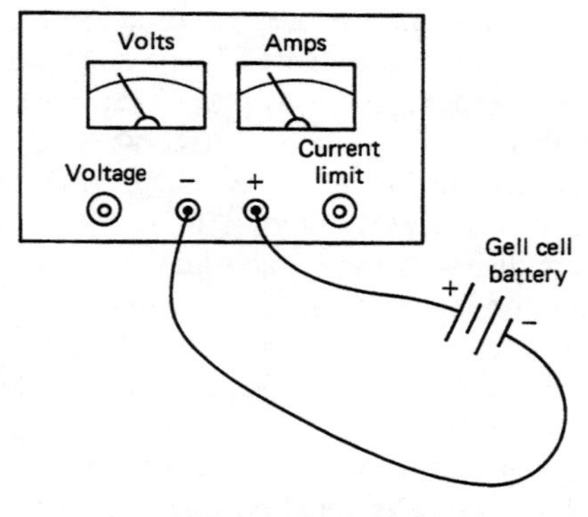

FIGURE 19-9

the fully-charged voltage of the battery, or perhaps a small amount higher (100–200 mV). Make sure S2 is in the shorting position and then close S1. Adjust the current limit control for a short-circuit current equal to the maximum permitted charge current of the battery (A-H/10 for many batteries). After the current and voltage are set, place switch S2 in the BATT position and charge the battery. When the battery voltage is less than the power supply output voltage, current flows into the battery. But when the battery voltage equals the power supply voltage, current flow ceases.

CONCLUSION

Batteries can provide freedom of operation for medical electronic equipment. But they can also be a nuisance if not maintained correctly. Proper maintenance of the battery will provide long and reliable life.

20

Computers in Medical Instruments

The modern digital computer is well known to nearly everyone in our culture because it is so utterly widespread. The computer is, however, a relatively new technology in that it did not exist prior to World War II. Although there were programmable "analytic engines" that were based on mechanical devices, the concept of the digital computer had to await the development of electronic switches that could carry on the switching functions that are required in a computer at ultrahigh speeds.

Although companies like IBM and certain advanced universities worked on computers in the 1930s, it took the necessities of war to stimulate the development of the computer. The first practical computers were developed under the auspices of military and naval authorities who needed fire control computations for their big guns. The calculations for a large cannon are not very difficult on the mathematical scale of things, but they have to be made and are "labor intensive" (as the saying goes). The computer could make the calculations based on inputs from observers, the number of rounds fired (barrels warp as they heat), and other factors, and then direct the crew where to point the gun.

The early computer pioneers were divided into two camps. On the one hand, some of them wanted to build special-purpose computers that were optimized for a specific job (like artillery). But the other faction, in one of the greatest insights and most far-reaching visions of the twentieth century, decided to build a *programmable* digital computer. The concept is simple, but at the time it was revolutionary: a single processor that would obey instructions that were stored in a memory bank (along with data). By writing a *program,* that is, a set of instructions that tell the computer what to do, the user could make the same machine do a lot of different chores. Thus, the same IBM-AT class machine that controls the patient monitoring system in an intensive care unit can also be used by the administrator's secretary as a word processor, by the administrator as a management information system, by central supply as an inventory and processes controller, and by the biomedical engineer to keep preventative maintainance records. And when the workday is over one can run games like *Flight Simulator*® on the same machine. All of this is possible because the computing machine is now a kind of "universal analytic engine." That is, it can be reprogrammed to perform a wide variety of different chores.

It was only three decades ago that the computer was a large mainframe unit sold by industrial giants such as IBM and Honeywell. These machines took up entire rooms (sometimes more than one) and were housed in a series of large metal cabinets. They were used for large-scale data processing chores only, and were not well suited for smaller tasks. In fact, at one hospital where I worked—a university medical center—the only computers it used in the 1960s were the IBM-1401 and later an IBM-360 down the street at main university data processing. The same institution is now overrun with computers of several sizes and employs its own in-house programmers.

In the 1960s a new form of computer appeared on the market. The *minicomputer* was housed in a single cabinet that was 19 inches wide and about 7 feet high. The unit still required special facilities such as a separate high-current electrical circuit and a large capacity air conditioner to carry off the large amount of heat generated by the machine.

In 1972 a quiet revolution took place in California's now-famous Silicon Valley. The Intel Corporation was contracted to build a small digital processor integrated circuit ("chip"). That simple unit was the start of the *microprocessor* industry. A microprocessor is a chip that contains all of the arithmetic and logic elements required for a programmable digital computer. All the designer needs to do to make a real computer is add external memory and input/output circuits. A *microcomputer* is a small desktop computer that is based on a microprocessor chip. Today, one can buy microcomputers that sit on a desktop—with plenty of room left over—and still have substantially more computing power than the roomful of equipment that I used in engineering school (1967). In fact, the abilities of the IBM-XT that I'm using to write this chapter are considerably greater than the IBM-1601 that I used at Old Dominion University in 1967.

The microcomputer has literally revolutionized medical (and other) instrument and control system design. Where designers were once strictly analog engineers, the instrument designer today has to be a synergist who can integrate the principles of sensor selection, analog circuit design, computer hardware selection and/or design, and software. Today, even small instruments are based on microcomputer chips, and for that reason we are going to consider these devices in some detail.

At one time, definitions were simpler. As a freshman engineering student at Old Dominion University in Norfolk, Virginia, I was allowed to use that old IBM 1601/1602 machine. *That* was a computer! No doubt about it. It took up an entire room on the second floor of the engineering school's building. But, today, an engineering student can sit at a small desk with an IBM PC/XT (complete with video CRT display, printer, 40-megabyte or larger hard disk drive, and two floppy disk drives) that has more computing power than that old 1601. Many engineering school students find that the cost of the typical small system is affordable and now they own their own computer. Indeed, while engineering students a generation ago treated the computer room with fear and awe approaching reverence, today many engineering schools require students to bring at least an XT-class machine to school with them. The cost of the modern microcomputer is less than one-tenth what one of the lesser machines of only a decade ago cost, not counting the fact that the dollar ten years ago had more value than the dollar today.

TYPES OF COMPUTER

Before attempting to define the role of the microcomputer, let's first try to define the microcomputer. Terminology tends to become sloppy both from our own laziness and from the fact that once genuine distinctions have become blurred as the state-of-the-art advances; terminology in the computer field is often overcome by events. For example, consider the terms *microcomputer* and *minicomputer*. Laziness tends to make some people use these terms interchangeably, while modern chips (for example, 80286, 80386, or 68xxx) makes such usage reasonable. But, for our purposes, we require sharply focused meanings for these two terms and others: microprocessor, microcomputer, single-chip computer, single-board computer, minicomputer, and mainframe computer.

Microprocessor

The microprocessor is a large-scale integration (LSI) integrated circuit (IC) that contains the *central processing unit* (CPU) of a programmable digital computer. The CPU section of a computer contains the *arithmetic logic unit* (ALU), which performs the basic computational and logical operations of the computer. The CPU also houses the *control logic* section (which performs housekeeping functions) and may or may not have several *registers* for the temporary storage of data. All CPUs have at least one temporary storage register called the *accumulator* or *A-register*. The principal attribute of a microprocessor is that it will execute instructions sequentially. These instructions are stored in coded binary form in an external *memory*.

Microcomputer

A microcomputer is a full-fledged programmable digital computer that is built around a microprocessor chip (i.e., integrated circuit); the microprocessor acts as the CPU for the computer. In addition to the microprocessor chip, the microcomputer typically will have some additional chips, the number varying from two to hundreds depending upon the design and application. These external chips may provide such functions as memory (both temporary and permanent) and input/output

(I/O). The microcomputer may be as simple as the old KIM-1 or as complex as a 30-board industrial machine with all the electronic data processing (EDP) and data collection options. The trend today in IBM-PC/XT/AT compatible machines is to stuff more and more capability into less and less space.

Single-Chip Computer

For several years we had no excuse for interchanging the terms *microprocessor* and *microcomputer*; a microprocessor was an LSI chip and a microcomputer was a computing machine. But the 8048 and similar devices dissolved previously well-defined boundaries because they were both LSI ICs and a computer. A typical single-chip computer may have a CPU section, two types of internal memory (temporary and long-term permanent storage), and at least two I/O ports. Some machines are even more complex. The single-chip computer does, however, require some external components before it can do work. By definition, the microcomputer already has at least a minimum of components needed to perform a job.

Single-Board Computer

The single-board computer (SBC) is a programmable digital computer, complete with input and output peripherals, on a single printed circuit board. Popular examples are the Rockwell AIM-65 and Z80 family of machines. The single-board computer might have either a microprocessor or a single-chip computer at its heart. The peripherals on a single-board computer are usually of the most primitive kind (AIM-65 is a notable exception).

Most single-board computers have at least one interface connector that allows either expansion of the computer or interfacing into a system or instrument design. The manufacturers of early SBCs, such as the KIM-1 and others, probably did not envision their wide application. These computers were primarily touted as trainers, that is, for use in teaching microcomputer technology. But for simple projects such computers also work well as a minidevelopment system. More than a few SBC trainers have been used to develop a microcomputer-based product, only to wind up being specified as a "component" in the production version. In still other cases, the commercially available SBC was used as a component in prototype systems, and then, in the production version, a special SBC (lower cost) was either bought or built.

Minicomputer

The minicomputer predates the microcomputer and was originally little more than a scaled-down version of larger data processing machines. The Digital Equipment Corporation (DEC) PDP-8 and PDP-11 machines are examples. The minicomputer uses a variety of small-scale (SSI), medium-scale (MSI), and large-scale integration (LSI) chips.

Minicomputers have traditionally been more powerful than microcomputers, although that distinction is also blurred. For example, they had longer-length binary data words (12 to 32 bits instead of 8 bits found in microcomputers) and operated at faster speeds of 6 to 12 megahertz (mHz) instead of 1 to 3 mHz. But this is an area of past distinctions now that 33-MHz 80386 machines are available and 10-MHz 8088 machines are considered the "low-end" of high technology. Digital Equipment Corporation, for example, offers the LSI-11 microcomputer that acts like a minicomputer. Similarly, 32-bit microcomputers are available, as are 20- to 33-mHz devices. It is sometimes difficult to draw the line of demarcation when an 80386-based microcomputer is in the same-sized cabinet as a minicomputer, and minicomputers can be bought in desktop configurations.

Mainframe Computer

The larger computer that comes to mind when most people think of computers is the *mainframe computer*. These computers are used in large-scale data processing departments. Microcomputerists who have an elitist mentality sometimes call mainframe computers "dinosaurs." But, unlike their reptilian namesakes, these dinosaurs show no signs of extinction and are, in fact, an evolving species.

Advantages of Microcomputers

That microcomputers have certain advantages is attested to by the fact that so many are sold. But what are these advantages, and how are they conferred?

The most obvious advantage of the microcomputer is *reduced size*; compared with dinosaurs, microcomputers are mere lizards! A 16-bit IBM-XT microcomputer with 640 Kbytes of random access memory (plus a hard disk drive) can easily fit inside a tabletop cabinet. Prices have dropped precipitously in the last few years. While the early microcomputers (circa 1977) were both very expensive and had limited capability, the machine today is a tremendous advance in technology at a low cost. It is now reasonable for nearly everyone to own personal or desktop computers (and indeed they do), and their spread throughout industry and science has set records.

The LSI microcomputer chip is more complex than a discrete-components circuit that does the same job. The interconnections between circuit elements, however, are much shorter (micrometers instead of millimeters). Input capacitances are thereby made lower. The metal-oxide semiconductor (MHOS) technology used in most of these ICs produces very low current drain; hence the overall power consumption is reduced. A benefit of reduced power requirements is reduced heating. While a minicomputer may require a pair of 100 cubic feet per minute (cfm) air blowers to keep the operating temperature within specifications, a microcomputer may be able to use a single 40-cfm muffin fan or no fan at all.

Another advantage of the LSI circuit is reduced component count. Although this advantage relates directly to reduced size, it also affects reliability. If the LSI IC is just as reliable as any other IC (and so it seems), then the overall reliability of the circuit is increased dramatically. Even if the chip reliability is lower than for lesser

ICs, we still achieve superior reliability due to fewer interconnections on the printed circuit board, especially if IC sockets are used on the ICs. Some of the most maddening troubleshooting problems result from defective or dirty IC sockets.

MICROCOMPUTER INTERFACING

The design of any device or system in which a microcomputer or microprocessor is used is the art of *defining* the operation of the system or device, *selecting the components* for the device or system, *matching and integrating* these components (if necessary), and *constructing* the device or system. These activities are known collectively as *interfacing*.

MICROCOMPUTERS IN INSTRUMENT AND SYSTEM DESIGN

Designers in the past used analog electronic circuits, electromechanical relays (which sometimes precipitate a maintenance nightmare), and other devices in order to design instruments, process controllers, and the like. These circuit techniques had their limitations and produced some irritating results; factors like thermal drift loomed large in some of these circuits.

In addition, the design was cast in cement once the final circuit was worked out. Frequently, relatively subtle changes in a specification or requirement produced astonishing changes in the configuration of the instrument; analog circuits are not easily adaptable to new situations in many cases. But, with the advent of the microcomputer, we gained the advantage of flexibility and solved some of the more vexing problems encountered in analog circuit design. The software stored in the memory of the computer tells it what to do and can be changed relatively easily. We can, for example, store program code in a *read-only memory* (ROM), which is an integrated circuit memory. If a change is needed, the software can be modified and a new ROM installed. If the microcomputer was configured in an intelligent manner, then it is possible to redesign only certain interface cards (or none at all) to make a new system configuration. An engineer of my acquaintance built an anode heat computer for medical X-ray machines. A microprocessor computed the heating of the anode as the X-ray tube operated and sounded a warning if the limit of safety was exceeded, thus saving the hospital the cost of a $10,000 X-ray tube. But different X-ray machines require different interfacing techniques, a problem that previously had meant a new circuit design for each machine. However, by intelligent engineering planning, the anode heat computer was built with a single interface card that married the "universal" portion of the instrument with each brand of X-ray machine. Thus, the company could configure the instrument uniquely for all customers at a minimum cost.

Another instrument that indicates the universality of the microcomputer is a certain cardiac output computer. This medical device is used by intensive care physicians to determine the blood-pumping capability of the heart in liters per minute. A bolus of iced or room temperature saline solution is injected into the patient at the "input" end of the right side of the heart (the heart contains two pumps, a right and left side, with the right side output feeding the left side input via the lungs). The temperature at the output end of the right side is monitored and the time integral of temperature determined. This integral, together with some constants, is used by the computer to calculate the cardiac output. These machines come in two versions, research and clinical. The researcher will take time to enter certain constants (that depend upon the catheter used to inject saline, temperature, and other factors) and will be more vigorous in following the correct procedure. But in the clinical setting, technique suffers owing to the need of caring for the patient, and the result is a perception of "machine error," which is actually operator error. To combat this problem, the manufacturer offers two machines. The research instrument is equipped with front-panel controls that allow the operator to select a wide range of options. The clinical model allows no options to the operator and is a "plug and chug" model. The interesting thing about these instruments is that they are *identical* on the inside! All that is different is the front panel and the position of an onboard switch. The manufacturer's program initially interrogates the switch to see if it is open or closed. If it is open, then it "reads" the keyboard to obtain the constants. If, on the other hand, it is closed, the program branches to a subprogram that assumes certain predetermined constants. The cost savings to the company of using a single design for both instruments are substantial.

SELECTING THE RIGHT MICROCOMPUTER

The terms *microcomputer* and *microprocessor* cover a variety of different devices that have different capabilities. There is no such thing as a "universal" computer, or computer configuration, that is all things to all applications. Matters to consider when buying a microcomputer for instrumentation purposes are the architecture of the machine (that is, register, memory, or I/O oriented), the instruction set (computationally strong or I/O operations strong), and the associated hardware requirements. If the IBM-PC/XT series of machines is selected, then a wide variety of software products and add-on circuit cards are available. Indeed, the IBM-PC class of machine is now the standard for the industry.

Which of these do you select for *your* application? All are microcomputers, yet they have vastly different properties. Obviously, one would not use the same machine for such vastly different chores as data processing and, say, burgler alarm or environmental systems monitoring.

It is, therefore, essential that you evaluate the task to be performed and also discern any *reasonable* future accretions to the system. Keep in mind that all projects tend to grow in scope as time passes. Some of this growth is legitimate; some growth occurs because people tend to enlarge a project to include additional functions that were neither intended nor advisable; some growth is due to *your* poor planning in the early stages of the project. Try to anticipate future needs and plan for them. A more or less valid rule of thumb is to follow the 50 percent rule regarding initial capacity: the current requirements should occupy only *one-half* of the machine resources (memory size, processing time, and number of I/O ports).

It is claimed that a smart designer will provide twice or three times the memory actually required for the presently specified chore, but will not under any circumstances tell the programmer. Programmers tend to use up all the memory available. Perhaps, if they think there is somewhat less memory available to them, they can find more efficient means to solve their problems.

The decisions made during planning phases of a project will affect future capabilities in large measure. If adequate means for expansion are not provided, extraordinary problems will surface later. One sure sign of poor planning in a microprocessor-based instrument is the use of extra "kluge boards" hanging onto the main printed circuit board.

The key to good planning is evaluation of system requirements. How many I/O ports are needed? How much memory (guess and then double the figure if cost will allow)? How fast will the processor have to operate? What kind of displays and/or input devices are needed? How many? What size of power supply is needed? In a small system, a bank of seven-segment LED numerical readouts can draw as much current as the rest of the computer.

Perhaps one of the earliest hardware decisions regards the microprocessor chip that will be selected. You will find such decisions are often made more or less on emotional grounds rather than technical; one gets attached to a type, often the first type you learned to program. Just as it is in photography and high-fidelity equipment, microprocessors and microcomputers attract "true believers." Sometimes, however, an emotionally satisfying choice made turns out later to have been utterly stupid for the need at hand.

Typical of the factors that must be considered, especially if the microcomputer is being used as a part of another instrument, are the following: power consumption, speed-power product, size, cost, reliability, and maintainability. These factors are not here arranged in any hierarchy, but they should be ranked by importance in your design planning. For example, if you are designing a computerized bedside patient monitor for a hospital or other medical user, power consumption and speed-power product assume less important roles than in, say, a space shuttle computer where available power is limited, heat dissipation tightly controlled, and data rates extremely high. Similarly, in the bedside monitor we can tolerate lower-reliability (hence lower-cost) equipment because repair service is readily available, and replacement units can be procured and stocked against the possibility of a failed unit. For a NASA satellite, on the other hand, once launched there is slim or no possibility of repair. For that computer, it might be worthwhile to build according to high-reliability specifications. Maintainability is less important to the satellite, but of critical importance to the hospital's biomedical equipment technician or clinical engineer. Cost, of course, is also very important to the hospital user.

Speed-power product can become important in many applications. Processing speed, as measured by system clock frequently, is usually related to power consumption. In most semiconductor devices, the operating speed relates to internal resistances and capacitances that form frequency-limiting RC time constants. Reducing internal resistance in order to increase operating speed (i.e., a short RC time constant) also causes increased power consumption.

Processing speed as measured from program execution time, however, is another matter. This time limitation depends upon the efficiency of instruction execution and the nature of the instructions available to the programmer. There are cases, for example, where the 1-mHz 6502 device (used in the Apple II series of machines) will execute a program slightly faster than the 2-mHz Z80 machine that is used in some controllers or single-board computers used today (in addition to obsolete CP/M machines).

A measure of programming speed is the *benchmark program* such as the often-touted Norton rating. Such a program attempts to standardize evaluation comparisons by having the different microcomputers under test perform some standard task and noting amount of time required. There are numerous pitfalls in this approach, however, because the selection of the task and the programming approach used to solve the problem or task can significantly affect results through bias in favor of one machine over another. The benchmark program should, therefore, be representative of the tasks to be performed by the end product.

Factors that can seriously affect processing speed are the nature of the instruction set and the architecture of the microcomputer. If the task is heavy on I/O operations, for example, it may be wise to use a microprocessor with a good repertoire of input/output instructions. A number-crunching data processing task, on the other hand, requires strong shift-left and shift-right instructions and a coprocessor capability. Some microcomputers have hardware multiply and divide coprocessing capability that is much faster than software implementations of these functions. Since these arithmetic functions tend to be time consuming in software, they are a major consideration if your computer will have to make many such computations.

If the application requires a 16-bit word (or anything greater than the 8 bits normally found on "traditional" microprocessors), the computer will have to be either a 16-bit machine or be programmed to process 16 bits by sequentially grabbing 2 bytes at a time. The IBM-PC and IBM-XT machines are based on the 8088 chip, so are 16 bits, while the IBM-AT class machines are 32 bits.

Support can also be a driving factor in the selection of the microcomputer. First, there is the matter of software and/or hardware available on the open market for that microcomputer. IBM-PC/XT/AT, MacIntoshes, plus the Z80 and 6502 machines, for example, have immense amounts of software available. The old CP/M operating system worked on Z80 machines, but it is now obsolete. It was, however, seminal for modern operating systems such as the MS-DOS (or PC-DOS).

If you are going to include either a microcomputer or microprocessor in the design of a product, be sure to consider second sourcing. Most major microprocessor chips are now multisourced, as are products such as motherboards and plug-in boards. There are also supposedly improved alternate chips. For example the NEC V-20 series of devices replaces the slower 8088 devices used in the IBM-PC. The reason for requiring a second source is that all companies from time to time have problems that prevent timely deliveries. If you are locked into a source that is a sole source, and it has such problems, you will be in a bind that is difficult to resolve. Your own production will be brought to a halt by someone else's problems.

It is often more difficult to obtain single-board computers that are second sourced. These products are often highly unique in their design, so only one company will make them. There are options, however, and these should be considered. Some standard bus single-board computers are made by several companies, so even if the products are not exactly interchangeable, they are close enough to make conversion less damaging to your schedules. Also, some single-board OEM manufacturers advertise that they will give you the drawings to allow you to become your own second source once you purchase a minimum number of machines (usually 100 to 200).

21

Electromagnetic Interference to Medical Electronic Equipment

Electromagnetic interference (EMI) is the general term covering a wide variety of problems of interoperability of electronic equipment. In one class of EMI problems, a device that produces a large amount of radio frequency (RF) energy (for example, an electrosurgery machine) interferes with other equipment (such as the ECG monitor). In other cases, unintentional radiation from one piece of equipment affects another. For example, following is the story of how an FM broadcast radio receiver used by nurses in a postcoronary care (telemetry) unit grossly interfered with the operation of the telemetry system. In still other cases, we find that TV or radio reception is affected by nearby radio transmitters that are operating completely legally. In this chapter we will deal with these problems.

EMI problems are surfacing in more and more different forms in medical settings. Part of this problem arises from the fact that there are increasingly large numbers of instruments and other electronic devices used in medicine. Coupled with the proliferation of electronic devices in the medical setting is a tremendous increase in the use of computers and word processors in the hospital. If you doubt that these devices are capable of interference, then try using an AM broadcast band radio receiver in close proximity to a desktop computer. Even further complicating the problem is the fact that there are many different forms of radio transmitter on the premises, or nearby. In addition to the walkie-talkies used by the security department, there may also be a hospital page system transmitter on the roof. Nearby buildings and businesses may also have powerful radio transmitters on their own premises. These are capable of interfering with medical equipment. And don't forget the potential interference from nearby broadcasting stations. Those stations are potentially the most powerful emitters of radio frequency energy around.

The first problems that we will consider are those that derive from the mixture of a large number of radio signals in the local vicinity.

"INTERMOD" PROBLEMS

There are two interrelated problems that often deteriorates radio reception in communications systems: *intermodulation* and *cross modulation*. Although there are fine technical differences between these two problems, their cures are about the same, so the author will take the liberty of calling them all "intermod problems." These problems result in interference on a given frequency due to heterodyning (mixing) between two other unrelated signals.

"Heterodyning" is a fancy term that refers to the nonlinear mixing of two signals. Consider the guitar analogy. Pick one string and make it vibrate to produce a tone. That tone has a frequency of $F1$. After that tone dies out, pluck another string and cause a new tone ($F2$). Now pluck both strings simultaneously. What happens? How many tones are present? The initial answer might be "$F1$ and $F2$," but that is wrong. In a nonlinear system (such as hearing) there are additional frequencies created. In addition to $F1$ and $F2$ there will be the sum frequency ($F1 + F2$) and the difference frequency ($F1 - F2$). It is the difference frequency, $F1 - F2$, by the way, that some guitar players use to tune the instrument. When two frequencies are close, but not exact, the difference frequency is very low, almost subaudible. It is this low frequency that accounts for the slow wavering tone that one hears as the strings are tuned closer to the same pitch. Exact tune is indicated by the wavering disappearing. This, then, is heterodyning.

There are other combinations also produced according to the expression $mF1 \pm nF2$, where m and n are integers. For most purposes, however, these additional frequencies are unimportant (a distinctly important problem with these additional frequencies is discussed here; "intermod problems" need not work on only $F1$ and $F2$).

There is a hill locally that radio technicians and engineers call "Intermod Hill." It happens to be one of the higher locations in the county, so several broadcasters and AT&T have seen fit to build radio towers there. In addition, both of the two main radio towers bristle with landmobile antennas whose owners rent space on the tower in order to get better coverage. In total, there are two 50,000-watt FM broadcast stations, a 1000-watt AM broadcast station, a many-frequency microwave relay station, and several dozen 30-mHz to 950-mHz VHF/UHF landmobile stations and radio paging stations. Nearby is a major community hospital that operates its own security system radio station and a hospital pager. They also have a coronary care unit that uses UHF radio telemetry to keep track of ambulatory heart patients. All of those signals can heterodyne together to produce apparently valid signals on other channels.

The frequencies produced in a signal rich environment are many, and roughly follow the preceding rule $F_{unwanted} = (mF_1) \pm (nF_2)$, where m and n are integers (1,

2, 3, . . .) and F_1, F_2 are the frequencies present. If the receiver system is linear, then there is little chance for a problem. But nonlinearites do creep in, and when the receiver is nonlinear in a case where extraneous signals are present, then "intermods" show up. Being in the fields of so many radio transmitter signals almost ensures nonlinearity; hence, intermod problems abound on and around Intermod Hill.

Imagine the number of possible combinations when there are literally dozens of frequencies floating around the neighborhood! My wife is a nurse, and she works in that hospital mentioned earlier. I used to wait for her in our car at the end of the shift and listened to my 2-meter ham radio set to pass time. I could hear the hospital security department and the local telephone company mobile telephone frequency clear as a bell on the amateur repeater frequency because of "intermods"!

The ability (or lack of same) to reject these unwanted signals is a good measure of a receiver's performance. A quality, well-designed radio receiver doesn't respond to either out-of-band or in-band off-channel signals, except in the most extreme cases of overload. The ability to discriminate against these spurious signals is a necessary requirement to specify when requesting quotations and estimates from industry for a new installation.

The linearity or dynamic range of the input RF amplifier of the receiver is the cause of most cases of intermodulation interference. There are other causes, however, and one must consider anything that can cause nonlinearity. For example, a well-known car radio had problems with the AGC rectifier diode. It was leaky, and the radio was easily overdriven by external signals. In some sets, the manufacturer used a pair of back-to-back small-signal silicon diodes across the antenna terminals to shunt high-voltage potentials to ground. This method was especially popular a few years ago. A large signal could drive these diodes into conduction and produce nonlinearity.

One of the funniest "intermod" situations I know of happened to me when I worked in another hospital as a bioelectronics engineer. We used a telemetry unit to monitor patient ECGs in the "PCCU," which is the unit that coronary care unit patients go to after they are no longer acute, but still bear watching. The portable ECG transmitters generated 1 to 4 milliwatts of VHF RF energy that was frequency modulated with the patient's electrocardiogram (ECG) signal. The signal level was so low that five 17-in. whip antennas sticking down from the ceiling were needed to cover an area that consisted of two corridors approximately 150 feet in length. Each antenna was connected directly to a 60-dB master TV antenna amplifier (the ECG transmitter channels were located in the "guard bands" between TV video and audio carriers of commercial VHF TV channels); one of the whip/amplifier assemblies was right over the receiver console.

One morning about 2 A.M, a nurse called me at home complaining that Mr. Jones's ECG was riding in on Mr. Smith's channel. Not quite believing her, I nonetheless went to the hospital and checked the situation out. Swapping receivers, telemetry transmitters, and amplifiers did no good. Finally, after two hours of trying (and almost to the point of looking silly to nurses who don't easily tolerate other's failures regarding their equipment), I noticed the FM broadcast receiver sitting on top of the telemetry receiver cabinet less than 18 inches from the antenna/amplifier

(Figure 21-1), and it was playing. On a sheer hunch, I turned off the receiver and Mr. Jones went back to his own channel! Previously, his signal was showing up on both his own channel and Mr. Smith's channel, but was now only where it belonged. Turning the FM receiver back on caused the situation to return. Also, tuning the radio to another channel made the problem go away.

What happened in that situation? The local oscillator in the FM broadcast receiver was heterodyning with Mr. Jones's signal to produce an "intermod" signal on Mr. Smith's channel. The situation is shown graphically in Figure 21-1. The six VHF receivers used in the system were installed in a mainframe rack that forms the nurses' station console (along with an oscilloscope and strip-chart recorder). The FM receiver was placed on top of the receiver rack such that its telescoping whip antenna was only a short distance from the telemetry receiver antenna.

Because the FM receiver is a superheterodyne, it produces a signal from the internal local oscillator that is 10.7 MHz higher than the received frequency. If the radio is tuned to the station at 99.7 MHz on the FM dial, then the local oscillator operates at 99.7 MHz + 10.7 MHz, or 110.4 MHz. This signal is radiated, and picked up by the telemetry antenna. Because of its close proximity, it is the strongest signal seen by the input of the 60-dB amplifier. The other signals imping-

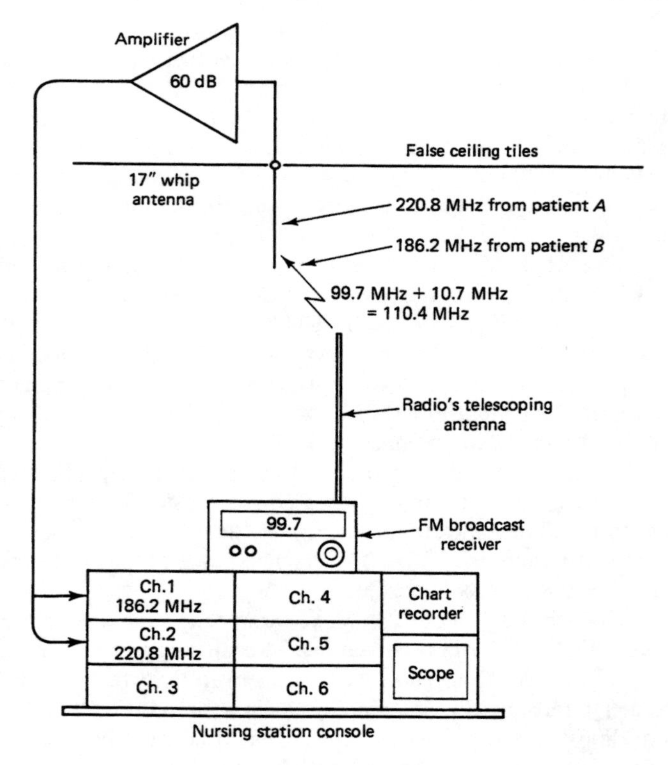

FIGURE 21-1

ing the antenna are weak signals at 220.8 MHz from Patient A and 186.2 MHz from Patient B. The mixing action at the input of the 60-dB amplifier, then, consists of 110.4 MHz, 186.2 MHz, and 220.8 MHz.

In the case cited, it was apparently the second harmonic of the FM radio local oscillator signal (i.e., 110.4 MHz × 2, or 220.8 MHz) that caused the problem. Consider the mathematics: 186.2 MHz + 220.8 MHz = 407 MHz. And, also, 407 MHz − 186.2 MHz = 220.8 MHz. In this scenario, the 186.2 MHz transmitter signal will appear on the 220.8 MHz channel!

The general rule of thumb for which signal will appear is based on the "capture effect." Telemetry transmitters and receivers are actually frequency modulated (FM). An FM receiver will generally "capture" the strongest of two competing cochannel signals and exclude the other. As a result, the strongest of the two signals, in this example 186.2 MHz translated to 220.8 MHz by mixing in the 60-dB amplifier, predominates.

Following that night the hospital banned FM radio receivers, patient-owned TV receivers, CBs, and ham radio sets in the CCU/PCCU area for exactly the same reason they are banned on commercial airliners: interference with the electronic equipment.

SOME SOLUTIONS

There are a number of ways to overcome most intermod problems. Modification of the receiver is possible, especially since poor design is a basic cause of intermods. But that approach is rarely feasible except for the most technically intrepid. There are, however, a few pointers for the rest of the people.

First, make sure that the receiver is well shielded. This problem rarely shows up on costly modern rigs, but is a strong possibility on lower-cost receivers. Most radio transceivers have adequate shielding because of the requirements of the transmitter in the same cabinet with the receiver. But if there are any holes in the shielding, then cover them up with sheet metal or copper foil (available in hobby shops). For others, the best approach is to use one of the methods shown in Figures 21-2 through 21-4. In all cases, you must identify one of the interfering frequencies, or (in some cases) at least the band.

Half-Wave Shorting Stub A nonmatching load impedance attached to the business end of a transmission line repeats itself every half wavelength back down the line toward the input end. For example, if a 250-ohm antenna is attached to the load end of a half wavelength piece of 50-ohm coax, an impedance meter at the input end will measure 250 ohms. Lengths other than integer multiples of half wavelength will see different impedances at the input end. This phenomenon is the basis for transmission line transformers used in antenna matching. Therefore, if the end of a piece of coax is shorted (see Figure 21-2), then the input end will see a short-circuit at the frequency for which the coax is a half wavelength. The interfering frequency will be shorted to ground, while the desired frequency sees a high impedance—provided that the two are widely separated. The length L is found from

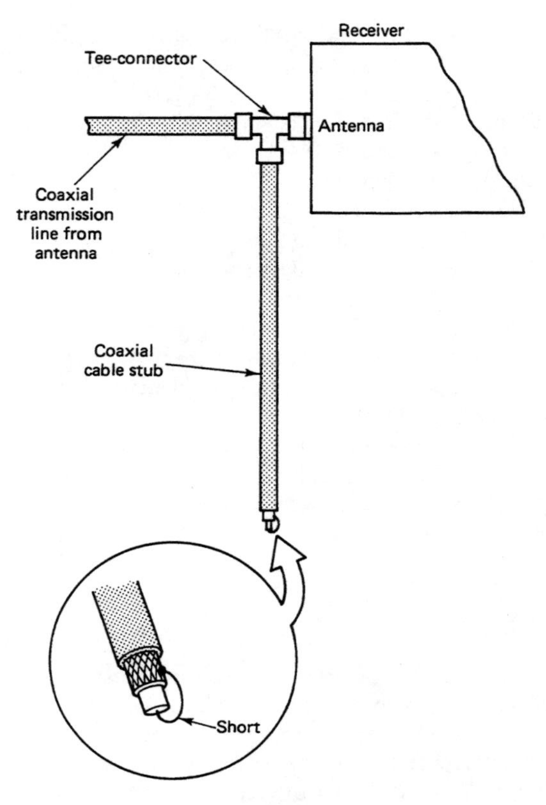

FIGURE 21-2

$L_{ft} = 492V/F_{MHz}$, where L is in feet, F is in MHz, and V is the velocity factor of the the coax (usually 0.66 for regular coax and 0.80 for polyfoam coax).

The method of Figure 21-2 is best suited to cases where the interfering signal is in the VHF region or lower. Because the length of the coax stub is very short relative to the HF wavelength of the desired band, some very untransmission line–like behavior might take place when transmitting. Therefore, for transceivers some engineers recommend adding a second antenna jack especially for the stub, but connected to the receiver circuitry (RX CKT).

Another method (Figure 21-3) is to use a frequency selective filter. The selection of type of filter, and the cutoff frequency, is determined by the case. In a maze of frequencies like "Intermod Hill," it might be wise to use a bandpass filter on the band of choice. Otherwise, use a low-pass filter if the interfering signal (at least one of them) is higher than the desired band, and a high-pass filter if the interfering signal is lower. For most cases, a low-pass TVI filter is desirable on HF, so this solution is automatically taken care of—the 35–45-MHz cutoff point of most such filters will attenuate most VHF signals trying to get back in.

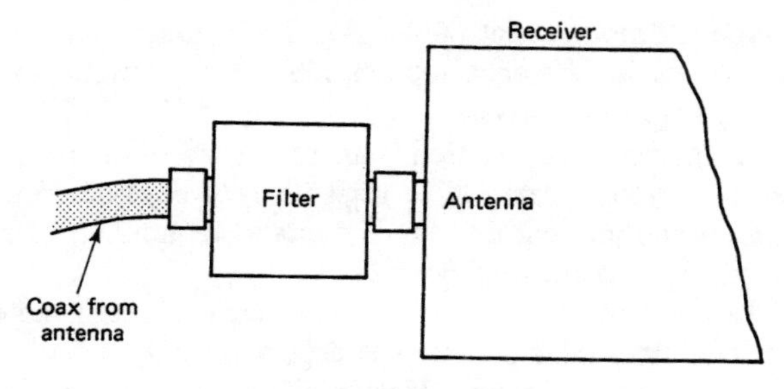

FIGURE 21-3

Figure 21-4 shows some of the different types of filter configuration that might be used. The first wavetrap is a parallel resonant circuit (Figure 21-4A) in series with the signal line. A parallel resonant trap has a high impedance at the resonant frequency, but a low impedance on other frequencies, so it blocks the undesired frequency. Figure 21-4B shows a series resonant trap across the signal line. The series resonant circuit is just the opposite of the parallel case: it offers a low impedance at its resonant frequency and a high impedance elsewhere. Thus, it serves much like the coax stub in Figure 21-2. In Figure 21-4C we see a combination wavetrap that uses both series and parallel resonant elements. Several editions of the ARRL *Radio Amateur's Handbook* had construction projects for AM broadcast band wavetraps of

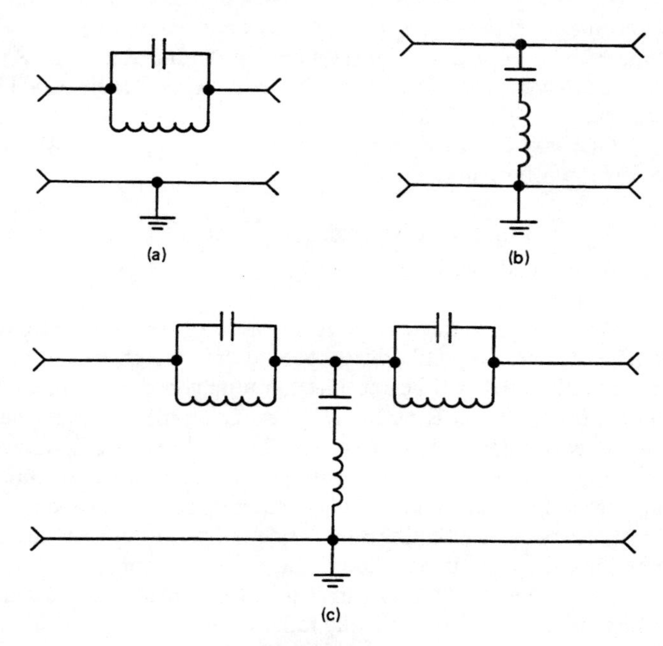

FIGURE 21-4

this type. Although that publication is for amateur radio operators, the techniques presented for interference suppression are quite useful for the hospital-based technician and engineer.

If the interfering station is an FM broadcaster, then most video shops and electronic parts stores carry "FM traps" for 75-ohm antenna systems. These traps cost only a few dollars but provide a tremendous amount of relief from the interference produced by broadcast stations.

It might be the case that the interfering signal is entering the equipment on the AC power line. This situation is especially likely if you live very close to a high-power broadcasting station. If there is space in the rig, then it might pay to install an AC line filter. Electronic parts distributors sell EMI AC line filters suitable for equipment up to 2000 watts or so (look at the ampere rating of the filter). Also, it is possible to install ferrite blocks on the line cord to serve as RF chokes. Some computer stores sell these to reduce EMI from long runs of multiconductor ribbon cable. It is sometimes possible to reduce the EMI pickup by either reducing the cord length or rolling it up into a tight coil. This solution works well where the cord is of a length nearly resonant (quarter wavelength) on the interfering signal's frequency.

DEALING WITH TVI/BCI

Television interference, TVI, is the bane of the radio communications and broadcasting communities. True TVI occurs when emissions from a transmitter interfere with the normal operation of a television receiver. Except for solo explorers on the North Slope of Alaska, and missionaries among the Indians of the Amazon basin, all radio operators have a potential TVI problem as close as their own TV set—or their neighbors' sets.

One way to classify TVI is according to the cause. All electronic devices must perform two functions:

1. Respond to desired signals.
2. Reject undesired signals.

All consumer devices perform more or less in accordance with the first requirement, but many fail with respect to the second. It is often the case that a legally transmitted signal will be received on a neighbor's TV or hi-fi set even though the transmitter operation is perfectly clean. On some TV sets, the high-intensity signal from a nearby transmitter drives the RF amplifier into nonlinearity, and that creates harmonics where none existed before. In other cases, we find that audio from the transmission is heard on the audio output of the set, or seen in the video, as a result of signal pickup and rectification inside the set. Improper shielding can cause signals to be picked up on internal leads and fed to the circuits involved.

Remember two rules of thumb: (1) if transmitter emissions are not clean, then getting rid of the TVI/BCI is the radio operator's responsibility, and (2) if the transmitter emissions are clean, and the TVI/BCI is caused by poor medical equipment design, then it is the medical equipment owner's responsibility to fix the problem—

not the radio operator's. Unfortunately, in a society that depends too much on lawyers, the solution opted for by some ill-advised administrators is to hire lawyers to intimidate the radio owner into silent submission. Wise managers will shun the lawyers and hire an engineer to solve the problem in a manner that would allow both parties to operate compatibly.

On the other hand, radio transmitter owners must respond responsibly to EMI complaints for several reasons. First, they have a legally imposed responsibility to keep transmitter emissions clean and free of spurious or unnecessary components. They must operate the transmitter legally. Second, it makes for good neighborhood relations if they attempt to help solve the problem. After all, we live in a society where more people seem willing to go running to lawyers than to engineers to solve technical problems. Even though they may win, a lawsuit brought by some lawyer who is either too greedy for a client's money to question the merits of the case, or too ignorant to research the matter properly, can break the radio owner financially. Also, some neighbors who don't bring suit will, nonetheless, run to local regulatory bodies even though they don't have jurisdiction over the matter (only the Federal Communications Commission may legally regulate radio stations, a position that the courts have affirmed).

Step 1 Make sure that the transmitter emissions are clean. Although it requires a spectrum analyzer to be sure that the harmonics are down 40 dB or more below the carrier, a few simple checks will tell the tale in many cases. An absorption wavemeter is an elderly device that can spot harmonics that are way too high. Also, listening on another receiver from a long distance (1 mile or more) away will give some indication of problems: at that distance, if you can hear the second or third harmonic, then so can the next-door neighbor. Finally, if you own an RF wattmeter, or forward-reading VSWR meter, and a dummy load, then you can make a quick check by measuring the ouput power with and without a low-pass filter (Figure 21-5) installed in the line. If the power varies between the two readings by appreciably more than the insertion loss of the low-pass filter, then suspect harmonics are present.

The techniques for making the transmitter output signal clean are simple: a low-resistance earth ground and adequate filtering. In the station shown in Figure

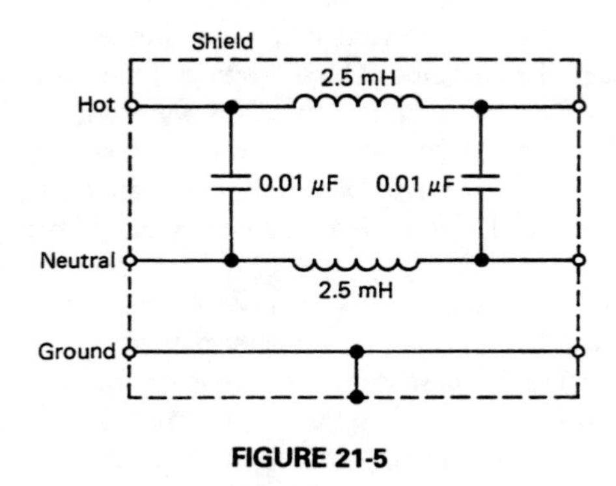

FIGURE 21-5

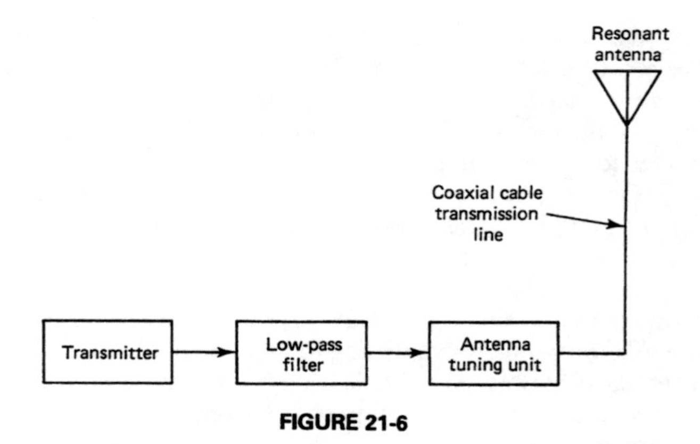

FIGURE 21-6

21-6, there are three frequency selective elements after the transmitter: low-pass filter, antenna tuning unit (in lower-frequency stations), and a resonant antenna. All of these will help in reducing whatever harmonics the transmitter puts out.

Step 2 Determine that you really have a TVI problem. Check for TVI both with the transmitter turned on and turned off. Also, make sure the TV is properly adjusted.

Also make sure that the interference is not coming from another source! Once an antenna goes up, all the neighbors will assume the worst and blame every flicker of the set on the radio operations. Local broadcast stations, landmobile radio stations, and all manner of electronic devices can generate TVI—it's not just an amateur radio problem. In my own house (which we just moved into) I am going to have to change those dimmer switches the former owners installed: they produce "salt and pepper" snow on the TV and make 75/80 meters on my ham radio receiver almost unusable.

Step 3 Try adding a high-pass filter to the TV set. These filters will only pass signals with a frequency greater than about 50 MHz, and severely attenuate HF amateur or CB signals. As shown in Figure 21-7, the high-pass filter must be installed as close as possible to the antenna terminals of the TV set. Make the connection wire as short as possible to prevent it from acting as an antenna in its own right.

Counsel the affected TV set owner to install an antenna that uses a coaxial cable transmission line, rather than 300 ohm twin-lead. Although theory tells us that there should be no difference, it is nonetheless true that 75 ohm coax systems are less susceptible to all forms of noise—including TVI. Install a high-pass filter and a 75- to 300-ohm TV-type BALUN impedance transformer at the TV's antenna terminals.

Many, perhaps most, TV receivers have very poor internal shielding, so signal can bypass the high-pass filter and get picked up on the leads between the TV tuner (inside the set) and the antenna terminals on the rear of the set. That situation makes the high-pass filter almost useless. A solution for this dilemma is to mount the filter directly on the tuner, inside the set, making the lead length essentially zero.

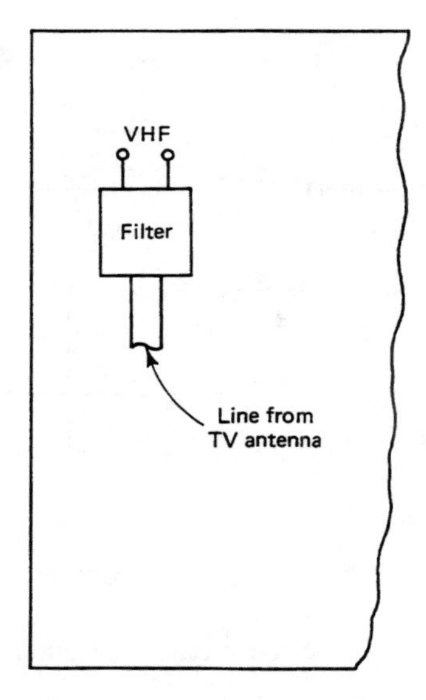

FIGURE 21-7

MEDICAL EQUIPMENT AND EMI

Medical equipment seems especially sensitive to picking up interfering signals. The ECG electrode wires are exposed at the ends. In addition, the patient's body is basically an electrical conductor, so it makes a relatively decent "antenna" to pick up signals that exist in the air. The solution to that problem is a low-pass filter (Figure 21-8) that blocks radio signals but not the ECG. These filters are not like the 60-Hz filter that is used in the ECG machine to eliminate power line artifact. Those filters take out a segment of the 0.05- to 100-Hz spectrum that is normally part of the ECG waveform, so will always affect the shape of the waveform presented to the medical person using the machine. The RF low-pass filter has such a high cutoff frequency that the ECG waveform is not affected.

One word of utmost caution! Do not, under any circumstances, install the filter on or in a neighbor's set. Do not allow hospital technicians to do the job, even though they are probably well qualified to do so. If you do, then your neighbor will blame you for every repair the set needs from then on. I once did volunteer work for a local TVI Committee (a voluntary body that tried to mediate interference problems) that was investigating interference from a CB operator (who was operating completely legally, by the way). The CBer had personally installed a high-pass filter on the TV receiver's external antenna terminals (he had not even opened the back of the set). Unfortunately, the vertical/horizontal/sync module went out a few days later. The upset neighbor then complained to just about everyone who would listen that this "ham operator" (she didn't know the difference) fouled up her TV set.

While some neighbors will blast you for every little problem, others are not so bad and may actually respond in a positive manner if you point the way to a TVI/

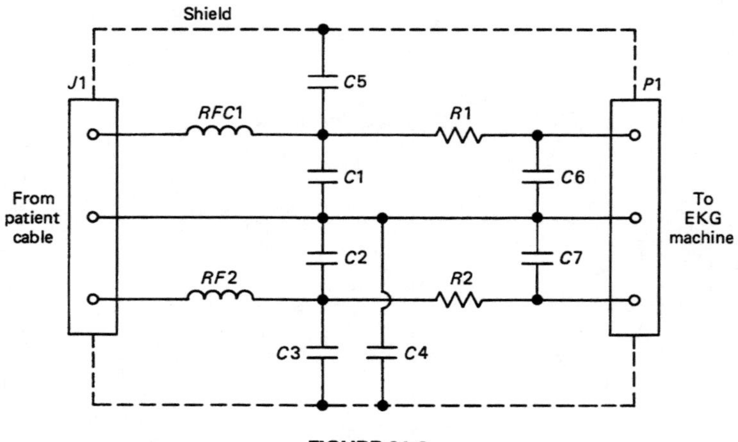

FIGURE 21-8

BCI solution even where the offending station is not yours. Let's revisit intermod hill.

A common problem for TV viewers in the area is FM interference. That form of TVI forms a herringbone pattern, which characterizes it as FM, not AM/SSB, interference. This form of interference often succumbs to either a bandstop filter or a shorted halfwave stub (refer again to Figure 21-2). FM broadcast band bandstop or "notch" filters are available from most electronics parts distributers, as well as many video stores and TV outlets. Both 75-ohm and 300-ohm forms are available (use the right kind). The shorted stub of Figure 21-2 can be built from either twin-lead or coax, depending upon the type of transmission line used. It is connected directly to the TV antenna terminals, and has a length of

$$L_{\text{inches}} = \frac{2952V}{F_{MHz}}$$

where

L = the length in inches

F_{MHz} = the offending transmitter frequency in megahertz

V = the velocity factor of the line (use 0.82 for TV-type coax)

Example

Find the length required for a shorting stub to suppress an FM broadcast signal on 101.1 MHz. Assume a 75-ohm coax transmission line.

$$L = \frac{(2952)(V)}{F_{MHz}}$$

$$= \frac{(2952)(0.82)}{101.1}$$

$$= \frac{2421}{101.1}$$

$$= 23.9 \text{ in.}$$

22

Selecting the Right Solid-State Replacement Components

Every technician who spends at least some time at the workbench repairing or building electronic equipment will eventually need a transistor that he or she does not have on hand—and maybe can't easily obtain. In some cases, the type number will be found in one of the standard transistor replacement catalogs. In other cases they are on their own. The subject of transistor substitution is one that has been talked about to the point of exhaustion among communications and service technicians, yet serious problems continue to reappear. The tips given in this chapter, while most appropriate to the types of transistors normally used in radio communications and broadcast equipment, are also applicable to a wide variety of other situations as well.

The main premise is that we are *servicing* radio equipment that *once worked properly and then failed*. This idea is terribly important. Much of what is discussed is also applicable to new construction projects and engineering laboratories, however, but construction project debugging is something of an arcane engineering art and is thus not suitable for general, too-broad, guidelines. Some poorly engineered equipment depends for proper operation on selected parameters of specific transistors, and would not even work with all otherwise working versions of the same "2N" number devices.

There are even cases on record where only those devices made by certain manufacturers will work properly in the circuit. Ancient history note: Those of us who go back to vacuum tube days recall certain very costly commercial HF receivers—the 51J4 and 51S4—that would retain their reputed "frequency meter" dial calibration accuracy only when RCA-branded tubes were used for the local oscillator. It seems that the interelectrode capacitance was critical. And because there are transistor equivalents to that situation, we must limit our consideration to repair of working—properly designed, we hope—equipment.

EXACT REPLACEMENTS

The easiest way to obtain a replacement solid-state device that will install easily and operate correctly is to order it from the original equipment manufacturer or an authorized distributor. As we are all painfully aware, however, this is not always either possible or practical. Some manufacturers do not sell to individuals, while others have an unrealistic minimum factory order (for example, $100–$500). In still other cases, the manufacturer will sell to independent shops, but wants a ridiculous amount of money for the part. Unless it is hand selected from the general population of the same type (for example, for some specific parameter), then this costing practice is unjustified.

INDUSTRY-STANDARD–TYPE NUMBERS

If the defective transistor has a standard "2N"-type number, then you just obtain a replacement device having the same number, and disregard the brand of the replacement. Unfortunately, some original equipment manufacturer (OEM) transistors are not marked with these standard numbers. They often have a house code number that is meaningless to anyone except the original equipment manufacturer. Sometimes, the house number is created because the transistor is specially selected from others of the same "2N" series, so only a similarly tested device will work properly in the circuit. In other cases, the house number is used because it becomes easier to control the parts inventory, and in some cases to ensure themselves replacement parts business.

CROSSOVER GUIDES

Crossover guides would seem to be a nearly perfect source of replacement numbers. They *should* be used whenever possible. But many are the gremlins that can pop up unexpectedly. Theoretically, the cross-matching has been done in advance by the use of an "infallible" computer. When we follow those recommendations, however, we sometimes find some suggested replacements that have insufficient power or voltage ratings, too narrow a bandwidth, a different physical shape causing mounting or space problems, or wrong mounting dimensions requiring modification of the chassis. Many of these discrepancies occur because the crossovers are compiled from printed lists that sometimes contain errors. It's an open secret that the recommended substitutes are seldom tried in any kind of equipment or circuit. It is a good policy to test the reasonableness of the selection by looking at the crossover devices specifications and compare them with what you know about the circuit and its requirements.

It is a good policy to return, along with a note of explanation, any crossover transistors that either don't work properly or require major reworking of the chassis or rewiring of the circuit. If everyone did this, then the supplier might take the hint. The economic power of a service shop's annual semiconductor purchases makes it relatively easy to obtain a refund on bad crossovers—consumers rarely have such clout.

Another problem has nothing to do with electrical specifications, but rather with identification. Most manufacturers of radio equipment use their own "house numbers" on solid-state components. This practice causes no problems if the crossover guides list suitable replacements. In other cases it is relatively easy to guess the required transistor type. But what about the possibility that each of two manufacturers accidentally assigned the same designation to two completely dissimilar devices? It's not likely that a crossover guide will solve all such problems (although some do accommodate such ambiguities).

Remember the old rule from high school math: "things equal to the same thing are (hopefully) equal to each other." Or, if $A = B$, and $B = C$, then $A = C$. We can use this observation to make crossover selections. Furthermore, we can use this technique in at least two ways. First, we can look up the device needed to find the replacement type number. For example, suppose a 2N5xxx is found in the crossover guide as a "ZE-234." We can look for other "2N" series devices also equal to ZE-234, and then use one of those.

This method is *especially useful* when crossing house numbers to 2*N* numbers—which is our second way to use the "$A = C$" theory. Suppose that your Wombat Thunderbolt VI transceiver uses a transistor with the part number "8501234." What is an "8501234"? Well, the guide calls it a ZE-234. By looking over the "2N" series columns in the crossover guide you find a 2N5xxx is also equal to a ZE-234. Chances are good that the Wombat engineers selected the 2N5xxx, and then relabeled it "8501234." It may not be the exact transistor, but it is a fair bet that it will work unless the 8501234 is a specially selected 2N5xxx (no guarantees, however—you still have to check specs and make an educated guess).

MOBILE PROBLEMS

Up to this point, the problems of obtaining suitable replacements for transistors in mobile rigs are identical with those for base station rigs. But there is one special problem that is more serious in mobile applications: environmental heat.

One car manufacturer became concerned about the excessive number of failures in its first all solid-state car radio models (c. 1962) and decided to investigate passenger cabin heat as the culprit. The company asked its electronics plant employees to leave their car doors unlocked for one day. During that day of 90°F weather, the engineers measured the temperatures inside many of the closed cars. They were surprised to find the average reading was 160°F on the seat and 180°F behind the dashboard.

DERATING THE SPECS

Published transistor power ratings are usually specified at room temperature, generally accepted to be 25 degrees Celsius (77°F). If transistors are used at higher temperature, as in mobile applications, then the maximum collector dissipation (in watts) must be reduced to prevent extra failures, which could occur even when all the electrical specifications are fulfilled.

A curve typical of those used for derating is shown in Figure 22-1. Notice that a transistor having a collector dissipation of 550 milliwatts (mW) at 25°C can safely dissipate only 375 mW at 65°C (142°F). This explains why a transistor that is operating below its maximum published wattage rating could be destroyed by using it in a hot car. Watch for such hazards, especially if you attempt to use "five-for-a-buck"

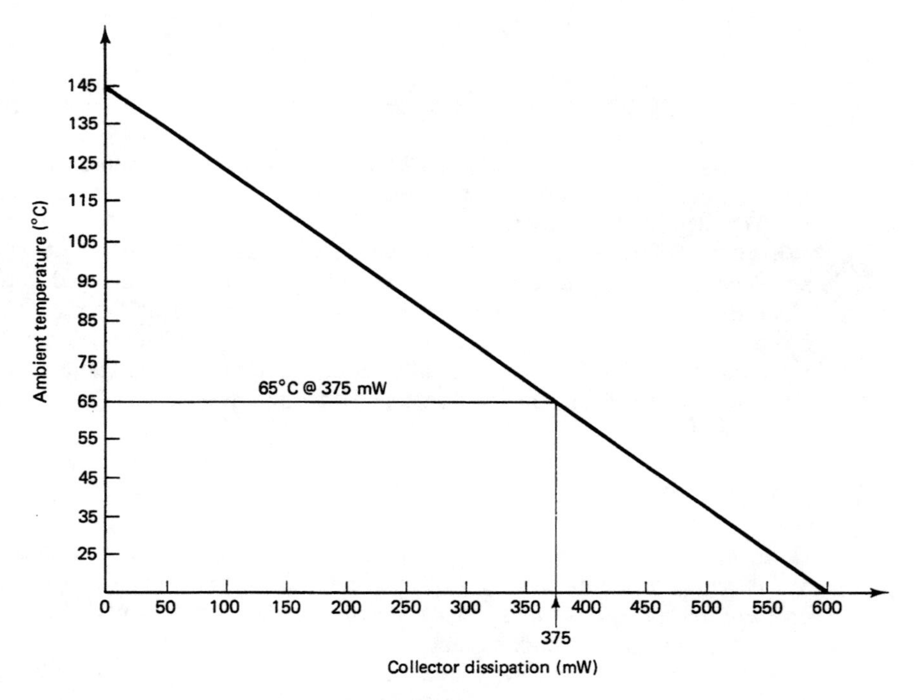

FIGURE 22-1

bargain basement replacements in which the collector dissipation rating was "optimistic."

BEYOND CROSS-MATCHING

Often the numbers on a bad transistor seem meaningless. There is no way to cross match, and you can't locate an OEM replacement from the equipment maker. The next step is to find a universal replacement from one of the many convenient sources. You must become an electronic detective and find out these things about the transistor:

1. Is it a silicon or germanium type?
2. Is it a PNP or NPN?
3. What is the gain (alpha or beta)?
4. What frequencies must it amplify?
5. What are the collector power dissipation requirements?
6. Are there any special mechanical mounting requirements?

After you have answered those questions, you can make a satisfactory selection from almost any brand of universal replacement.

SILICON OR GERMANIUM

Silicon transistor junctions measure higher DC resistances than do germanium junctions. In fact, silicon transistors usually read "open" on all measurements except with base/emitter and base/collector forward biasing polarity. If even one junction remains intact on a blown transistor, you can tell which material it is by comparing readings with those of known types in the same size and power category.

Forward-biased voltages for all stages other than oscillators (and certain pulse circuits used in video equipment) should be 0.2 to 0.3 volts for germanium transistors and 0.5 to 0.7 volts for silicon transistors. Check the schematic, or another of the intact junctions (or a similarly numbered good transistor in the circuit), to see which voltage levels are found. The answer will tell you whether to look for Ge or Si transistor replacements.

PNP OR NPN?

When the collector voltage is more positive (or less negative) than the emitter, then the transistor is an NPN type, and if the collector is more negative (or less positive) than the emitter, then the transistor is a PNP type. Most schematics give these voltage readings. On the other hand, you can measure the collector/emitter voltages accurately enough for this purpose, right in the circuit in most cases.

If even one junction of the defective transistor is intact, then you can determine the polarity by using an ohmmeter. If you obtain a normal low-resistance diode-type reading with the positive ohmmeter lead on the base and the negative lead on the collector or emitter, then it is an NPN type. If you must reverse the leads to obtain a low-resistance reading, the transistor is a PNP type. This measurement must be made with an old-fashioned VOM/VTVM, or a modern digital meter with a "diode" or "high-power" ohmmeter function.

FREQUENCY RESPONSE

Suppose you have installed a "universal" small-signal replacement transistor and it doesn't amplify. According to the DC voltages, however, it's drawing normal current and it doesn't heat excessively—yet it still fails to operate. Chances are good that the transistor selected has a bandwidth that is too narrow, and so the amplification is insufficient.

There is no one way of measuring the frequency response of transistors. Worse yet, the manufacturers can't seem to agree on the correct method of rating the frequency response. In fact, in one case three different methods are all used in the same crossover guide!

Probably that's the reason you can install a transistor rated simply as "50 MHz" and yet find it won't properly amplify a signal in a 10.7-MHz IF amplifier in a VHF FM radio receiver. Of course, the manufacturer didn't lie, but he may have inadvertently used a rating system that doesn't fit your circuit.

As shown in Figure 22-2, one factor is the capacitances between the junctions. Another factor is the thickness and geometry of the base region and the time it takes for the majority electrical carriers to cross the base region. If the capacitances of the replacement are too far out of tolerance, then the gain will be reduced at high frequencies (and any LC tank circuits in the transistor amplifier will be mistuned).

In addition, there is the Miller effect, which is the effective capacitance produced by internal feedback from the output signal back to the input "amplifying" the actual capacitance. A small difference of internal capacitance can create a larger change of effective capacitance because of the Miller effect.

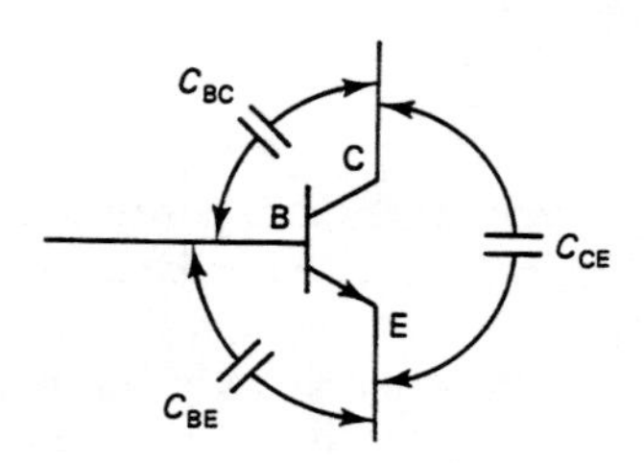

FIGURE 22-2

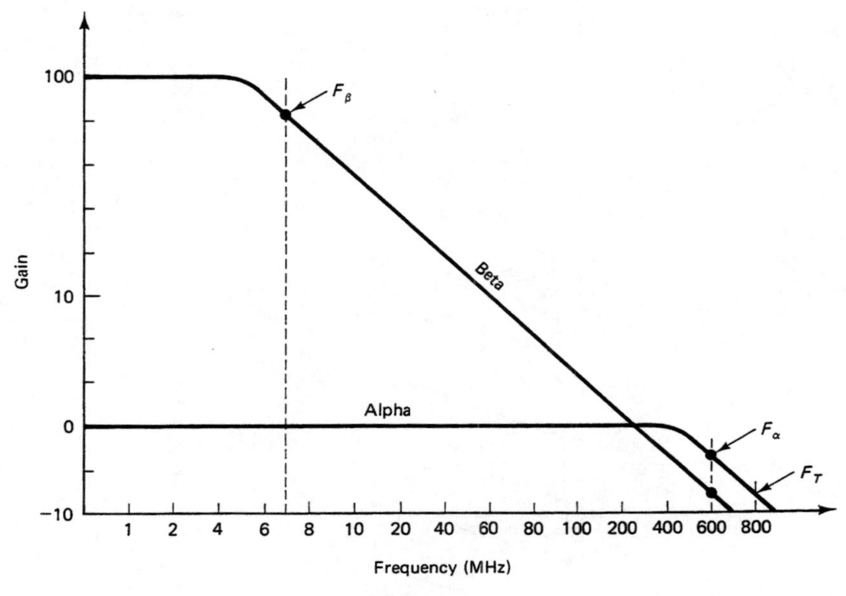

FIGURE 22-3

ALPHA AND BETA GAIN

Transistor alpha gain is the ratio of the collector current to the emitter current, and can never exceed one. Alpha gain is often measured in a common-base circuit. Beta gain is the ratio of collector current to base current and is usually measured in the common-emitter configuration. The frequency cutoff point is greatly different for these two kinds of ratings, as illustrated in Figure 22-3. A manufacturer who rates his transistors by the common-base method might correctly list them as having a far wider response than is possible by the common-emitter method. Of course, the common-base rating can provide you with a no-gain 10.7-MHz IF stage!

GAIN-BANDWIDTH PRODUCT

Another way of rating frequency response is the gain-bandwidth product method. It is defined as the frequency at which the common-emitter gain drops to unity. For an example, let's assume a transistor with a low-frequency (1000-Hz) beta rating of 50 and a gain-bandwidth product of 50 MHz. The gain-bandwidth product equals the beta times the common-emitter cut-off frequency, so the common-emitter cutoff frequency is found to be only 1 MHz. That's why you can act on some of the short-form specifications and still obtain a dud that won't amplify.

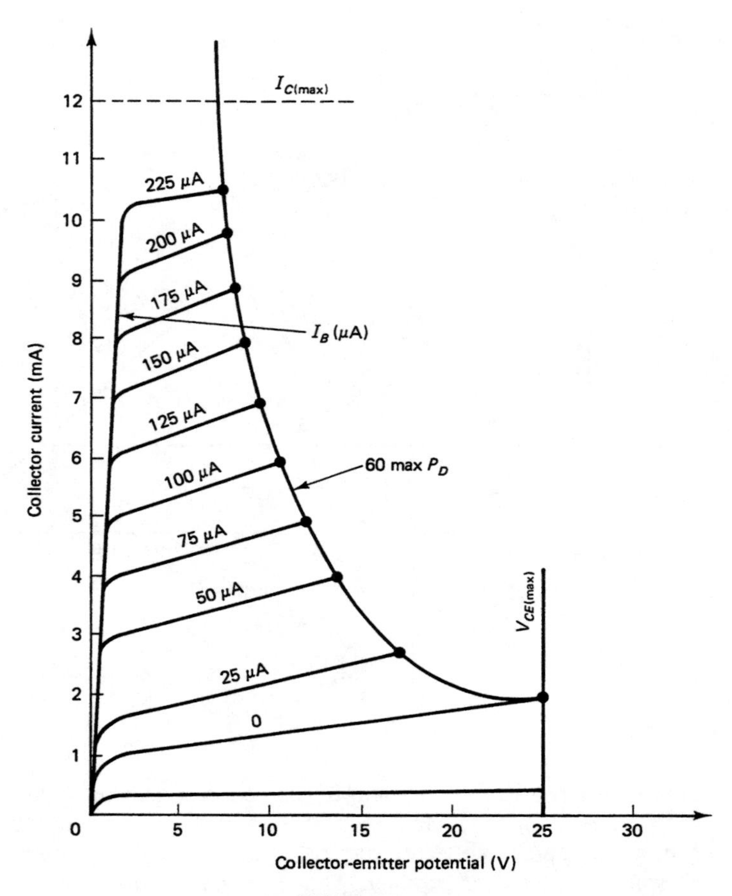

FIGURE 22-4

ANALYZING MAXIMUM RATINGS

Care must be used in analyzing the manufacturer's maximum voltage and current ratings. Just because a transistor is listed for certain maximum collector voltage and current doesn't mean it can always operate safely at those levels. The graph in Figure 22-4 shows that the transistor can safely stand either high current or high voltage, but not both at the same time. Maximum collector dissipation, the *product* of both voltage and current (watts), must not be exceeded.

MECHANICAL PROBLEMS

Problems of physical size, connecting leads, and methods of mounting some substitute transistors are equally as vexing as those of finding a suitable electrical characteristic.

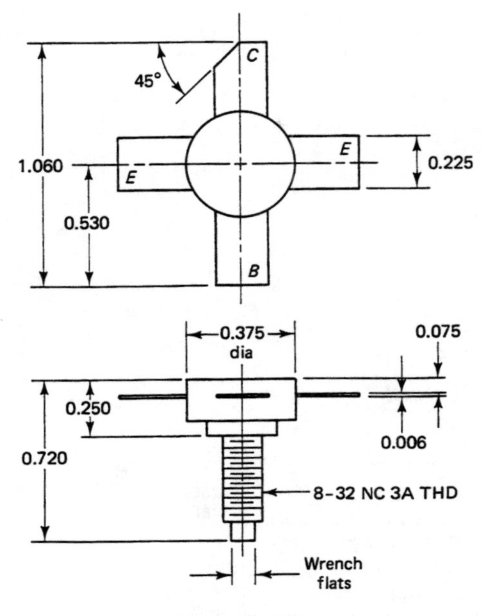

FIGURE 22-5

Our first transistor package is the RF power transistor in Figure 22-5. This device uses thin, flat, "low-inductance" leads. Several sizes are available, and size doesn't always indicate relative power dissipation rating (although it usually does). There was one 150-MHz FM mobile power amplifier that came with either of two different types of power transistor. The hole in the printed wiring board was cut for the larger type, and rubber "O-rings" were placed around the smaller to make them fit.

Figure 22-6 shows several types of power transistor package. The TO-3 transistor in Figure 22-6A is the so-called "standard" power transistor in a diamond-shaped package. A smaller diamond-shaped package is the TO-66 shown in Figure 22-6B. There is also a Japanese "similar-to-TO66" package that looks at first blush like the TO-66, but has slightly different pin spacings. Finally, the big horse shown in Figure 22-6C is the TO-36. This high-power transistor is used extensively in automotive audio applications, mobile solid-state HV multivibrator DC power supplies, and industrial electronics applications; older tube-type mobile transmitters often used these transistors in the 13.6-V DC-to-HV power supply.

Figure 22-7 shows several popular plastic power transistor packages. Some of these are listed as replacements for TO-3 or TO-66 diamond shaped power transistors. The package in Figure 22-7A is the TO-220 (once also called "P-66") and is common in small, low- to medium-powered audio applications (and most car radios). Two additional tab-mounted plastic power transistors are shown in Figures 22-7B and 22-7C. Finally, the device shown in Figure 22-7D is representative of a

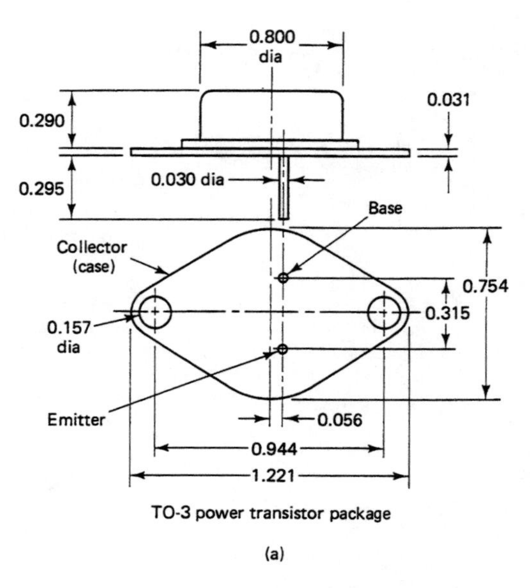

TO-3 power transistor package

(a)

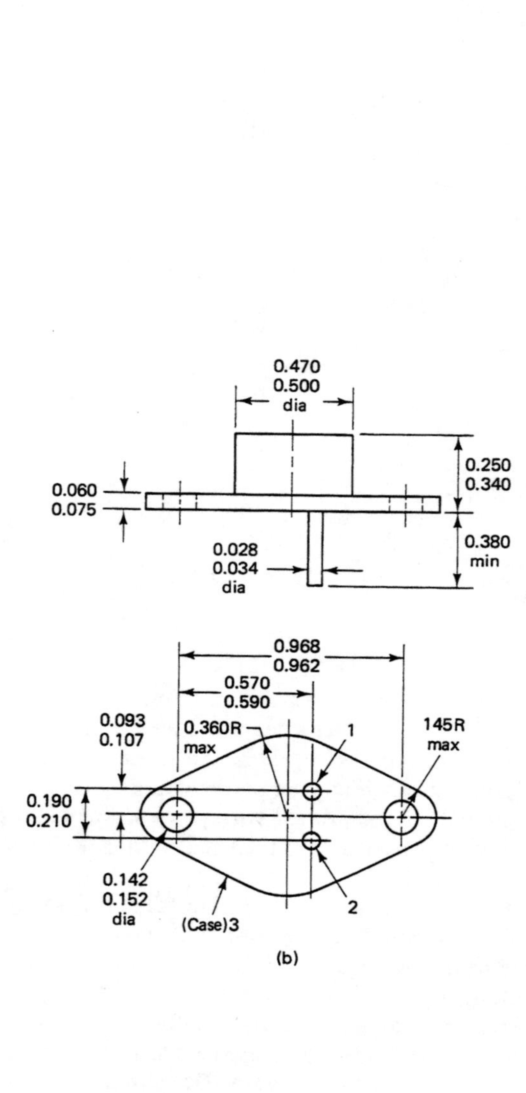

(b)

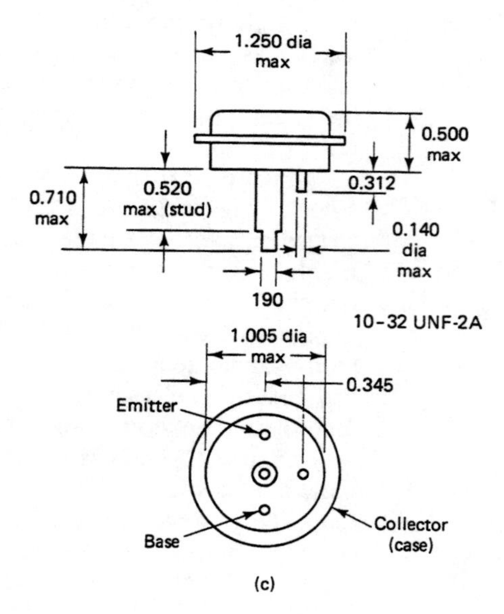

(c)

FIGURE 22-6

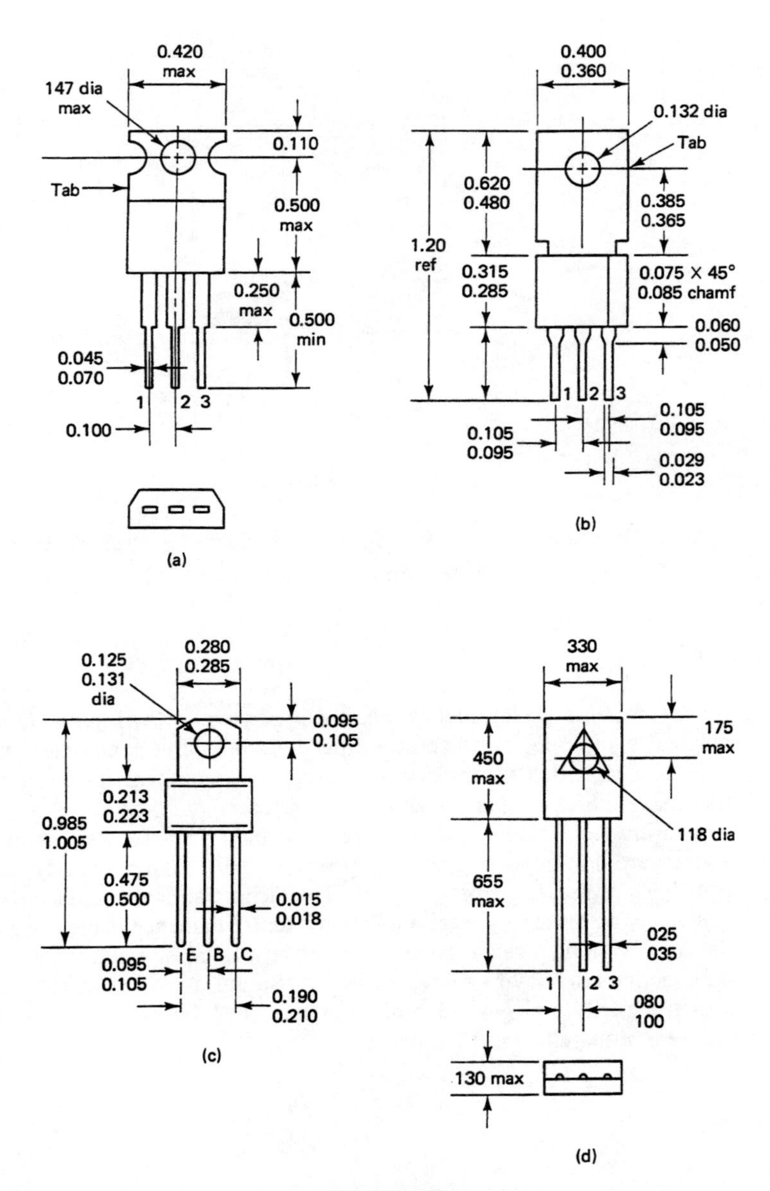

FIGURE 22-7

class of Motorola power transistors. These devices are not tab mounted, but instead have a mounting hole through the body of the transistor.

Figure 22-8 shows how a plastic, tab-mounted TO-220 power transistor can replace a TO-3 power transistor. The center terminal (collector) is cut off the TO-220 (it won't be needed, the tab mount is also connected to the collector), and the

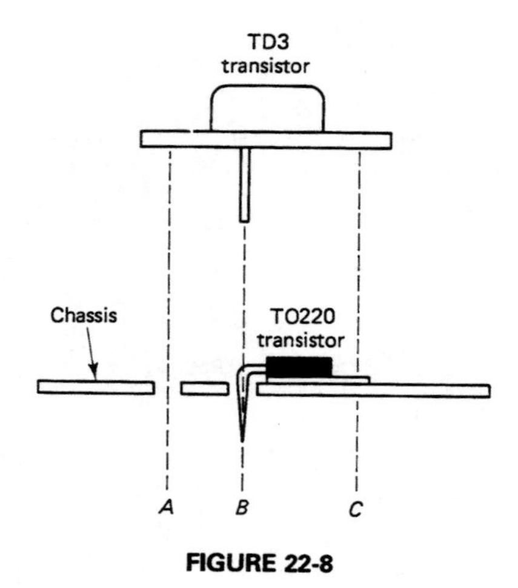

FIGURE 22-8

base and emitter leads are bent down. The mounting screw is passed through the tab hole into the original mounting hole for the TO-3 tansistor.

CONCLUSION

Ideally, when a replacement transistor is needed, we will have an original from the original equipment manufacturer's parts catalog. But sometimes, we are either unable to obtain such a transistor, or the cost is prohibitive. In those cases we can usually make educated guesses at a proper replacement type.

Warning: Transistor and IC replacements must be done with extreme caution and regard for good engineering practice. This chapter merely lays out the basic principles of making cross-matches. The technician who makes a modification, however, may be assuming legal liability for future damages if the device fails. Knowing the legal system, even a good match not involved in a failure will be twisted by a malpractice attorney to show evil intent. So unless you want to be a made out to be a dirty, smelly bad guy, regardless of the truth, be careful of making substitutions and seek a manufacturer's advice.

23

Radio Communications for Medical Emergency Units

The most significant step forward for emergency units of all types, including medical, in the past 60 or 70 years is the two-way radio. More than just a "talk-toy," the modern emergency service communications system can be a complex data transfer network. Some networks have voice, video, digital data (including computer terminals in the vehicle), analog waveform (e.g., electrocardiograph) data, and other forms of information transfer. But there are problems that one must be aware of when using radio communications equipment.

Radio communications depends upon getting the radio wave from the transmitting antenna to the receiving antenna in an effective and efficient manner. Sound like a question that begs the obvious? Well, it is begging the obvious, but nonetheless the transmission path is very important in communications. Your ability to deliver care to victims of accidents and illness depends upon the radio! Many problems faced by communications users derive directly from radio propagation problems. Before looking at some examples, let's first take a look at the basics of radio waves.

THE ELECTROMAGNETIC FIELD

Radio signals are *electromagnetic* (EM) waves exactly like light, infrared and ultraviolet, except for frequency. The EM wave consists of two mutually perpendicular oscillating fields (see Figure 23-1A) traveling together. One of the fields is an *electric* field; the other is a *magnetic* field.

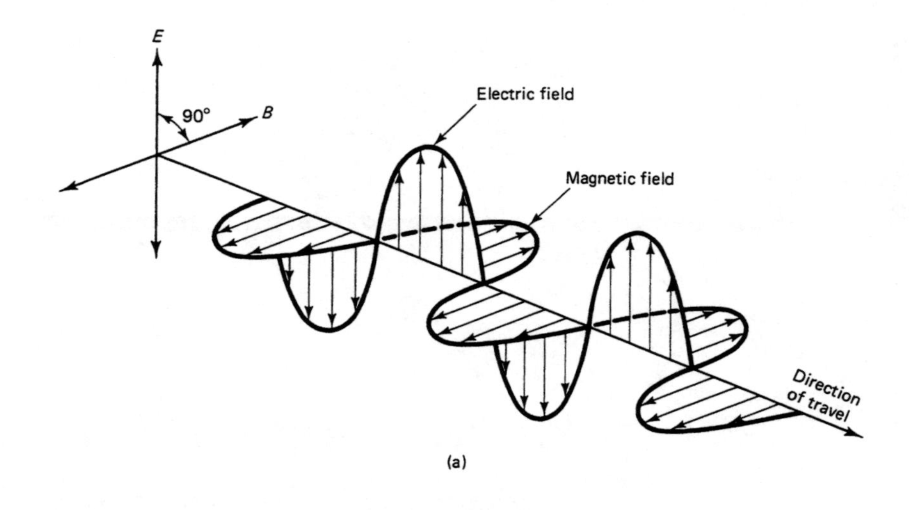

(a)

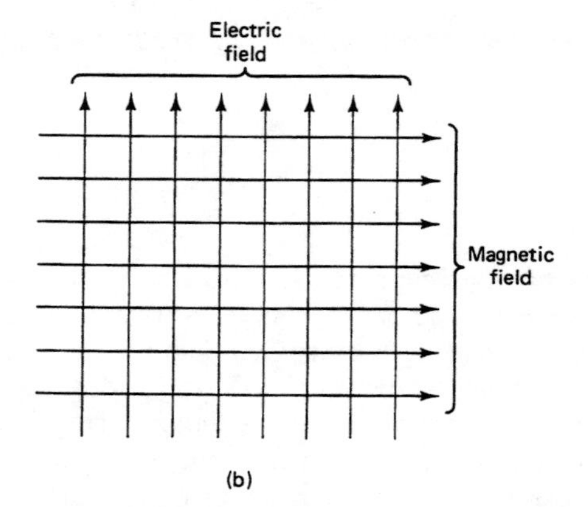

(b)

FIGURE 23-1

In dealing with radio wave propagation we sometimes make use of a textbook construct called an *isotropic source* for the sake of comparison and easy arithmetic. An isotropic source assumes that the radiator (i.e., "antenna") is a very tiny spherical source that radiates equally well in all directions. The radiation pattern is thus a sphere with the isotropic antenna at the center. As the wave propagates away from the source, that sphere gets ever larger. If, at a great distance from the center, we take a look at a small slice of the advancing wavefront, we can pretend that it is a flat plane, as in Figure 23-1B. This phenomenon is similar to the fact that the nearly spherical Earth looks nearly flat on the surface. In such a situation, we would be able to "see" the electric and magnetic field vectors at right angles to each other (Figure 23-1B).

The *polarization* of an EM wave is, by definition, the *direction of the electric field*. In Figure 23-1 we see vertical polarization because the electric field is vertical with respect to the earth. If the fields were swapped, then the EM wave would be horizontally polarized.

These designations are especially convenient because they also tell us the type of antenna used: vertical antennas produce vertically polarized signals, while horizontal antennas produce horizontally polarized signals. Some texts erroneously state that antennas will not pick up signals of the opposite polarity. That claim is nonsense, although up to ten times or so cross-polarization loss might be observed at the VHF through microwave frequencies typically used by emergency radios.

An EM wave travels at the speed of light (designated by the letter c), which is about 186,000 miles per second (or 300,000,000 meters per second if you prefer metric). To put this velocity in perspective, a radio signal originating on the Sun's surface would reach Earth in about 8 minutes. A terrestrial radio signal can travel around the Earth seven times in 1 second. The velocity of the wave slows in dense media, but in air the speed is so close to the "free-space" value of c that the same figures are used for both air and outer space.

PROPAGATION PHENOMENA

Because EM waves are waves, they behave in a wavelike manner. Figure 23-2 illustrates some of the wave property phenomena associated with light and radio waves: *reflection, refraction,* and *diffraction*. All three play roles in radio propagation. In fact, many practical radio propagation situations involve all three in varying combinations.

Reflection and refraction are shown in Figure 23-2A. Reflection occurs when a wave strikes a denser medium, as when a light wave strikes a glass mirror. The incident wave (shown as a single ray) strikes the interface between less dense and more dense mediums at a certain angle of incidence (a_i) and is reflected at exactly the same angle (now called the angle of reflection, a_r). Because these angles are equal, we can often trace a reflected radio or TV signal back to its origin.

Refraction occurs when the incident wave enters the different density region and thereby undergoes both a velocity change and a directional change. The amount and direction of the direction change is determined by the ratio of the densities between the two media. If Zone B is much different from Zone A, then bending is great. In radio systems, the two media might be different layers of air with different densities. It is possible for both reflection and refraction to occur in the same system.

Diffraction is shown in Figure 23-2B. In this case, an advancing wavefront encounters an opaque object (e.g., a steel building). The "shadow zone" behind the building is not simply perpendicular to the wave, but takes on a cone shape as waves bend around the object. The "umbra region" (or "diffraction zone") between the shadow zone ("cone of silence") and the direct propagation zone is a region of weak (but not zero) signal strength. In practical situations the cone of silence is never really zero. A certain amount of reflected signals scattered from other sources will fill in the shadow a little bit. However, emergency medical, fire, and police units often experience reduced or interrupted radio communications caused by this effect.

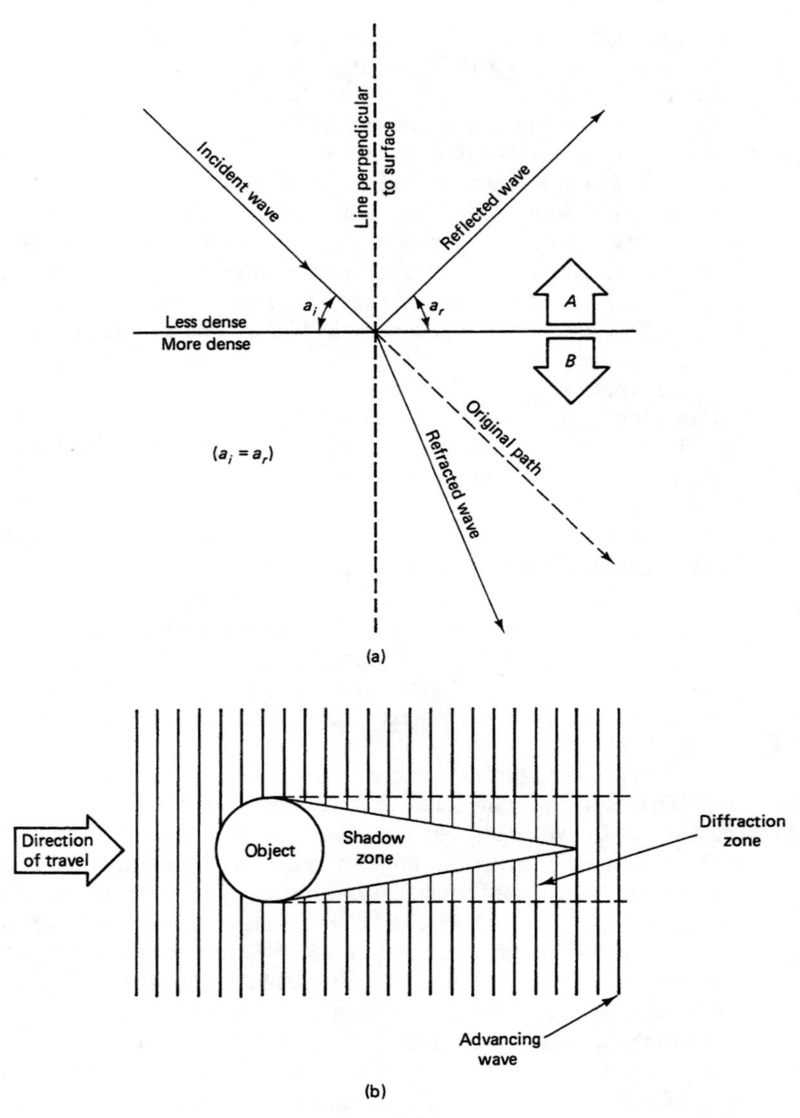

FIGURE 23-2

PROPAGATION PATHS

There are four major propagation paths for emergency radio systems: *surface wave* and *space wave*. Long-distance communications involve "ionospheric" propagation and is only important for most emergency medical units for the trouble it can cause. Ionospheric propagation is the mechanism for "skip," that is, the phenomena seen in the citizen's band, amateur radio bands, and the international shortwave broadcast bands under which signals can travel from continent to continent.

For emergency units, "skip" can cause disruption to local operations when very strong "skip" signals from distant locations interfere with local signals. The author recalls a police situation on the old 38-MHz "low-band VHF" band. A call indicating a bank robbery in progress was heard by police patrol cars, and they went off in response with sirens screaming, guts tight, and the professional willingness to confront the dirty, smelly bad guys. But at the county line they realized that there *was no 8000 block of Wilson Blvd!* It turns out that this Virginia police department used the same 38.17-MHz radio frequency as a police department in Texas—where there was also another "Wilson Blvd."

The space and surface waves are both classed as "ground waves," but behave differently enough from each other to warrant separate consideration. The surface wave travels in direct contact with the earth's surface. It suffers a frequency-dependent attenuation due to absorption into the ground. Because the absorption increases with frequency, we observe much greater surface wave distances in the AM broadcast band (540–1620 KHz) than in the 11-meter citizens band (27,000 KHz).

The space wave is also a ground wave phenomena, but is radiated from an antenna many wavelengths above the surface. No part of the space wave normally travels in contact with the surface; VHF, UHF, and microwave frequencies used by emergency services usually produce space waves. There are, however, two components of the space wave in many cases: *direct* and *reflected* (see Figure 23-3).

The ionosphere is the region of earth's atmosphere that is above the stratosphere, and is located 30 to 300 miles above the surface. The peculiar feature of the ionosphere is that molecules of air gas (O_2 and N) can be ionized by stripping away electrons under the influence of solar radiation and certain other sources of energy. The electrons are negative ions, while the formerly neutral atoms they were removed from are now positive ions. In the ionosphere the air density is so low that ions can travel relatively long distances before recombining with oppositely charged ions to form electrically neutral atoms. As a result, the ionosphere remains ionized for long periods of the day—even after sunset. At lower altitudes, however, air density is greater, and recombination thus occurs rapidly. At those altitudes solar ionization diminishes to nearly zero immediately after sunset and never achieves any significant levels even at local noon.

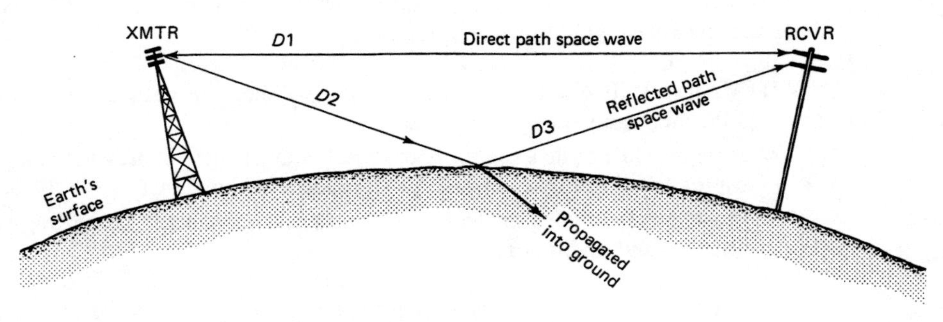

FIGURE 23-3

Ionospheric propagation is seen in the form of a "sky wave," which is responsible for the so-called "skip phenomenon" seen in the MW-, HF-, and lower-VHF-frequency regions. It is skip that makes these signals propagate over long (even intercontinental) distances. To the emergency radio user on low-band VHF frequencies, "skip" produces the interference described earlier. There are many cases on record of emergency units responding to nonexistent addresses—obviously expensive and very dangerous when the unit is needed for a real emergency locally.

GROUNDWAVE PROPAGATION

The ground wave, naturally enough, travels along the ground (or at least in close proximity to the surface). There are two forms of ground wave: space and surface. The space wave does not actually touch the ground. As a result, space wave attenuation with distance in clear weather is about the same as in free space. Of course, above the VHF region weather conditions add attenuation not found in outer space. The surface wave is subject to the same attenuation factors as the space wave, but in addition it also suffers ground losses. These losses are due to resistive loss in the conductive earth. In other words, the signal heats up the ground!

The surface wave attenuation is a function of frequency, and increases rapidly as frequency increases. In the AM broadcast band the surface wave operates out to about 100 miles or so. In the citizens band, however, attenuation is so great that communications is often limited to less than 20 miles. It is common in the upper HF region to be able to hear stations across the continent, or internationally, while "local" stations only 20–30 miles distant remain unheard, or are very weak.

For both forms of ground wave, communications is affected by these factors: frequency, height of both receive and transmit antennas, distance between antennas, and terrain and weather along the transmission path.

Ground wave communications also suffers another difficulty, especially at VHF and above. The space wave is made up of two components: direct and reflected waves. If both components arrive at the receive antenna, they will add algebraically to either increase or reduce total signal strength. There is always a phase shift between the two components because the two signal paths have different lengths. In addition, there may be a 180-degree phase reversal at the point of reflection (especially if the incident signal is horizontally polarized), as in Figure 23-4. The following general rules apply in these situations:

1. A phase-shift of an odd number of half wavelengths causes the components to add, increasing signal strength.
2. A phase-shift of an even number of half wavelengths causes the components to subtract (for example, Figure 23-4), reducing signal strength.
3. Phase-shifts other than half wavelength add or subtract according to relative polarity and amplitude.

A practical result of these general rules is the existence of radio dead spots even in places where shadowing is not a factor. An emergency medical technician in

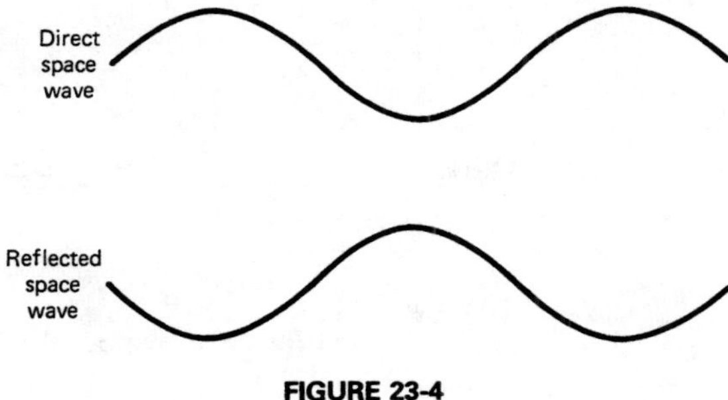

FIGURE 23-4

one of these spots need only move the antenna (which means whole vehicle in mobile units) a few inches to get out of a rule 2 dead zone to a rule 1 hot zone.

At VHF and above, the space wave is limited to so-called "line-of-sight" distances. The horizon is theoretically the limit of communications distance. But as any radio user will testify, the radio horizon is about 60 percent farther than the optical horizon. This phenomenon is due to bending in the atmosphere. Although more sophisticated models are available today, we can still make use of the traditional model of the radio horizon shown in Figure 23-5. The actual situation is shown in Figure 23-5A. Distance d is a curved path along the surface of the earth. But because the earth's radius R is about 4000 miles and is thus very much larger than practical antenna height h, we can simplify the model to that shown in Figure 23-5B. The underlying assumption for trigonometry buffs is that the earth has a radio radius equal to about four-thirds its physical radius.

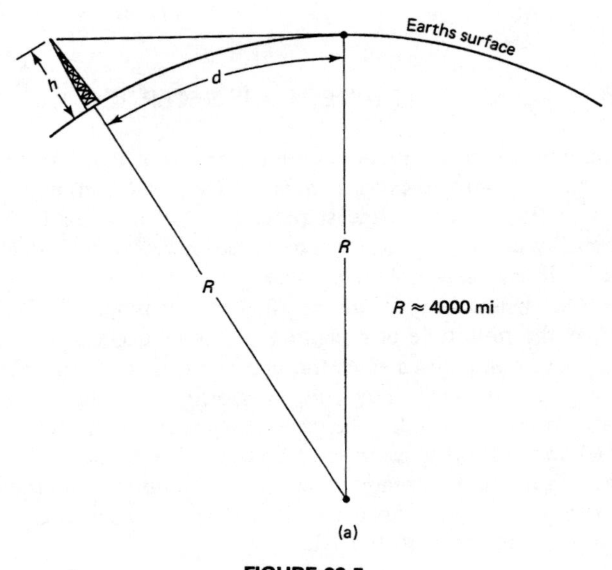

FIGURE 23-5

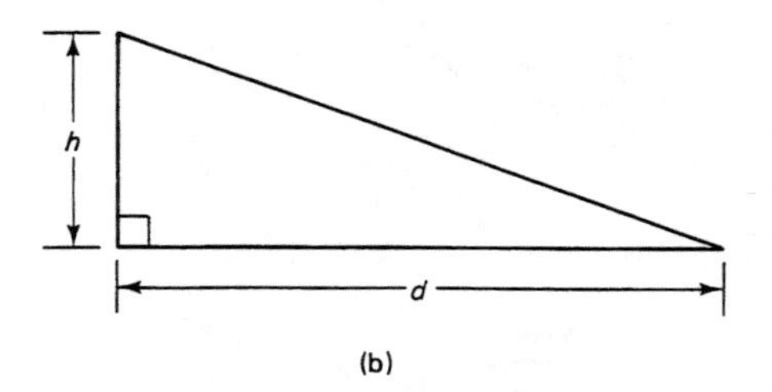

(b)

FIGURE 23-5 (continued)

The value of distance d is found from the expression

$$d = 1.42(h)^{1/2}$$

where

d = the distance to the radio horizon in miles
h = the antenna height in feet

Example

A radio tower has a 150-MHz radio antenna mounted 150 feet above the surface of the Earth. Calculate the radio horizon (in miles) for this system.

Solution:

$$\begin{aligned} d &= 1.42(h)^{1/2} \\ &= (1.42)(150 \text{ ft.})^{1/2} \\ &= (1.42)(12.25) \\ &= 17.4 \text{ miles} \end{aligned}$$

PECULIAR PROBLEMS THAT AFFECT VHF RECEPTION

Communications receivers have long been hot items in the automobile electronics and mobile communications market. The most common receivers, of course, are FM and FM stereo broadcast receivers, but now many thousands of vehicles are equipped with communications receivers either as individual monitors or as part of a VHF/UHF two-way FM transceiver.

One headache that affects all forms of mobile FM VHF/UHF receiver, however, is the multitude of reception problems experienced. Technicians in the repair shops have complained since the late 1950s that salespeople create a lot of the complaints because they sell too much performance. While every good salesperson "sells the sizzle, not the steak," the customer sometimes finds that the sizzle is from greasy fatback instead of the promised prime rib! The purpose of this section is to show you some of the more common reception problems seen on mobile FM receivers so that you can tell whether some specific difficulty is normal or is a defect that needs correcting by the repair technicians.

NOISE REJECTION

Advertising and salespeople often make the claim that FM reception is "noise free." While this claim is most often heard in the context of FM broadcast band receivers, the same idea also carries over to other FM receivers (e.g., mobile and portable communications receivers) as well. Without some qualification, however, this claim is patently false. FM reception is more noise free than AM reception, but only under certain specific conditions will FM reception be virtually noise free. It is not true that you will never be bothered by noise when monitoring an FM receiver. The FM receiver's "limiter" circuit is the key to this phenomena.

Figure 23-6 illustrates graphically how an FM receiver reduces or eliminates noise signals. Notice that when a strong signal is passed through a limiter stage, its amplitude peaks are clipped. Because most fabricated and natural types of static noise tend to *amplitude modulate* the signal (true frequency modulation of the signal by noise does occur, but it is rare), it is removed along with the signal peaks. Under conditions where the signal is subject to maximum limiting, little or no noise will get through to the detector.

Figure 23-7 illustrates the situation in which the noise *will* get through to the detector, and subsequently appear in the audio output. Suppose the receiver is tuned to either a very-low-power station or a distant station. If the received signal is below the limit sensitivity of the receiver, the limiter circuit will have no effect. When a signal is tuned in that has less than the level required to initiate limiting, then the limiter will fail to act and will perform merely as an amplifier. Those noisy signal peaks will pass through the detector to the audio amplifiers. Even when inadequate or no limiting occurs, the noise produced by an FM receiver may be less severe than that produced by an AM receiver. This is attributable to several factors that aid in reducing any noise that gets by the limiter.

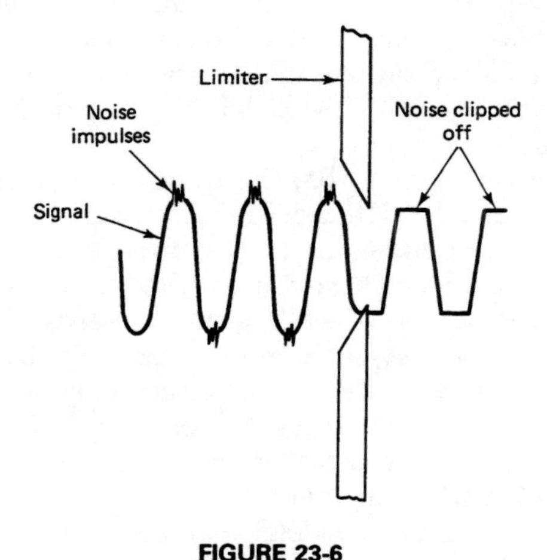

FIGURE 23-6

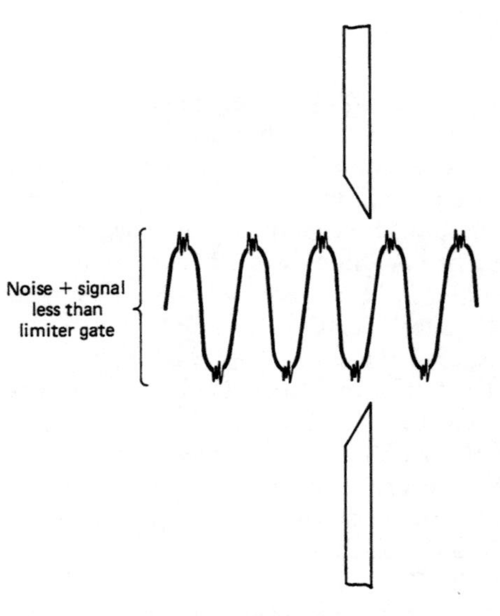

FIGURE 23-7

SENSITIVITY

Mobile radio and automobile radio technicians routinely receive complaints that the FM receiver seems unable to receive distant stations. A user once complained to the author that he was told that he could easily monitor a station that was some 40 miles distant, if he would only buy the VHF-FM radio offered by that particular dealer. A demonstration was given in the showroom, and sure enough, the station was loud and clear. The chap was naturally upset when he discovered that the "sizzle" sold by the salesman was coming out the loudspeakers! That $1400 receiver was incapable of giving him local performance on signals received from 40 miles away. The problem was sensitivity. Sensitivity is a measure of the radio's ability to pick up weak signals. The reliable range of most radios at that time was about 20 miles or so.

The reception of any FM signal, whether communications or broadcast, is limited by the fact that VHF and UHF frequencies used for these signals are "line of sight." At lower frequencies, such as those occupied by AM and shortwave-band broadcasters, the ionosphere will bend the radio signals back to earth so that they land some distance away—often many thousands of miles away. At VHF/UHF the degree of refraction is insufficient to reflect them back to earth. Those waves travel out into space. In the VHF/UHF spectrum, only the ground wave is useful.

Because the useful propagation of VHF/UHF signals is limited to the ground wave, the greatest distance that can be reliably used is a little farther than the optical horizon (4/3 earth's curvature). This is "line-of-sight" propagation, although the term itself is a little misleading. Stations are often received at distances that are greater than the "radio horizon." The reason for this discrepancy is that the radio

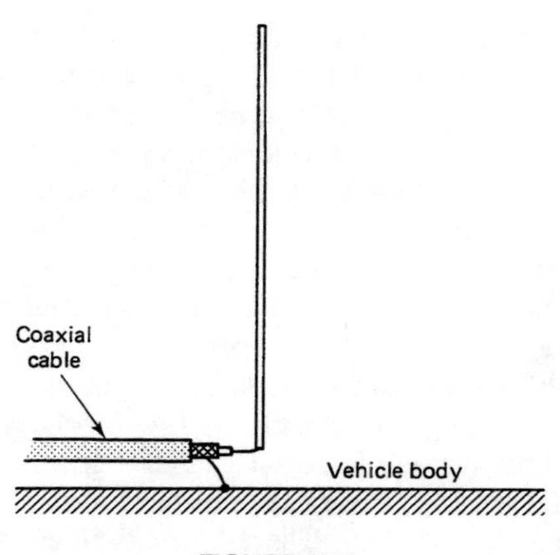

FIGURE 23-8

line of sight is a function of the height of the transmitter and receiver antennas above the earth's surface.

Because most mobile unit antennas are close to the ground, reception of VHF/UHF FM signals by a mobile radio receiver over longer than optical distances requires a very high transmitting antenna. That is why mobile radio operators typically rent space on top of buildings or on broadcast station towers for their base station antennas. People who typically have better reception at base stations than in the vehicle generally have either a prime location, a superior antenna, or both. The base station receiver is connected to a great antenna, while the mobile receiver will have either a simple quarter wavelength vertical or some minimum gain antenna. While base stations may have a 50- to 100-foot tower for their antennas, very few mobile installations can boast the same.

A fair improvement in apparent sensitivity can be realized if the antenna is tuned somewhere near reasonance. Figure 23-8 shows a typical quarter wavelength vertical antenna. The length of the quarter wavelength whip antenna is set at the height determined from the equation

$$L_{\text{in.}} = 2808/F_{\text{MHz}}$$

This formula will yield the height in inches of the radiator element, when the frequency is expressed in megahertz.

FADING

One Sunday afternoon the burglar alarm at a local bank went off. A covey of cops showed up and determined that the problem was an alarm failure. One of the officers remained behind to await the bank manager to come and disable the errant alarm. When he parked, he noticed that his radio reception was poor, so he called the dispatcher and requested a "slow ten count." As the radio crackled out "1, 2, 3 . . ." the officer moved the car *a few inches* and restored reception. It is interesting that, because of the short wavelengths in the VHF spectrum, the patrol car could move only a few inches and make such a profound difference in the reception!

Another well known phenomenon is the ability of VHF/UHF signals to penetrate tunnels where AM band radios fade out (although a VHF/UHF signal may fade out in a tunnel just as badly as the AM signal if the tunnel is long enough or if the "propagation" inside the tunnel is wrong). The downtown areas of many cities provide many examples of fading and reception irregularities similar to both of our examples. The causes are "dead zones" and "multipath cancellation" of the signal.

A dead zone exists where there is little or no signal. It can be caused either by the multipath problem or by shadowing. One type of shadowing was shown in Figure 23-2B. The longer waves in the AM broadcast band can bend around obstructions. The short waves of the VHF/UHF bands, however, cannot. An obstruction, such as a tall building, therefore, creates a shadow zone on the side that is opposite of the transmitter antenna. There can exist many hundreds of shadow zones in a downtown area.

Unfortunately, shadow zones tend to increase as the angle between the receiving and the transmitting antennas is reduced. This effect is similar to the effect of the setting sun on your own shadow. With the sun directly overhead at noontime, there is little or no shadow. However, as the sun sets, your shadow tends to become both deeper and longer. Likewise, in a radio system, the shadow zones will become more severe as the distance between the receiving and transmitting antennas increases, or the antenna heights decrease.

Multipath reception is illustrated in Figure 23-9. It occurs when a signal bounces off an obstruction, such as a building or water tower, and arrives at the receiver a few microseconds later than the direct signal. This is the same phenomenon

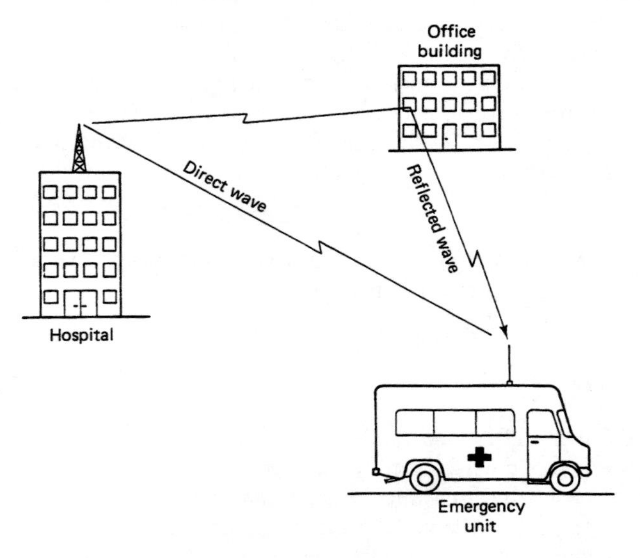

FIGURE 23-9

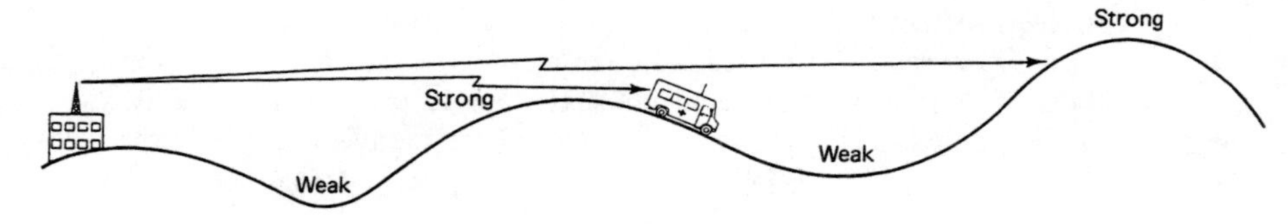

FIGURE 23-10

that causes "ghosts" in TV reception. Because this late-arriving signal is out of phase with the direct signal, there will be at least some partial cancellation of both signals when they meet at the receiver antenna (this effect is a function of their wave nature). The listener hears a "ffft ffft ffft" sound as the car moves from one multipath zone to another. Technicians who work on FM broadcast auto radios receivers sometimes call this effect "picket fencing." Note that picket fencing can mimic the sound of a defective radio, so one should be certain that the radio is operating properly. Those defects will occur whether or not the vehicle is moving, while the multipath effect only occurs when in motion, and it is not found in all locations. It was a multipath effect that caused the police officer in my earlier story to move his car. This effect depends upon the wavelength of the signal and can be expected to change every quarter wavelength or so. In the case of the 157-MHz police radio, quarter wavelength was on the order of 18 inches, which explains why the officer moved the car only a foot or so and found reception a lot better.

Although most VHF/UHF shadow zones are in what might be called overcivilized areas where there are lots of buildings, it is not unusual to encounter them also in the open countryside. The obstruction that causes either a reflection or shadow can be located many miles from where the reflected and direct signals recombine at a receiver. Either type of zone can be located anywhere, and might be only a few inches across.

Another example of VHF/UHF fading out on the open road is the phenomenon of "hilltopping" (see Figure 23-10). On top of the hill, the received base station signal is loud and clear to the mobile unit, and the low-power mobile transmitter has no trouble getting into the base station (or repeater) receiver. In the troughs, however, the signals are weak (or nonexistent) and the mobile transmitter won't even "key up" the repeater transmitter.

INTERMODULATION PROBLEMS

Remember "Intermod Hill" in the author's hometown? It happens to be one of the higher locations in the county, so several broadcasters and AT&T have seen fit to build radio towers there. In addition, the two main radio towers bristle with landmobile antennas whose owners rent space on the tower in order to get better coverage. We have, then, two 50,000-watt FM broadcast stations, a 1000-watt AM broadcast station, a many-frequency microwave relay station, and several dozen 150-mHz to 950-mHz landmobile and radio paging stations. Nearby is a hospital that operates its own security system radio station and a hospital pager system. They also have a coronary care unit that uses radio telemetry to keep track of ambulatory patients. All those signals can combine in unusual ways to produce apparently valid signals on other channels. The frequencies produced are many, and follow the rule

$$F_{unwanted} = mF_1 \pm nF_2$$

where m and n are integers (1, 2, 3 . . .) F_1 and F_2 are the frequencies present.

Imagine the number of possible combinations when there are literally dozens of frequencies floating around the neighborhood! The ability (or lack of same) to reject these intermods is a good measure of a receiver's performance. Linearity and dynamic range of the receiver's input RF amplifier is a factor in intermodulation cases.

INTRABUILDING COMMUNICATIONS

Radio communications systems are increasingly being used inside of buildings. While previously it was the case that radio equipment was not considered unless the system had to cover more than a single building, there are an increasingly large number of systems in which employees inside a single building are kept in radio communications. Such a building might be a factory or warehouse in which key or critical employees are kept in touch by radio. In other cases, the building "engineer" is kept in contact with the building manager's office by walkie-talkie. A large number of construction workers and craftspeople keep in touch with radios. In my own office building there are emergency medical technicians on every second floor, and they carry portable radios on their belts. When the author worked in a major hospital, we operated several radio systems: the medical pager system, the security system, and a central supply system. All radios operated in either VHF or UHF bands.

But there are problems that show up on intrabuilding systems. Shielding, shadowing, and multipath problems persist despite the efforts of engineers to resolve them. But there are some solutions.

One common problem is that the low-power handheld transmitters cannot be received at the base station. A solution is to install either a multiple receiver system (Figure 23-11) or a multiple-RF amplifier system such as used in the ECG telemetry system. A voting system is used on the multiple receiver system in order to keep the audio constant. The receiver with the strongest signal from any given source is used as the system audio.

It almost goes without saying that a repeater (Figure 23-12) is needed in the intrabuilding system. The handheld units transmit on F1 and receive on F2, while the main base station does just the opposite: it transmits on F2 and receives on F1. In some areas of the building, where particular dead zones are located, a supplementary antenna is placed to radiate signal into that region. Care must be exercised, however, to prevent this secondary signal from interfering with the main signal and thereby causing other dead zones.

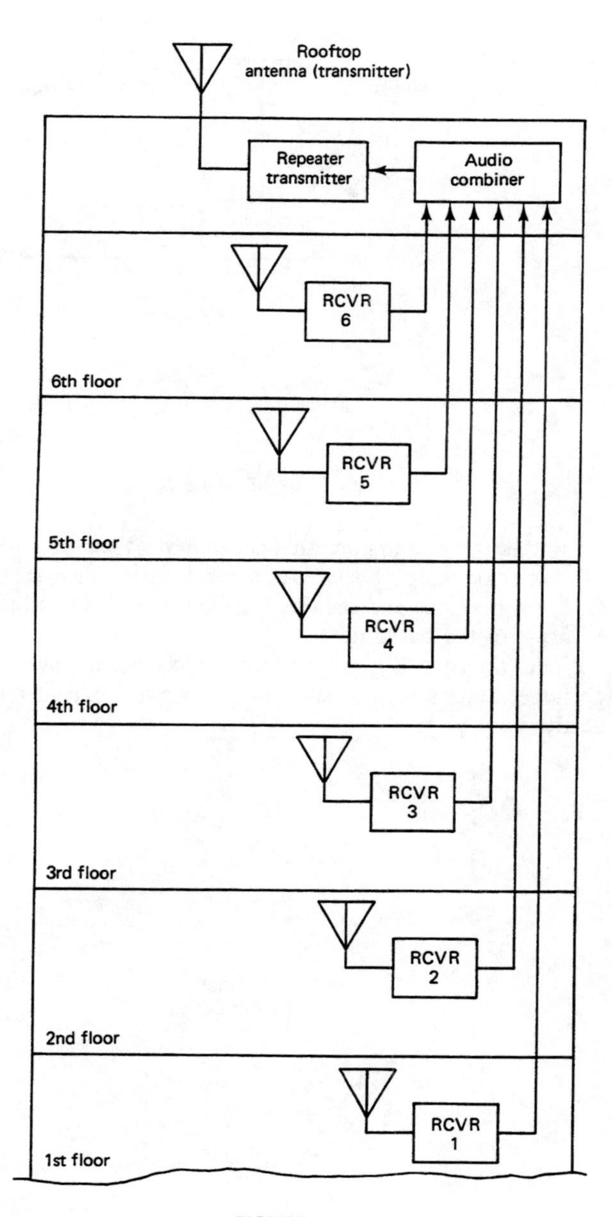

Rooftop
antenna (transmitter)
Repeater
transmitter
Audio
combiner
RCVR
6
6th floor
RCVR
5
5th floor
RCVR
4
4th floor
RCVR
3
3rd floor
RCVR
2
2nd floor
RCVR
1
1st floor

FIGURE 23-11

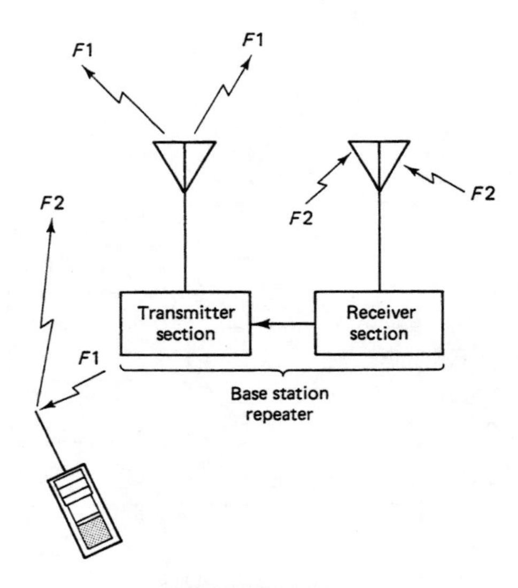

FIGURE 23-12

Another option, and one that is often overlooked, is to place the repeater on an off-site tower or building roof. As a result of the displacement from the main site, downtown reflections and multipath have the result of filling in most of the shadow zones inside of the building.

Where the need is great, and the frequencies are available, then it is possible to design larger and more sophisticated systems that permit reliable intrabuilding communications.

24

Selecting the Right Desktop Personal Computer for Biomedical Systems

Personal computers are now ubiquitous in all areas of commerce, industry, medicine, science, and other fields. These little machines, which fit easily onto a desktop with plenty of room to spare, are computational powerhouses that offer considerably more power than the mainframe units of a couple decades ago. There is a wide variety of options available, and those which should be selected depend on the application and growth patterns required for the application at hand.

Biomedical engineering personnel might use these machines for record keeping (for example, the preventative maintainance system), or they might use them as part of an analog data acquisition system in a laboratory setup. While the fundamental machine used for such disparate tasks are very similar—indeed may be identical—there is no such thing as a truly "universal" computer or computer configuration—that is, a machine that is all things to all people in all applications.

Matters to consider when buying a microcomputer for biomedical purposes are the architecture of the machine (that is, register, memory, or I/O oriented), the instruction set (computationally strong or I/O operations strong), and the associated hardware requirements. If the IBM-PC/XT series of machines is selected, then a wide variety of software products and add-on circuit cards are available. Indeed, the IBM-PC class of machine is now the standard for the industry.

Which of these do you select for *your* applications? All are microcomputers, yet they have vastly different properties. Obviously, one probably would not use the same machine for such vastly different chores as number crunching data processing, control systems, maintenance record keeping, or data acquisition.

It is, therefore, essential that you evaluate the task to be performed and also discern any *reasonable* future accretions to the system. Keep in mind that all projects tend to grow in scope as time passes. Some of this growth is legitimate; some growth occurs because people tend to enlarge a project into additional functions that were neither intended nor are advisable; some growth is due to *your* poor planning in the early stages of the project. Try to anticipate future needs and plan for them. A more or less valid rule of thumb is to follow the 50 percent rule regarding initial capacity: the current requirements should occupy only one-half of the machine resources (memory size, processing time, and number of I/O ports).

It is claimed that a smart designer will provide twice or three times the memory actually required for the presently specified chore, but will not under any circumstances tell the programmer how much is available. Programmers tend to use up all the memory available. Perhaps, if they think there is somewhat less available to them, they can find more efficient means to solve problems.

The decisions made during planning phases of a project will affect future capabilities in large measure. If adequate means for expansion are not provided, extraordinary problems will surface later.

The key to good planning is evaluation of system requirements. How many I/O ports are needed? What *kind* of I/O ports are needed (parallel? serial?)? How much memory (guess and then double the figure if cost will allow)? How fast will the processor have to operate? What kind of displays and/or input devices are needed? How many? What size of power supply is needed?

The basis for any personal computer is the central microprocessor chip used in the computer. On many machines, there is no real choice for the end user, but on machines that are considered IBM compatible, there are several options. The original chip used was the Intel 8088, which was used in the original IBM-PC, IBM-XT, and their clones. The NEC V-20 is a variant of this chip and is said to be faster than the 8088 in some forms of operation. Later machines, that is those that are IBM-AT clones, are based on the 80286 (aka '286) chip. This chip is more powerful than the 8088. The next chip to enter the fray is the 80386, and a very expensive 80486 is said to be on the near horizon.

If your needs are modest, then a simple 8088-based machine is sufficient. However, one should be aware that the 80286 is now the de facto standard in the commercial world and occupies the place previously occupied by the 8088. At one time, the cost of an 80286 machine was prohibitive, so one only specified these machines if a pressing need arose. However, the current cost of 80286 machines is quite low (compared with previous levels), so is the best choice for a basic machine. Advanced machines, or where finances permit, should be based on the 80386 ('386) microprocessor chip.

Speed-power product can become important in many applications. Processing speed, as measured by system clock frequency, is usually related to power consumption. In most semiconductor devices, including microprocessor chips, the operating speed relates to internal resistances and capacitances that form frequency-limiting RC time constants. Reducing internal resistance in order to increase operating speed (i.e., a short RC time constant) also causes increased power consumption. A problem seen with some *turbo* machines is that they use lower speed chips at a higher speed, in order to save cost, but that design has the effect of heating up the chip and therefore reducing reliability. A basic guideline is to assume that a 10°C increase in internal junction temperatures reduces the mean time between failure for the chip to one-half. The lesson to take from this discussion is to be sure that the chip in a turbo machine is capable of the advertised speed—otherwise, the machine is truly "turbo" only on its advertising brochure.

Processing speed as measured from program execution time, however, is another matter. This time limitation depends upon the efficiency of instruction execution and the nature of the instructions available to the programmer. A measure of programming speed is the *benchmark program* such as the often-touted Norton rating. Such a program attempts to standardize evaluation comparisons by having the different microcomputers under test perform some standard task and noting the amount of time required. There are numerous pitfalls in this approach, however, because the selection of the task and the programming approach used to solve the problem or task can significantly affect results through bias in favor of one machine over another. The benchmark program should, therefore, be representative of the tasks to be performed by the end product.

If the application requires a 16-bit word (or anything greater than the 8 bits normally found on "traditional" microprocessors), the computer will have to be either a 16-bit machine or be programmed to process 16 bits by sequentially grabbing 2 bytes at a time. The IBM-PC and IBM-XT machines are based on the 8088 chip, so are 16 bits, while the IBM-AT class machines are 32 bit.

Software support can also be a driving factor in the selection of the microcomputer. The IBM-PC/XT/AT machines, and the Macintoshes, have immense amounts of ready-made software available. Other machines, however, may have considerably less software available, so are not too much of a value when offered at a lower cost than a more standard machine.

Available hardware is another consideration. Both IBM-based machines and the "Mac" are well regarded and have a number of different hardware options, both at the time of purchase and in the after market. The IBM series of machines (and their clones) are particularly well suited to customizing because of the six to eight plug-in slots available on the motherboard inside the machine.

Finally, you must select the data storage media for the machine. There are two sizes in each of two formats of floppy disk. The 5.25-inch disk is available in either double density (360-kilobyte) or quad density (1.2-megabyte), while the 3.5-inch disks are available in 720-kilobyte and 1.44-megabyte formats. In most cases, one should have the A drive outfitted with a 5.25-inch floppy disk, and then either another 5.25-inch or a 3.5-inch in the B drive slot.

Hard disks are available in sizes from 10 megabyte (which are fast disappearing) up to more than 100 megabytes. As a general rule, one should obtain the largest hard disk that can be afforded. Although one must consider that large-capacity hard disks often show poorer reliability than lesser forms, the extra memory is well worthwhile.

The type and number of output ports on the computer is also a consideration. The well-equipped machine will have a parallel printer port and at least one serial RS-232C communications port. It is also a good idea to include an internal modem (telephone communications device) in 300-, 1200-, and 2400-baud speeds.

25

Repairing Water Damage to Medical Equipment

Five full days of heavy rains pelted the East Coast. In our area the river crested 11 feet above flood stage, but 80 miles upstream in the narrow mountain canyons it became a 54-foot-high wall of water that overwhelmed the best efforts of hundreds of bone-tired volunteers. Despite backbreaking heroic efforts, the sandbag wall at the edge of one town gave way under the relentless pressure of an angry river. Over the next 24 hours the water rose, completely flooded basements and gushed into the first floor of most homes and businesses to a height of 6 feet. As the waters receded, the governor called out the National Guard to prevent looters, and people returned home to recover what they could. After cleaning out the water moccasins that inevitably come along with the flood waters, they found their possessions soaked and mud-caked. Among the damaged goods were electronic products, which they bring to the service shop in hopes that something could be salvaged. Could you help such a customer?

Or could you help yourself? Service businesses and MROs can be forced into bankruptcy if their critical test equipment and instruments are flood damaged—and the insurance is not enough. Economic survival might depend upon knowing how to handle flood-damaged electronic equipment!

Although most flood damage scenarios are not as dramatic as this one, we nonetheless hear of electronic equipment that has taken a bath: boating accidents, plumbing failures, and a variety of other problems splash equipment out of service.

The author recalls one incident where a hospital plumber burst a 3.5-inch water pipe that he was repairing (in a nurses' station workroom). Water came pouring out of the pipe at a high rate, causing a massive flood that damaged patient monitoring equipment in the operating room and postanesthesia recovery room on the floor below. After the smirks died over the announcement "All housekeepers STAT to 2 East," a major effort was undertaken to save nearly $50,000 worth of electronic equipment that was freshwater damaged. Fortunately, there are certain things that a skilled technician can do to restore operation.

If the insurance company pays off well enough, then one could go out and buy a new product. But if the insurance company refuses to pay ("sorry . . . wind-driven water damage excluded . . ."), or if there is no insurance, then the you might want to attempt restorative action. Even if the insurance company does pay, customers can often buy the equipment back from them for salvage value. I recall one customer, a doctor, who received $325 for a two-year old marine VHF-FM two-way radio and bought it back from the insurance company for $20. The company sent him a check for $305, and he kept (and paid to restore) the "carcass."

Some of the steps recommended may sound a little bizarre to you from a normal perspective, but are capable of restoring an expensive piece of equipment. Some of the steps might cause a little damage that will also have to be repaired (especially those involving baking the moisture out or using chemicals for cleaning). If that makes you nervous, then please remember that in the case described, you cannot harm the equipment anymore: *it is already a total loss!* Any restoration is therefore pure gain.

Before making any wild promises, however, make sure that the customer understands that you are undertaking heroic measures that may not be successful. One of the most frequently cited causes of bitter customer dissatisfaction is not your poor performance but, rather, *dashed expectations*. If your customer is led to believe that the job will turn out much better than is possible, then he or she will not be in a forgiving mood when you fail to catch the bullet in your teeth. The fact is especially true in medical service where egos are large and memories long. But if the job is a lot better than their expectations, then you will probably hear word-of-mouth "advertising" around town about your ability to walk on (or at least get rid of) water.

The first thing to do is *refrain from turning the equipment on,* even for a brief test to see if it is broken. Satisfy yourself right now that even a short dunk will cause fatal damage! Still the all-too-natural urge is to see if the equipment survived the flood: *if it was immersed in water, then it did not survive!*

The first job is to remove the covers and give the equipment a bath. A shop in a seaport town finds saltwater damage to electronic equipment common. One such shop received an $1800 UHF-FM radio-telephone set (the kind typically used in taxicabs, police cars, fire trucks, and ambulances) that had been immersed the night before during a storm. A saltwater river tributary overflowed its banks just high enough to cover the radio mounted in the equipment well! The first thing the technician did was take the transceiver out on the back parking lot and give it a ten-minute shower with a garden hose. He had lived in that town all his life, and therefore had much experience with water-damaged radio gear. Incidentally, if the damage is due to saltwater, then do the cleaning job immediately. The longer salt residue remains in the equipment, the greater will be the corrosion damage, and the lower the chance of successful restoration.

In some cases it will be necessary to follow the shower with an immersion bath. One technician uses a 25-gallon tub, the kind you might use to bathe a large dog. He mixes together in the tub 2 to 4 quarts of a product like *Lestoil,* a small bottle (2–4 fluid ounces) of either fingernail polish remover or acetone (same chemical), and enough tap water to fill the tub all the way to the rim. Leave the set in the bath for an hour, and then pour out the solution; rinse the tub out thoroughly and refill with plain tap water (some people prefer distilled water, which is available in bottles in some areas). This second bath removes the residue left by the chemicals in the first bath.

Note: This bath may damage some plastics. If this worries you, then use plain soapy water. It isn't quite as effective a solvent, but it works somewhat. Keep in mind that most plastic pieces can be replaced, and the damage will not usually prevent the set from operating: it is already a total loss, so don't worry about trivial secondary damage!

The next step is drying the unit out *thoroughly*. If you live in Arizona (yes, they have floods in the desert!), then simply leave the equipment out in the sun for about a week; everyone else will have to use some other method. The kitchen oven is a good bet, provided that it can be regulated to maintain a temperature of 125 to 130° F. That range is low for a kitchen oven, and some might not be able to remain that cool. Higher temperatures will dry the set out faster, but they will also melt some of the plastics used in it—so beware. The drying process takes several days, perhaps as long as a week.

Another alternative is to build a cardboard (or other material) box and use several hundred watts of incandescent lamps to provide heat. Use a thermometer inside the enclosure to ensure that (1) the 130°F "melt limit" is not exceeded and (2) the box doesn't catch fire from neglect (cardboard burns). Again, up to about a week is needed—although in one case a car radio that was dropped in a freshwater lake for a few minutes dried out in only one day.

Now comes the big test! In some cases, the only way to test the equipment is to turn it on and look for smoke. The more conservative approach sneaks up on it one step at a time. The first step in the test is to disconnect the DC power supply; this step can be absolutely essential to the future health of the set being repaired—especially those with high-voltage (HV) power supplies.

Without connecting the set to AC power, connect a bench power supply to the circuitry that was previously connected to the rig's internal power supply. It is essential that you use a DC power supply that will provide the same voltage as the original internal supply, and additionally (this is important) has a *current limiter* control. The output voltage is set to the DC voltage normally supplied by the rig power supply, and the current limiter control is set for a short-circuit current only a little above the normal operating current of the circuit under test.

Why go to such trouble? The reason is prevention of secondary damage. There is almost inevitably a short circuit or other condition that draws loads of current. If such a condition exists in the equipment, then the internal power supply normally used probably produces enough current to burn up components, printed wiring board tracks, and other components. After the circuit is checked out, then check out the power supply and (if working) reconnect it.

The low-voltage DC power supply should be checked out separately, especially if it uses a series-pass regulator (most equipment does these days). If the voltage regulator circuit is not working, then several possible faults allow the rectifier output to be connected to the regulator output; this occurs when the series-pass transistor is either shorted or hard biased to full turn on. Since the rectifier voltage is always higher than the regulator output voltage, it can damage circuits that were just pronounced healthy.

High-voltage power supplies have special problems all their own. These supplies are common in CRO monitors and electrosurgery equipment. Small amounts of moisture that are no problem in low-voltage supplies will permanently damage an HV supply. The special problem is the HV transformer. If moisture has penetrated the transformer, then the unit may have to be replaced. It may help to provide some extra drying for the transformer, but be prepared to replace it. Figure 25-1A shows a method for drying a power transformer. A 115-volt AC lamp in series with the primary of the HV transformer. The current flow is enough to cause internal heat build up, but not enough to destroy the transformer if it is shorted. If the HV power supply uses a 220-volt AC primary circuit, then place one lamp in series with each AC hot line (see Figure 25-1B).

Some remaining areas of concern (and probable damage) are those components where moisture can get in and remain hidden. Candidates include trimmer ca-

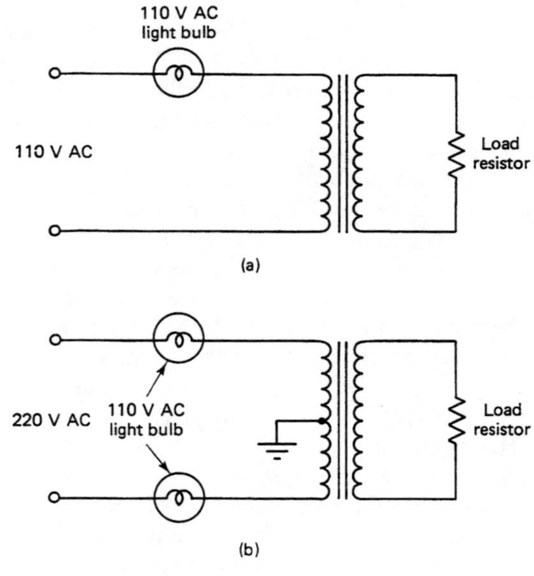

FIGURE 25-1

pacitors, air variable capacitors, IF and RF transformers, switches and potentiometers, paper capacitors, and electrolytic capacitors.

With regard to trimmer capacitors, we can open the capacitor up to the minimum capacity position (screw all the way out) and apply a hair dryer or incandescent lamp for 10 or 15 minutes. Whether or not this step is needed can be determined after the initial power-on test shows a specific problem. Otherwise, you will destroy the alignment of the set for nothing. This step should not, therefore, be used merely as a matter of course—only in response to a specific symptom.

Similarly, air variable capacitors may have corroded contact wipers between the rotor and stator, and this will be apparent when the rig is turned on.

Paper and electrolytic capacitors can absorb water, especially if they have a fiber or cardboard end cap. If the capacitor shows signs of being soggy, then replace it; capacitors are, after all, relatively low-cost items.

If there remains a lot of scum on the printed wiring board, then spray clean it with Freon TF or some similar solvent. Some technicians prefer to use a small paintbrush or "cheese cloth" to help remove the material.

Flood-damaged equipment is often salvageable. The methods described have been used by professional service technicians for a lot of years—and are proven successful.

Recently the author heard from a reader who added some advice of his own. He was a former naval officer who used to have electronics technicians working for him on board a naval ship. He said they used to repair saltwater soaked equipment in an unusual manner. A sailor would take the equipment into the shower, and slosh it down with warm water. They then took the desalinated equipment to the galley (kitchen to landlubbers) and dried it out in the ovens with low heat and good air circulation. The retired officer also advised that distilled water is best, and that tap water in some locations is too hard (i.e., contains minerals); anyone using this method must either buy distilled water or use an in-line water softener.

For a chassis covered with oily dirt, the equipment can be cleaned with a mixture of 8–10 oz of household ammonia, 4–6 oz of a cleaner such as Mr. Clean or Lysol, 4–6 oz of acetone (the ingredient in some fingernail polish removers), and enough distilled (or soft) water to make 1 gallon of solution. The equipment is dunked into this mess. For larger equipments, proportionally larger amounts can be used. An old dental "Water Pik" can be used to hose off equipment that is too large to dunk. The equipment is then burned dry in an oven set to 140 to 150°F (as noted earlier, some plastics used in electronic equipment will melt at temperatures over 130°F, so beware) for 4–5 hours. All lubricants in switches, potentiometers, and air variable capacitors (where used) must be replaced after this treatment.

The black asphaltlike paste that oozes out of overheated transformers can be easily removed from chassis by using either freeze spray or a blast from a CO_2 fire extinguisher (use an underpressure one that already needs refilling; don't waste your protection on cleaning jobs). The frozen paste becomes brittle and can be flaked off using a dental tool or soldering aid tool.

Warning: Mixing other cleaners with Chlorox or other hypochlorite-containing liquids can release poisonous chlorine gas. Only do this job in a well-ventilated area or outdoors.

26

What Test Equipment and Tools Are Needed?

If you don't have a certain minimum set of test equipment and a proper kit of tools, then don't even think about attempting the repair of medical equipment. These items are so basic to the proper maintenance of equipment that they cannot be deleted from your plans. It is unfortunate that shortsighted hospital administrators and corporate managers sometimes short-shrift their technical staffs in the matter of test equipment and tools—but somehow never seem to also downscale their expectations of the shop.

TOOLS

Perhaps the first thing you need are the screwdrivers required to remove the covers. Be sure to have the correct size screwdrivers: improper size screwdrivers will tear up both the screw head and the screwdriver—or pop out of the screwhead and either scratch the cabinet paint job or cause other (more serious) damage.

Some medical equipment is made in Japan. The Phillips screws on many Japanese products have a different bevel angle than on U.S.-made Phillips screws. As a result, U.S.-made tools turn improperly inside the screw slots, and tear up the screw. This is a case where cheap imported screwdrivers work better than classy $4 U.S.-made models.

You will also want to have a couple of soldering devices on hand. For light work and printed circuit board (PCB) repairs use a 25-watt to 75-watt pencil iron; larger jobs require a 250-watt soldering gun.

Solder and desoldering aids are every bit as important as the soldering iron you select. The only type of solder to use is *resin core* solder marked for radio-TV or electronic use. Many experienced hands will smirk that this advice is a useless restatement of the obvious, but it is necessary nonetheless: every shop occasionally sees a set that is ruined from the use of the wrong solder. Do not use any solder such as acid core solder, plumber's solder, or "industrial solder." All those products use an acid core that will corrode your equipment into the junkyard! So remember, use only resin core solder marked for radio, TV, or electronic uses. Most professional technicians prefer either Kester or Ersin Multicore brands in either 50/50 or 60/40 lead/tin mixtures. In hospitals, where different trades work together (sometimes in the same department), sharing supplies is common. But don't let the plumber and the electronics technician share solder! Even electricians sometimes use acid core solder, so don't make a bad mistake in the electronics shop!

Solder size (or gauge) is also important. For light work on things like IC pins or other PCB points, use #22, #24, or even #26 solder. Larger work might require #14 to #20 size solder. Some shops keep rolls of #14, #18, and #24 solder on hand. Solder isn't cheap ($8/lb to $24/lb), by the way, so learn to use it sparingly.

Desoldering is a workbench skill that is just as important as soldering—but is all too often ignored in servicing circles. There are several aids available for desoldering, especially on printed wiring boards: desoldering tips, solder suckers, and solder wick.

Desoldering Tips These devices are special soldering iron (or gun) tips that are shaped like the pin pattern for the device being desoldered. For example, there are tips that fit over all 14 or 16 pins of a DIP integrated circuit. The tip is chucked up in Weller (or equivalent) soldering gun so that all pins can be heated simultatneously.

Solder Suckers These devices are vacuum tools that, when used in conjunction with a soldering iron, will suck melted solder off a joint. Really fancy (high-cost) systems are available that use a vacuum pump and a pneumatic plumbing system that is an integral part of the soldering iron. Such tools are for the largest commercial maintainance shops and industrial users. Smaller shops can get away with less fancy solder suckers.

There are at least two types of practical low-cost solder suckers. One type is a rubber squeeze ball with a nylon or Teflon desoldering nozzle. The squeeze ball is like those little ear irrigating syringes consumers can buy at the drugstore (not the medical variety).

The other type of solder sucker is a spring-powered piston device. The operator cocks it by engaging the spring, places the tip against the molten joint, and presses the spring release trigger: the solder zips up into the tool, leaving a cleaned joint. If you buy one of these devices, then also buy a spare tip. When tips wear out, they tend to splash solder around the PCB a little bit. A small file or penknife does wonders in repairing worn-out tips, but a spare tip is nice to have on hand.

A small collection of other handtools is also necessary. You should have a small pair of diagonal sidecutters, small long-nose pliers, midsize long-nose pliers, wire strippers, several sizes of nut-drivers, and some alignment tools suitable for the type of equipment that you own.

With that last comment the author feels compelled to issue a stern warning—please heed it: *Alignment or harmonization adjustments are never used in troubleshooting!* The mark of a neophyte servicer is the use of the "diddle stick" in troubleshooting. So-called alignment problems typically occur over a very long period, not suddenly. When alignment shifts suddenly it isn't an "alignment problem" at all, but rather a component failure. Alignment causes a certain amount of wear and tear trauma, so constant tweaking will put on more faults than it removes.

You might also want to lay in a small supply of certain service chemicals. Repair and maintenance jobs sometimes require cleaning of switches and potentiometers, so a spray can of cleaner (e.g., Blue Stuff) is handy. You will also need a small tube of either silicone grease or white grease (e.g., Lubriplate), some heat-transfer grease for power transistors, and a freeze spray for locating intermittents. For that really professional touch on equipment with PCBs, buy a bottle of PCB cleaner designed to remove solder resins. Cleaning cabinets can be done with special (expensive) cleaners, but moderate amounts of soapy water on soft sponges or cloths also works (and costs less).

SHOP MANUALS ARE TOOLS TOO!

Order the shop manuals for your equipment. Most units come with a manual that is fine for operating the set, and may even contain a schematic diagram, but is not much good for troubleshooting. The really nice shop manual must be purchased separately in most cases. One some units, a postcard or order form is packed with the unit's documentation to make ordering easier. In other cases, you will have to write to the manufacturer or importer and ask about the availability of the manual.

Also consider buying service aids such as PCB card extenders (allows you to operate a PCB out of the rig for troubleshooting), patch cords, and other things the company offers to professional servicers. It is good management practice to include a statement on all equipment purchase orders requiring manuals and service aids (if used) be included in the price of the equipment—and deliverable before payment for the entire system is made. Retaining the service information (or charging an obscene price for it) is a shabby trick used by some unscrupulous vendors to keep the service in their own hands and at high cost. While some equipment should be serviced by the manufacturer, that is not the case with most medical equipment.

TEST EQUIPMENT

Test equipment is used to measure, troubleshoot, and verify the performance of medical equipment. There are several different types of test equipment needed in the medical maintenance shop. Some of these are common equipment used in all such shops. Other items are high-precision versions of common equipment, and are used for special purposes. Still other items of test equipment are specialty items used only in the medical equipment maintenance shop. In the balance of this chapter we will take a look at some of the various types of equipment likely to be needed.

SELECTING AND USING A MULTIMETER

Everyone involved in electronics eventually looks at the many multimeters that are now on the market. Instruments that cost an arm and a leg only a half-decade ago are now reasonably priced. Even shops on a relatively low budget now own instruments with accuracies and capabilities that existed only in engineering laboratories—or not at all—only a few years ago.

These instruments are more than an aid in troubleshooting—they can be your right arm. A multimeter is a combination instrument that offers several meters in one: DC voltmeter, AC voltmeter, and ohmmeter (plus other functions on certain premium instruments). We are going to talk about the various instruments currently on the market, and what you should look for when selecting a model. Be careful, however, to survey the entire market when making a purchase decision, because capabilities change rapidly.

TYPES OF MULTIMETER

Over the years several different forms of meter have developed. Further, there is more than one way to classify meters. For example, we could classify them by their active elements: none (as in the classical VOM), vacuum tubes, FET, and so forth. We could also classify them according to the display mechanism: analog or digital. The analog meter uses a regular pointer-type meter movement based on either the D'Arsonval or Taut-Band designs (there are others, but are used rarely—if ever—in multimeters). The scale of the analog meter is printed on the panel behind the movable pointer. The digital meter uses digital circuit techniques to make the measurement and displays the result on digital numerical readouts (either LED or LCD).

Figure 26-1 shows a modern example of perhaps the oldest form of multimeter: the volt-ohm-milliammeter, or "VOM." This instrument is based on an analog meter movement, and has switch selectable ranges for DC volts, AC volts, DC milliamperes, and resistance (ohms). Classical VOMs do not contain any active devices, and don't require any power at all except for a single battery for the resistance scale. The sensitivity of the meter is a determining factor when purchasing such an instrument. The sensitivity figure is a measure of the voltmeter input impedance, and tells something about the load the meter places on the circuit being tested. In the case of Figure 26-1, the sensitivity is 20,000 ohms/volt. Multiply the full-scale voltage on any given range by the sensitivity to find the input impedance. For example, when the 50-volt scale is selected, the input impedance is (50 V × 20,000 ohms/V), or 1,000,000 ohms.

The disadvantage of the VOM is that it usually loads down modern solid-state

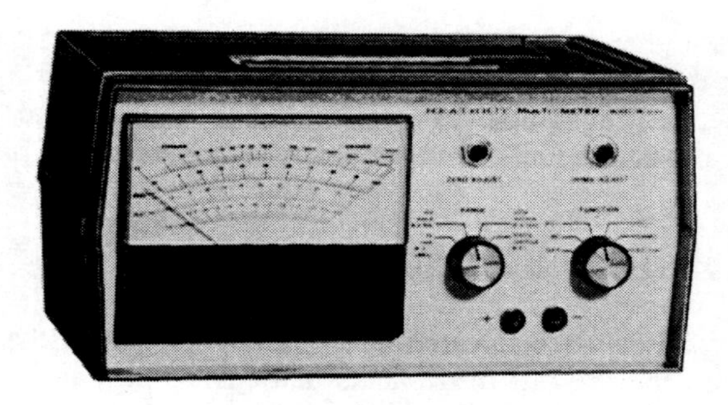

FIGURE 26-1

circuits too much for practical use. In vacuum tube circuits the meter worked well most of the time, but in solid-state circuits there are often problems. For example, when measuring the base voltage of an NPN common-emitter transistor amplifier (Figure 26-2) we expect to find a base-emitter voltage of 0.2–0.3 for germanium and 0.6–0.7 for silicon transistors. So, using the 1.5-volt DC scale, we know that the input impedance of the meter is (1.5 V × 20,000 ohms/V), or 30,000 ohms. Unfortunately, this resistance is of the same order of magnitude as bias resistances in many transistor circuits, so the application of the meter probes changes the bias conditions—and renders the measurement invalid.

The advantage of the VOM is that it is truly a "minimum hassle" instrument to keep, store, and use. In addition, it is very portable, and many models are reasonably tough. These factors make the VOM popular with people who work for long periods in remote areas without the possibility of easy resupply.

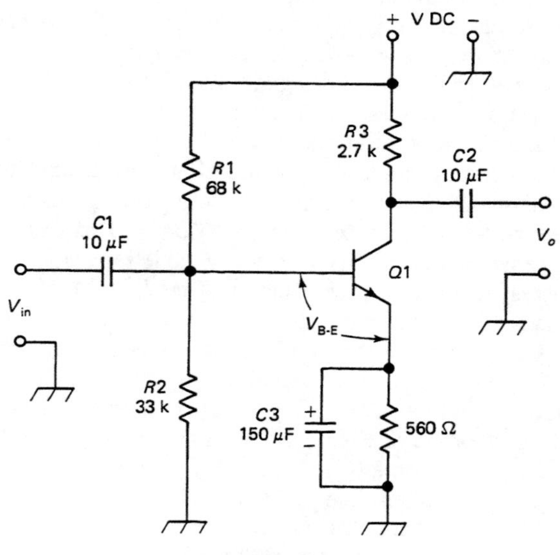

FIGURE 26-2

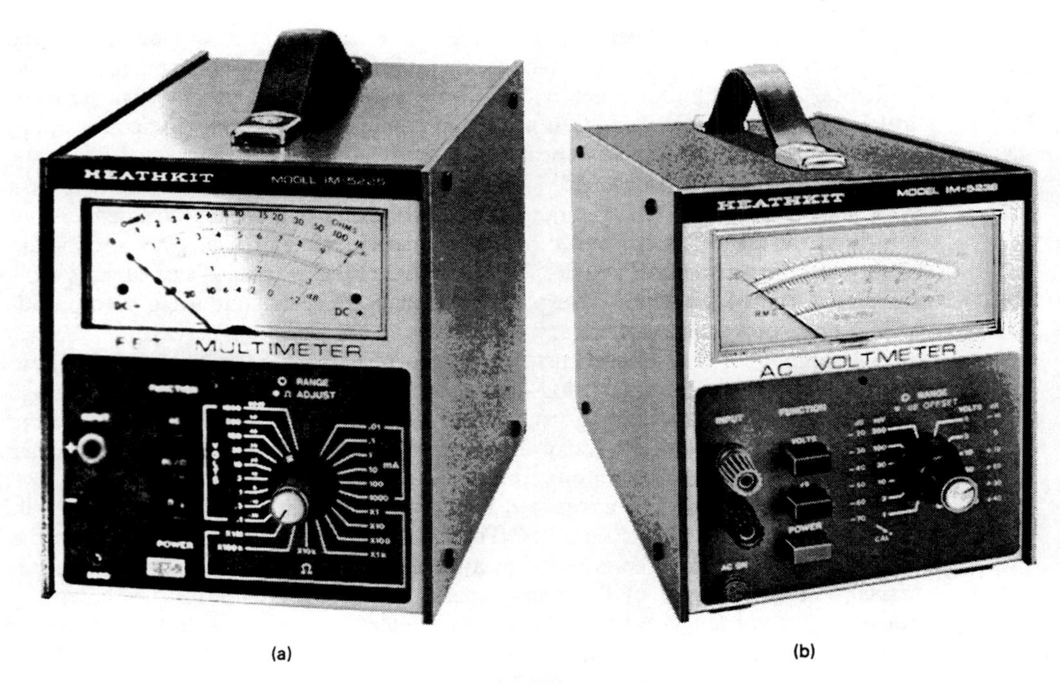

(a)

(b)

FIGURE 26-3

Finally, people who work around electrosurgery machines, some older diathermy machines, radio transmitters, and other high-power RF generators might want to keep a VOM in their toolkit even if they normally use a modern digital instrument. The classical VOM, without any active devices to be misbiased by strong RF fields, will work around electrosurgery machines where other (more expensive) instruments fail.

Figure 26-3A shows another form of multimeter. This type is representative of a larger class of electronic voltmeters and is a field effect transistor (FET) multimeter (FETVM or FETMM). Previous members of the class include vacuum tube voltmeters (VTVM) and transistor voltmeters (TVM). These devices are collectively sometimes called *electronic voltmeters,* or EVMs. The names for these instruments are derived from the input circuit device: vacuum tube, transistor, or field effect transistor. The purpose of the input amplifier device is to increase the input impedance, thereby reducing the circuit loading. For example, a typical specification for the VTVM is an input impedance of 10 megohms, with an additional 1 megohm in the probe, for a total of 11 megohms. Additionally, there is usually 20 pF to 50 pF of capacitance shunting the input resistance. Modern FETVM and other EVM types sometimes sport input impedances even higher than 11 megohms—100 megohm instruments have been advertised.

Like the VOM, the FETVM is a multirange meter that uses a front-panel switch to select range, although in this case the function (DC volts, AC volts, ohms, etc.), are selected by push-button switches. Unlike the VOM, the FETVM (and all

EVMs) require a DC power supply for the active devices. In most cases today, the DC power supply is battery, although some 115-V AC line-operated models are available. Also unlike the classical VOM, EVM instruments are somewhat sensitive to RF fields so will not work well around high-power RF generators (electrosurgery machines, diathermy, inductive heaters, etc.).

Both the FETVM and VOM have an *AC volts* scale. Even where there is a very-low-range scale on the AC ranges, the AC voltmeter in these instruments is not a substitute for the AC voltmeter required for measurement or alignment of audio circuits and type recorders (Figure 26-3B). The AC scales in these instruments typically have a limited frequency response. While they are accurate when used on 50- to 400-Hz AC power, the accuracy falls off badly as frequency increases.

Examples of digital multimeters are shown in Figures 26-4 and 26-5. These instruments use an internal analog-to-digital converter to convert the input voltage to seven-segment digital display output. These instruments are representative of the majority of multimeters sold today. Like the EVM and VOM, the digital multimeter (DMM) offers DC volts, AC volts, milliamperes, and ohms ranges.

You will see DMM's advertised as $2\frac{1}{2}$ digit, $3\frac{1}{2}$ digit, $4\frac{1}{2}$ digit, and so forth. Care to guess what a "half digit" is? The most significant digit (all the way to the left) can only be 0 or 1, so is billed as a "half-digit." Consider the $3\frac{1}{2}$-digit instruments. The basic range of these instruments is 0 to 999, with 100 percent over-range, for a total range of 0 to 1999 units. The number of digits is a rough measure

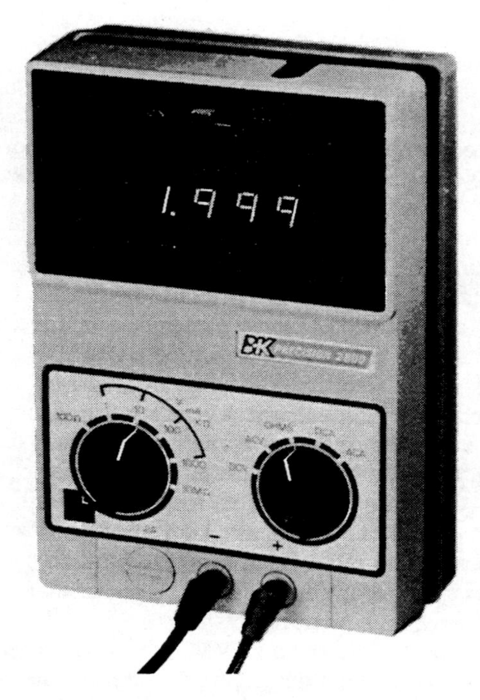

FIGURE 26-4

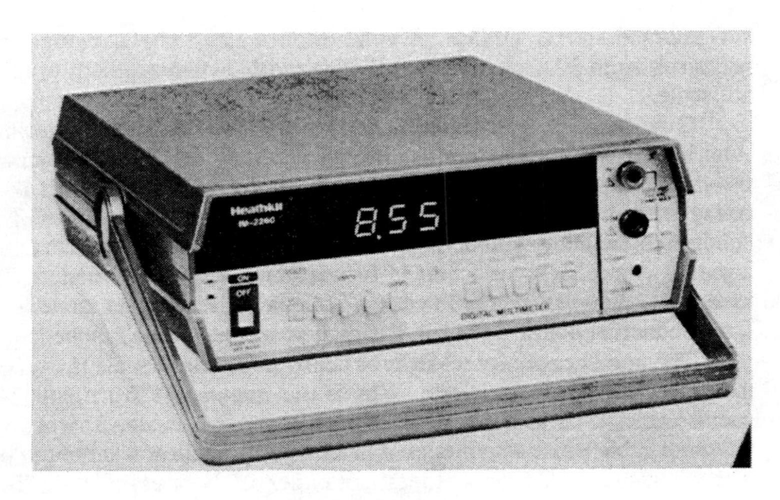

FIGURE 26-5

of precision, although lots of digits is no guarantor of goodness. Generally, most troubleshooting applications require $3\frac{1}{2}$ digits. There are cases where $2\frac{1}{2}$ digits isn't enough, and $4\frac{1}{2}$ digits is more expensive than warranted. Most technicians prefer to have as many digits as possible—dollar for dollar, quality for quality—but with due regard for the realities of measurement making. Only in the most precision cases are more than $4\frac{1}{2}$ digits required.

Does more digits mean more accuracy? In fact, isn't it true that DMMs are inherently more accurate than VOM and other EVM instruments? No! In both cases, the statement is false. The accuracy of the meter depends less on the number of digits than on the internal workings of the instrument. For example, the accuracy of the internal A/D converter voltage reference, and certain other components can affect accuracy. In general, ethical manufacturers don't display more digits then they can support, but the size of the display cannot be taken to be an absolute indicator of quality.

Now regarding the really big heresy: "Whatdya mean my digital DMM isn't necessarily more accurate than your crummy old VOM?!?" While it is true that DMMs have the *potential* for greater initial and long-term accuracy than VOMs, it depends on the implementation, the quality of internal circuits and other factors. There is also the fact the noisy signals tend to be integrated (low-pass filtered) by the inertia of an analog meter pointer, but can fool some DMMs.

As regards matters such as accuracy and resolution, always buy from a reputable source and *read the spec sheet* before committing to the purchase. Also, be wary of overspecing the instrument. When in the market for a troubleshooting instrument don't let the gleam in your eye over the high-priced superaccurate laboratory models reach down as far as your wallet.

Instruments such as those in Figure 26-5 are very much in evidence in any electronic parts store you visit. Various low-priced models are offered that not only make the classical measurements of the VOM, but also certain other things as well.

For example, some DMMs measure capacitance. The capacitance measurement scales run from 2000 picofarads full scale (with 1-pF resolution) to 2000 microfarads full scale.

Other features to look for in DMMs are *diode mode* and *continuity tester* with aural indication. The diode mode is used to test diodes and PN junction bipolar transistors (PNP and NPN). The normal ohmmeter mode in DMMs uses a very-low-voltage source that is too low to forward bias PN junctions. The *diode mode* (usually indicated by a diode symbol on the meter front panel) is a resistance mode but with a higher voltage that is sufficient to forward bias the PN junction. The DMM can be used to measure resistances in circuit while in the low-power mode, and then test the semiconductors out of circuit in the high-power or "diode" mode.

The aural continuity tester is basically a resistance scale that goes "beep" when the probes see a low resistance. Why is this important? Try ringing out a multiconductor cable, such as a computer printer or modem cable, or worse yet, a hospital intercom cable while standing on a ladder. You cannot watch both probe tips and the meter at the same time—at least not either safely or easily. The "beep" of the meter tells you when the connection is made, and its absence warns you of an open circuit.

HOW TO CONNECT METERS INTO CIRCUITS

The ways that meters are connected into the circuit are critical—failure to use them in the correct manner can (and will!) result in catastrophe. Figure 26-6 shows the methods for connecting the various forms of meter. Note that current, voltage, and

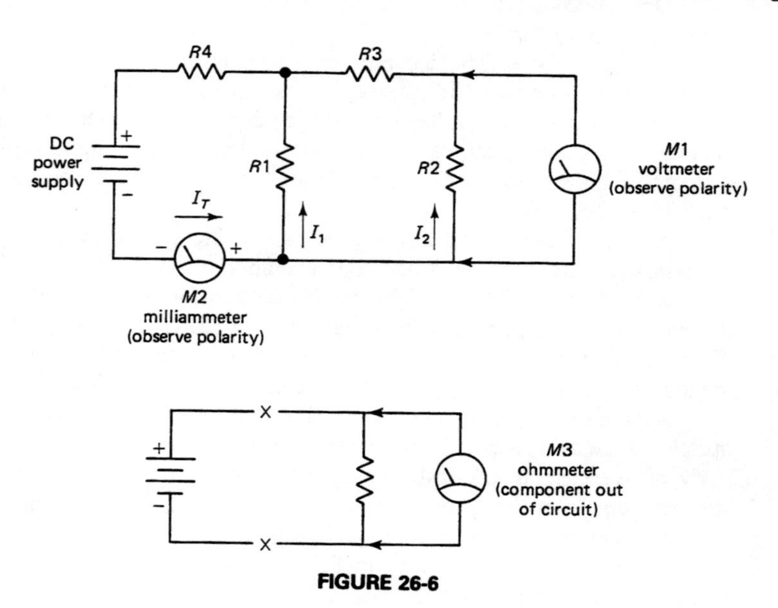

FIGURE 26-6

resistance are measured in different ways. This fact leads to a possibility of damage to multimeters, where the different functions are switch selected. It is all too easy to "misconnect" a multimeter simply by switching ranges without first changing the probes.

There are two rules for connecting meters:

1. Voltmeters are connected in parallel with the load.
2. Current meters are connected in series with the load.

Don't ever violate these rules! The current rule—always connect the ammeter in series, *never* parallel—is especially important. If an ammeter is connected across the load, then its low internal resistance will draw a large current from the power supply of the circuit under test—and that current will be very much larger than the full-scale range of the meter. On an analog meter, the pointer will often bend around the peg and a puff of smoke will waft out from around the edge of the case. The problem is decreased on some digital multimeters (DMM), but is still present. Fortunately, some manufacturers place fuses in series with their multimeter probes.

The rule for ohmmeters is to disconnect the resistance being tested from the circuit, even though the power is turned off. There are two reasons for this procedure. First, there may be parallel alternate paths for current that will cause an erroneously low reading. Second, there may be current stored in capacitors in the circuit, and that current can destroy certain meters. DC power supply filter capacitors are particularly dangerous to your meter. Although you will undoubtedly find even experienced professional electronics workers ignoring this rule, it is a good habit to follow—even if disconnecting components is annoying.

VOLTMETER "ERRORS"

I can recall an electrical engineering professor who could not tell a certain student why the voltages read in a lab experiment were considerably lower than called for in the lab manual. The reason turned out to be loading of the circuit by the voltmeter. A voltmeter has a certain input impedance. For a volt-ohm-milliammeter (VOM) type of instrument, the input impedance can be determined by the *sensitivity* in "ohms per volt." Most good meters have a sensitivity of 20,000 ohms/volt, and some especially fine meters are rated at 100,000 ohms/volt. A lot of very cheap imports have a sensitivity of 1000 ohms/volt, which is very bad. Incidentally, the sensitivity reflects the natural full-scale range of the meter movement used in the VOM. The 20 Kohm/volt uses a 50 μA meter movement, while the 1 Kohm/volt uses a 1-mA meter movement!

Figure 26-7 shows a sample circuit to illustrate graphically the problem of loading. The circuit consists of a 10-volt source, V, and two series-connected resistors R1 and R2. What is the voltage across resistor R2? The correct voltage will be

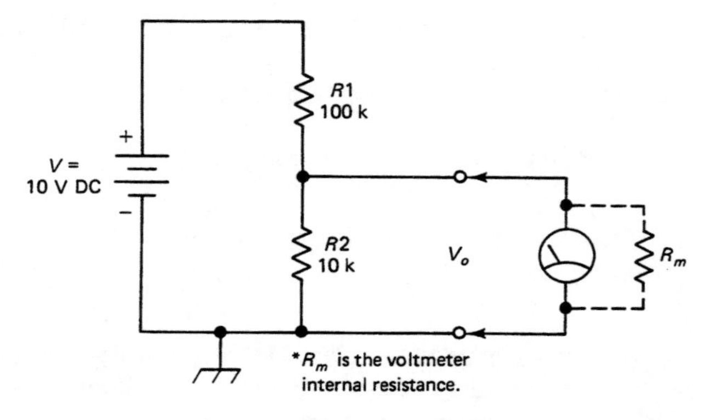

FIGURE 26-7

$$V = \frac{(V)(R2)}{(R1 + R2)}$$

$$= \frac{(10\ V)(10K)}{(100K + 10K)}$$

$$= 0.909 \text{ volts}$$

Now, consider what happens when the voltmeter is connected across resistor R2. The total resistance of this branch of the circuit is now the parallel combination of R2 and the internal resistance of the meter. Consider a 1.5-volt full-scale setting for the meter. At this setting, the 20-Kohm/volt model has an input impedance of 30 Kohms, and the 1-Kohm/volt model has an input impedance of 1.5 Kohms. When connected in parallel with R2 to measure the voltage drop across that resistance, the combination of R2 and the internal resistance results in new values of "R2" of 7.5 Kohms or 1.3 Kohms. These heavily loaded resistances reduce the measured voltage from 0.909 to 0.697 and 0.128 volts, respectively. These are substantial errors and show us the reason for using a voltmeter with a high internal resistance.

HIGH-VOLTAGE PROBES

Most high-voltage meters are ordinary meters with a multiplier resistor or voltage divider network added. Figures 26-8 and 26-9 show two methods for adding high-voltage capability to the standard multimeter. The HV probe of Figure 26-9 is used on those meters that have a specified input impedance of 10 megohms. When the series resistance inside the probe is 990 megohms, the voltmeter will read 1/100 the actual voltage. Thus, a 30,000-volt potential will read 300 volts on the meter. This type of probe is widely available from electronic supply stores, especially those that number a lot of television service technicians among their customers. The techni-

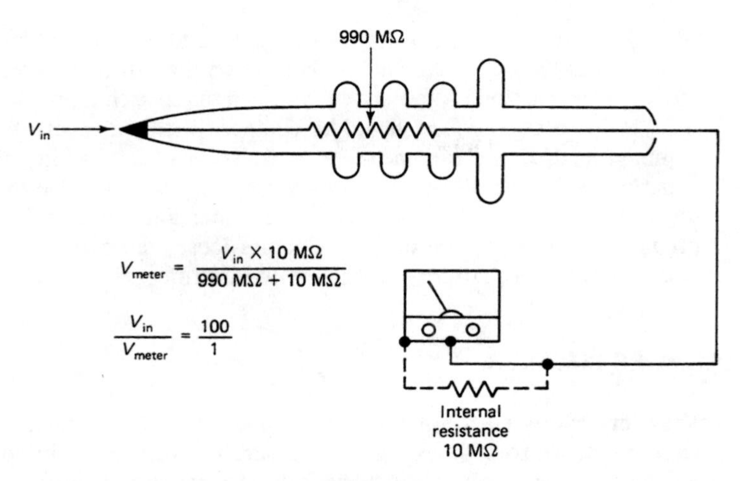

FIGURE 26-8

cians often use these probes ahead of a regular voltmeter for measuring the anode potential of color TV sets.

The basis for the probe of Figure 26-8 is a resistor voltage divider circuit, in which one element is the series resistance and the other is the voltmeter input impedance. These probes require an input impedance of 10 megohms. Modern electronic voltmeters, including FETVMs and DMMs, have input impedances much higher than 10 megohms. For those cases we use a circuit like Figure 26-9. Again,

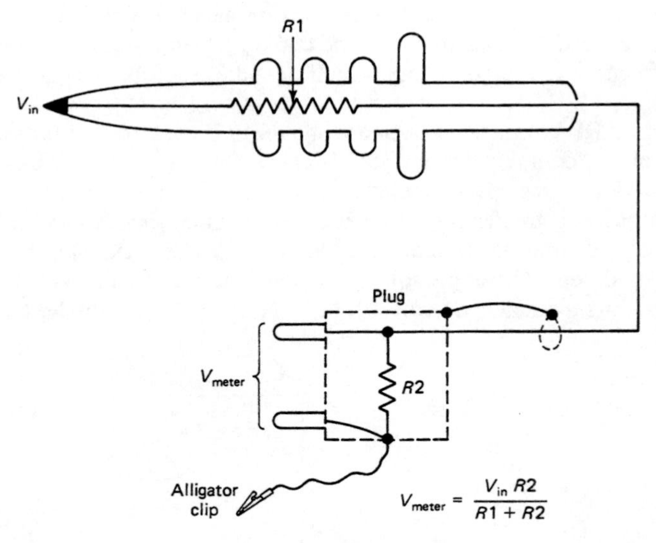

FIGURE 26-9

when you buy an HV probe for your model instrument it is likely to have this circuit in it—in fact, some "universal" probes are on the market that advertise "100 : 1" or "1000 : 1" reduction. Alternatively you can make such a probe yourself.

High-voltage probes should be equipped with a competent alligator clip for the common lead. If you use an ordinary probe, or a poor-quality alligator clip, for the common lead, then all bets are off—you could easily damage the meter. Damage to the meter is especially likely when the meter and the circuit under test are both grounded. When the common lead comes loose, the current from the high-voltage circuit will try to find ground through the instrument.

METERS IN RF CIRCUITS

Very few multimeters are designed to operate in RF circuits. There are two problems. First, we sometimes need to measure DC voltages in the presence of large RF voltages. Second, we might want at least a relative indication of the value of RF voltage present. It is possible to build probes that serve both functions.

The RF blocking probe shown in Figure 26-10 is designed to allow measurement of DC voltages in circuits where RF is likely to be present—such as in an electrosurgery machine. The circuit inside the probe is a low-pass filter consisting of a 2.5-mH RF choke and a 0.01-μF capacitor. This circuit will block enough RF in most cases to permit a reading. If there is still some problem, try two or three sections of the RFC/capacitor circuit to add additional attenuation.

There are problems to be aware of when using the RF blocking probe of Figure 26-10. The most obvious aspect is that the RF choke and the capacitor interact with tuned elements in the circuit, and could thus distort the readings. Another problem is that the RF choke has a resonant frequency which is a result of the inductance and interwinding capacitance of the choke. When using the probe at the natural resonant frequency, the combination will act like a resonant circuit and possibly destroy itself.

RF voltmeter probes are shown in Figure 26-11a thru c. These are sometimes called "demodulator probes" because they will demodulate AM signals. With the diodes shown, it is possible to measure RF potentials up to about 50- or 60-volt peak. For greater potentials use two or more diodes in series. The diodes, incidentally, can be old-fashioned germanium diodes. Although largely supplanted by silicon diodes, there are still many 1N60 diodes used in video detectors in TV receivers. As a result, you can still buy 1N60 equivalents under the universal replacement

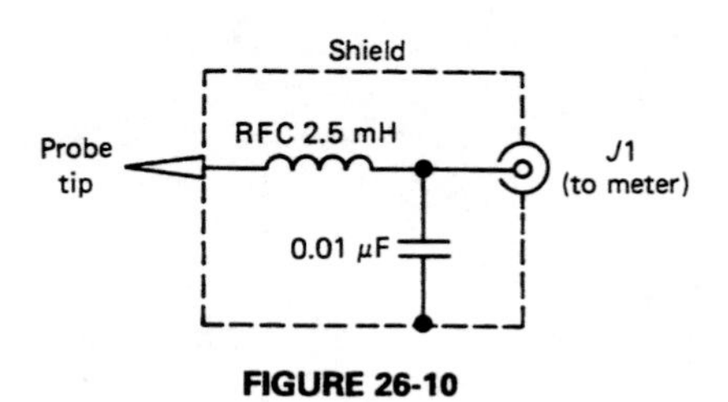

FIGURE 26-10

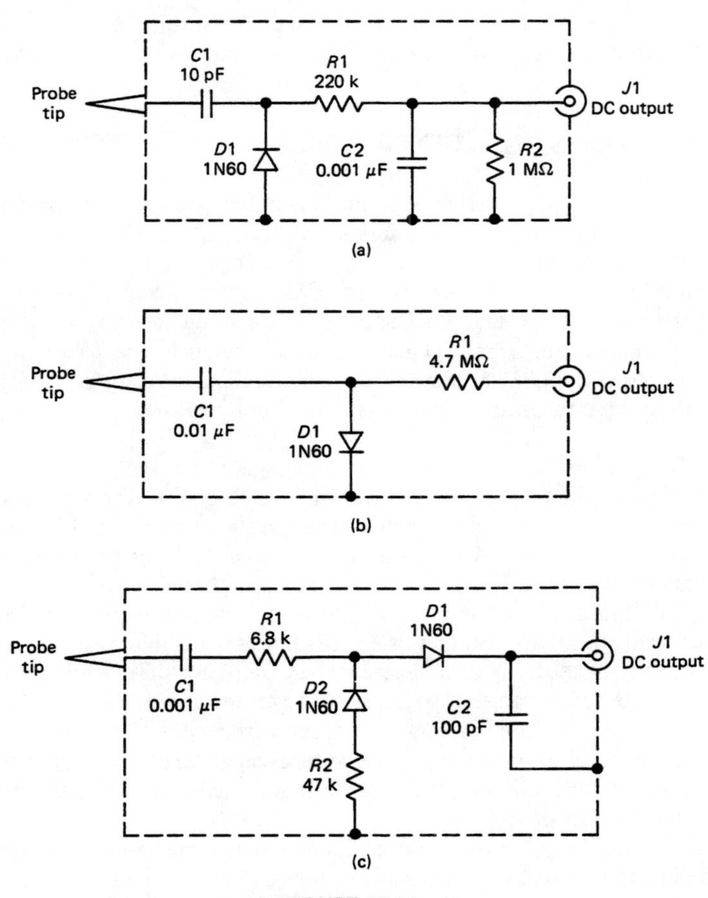

FIGURE 26-11

part numbers (several vendors of replacement semiconductors still offer 1N60 diodes). The germanium diode has a lower junction potential than silicon diodes, so can measure small-signal voltages.

The multimeter is one of the basic instruments that no one with a technical interest in electronics should be without. If you follow the rules given earlier, you will keep your instrument a long time. Some of the other material will allow you to extend the usefulness of the instrument.

SELECTING AND USING SIGNAL GENERATORS

The signal generator is an instrument used to provide a controlled and measured signal to the input of an electronic circuit or device being tested. There are several types of signal generator available, and they range in cost from a few dollars to a few kilodollars. In this section we will examine several different varieties of signal generator and discuss some applications and uses of the instruments.

WHAT KINDS OF SIGNAL GENERATORS?

There is a large variety of signal generators available on the market. Some of them are general-purpose instruments, while others are designed for highly specialized forms of work. Examples of the latter category are the specialized signal generators used to service, evaluate, or align FM stereo radio or TV receivers, video generators intended for TV and VCR service, and special medical signal generators. One way of categorizing signal generators is according to the following breakdown: *audio, function,* and *RF*. While these categories are overlapping and somewhat indistinct, they serve to differentiate the field for our purposes.

Audio generators. An audio generator will, as its name implies, produce signals in some part of the audio range. To qualify for the audio category the signal generator must output signals at least in the audio range (20 to 20,000 hertz). Most such generators sold today, however, are capable of producing signals at higher frequencies (typically 100- or 200-KHz upper limit).

Figure 26-12 shows two forms of common audio signal generator. The model shown in Figure 26-12A is a continuously tunable version. The exact output frequency is set by a variable-frequency oscillator dial, while a bandswitch selects the general output range. The version shown in Figure 26-12B is a step-variable model. This type of signal generator outputs a frequency that is set by a series of switches that control an internal RC (resistance-capacitance) oscillator circuit. The *multiplier* control is usually the capacitor in the RC oscillator, while the decade controls (100s, 10s, 1s) are the resistors.

Although some audio oscillators will output only sine waves, others (perhaps most today) will output both sine waves and square waves. Figure 26-13 shows several methods by which the waveforms are generated. In Figure 26-13A is a hetero-

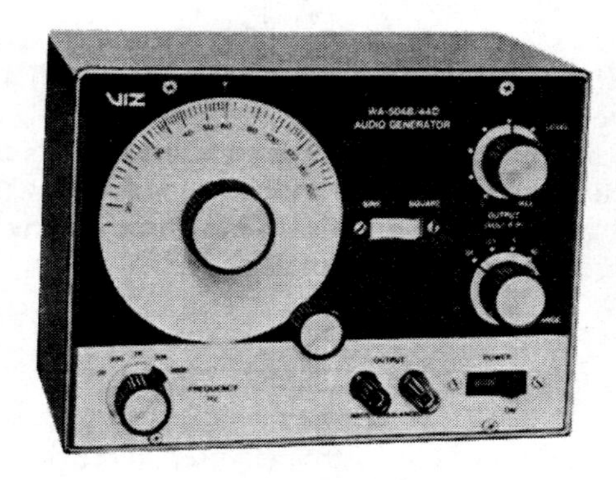

FIGURE 26-12

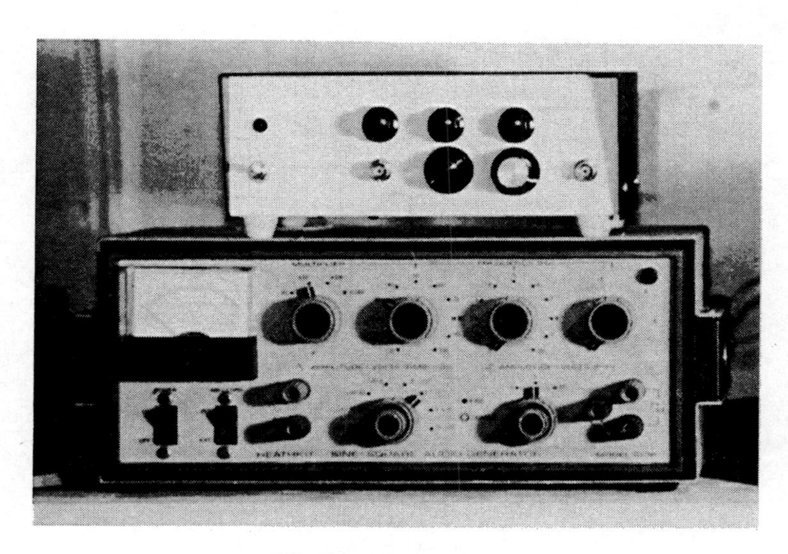

FIGURE 26-12 (continued)

dyne method that is used in some models to generate audio range signals. A fixed oscillator will operate on a single frequency in the vicinity of 100 KHz, while a variable-frequency oscillator operates over either 80–100 KHz or 100–120 KHz. The main tuning knob of the signal generator controls the variable oscillator. This method is typically used for continuously variable audio signal generators because it is difficult to achieve wide-range oscillator circuits at low cost.

The outputs of the fixed oscillator and the VFO are combined in a mixer circuit that produces both sum and difference signals. A low-pass filter selects only the difference signal. When the fixed oscillator is 100 KHz, and the VFO operates over 100–120 KHz, then the output of the low-pass filter will be 0–20 KHz. In actual practice, the dial calibration will be 20 Hz to 20 KHz.

The output of the sine wave generator can be converted to a square wave by any of several circuits. Perhaps the most common method uses a comparator (see Figure 26-13B) to make the conversion. The comparator shown here is ground referenced, so has a zero output only when the input sine wave is crossing the zero volts point. When the input sine wave is positive, then the output of the comparator is at $-V$, while a negative sine wave input produces a $+V$ output potential. Thus, the output of the comparator snaps back and forth from $+V$ to $-V$ as the sine wave input signal oscillates.

Most step-type signal generators (Figure 26-12B) use a square wave oscillator as the master signal source. These circuits offer two advantages. First, they produce a stable output amplitude (while sine wave oscillators produce an ouput that varies with frequency). Second, it is relatively easy to construct a multioctave square wave signal source from RC components. Sine wave oscillators often require a lot of attention to circuit detail in order to produce even a single octave of output frequencies. To convert the square wave to a sine wave a sharp roll-off low-pass filter is pro-

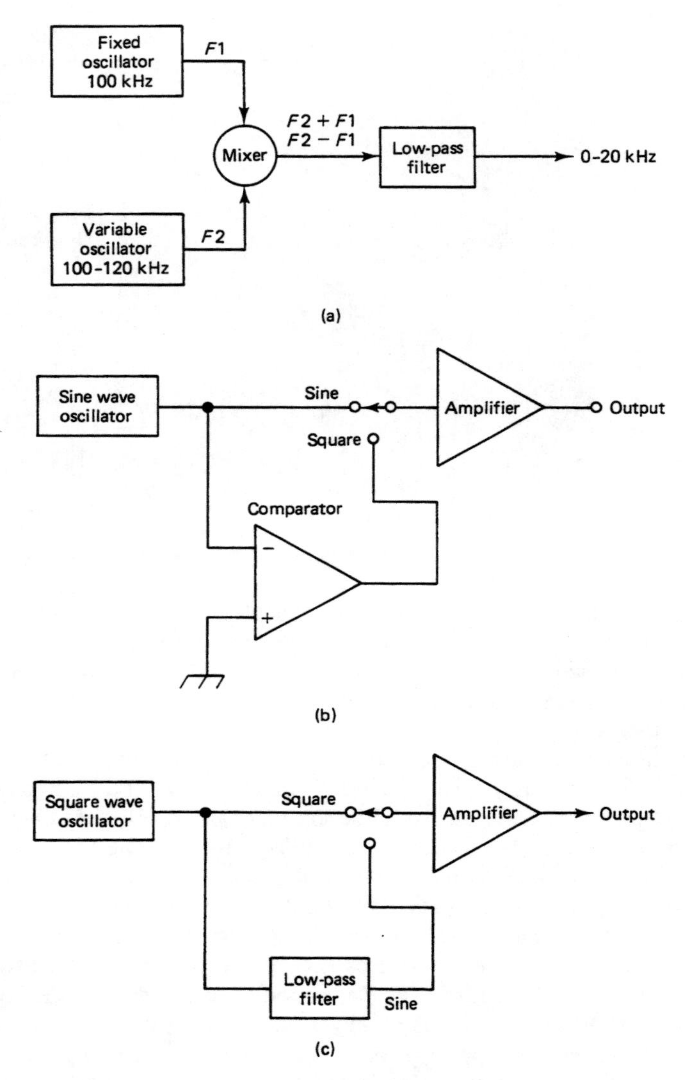

FIGURE 26-13

vided at the output of the square wave generator. The normal frequency spectrum of the square wave includes a fundamental spectral line and a large number of harmonics.

The standard output impedance for audio generators is 600-ohms resistive. Most modern instruments use a pair of binding posts spaced 0.75 inches center to center for the output connectors. Adapters are available to convert this output connector to BNC, RCA phono, or SO-239 fittings if required by some particular application.

Function generators The function generator is a little harder to categorize than the audio and RF generators because it operates over a frequency range that is typically both lower and higher than audio generators. It becomes more confusing because some audio generators operate at the same low frequencies as the function generator, and some function generators operate to 10 or 11 MHz (which is clearly "RF").

A typical function generator is shown in Figure 26-14A. This model produces from less than 1 Hz to 100 KHz and produces sine wave, square wave, and triangle

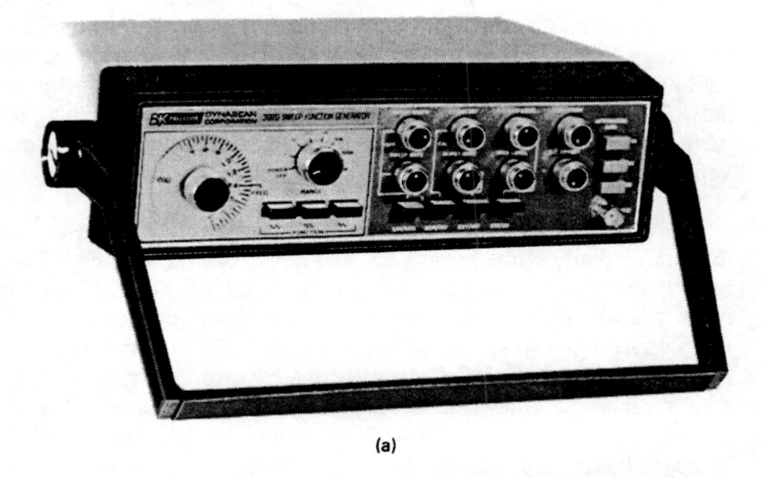

(a)

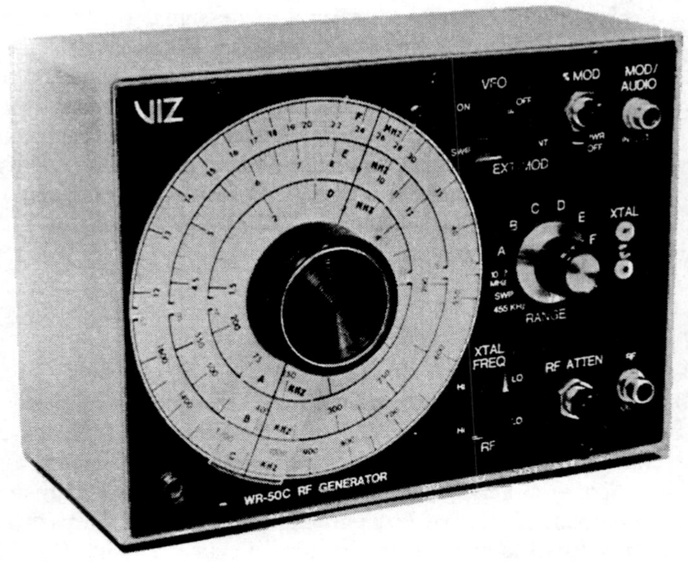

(b)

FIGURE 26-14

wave outputs. The one feature that makes a function generator different from audio generators is the availability of at least three waveforms: sine, square, and triangle. Some function generators also produce pulse outputs.

Another feature to look for on some instruments is the sweep function. The generator shown in Figure 26-14 is a sweep function generator. It will sweep a 10 : 1 to 1000 : 1 frequency range in response to either a sawtooth of DC voltage applied to the appropriate input connector. These instruments are usable for performing frequency response tests on electronic circuits and instruments.

The output of a function generator might have any of several impedance levels, and some have at least three different output impedances. In the model shown in Figure 26-14A, the output impedance is 50 ohms, while many other models offer the audio standard of 600 ohms. Several models on the market offer three different outputs: 50 ohms, 600 ohms, and TTL compatible. The TTL output is always square wave or pulse, and is compatible with TTL digital logic elements (low is 0–0.8 volts, high is 2.3–5.2 volts).

RF generators The RF generator produces RF signals—beyond that it is difficult to really home in on what an "RF signal" is or is not. For example, certain navy radio stations operate in the 10- to 20-KHz region, which some people would quickly label "audio." Other RF signal generators operate in the HF, VHF, UHF, or microwave regions—or all of same! Perhaps the intended use of the instrument is the telling difference: RF devices are intended to deal with or generate electromagnetic radiations, rather than acoustical waves heard in ears. A 12-KHz audio signal can be heard by most people with good hearing, while a 12-KHz RF signal cannot be heard by anyone without the aid of a demodulator or receiver of some sort.

Figure 26-14B shows a service-grade signal generator that operates over the VLF to low-VHF region, including the entire HF spectrum. The intended use of this signal generator is mostly troubleshooting. It can also be used for alignment of noncritical circuits, but is not entirely suitable for the alignment of precision receivers.

The RF output connector on this model is the same kind of binding posts normally associated with audio generators, while most other RF generators will have some form of RF connector (BNC, SO-239, Type-N, etc.). The usual output impedance for RF signal generators is 50 ohms resistive (for TV-only systems, the impedance will be 75 ohms).

OUTPUT ATTENUATORS

One of the principal differences between high-priced signal generators and lower-cost instruments is the controllability of the RF output. In low-cost instruments, the shielding is usually poor, and the output level control is not too effective. A problem with aligning either precision or very sensitive circuits with such a signal generator is the amount of RF that leaks around the shielding and past the attenuator. In this section we will look at some common attenuator circuits (see Figure 26-15).

The simplest and least effective form of output attenuator is the simple potentiometer system shown in Figure 26-15A. In this case, a 50-ohm or 100-ohm poten-

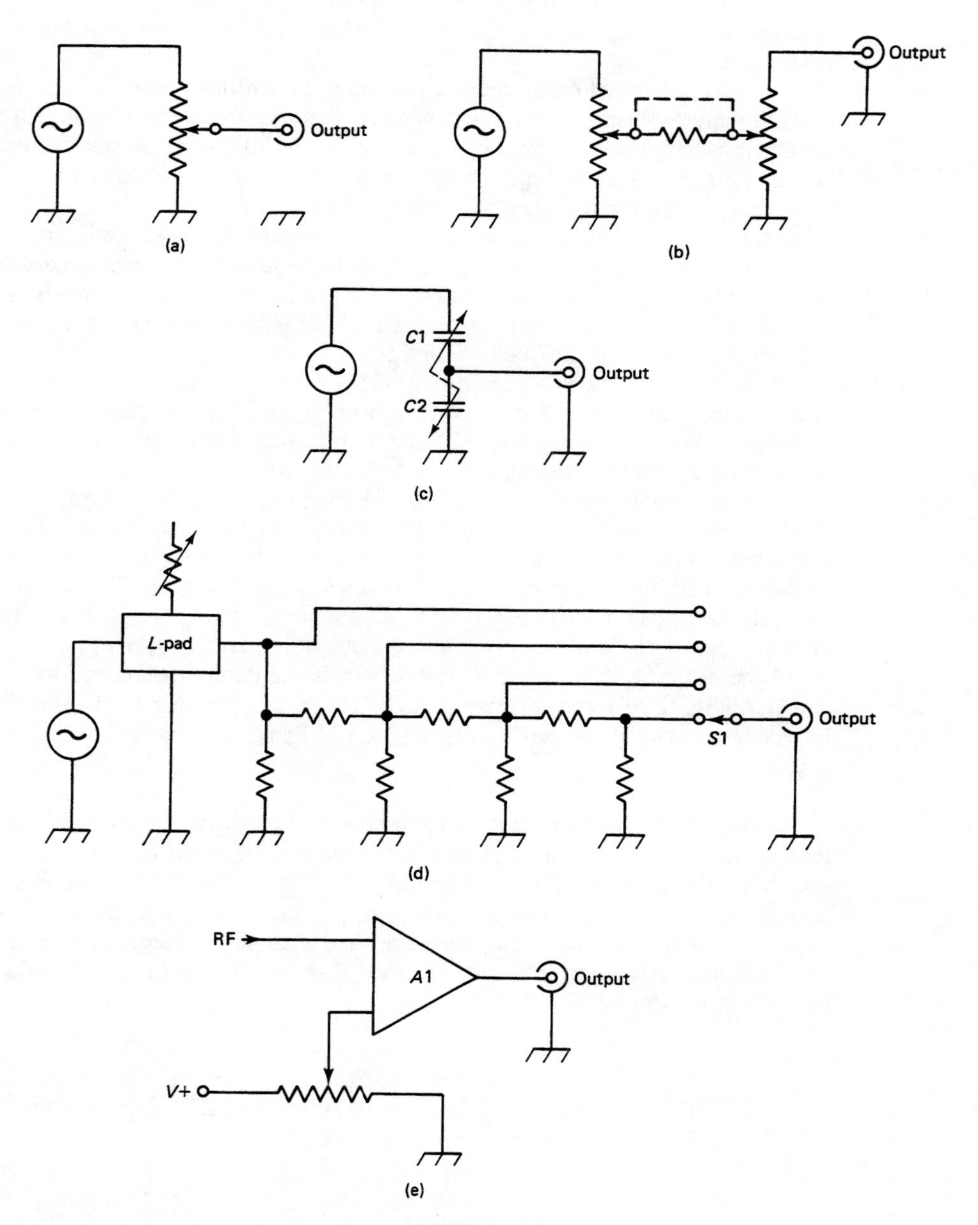
Output
(a)
Output
(b)
C1
Output
C2
(c)
L-pad
Output
S1
(d)
RF
A1
Output
V+
(e)

FIGURE 26-15

tiometer is used as a "volume control" to set the output level. A significant problem with this method is that the output impedance varies with the output level control setting. In addition, there is significant leakage across the potentiometer in most designs.

A method based on an attenuator pad is shown in Figure 26-15B. A pair of potentiometers sharing a common shaft are connected at their respective wiper terminals with a third resistor. In one design the third resistor is also a third potentiometer instead of a fixed resistor (as shown). The output impedance of this method is somewhat less variable than with the method of Figure 26-15A.

An attenuator that is based on a differential variable capacitor is shown in Figure 26-15C. This circuit is the basis for most high-quality RF signal generator output attentuator controls (although most are a little more sophisticated than shown here). This circuit works on the basis of the ratio of capacitive reactances between C1 and C2, which form an AC/RF voltage divider.

The attenuator shown in Figure 26-15D is typically found on audio generators and function generators. A variable ("vernier") control is provided in the form of a variable L-pad attenuator. Step attenuator following the L-pad form the basis for various signal level ranges, as selected by switch S1.

An electronic attenuator is shown in Figure 26-15E. This form of circuit is used in many high-quality instruments. There are two basic forms of electronic attenuator. The one shown in Figure 26-15E uses a gain-controlled wideband amplifier to set the output level. In some cases, a fixed 1- to 3-dB attenuator pad is used at the output to stabilize output impedance at 50 ohms. The DC reference potential set by the potentiometer sets the output level.

The other DC-controlled RF attenuator is the double-balanced modulator circuit normally used for other purposes. By using DC coupling to the diodes, and a DC control voltage as the "local oscillator" signal, a variable attenuator can be made.

Output level indicators There are two methods for metering the output level of a signal generator. The first is to measure the input level to the attenuator and then calibrate the dial relative to this level (Figure 26-16). In these instruments, a calibration mark is provided on the output meter. A vernier control is used to adjust the signal level to match this mark, and then actual output level is read from the calibrated attenuator. The other method (less popular) is to provide an audio (or RF, which is rarer still) voltmeter at the output.

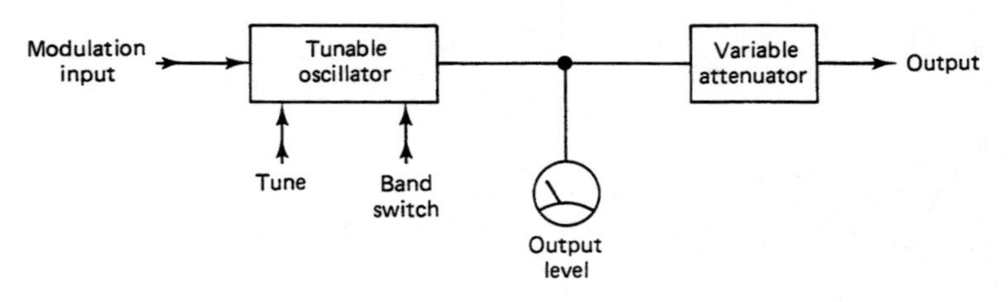

FIGURE 26-16

Output attenuator calibration may be in terms of either voltage or power. For audio generators, the voltage levels will be millivolts, while the power levels are in volume units (VU)—a decibels-based scale. For RF signal generators the output levels are in microvolts or (for power) "dBm" (decibels relative to 1 mW). In both RF and audio cases, the power measurement accuracy of the depends on seeing a fixed output impedance, usually 50 ohms for RF and 600 ohms for audio generators.

APPLICATIONS OF SIGNAL GENERATORS

In this section we will examine a few practical matters in the use of signal generators. Additional information of a more specific nature is given in chapters on troubleshooting types of equipment.

Combining instruments In many measurements it is necessary to combine two or more instruments to form a common signal. For example, in sweep alignment of FM communications receivers, we might want to combine the marker and main RF signals. In most cases, we will want to combine these signals linearly, so will need to use a resistive pad of some sort. Figure 26-17A shows the proper pad for combining two 50-ohm signal generators into one 50-ohm path, while Figure 26-17B shows the pad for three 50-ohm signal generators.

Why isn't the voltage what I set it to? There are several situations that can arise where the results of a measurement tend to indicate that the set output voltage from the signal generator is more or less than what the output control dic-

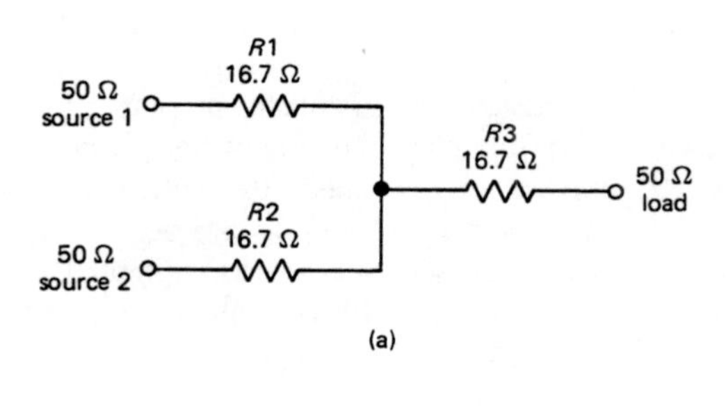

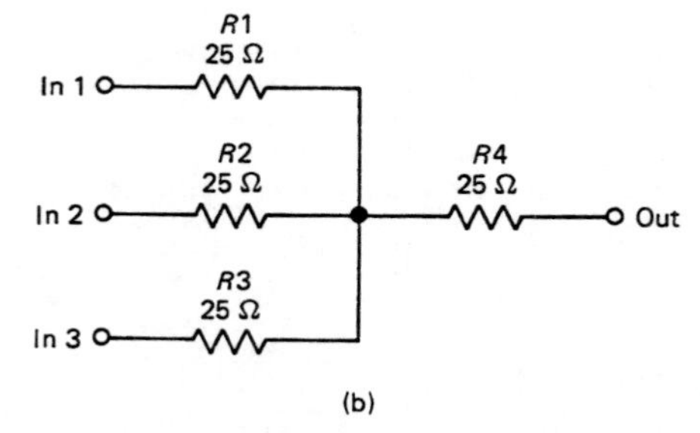

FIGURE 26-17

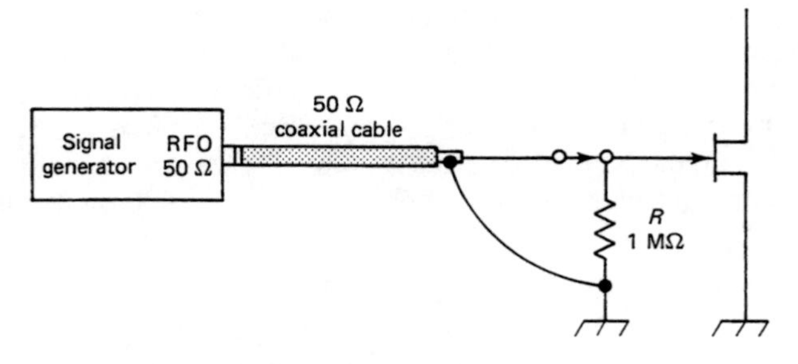

FIGURE 26-18

tates. There are at least two problems that cause these effects (see Figures 26-18 and 26-19).

First, it is possible to develop standing waves on an improperly terminated signal generator output cable. The coaxial cable at the output of the RF signal generator is a transmission line, especially at higher frequencies where its length is an appreciable fraction of a wavelength for the specific operating frequency. Figure 26-18 shows such a situation. Here we have a 50-ohm output signal generator feeding a 50-ohm transmission line, but the output of the transmission line is connected to a high-impedance load. The result of this mismatched transmission line is the same as for any other mismatched transmission line: standing waves. The VSWR of the signal generator line indicates that the measured voltage at specific points will be the algebraic sum of the forward and reflected components and most certainly not the output voltage set by the attenuator on the signal generator. One good "fix" for this problem is to use a fixed attenuator in the 1- to 3-dB range between the end of the cable and the load.

Second, it is possible to mismatch the output impedance of the signal generator. For example, in one class the school bought new function generators and used them for RF experiments because the instrument produced waveforms up to 11 MHz—but the generator had a 600-ohm output impedance (see Figure 26-19 for an equivalent circuit). The attenuator was calibrated assuming a 600-ohm load, not the 50-ohm load called for in the laboratory workbook. The actual output voltage can be found from the ordinary voltage divider equation

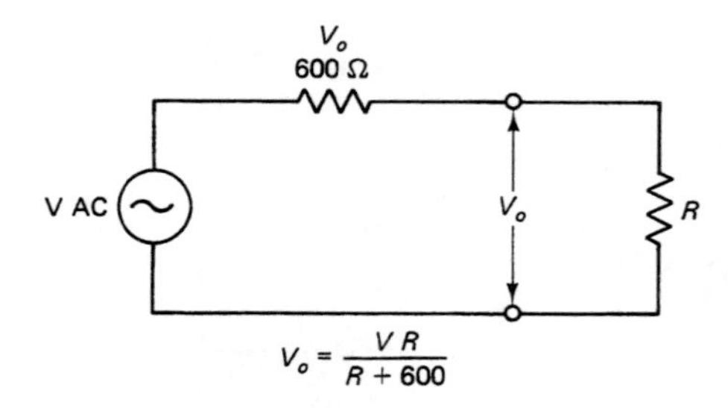

FIGURE 26-19

$$V_o = \frac{V \times R}{R + 600}$$

where

V_o = the actual output voltage
V = the indicated output voltage set on the signal generator
R = the load impedance
600 = the impedance of the signal generator

For our situation, with a 600-ohm signal generator driving a 50-ohm circuit, the output voltage was 50/650 of the indicated voltage.

RF WATTMETERS

A key instrument required in checking the performance of, or troubleshooting, electrosurgery machines and radio communications transmitters is the RF power meter (or "wattmeter") These instruments measure the output power of the transmitter, and display the result in watts, or some related unit. Closely related to RF wattmeters is the antenna VSWR meter. These instruments also examine the output of the transmitter and give a relative indication of output power. They can be calibrated to display the dimensionless units of *voltage standing wave ratio* (VSWR). Many modern instruments, a couple of which will be discussed as examples in this chapter, combine both RF power and VSWR measurement capabilities.

MEASURING RF POWER

Measuring RF power has traditionally been notoriously difficult, except perhaps in the singular case of continuous wave (CW) sources that produce nice, well-behaved sine waves. Even in that limited case, however, some measurement methods are distinctly better than others.

Consider the simplest case: the ordinary unmodulated CW waveform (typical on "CUT" mode in electrosurgery machines). It has a single-frequency spectrum and is easily measured. Suppose, as shown in the example, the peak voltage of the waveform is 100 volts (that is, peak-to-peak 200 volts). Given that the CW waveform is sinusoidal, we know that the RMS voltage is 0.707 times the peak voltage, or 70.7 volts. The output power is related to the RMS voltage across the load by

$$P = \frac{(V_{rms})^2}{Z_o}$$

where

P = the power in watts
V_{rms} = the RMS potential in volts
Z_o = the load impedance in ohms

If we assume a load impedance of 50 ohms, then we can state that the power in our hypothetical waveform is 100 watts.

We can measure power on unmodulated sinusoidal waveforms by measuring either the RMS or peak values of either voltage or current, assuming that a constant value resistance load is present. But the problem becomes more complex on modulated signals.

One of the earliest forms of practical RF power measurement was the thermocouple RF ammeter (see Figure 26-20). This instrument works by dissipating a small amount of power in a small resistance inside the meter and then measuring the heat generated with a thermocouple. A DC current meter monitors the output of the thermocouple device, and indicates the level of current flowing in the heating element. Because it works on the basis of power dissipated heating a resistance, *a thermocouple RF ammeter is inherently an RMS-reading device*. Because of this feature it is very useful for making average power measurements. If we know the RMS current and the resistive component of the load impedance, and if the reactive component is zero or very low, then we can determine RF power from the familiar expression

$$P = I^2 R_i$$

There is, however, a significant problem that keeps thermocouple RF ammeters from being universally used in RF power measurement: those instruments are highly frequency dependent. Even at low frequencies it is recommended that the meters be mounted on insulating material with at least ⅜-inch spacing between the meter and its metal cabinet. Even with that precaution, however, there is a strong frequency dependence that renders the meter less useful at higher frequencies. Some meters are advertised to operate into the low-VHF region, but a note of caution is necessary. That recommendation requires a copy of the calibrated frequency response curve for that specific meter so that a correction factor can be added or subtracted from the reading. At 10 MHz and higher, the readings of the thermocouple RF ammeter must be taken with a certain amount if skepticism unless the original calibration chart is available.

We can also measure RF power by measuring the voltage across the load resistance (see Figure 26-21). In the circuit of Figure 26-21 the RF voltage appearing

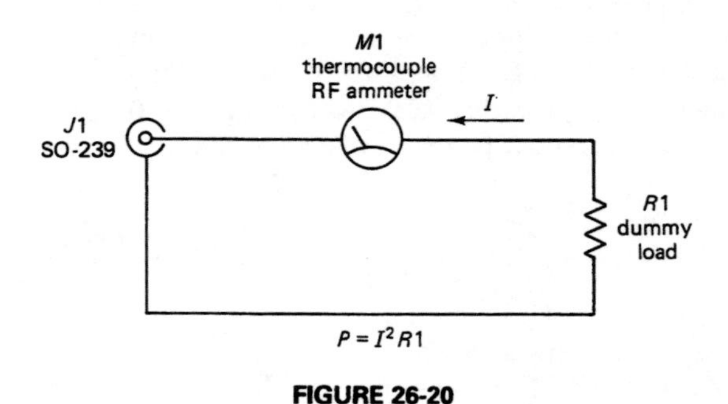

FIGURE 26-20

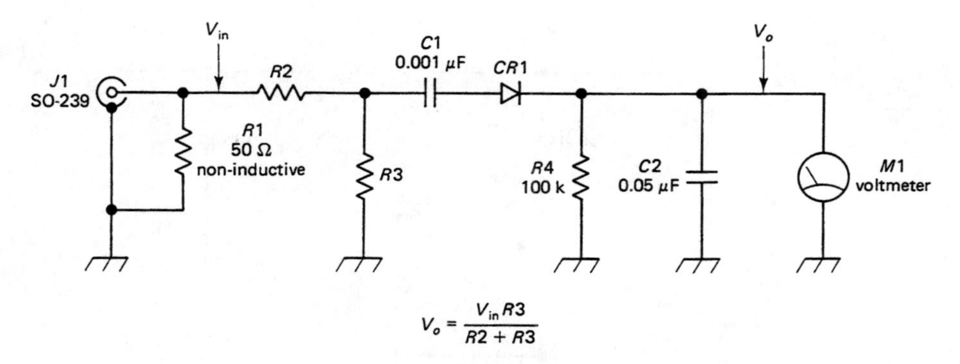

FIGURE 26-21

across the load is scaled downward to a level compatible with the voltmeter by resistor voltage divider R2/R3. The output of this divider is rectified by CR1 and is filtered to DC by the action of capacitor C2.

The method of measuring the voltage in a simple diode voltmeter is valid only if the RF signal is unmodulated and has a sinusoidal waveshape. While these criteria are met in many transmitters, they are not universal. If the voltmeter circuit is peak reading, as in Figure 26-21, then the peak power is

$$P = \frac{V_o^2}{R1}$$

The average power is then found by multiplying the peak power by 0.707. Some meter circuits include voltage dividers that precede the meter and thereby convert the reading to RMS, thus also convert the power to average power. Again, it must be stressed that terms like "RMS," "average," and "peak" have meaning only when the input RF signal is both unmodulated and sinusoidal. Otherwise, the readings are meaningless unless calibrated against some other source.

It is also possible to use various bridge methods for measurement of RF power. In Figure 26-22 we see a bridge set up to measure both forward and reverse power. This circuit was once popular for VSWR meters. There are four elements in this quasi–Wheatstone bridge circuit: R1, R2, R3, and the antenna impedance (connected to the bridge at J2). If R_{ant} is the antenna resistance, then we know that the bridge is in balance (i.e., the null condition) when the ratios R1/R2 and R3/R_{ant} are equal. In an ideal situation resistor R3 will have a resistance equal to R_{ant}, but that may overly limit the usefulness of the bridge. In some cases, therefore, the bridge will use a compromise value such as 68 ohms for R3. Such a resistor will be usable on both 50-ohm and 75-ohm antenna systems with but small error. Typically, these meters are designed to read relative power level rather than the actual power.

An advantage of this type of meter is that we can get an accurate measurement of VSWR by proper calibration. With the switch in the forward position, and RF power applied to J1 ("XMTR") potentiometer R6 is adjusted to produce a full-scale

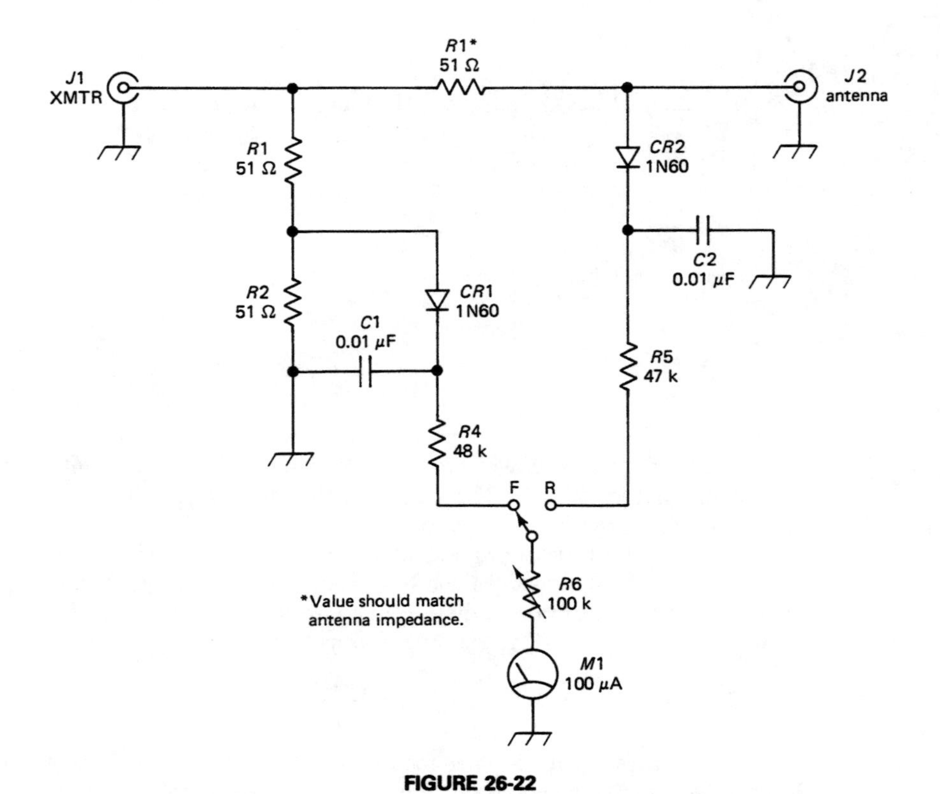

FIGURE 26-22

deflection on meter M1. When the switch is then set to the reverse position, the meter will read reverse power relative to the VSWR. An appropriate "VSWR" scale is provided.

A significant problem with the bridge of Figure 26-22 is that it cannot be left in the circuit while transmitting because it dissipates a considerable amount of RF power in the internal resistances. These meters, during the time when they were popular, were provided with switches that bypassed the bridge when transmitting. The bridge was only in the circuit when making a measurement.

An improved bridge circuit is the capacitor/resistor bridge in Figure 26-23; this circuit is called the "micromatch" bridge. Immediately we see that the micromatch is improved over the conventional bridge because it uses only 1 ohm in series with the line (R_i). This resistor dissipates considerably less power than the 51-ohm resistance used in the previous example. Because of this low-value resistance we can leave the micromatch in the line while transmitting. Recall that the ratios of the bridge arms must be equal for the null condition to occur. In this case, the capacitive reactance ratio of C1/C2 must match the resistance ratio R1/R_{ant}. For a 50-ohm antenna, the ratio is 1/50, and for 75-ohm antennas it is 1/75 (or, for the compromise situation,

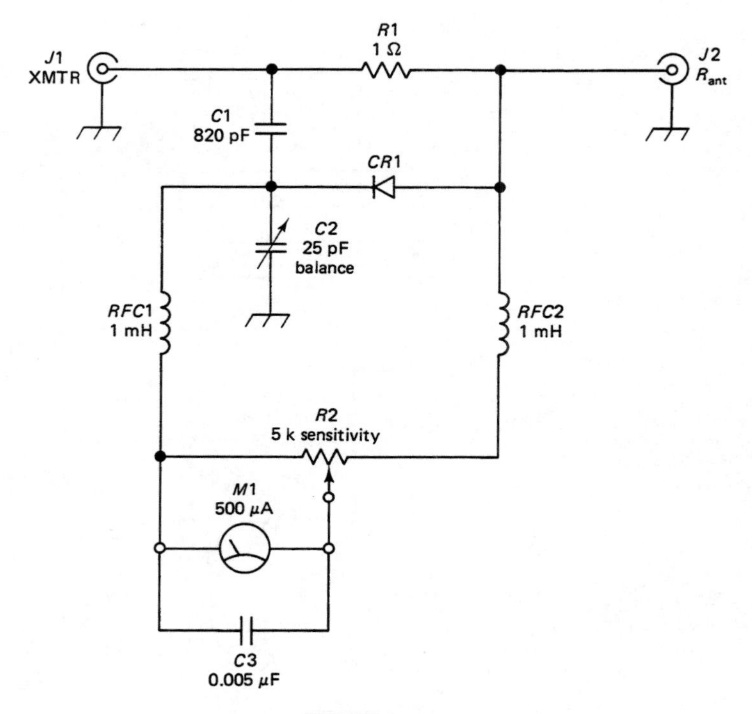

FIGURE 26-23

1/68). The small-value trimmer capacitor (C2) must be adjusted for a reactance ratio with C1 of 1/50, 1/75, or 1/68, depending upon how the bridge is set up.

The sensitivity control can be used to calibrate the meter. In one version of the micromatch, there are three power ranges (10 watts, 100 watts, and 1000 watts). Each range has its own sensitivity control, and these are switched in and out of the circuit as needed.

The monomatch bridge circuit in Figure 26-24 is the instrument of choice for HF and low-VHF applications. In the Monomatch design, the transmission line is segment *B*, while RF sampling elements are formed by segments *A* and *C*. Although the original designs were based on a coaxial cable sensor, later versions used printed circuit foil transmission line segments for *A*, *B*, and *C*.

The sensor unit is basically a directional coupler with a detector element for both forward and reverse directions. For best accuracy diodes CR1 and CR2 should be matched, as should R1 and R2. The resistance of R1 and R2 should match the transmission line surge impedance, although in many instruments a 68-ohm compromise resistance is used.

The particular circuit shown in Figure 26-25 uses a single DC meter movement to monitor the output power. With the addition of potentiometer R5 and switch

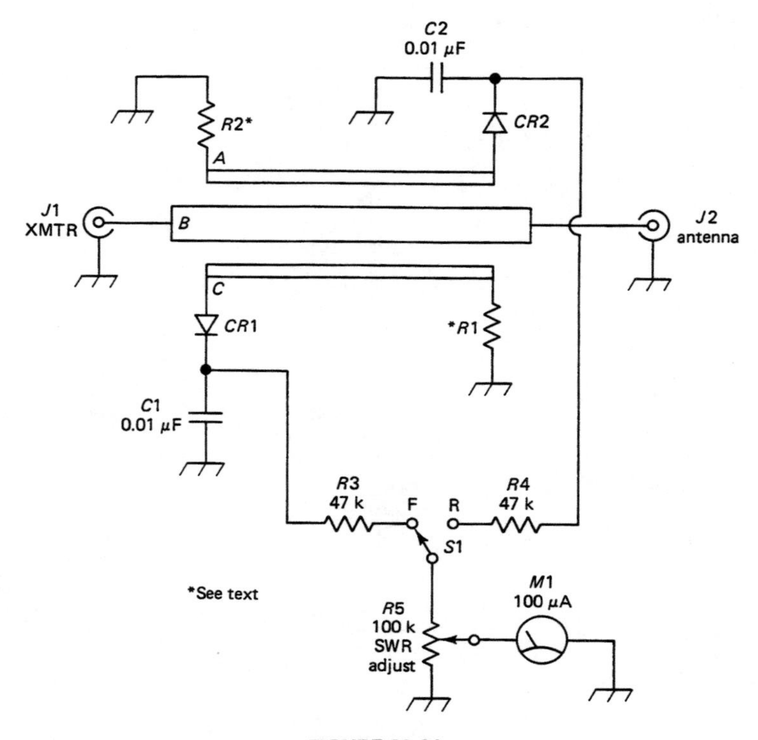

FIGURE 26-24

S1 the circuit becomes a VSWR bridge. Many modern designs use two meters (one each for forward and reverse power).

One of the latest designs in VSWR meter sensors is the current transformer assembly shown in Figure 26-25. This circuit is the basis of many common instruments, and was featured in a *Journal of Clinical Engineering* article by the author in the late 1970s. In this instrument a single-turn ferrite toroid transformer is used as the directional sensor. The transmission line passing through the hole in the toroid "doughnut" forms the primary winding of a broadband RF transformer. The secondary, which consists of 10 to 40 turns of small enamel wire, is connected to a measurement bridge circuit (C1 + C2 + load) with a rectified DC output.

The Bird Model 43 Thruline[R] RF wattmeter shown in Figure 26-26 has for years been one of the industry standards in communications service work. Although it is slightly more expensive that lesser instruments, it is also versatile, and is accurate and rugged. The Thruline meter can be inserted into the transmission line of an antenna system with so little loss that it may be left permanently in the line during normal operations. The Model 43 Thruline is popular with landmobile and marine radio technicians.

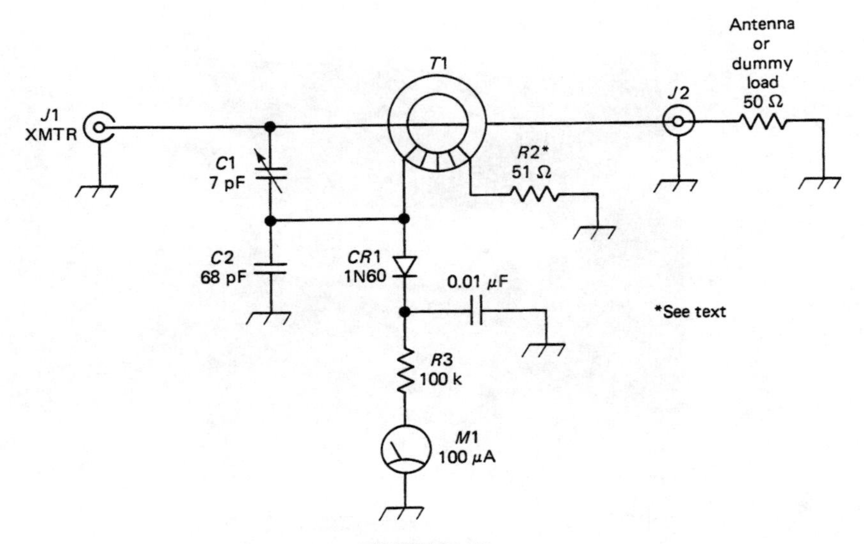

FIGURE 26-25

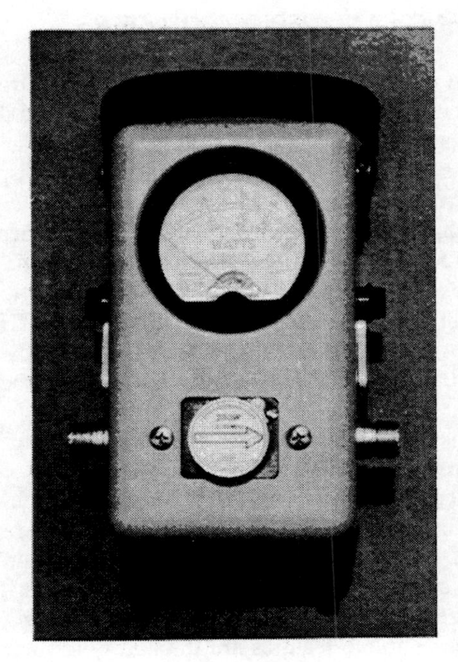

FIGURE 26-26

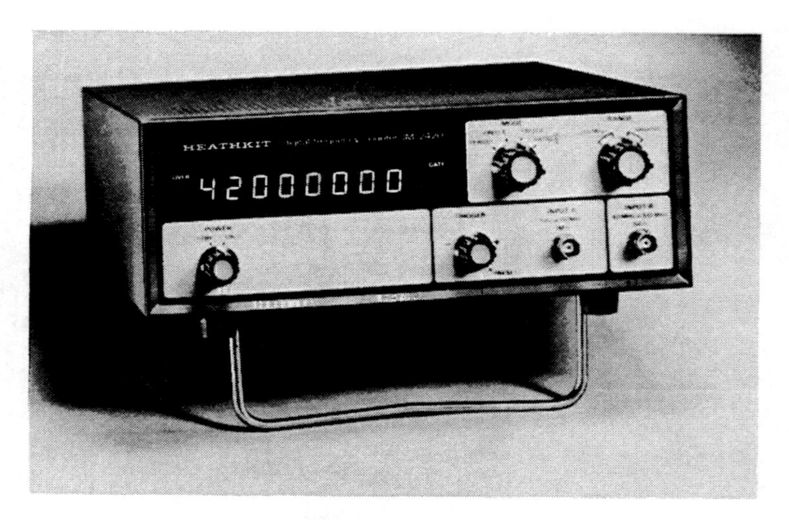

FIGURE 26-27

DIGITAL FREQUENCY AND PERIOD COUNTERS

The digital frequency meter, also called a digital frequency counter, is a device that counts the cycles of an input signal one by one and displays the result as a frequency. The counter is actually an events counter, but because the counter module is allowed to receive signals only through a timed gate, the display is actually events per unit of time or frequency. Figure 26-27 shows a basic digital counter, the Heath/Zenith IM2420, that is suitable for much medical equipment service.

Features to look for on a service shop–grade counter is a frequency counter that works from low audio to well into the RF region. On the high end, the telemetry units in the cardiac care area, or the 900-MHz "ultrasonic" (they are reallly microwave) diathermies will set the upper frequency limit. Very desirable on the unit that you obtain is a variable trigger control, and both 50-ohm and high-impedance inputs.

The selected counter should also offer the ability to measure period. Because period is merely a measure of the time required for each cycle to pass, it is the reciprocal of frequency. It is thus easy to measure with the same digital circuits as frequency. You might want the counter to measure period from microseconds to 10 seconds or so. The period counter is used in adjusting a number of different circuits, and can also be used to indirectly measure the frequency ($F = 1/t$) of the very-low-frequency signals encountered in medical electronics.

Other desirable features are the ability to measure the ratio of two frequencies and the ability to count events (rather than either period or frequency).

OSCILLOSCOPES

The oscilloscope is the single most valuable instrument in the service shop or electronics laboratory. The 'scope is an instrument that displays the waveform of a time varying electrical signal on a cathode ray tube (CRT). An electron beam inside the CRT strikes the phosphor-coated viewing screen to create a spot of light. When the electron beam is deflected, the light spot paints a line on the viewing screen. An internal sawtooth deflects the electron beam in the horizontal (X) direction, creating a time base for the instrument. The input signal is used to deflect the electron beam in the vertical (Y) direction. Thus, the light on the CRT describes the shape of the time-varying waveform applied to the input connectors.

Figure 26-28A shows a service-grade oscilloscope. This instrument is used primarily for troubleshooting and is quite adequate for most medical electronics shops. The only thing that might be desired that this model lacks is a second vertical channel. Dual-beam (two-channel) oscilloscopes have a larger usefulness in that they permit comparison of two time-related signals. Figure 26-28B shows a more expensive, but also more flexible, oscilloscope that is used for the more critical applications in medical equipment servicing and in electronics laboratories. The key feature of this class of 'scope is that the main controls and oscilloscope functions are contained within the main frame, while the plug-in unit determines what the 'scope actually does. A large number of plug-in modules allow the user to configure the mainframe for a large number of applications.

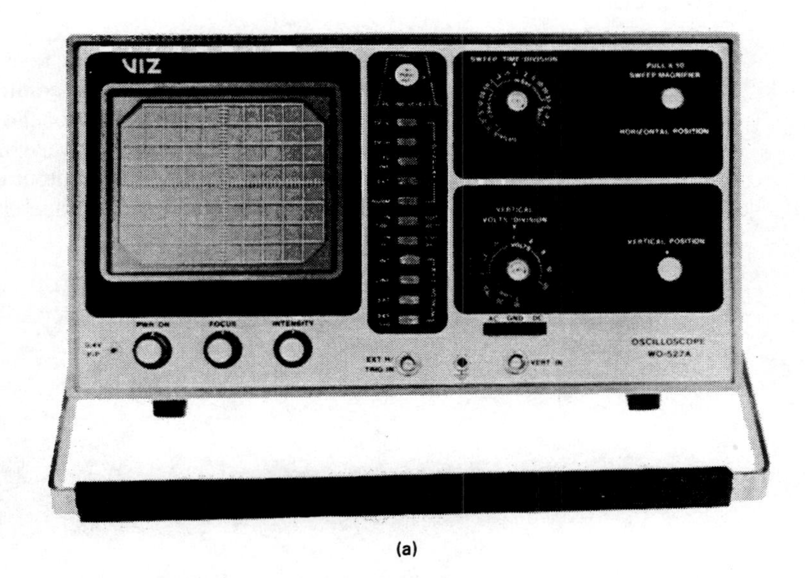

(a)

FIGURE 26-28

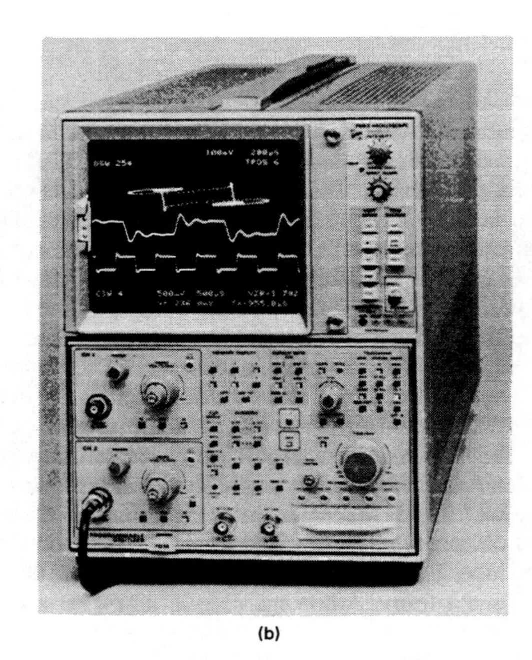

(b)

FIGURE 26-28 (continued)

BENCH POWER SUPPLIES

DC power supplies are used on the service bench in order to substitute for the DC power supply within the equipment being serviced. It is common to substitute the internal supply with a bench supply in order to troubleshoot the set even though the internal supply is defunct. The supply should at least have variable output voltage (as in Figure 26-29) and a current meter. Also desirable is output current limiting. This last feature is useful to prevent secondary damage to the supply itselt in the event that the load is short-circuited to ground.

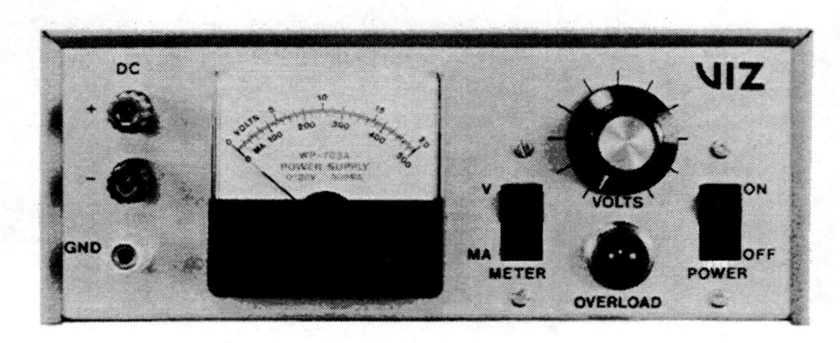

FIGURE 26-29

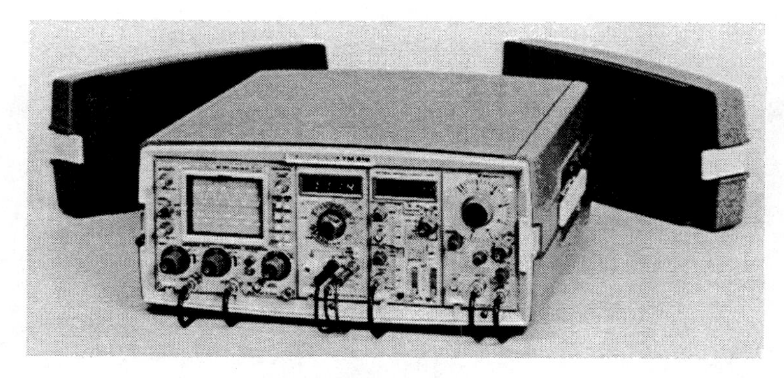

FIGURE 26-30

SELF-CONTAINED INSTRUMENT PACKAGES

Much of medical equipment servicing is actually field servicing. This is even true of in-house service departments. Technicians from biomedical engineering (or some equivalent department) will often be required to tote instruments to a unit within the hospital in order to test or troubleshoot a problem. For these cases the transportable instrument package such as the Tektronix TM-500 series shown in Figure 26-30 is invaluable. The individual instruments are plug-in units that can be installed in either a bench rack or portable rack (as shown). The technician or engineer can configure the portable rack as needed for the specific job. In the specific rack-up shown in Figure 26-30, the instruments selected are (left to right) an oscilloscope, a digital multimeter, a digital frequency/period counter, and a function generator.

SPECIALIZED MEDICAL DEVICE TEST EQUIPMENT

Most of the electronic instruments used in testing medical devices is the same common equipment used in other electronic servicing. These instruments were discussed earlier. There are, however, several instruments that are necessary in a specifically medical context.

Electrical safety is of paramount importance in the medical environment. One of the principal issues (see Chapter 17) is AC leakage current from the case or cabinet of the medical device. The technician must test and certify that the equipment is free of such defects. An adapter such as the millidapter shown in Figure 26-31A allows the use of an ordinary VOM or multimeter to measure the leakage current. One might prefer, however, to use a more comprehensive tester such as the unit shown in Figure 26-31B.

A defibrillator energy tester is shown in Figure 26-32. A defibrillator is a capacitor discharge instrument that is used to resuscitate heart patients who go into ventricular fibrillation. These devices are high voltage, so tend to be hard on their

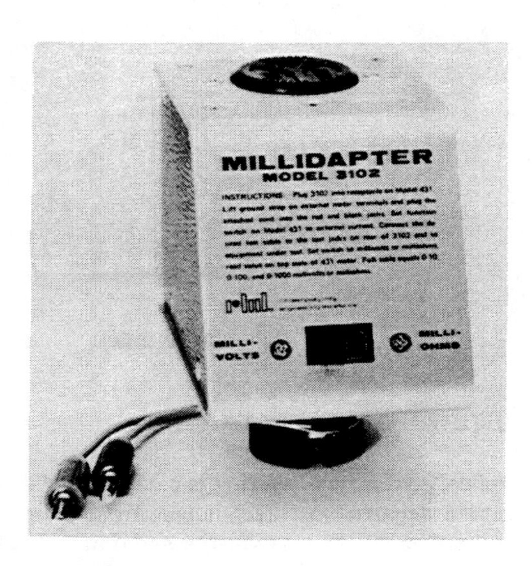

(a)

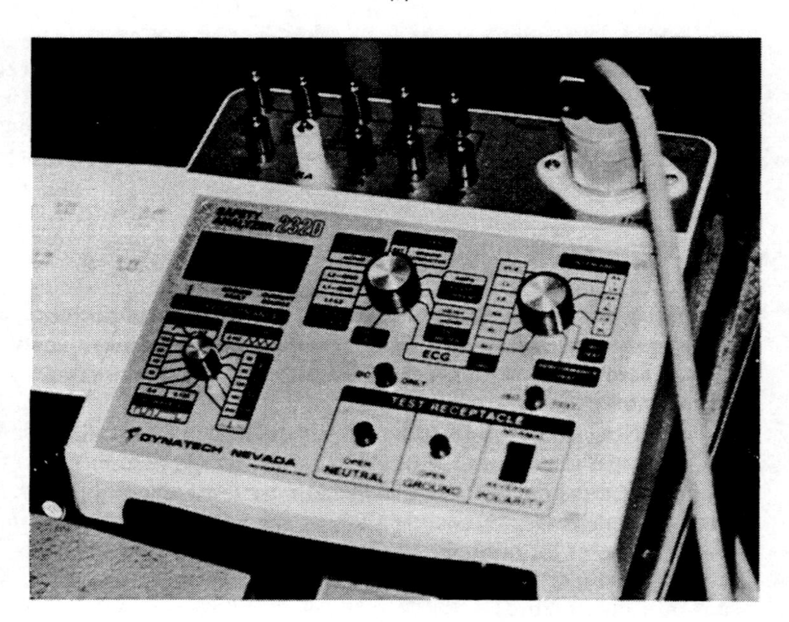

(b)

FIGURE 26-31

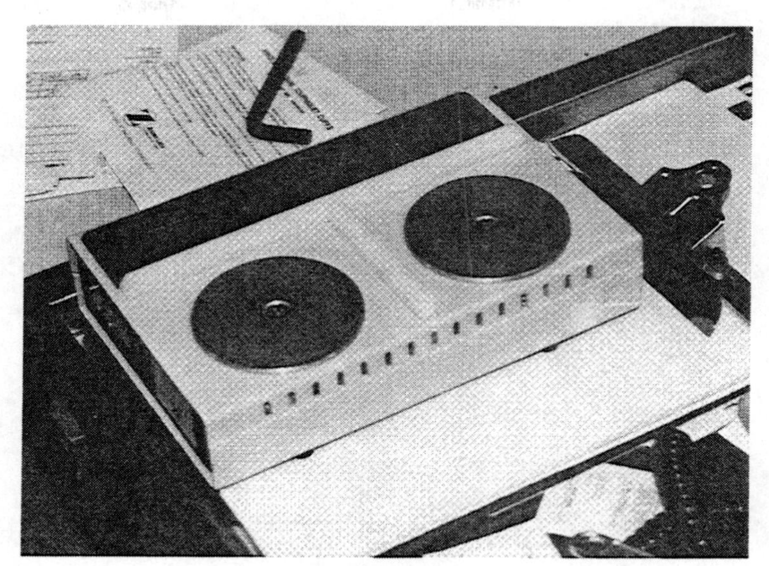

FIGURE 26-32

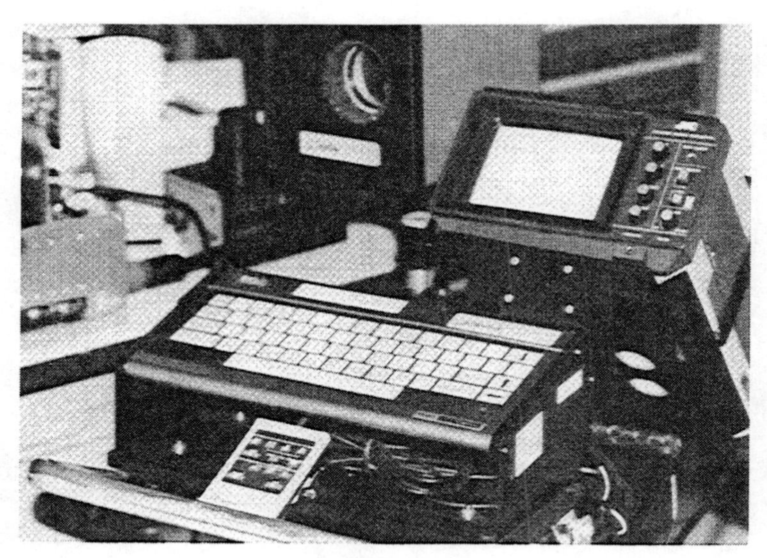

FIGURE 26-33

own components. Two issues are of importance: the amount of energy delivered (related to the set energy) and the waveshape of the output pulse. An integrating voltmeter or similar instrument can be used to measure the energy content of the defibrillator output wave.

The waveshape is a little more difficult to measure. There are two alternatives. First, some analyzers have an oscilloscope output. The waveshape is either displayed on a storage 'scope or photographed on the CRT screen of an ordinary 'scope. Second, the digital form of instrument records the waveform in a digital memory, and then allows it to be read out on an ordinary strip-chart recorder.

Some instruments are impromptu and ad hoc. The technician in Figure 26-33 is testing a thermographic television camera used in mammography and to explore vascular problems. The "test equipment" used is an ice-cold diet Coke in a can!

27

Preventative Maintenance and Proper Program Design

Preventative maintenance (PM) is both *the* proper tool for managing an equipment system, and a fraud perpetrated on the unknowing. How is this apparent paradox resolved? First the fraud part.

Subordinates with any sense want to please higher authority. Similarly, hospital administration wants to please regulatory agencies and malpractice insurance carriers. When authority mandates a PM program, some people "knee jerk" and produce a supposed preventative maintenance regime for every piece of equipment in the house, regardless of whether or not it makes sense. Under such circumstances, the PM program is at the least fraudulent or ill advised and at worst downright harmful.

The purpose of a properly designed PM program is to (1) extend the service life of the equipment and (2) prevent downtime from unforeseen failures. The nature of a proper PM program depends on the nature of the system or equipment that it serves. There are some criteria to consider, and not all of them are technical.

First, what are the requirements of accreditation, legal, and insurance authorities? Any program to PM medical equipment must, at a minimum, meet the requirements of these groups. It is not relevant that these requirements sometimes make little sense from an engineering point of view. A driving factor is the perception of taking all "reasonable" and "prudent" steps to ensure the equipment is operating in a safe and efficacious manner. To a lawyer presenting a malpractice claim, it does not matter that PM is not required on an item if a jury can be convinced otherwise.

Second, does something on the equipment wear out with time and use? Certain mechanical parts such as rollers, drives, and motors wear out within a predictable time window. Once a certain number of operating hours are accumulated a failure can be expected.

Third, do adjustments and alignments degrade with time? Does this degradation affect performance?

Fourth, do certain components degrade with time but without affecting performance until a critical failure occurs?

The nature of the PM program created depends on the nature of the equipment and the answers to these questions. It is likely that several methods will be blended into a custom-tailored package that meets the needs and expectations of the organization. For example, an appropriate PM program for an entirely electronic device (that is, no rotating mechanical components) might be simple operations checks. If the device has a built-in test (BIT) capability, then the PM technician need only run the test and then examine and *document* the results.

At one time a hospital where I worked owned a helium (He)-driven aortic balloon pump. The PM program required mechanical devices to be periodically taken apart and cleaned, inspected, and tightened up. Unfortunately, that was not prudent on the He-driven IABP. Helium is a very light gas consisting of only two protons and two electrons for each molecule. That fact is very important to mechanical designers because helium will escape through fittings that are tight to other gases. The closed-loop gas system could be pressure tested with room air or nitrogen and found good. However, when the test gas (which is heavier) is replaced with helium, the system sometimes would not hold pressure. Even small leaks that are impassable to air will leak helium rapidly. The problem with the PM program is that it caused the fittings to wear out much faster (for use with helium) and thereby actually reduced reliability.

There is also the problem of putting more faults on the system than are taken off. Many years ago a Canadian telephone system noted that the two most failure-prone days for relays were the second and sixteenth of the month. This result is counterintuitive: faults should either be distributed more or less equally across the month if usage is constant, or distributed about days of heavy usage. The second and sixteenth did not follow particularly heavy usage days. The problem was traced to an inappropriate PM program: technicians regularly cleaned and burnished the relays on the first and the fifteenth. The faults that their errors created showed up on the next working shifts, which were on the second and sixteenth of the month.

Nobody ever "PMed" reliability into equipment that is poorly designed. The time for a manager to build the reliability into a system is at the "front end," when the various manufacturer's proposals are being evaluated. However, there are some things that a good PM manager can do to improve the performance of equipment from the reliability point of view. For example, if the equipment runs too hot, it will fail frequently. The PM manager can evaluate the problem and recommend corrective action. Following is material on managing overheating problems. This material comes from articles and lectures the author has delivered.

KEEPING IT COOL

Solving Overheating Problems in Electronic Equipment

Some electronic equipment seems to always go back to the service shop for additional repairs, often of the same original defect. Some equipment just seems naturally failure prone, and the shop is said to be "married" to such gear. When you face such a situation be sure to consider *overheating* as a possible cause. It is well recognized that heat is the great killer of electronic equipment. For decades reliability engineers have identified heat as a principal cause of electronic component failure.

Many electronic device ratings or specifications are based on maintaining certain operating temperatures. One "bargain pack" replacement audio power transistor, for example, offers a seemingly tremendous collector power dissipation (which is prominently advertised), but the full power is only available at room temperature (25–30°C). At temperatures above 30°C the transistor must either be derated substantially or replaced frequently. Almost *anyplace* that the transistor is used inside a cabinet or box the temperature will exceed 30°C!

Similarly, the RF power transistors used in radio communications transmitters fail as often from overheating as from antenna faults (the traditional cause of transistor failure in that type of equipment), but the heat problem is less well recognized in many service shops. In one case there were constant failures of the RF power transistors in a trunk-mounted 100-watt VHF power amplifier used in an ambulance radio. Technicians repaired the rig several times before they drew the connection with heat. The trunk or equipment well of a vehicle during the summer months is extremely hot while the passenger cabin cools off with air conditioning in only a few minutes. Moving the amplifier to behind the dashboard cured the problem.

Reliability experts measure equipment performance in terms of "mean time between failure" (MTBF), which is usually expressed in hours. For example, an MTBF of 1000 hours implies that, for a large number of samples of the equipment, the average will be one failure per thousand hours of operation. One source claims that a 10°C rise in operating temperature will cut the MTBF almost in half.

How important is cooling in electronic equipment? Let's consider some examples. The author worked in a university hospital repairing patient monitoring equipment. The slave ECG oscilloscopes at the nurses' central station were a reliability nightmare. About once a week, usually at 3 AM, the staff would call me to come repair one of the four 'scopes. Yet the same model 'scopes at bedside operated with better reliability. The problem was overheating of the central station 'scopes, which were mounted inside a completely closed wooden desk/console. The hospital carpenter had done his job well, but he was an artist, not a reliability engineer. After cutting ten 1-inch ventilation holes, and installing a pair of 100-cfm "whisper fans," the central station 'scopes became as reliable as the bedside 'scopes.

In another case, a certain bedside monitor had problems with the ±200-volt DC power supply module. Examination revealed that the transistor used for the voltage regulator was overheating so badly that the leads crystalized and broke off.

The data sheet showed the same device available in a heavier, more heat dissipative, package. Using the new transistor style plus adding a "top-hat" heatsink reduced the failure rate to nearly zero. Incidentally, the net price of the old transistor was $1.36, while that of the heavier version of the same type number was $1.52—so what prompted the use of the lesser one (it certainly could not have been price)?

No one with any professional electronics experience will deny that heat is the great killer of electronic devices. Equipment that passes or delivers large amounts of either current or power must be kept cool for proper operation. The methods given in this chapter are simple and sufficient for most servicer's applications. While reliability engineers and the thermodynamicists will flinch at the lack of mathematical elegance, the methods are nonetheless effective for most practical applications faced by service technicians.

There is only one simple rule: *where there is excessive heat, remove it*. What does "excessive" mean? If the equipment feels too hot to the touch, or has a history of unexplained failures and/or repairs, then it is probably running too hot. An engineer will have specifications to meet and calculations to make, and but they are beyond the scope of this book. The practical "skin of the thumb" rule suffices for our needs.

There are three basic tactics which can be used either singly or in combination: (1) radiate more of the heat, (2) improve natural ventilation, or (3) add or increase forced-air cooling. Water cooling is not an issue for some readers although some commercial broadcast transmitters and high-power industrial electronics devices use circulating water for cooling. (Some broadcasting stations use the waste heat from the transmitter's water radiator to heat the transmitter building.)

PROTECTING TRANSISTORS AND IC REGULATORS

On small equipment it is not practical (or possible) to use forced-air cooling, so you will have to provide heatsinking for the semiconductors. In fact, even in most forced-air cooled equipments the semiconductors will need these metal radiators. Figure 27-1A shows the metal TO-5 transistor package. Most of these transistors are mounted on printed wiring boards and are low-signal (and low-heat) devices. But certain TO-5 transistors, such as the 2N3053 and certain 3- to 10-watt RF power transistors, operate at moderate power levels. A "top-hat" finned heatsink such as Figure 27-1B is mounted on the TO-5 package to radiate heat. There are also cer-

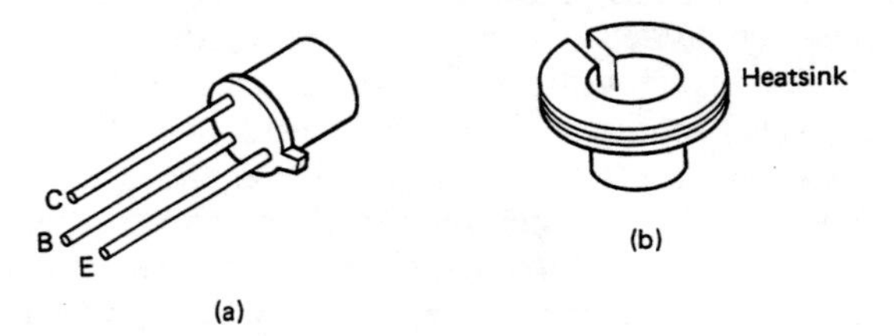

FIGURE 27-1

tain other "spring clip" versions of this same kind of heatsink. These are the heatsinks the author used in modifying the monitors mentioned.

Figure 27-2A shows two forms of plastic power device package. You will find these packages in audio power transistors (for example, 2N5249), thyristors, and three-terminal IC voltage regulators. In the regulator case, the devices are usually rated at 750 mA in free air and 1000 mA when heatsinked. These devices are frequently used at higher power than they are rated for! Either vertical or horizontal finned sheet metal heatsinks such as in Figure 27-2B are used to provide heat dissipation. Be sure to use a thin layer of silicone heat transfer grease between the metal tab surface on the transistor (or regulator) and the heatsink. Also be sure to tighten the mounting screw properly to facilitate heat transfer to the heatsink.

Sheet metal heatsinks for TO-3 transistors and three-terminal regulators that are mounted on a printed circuit board. The bent sheet metal heatsinks are good for up to about 10 watts of power or voltage regulators up to 1.5 amperes. For the 3-ampere, 5-ampere, and 10-ampere voltage regulators that also use a TO-3 package it would be better to use a larger finned heatsink.

In many equipments the metal chassis is used for heatsinking. In those cases the transistors are bolted either directly to the metal chassis or mounted via mica in-

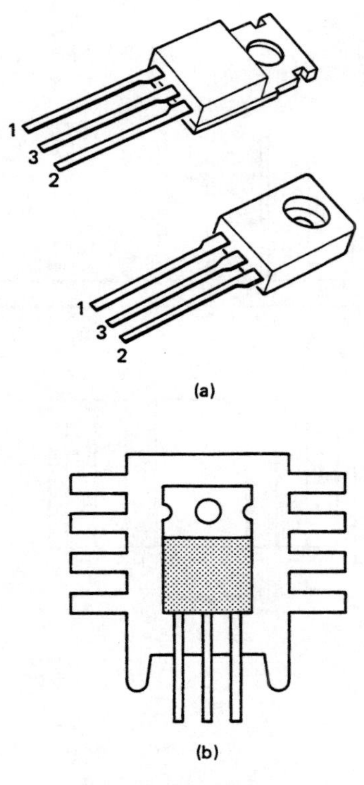

FIGURE 27-2

sulators if electrical isolation is required. In both cases, silicone heat transfer grease is used between the semiconductor device and the chassis. This method is especially successful when the chassis is large or when it is particularly thick (that is, has a high "thermal mass").

Some printed wiring boards (PWB) use large areas of unetched copper foil and/or large metal ridges or blocks to provide better heatsinking. This method is used especially where there are no single devices that can be individually heatsinked (for example, a TO-220 transistor), but rather when there are a large number of heat-producing devices such as TTL ICs.

There are many different forms of large, finned heatsink used for TO-3 (and other) transistors, high-current voltage regulators, and high-current diodes and SCRs; Figure 27-3A shows a side view of one of these heatsinks. In this case, the TO-3 transistor (or other device) is mounted on the flat central surface of the heatsink with screws. In most situations, it is wise to use a thin smear of silicone heat transfer grease between the device and the heatsink. This grease is especially needed when a mica insulator is placed between the semiconductor device and the heatsink. Again it is necessary to make sure that the mounting screws are cinched down tight enough to allow maximum heat transfer (but not enough to distort the

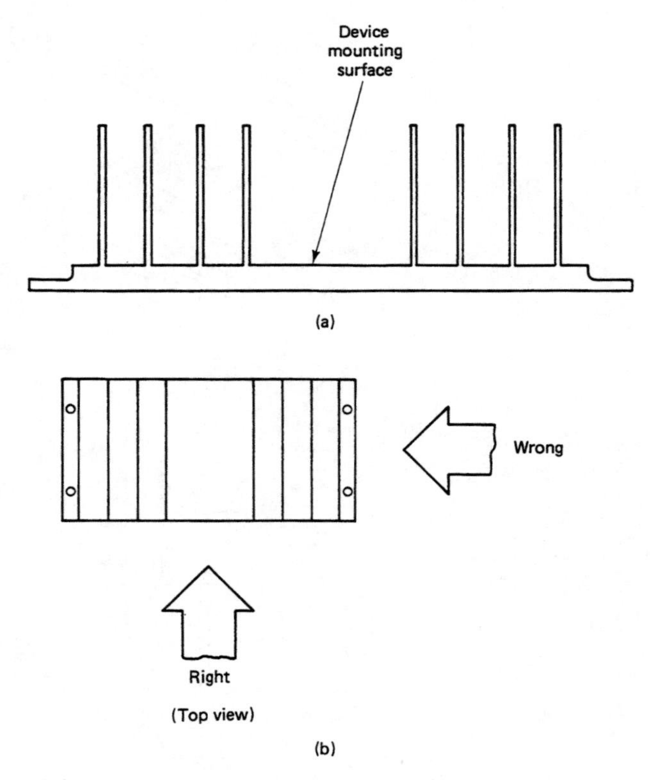

FIGURE 27-3

device package). The big issue in selecting a heatsink is the surface area in square inches.

When forced air is used to cool a heatsink—a good idea when the power and/or current is high—then the orientation of the heatsink with respect to the airflow is sometimes important. Figure 27-3B shows the right and wrong ways to force air over the finned surfaces. Keep in mind, however, that orientation is not always critical, especially when air from the "wrong" direction is sufficient or blows over the entire surface. The designations "right" and "wrong" are merely general considerations for some critical applications.

OTHER COMPONENTS

Certain components other than power transistors generate heat. Rectifier diodes and power resistors should be mounted with their bodies 0.125 to 0.250 inches off the PWB (see Figure 27-4). This procedure allows the heat to dissipate into the air instead of the PWB material. Many phenolic and some fiberglass printed wiring boards are badly damaged from the effects of a 10-watt power resistor mounted flush to the surface. Some "bargain basement" rectifier diodes can meet their rated forward current only when the rectifier is (1) mounted 0.50 inches off the board and (2) have the axial leads cut to 0.75 inches or longer. Those diodes are overrated and should be either used only in lower than the rated current applications or shunned entirely. For medical equipment, the latter is the proper choice.

Besides reducing the operating life or limiting the power output of circuits, overheating can also decrease performance in other ways. Certain circuits, oscillators, for example, are inherently sensitive to heat. There was once a popular two-way radio transceiver that suffered terrible frequency drift because the master oscillator was located right next to the RF/IF strip vacuum tubes. Although that was such a bad design error that nothing would really "fix" the situation, a lot of technicians improved the frequency stability markedly by adding some thermal insulating material between the RF/IF PWB and the aluminum oscillator shielded housing.

LARGE MULTIBOARD EQUIPMENT

Figure 27-5A shows a typical piece of large-scale multiboard equipment—such as a microcomputer—in which plug-in printed wiring boards are installed on a socketed motherboard. Usually, these PWBs will be mounted in a closed cabinet for both

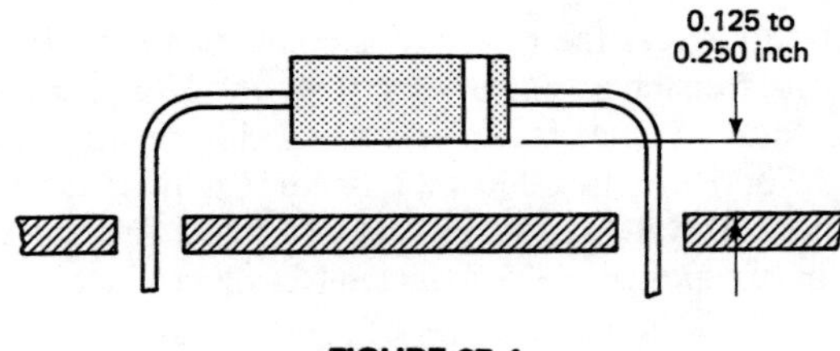

FIGURE 27-4

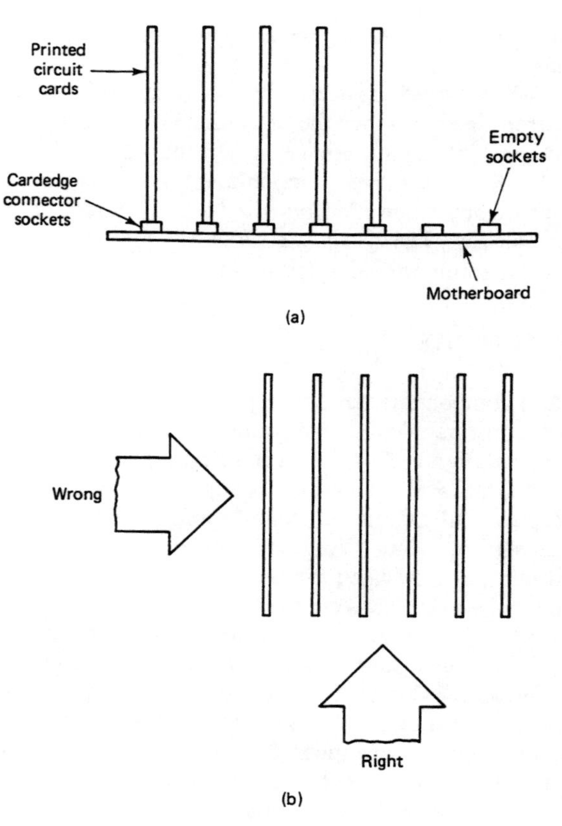

FIGURE 27-5

EMI and aesthetic reasons. If we apply air broadside to the PWBs, then only the first one in the lineup will benefit. Figure 27-5B shows a top view that permits you to see right and wrong airflow directions. Obviously, air coming in from the sides is able to remove heat from more of the PWBs more effectively.

Figure 27-6 shows a method used in a microcomputer. There is a large metal chassis with a motherboard mounted on it to hold the PWBs. There were 0.75-inch holes cut in both the chassis top and the motherboard to admit air between the boards. Although only one hole is shown between each board in this sideview, there were four per row in the actual computer. Air from the blower flowed up through the holes and across the electronics components on the PWBs.

Radio frequency power amplifiers and high-power transmitters pose special heat problems. Some linear power amplifiers, for example, are only 45 percent efficient. Therefore, a 1000-watt linear amplifier delivers 450 watts of usable RF power and 550 watts of waste heat. To make matters even worse, the necessity of keeping harmonics inside the transmitter means buttoning up all that heat inside of a shielded metal cabinet.

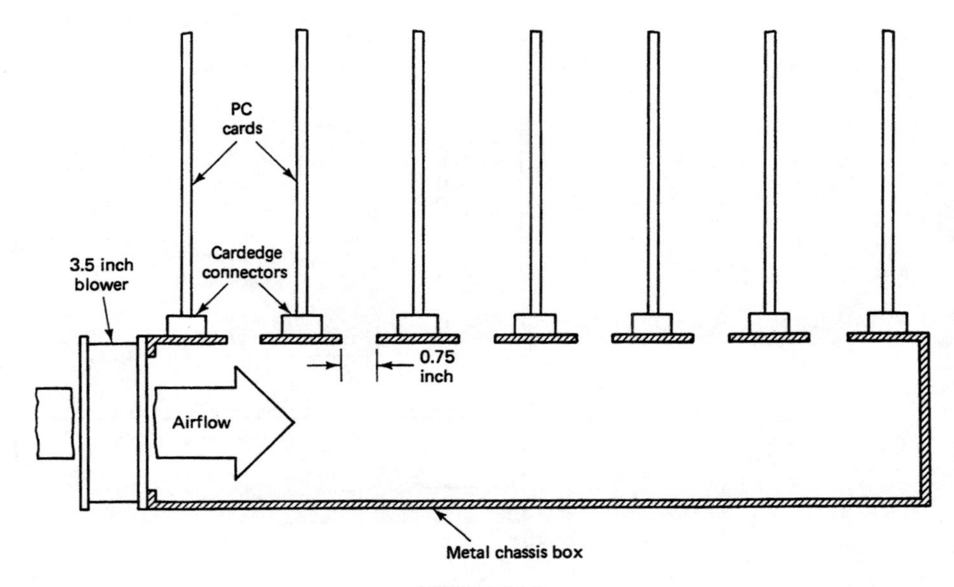

FIGURE 27-6

Most RF power amplifier tubes used in medical diathermy and electrosurgery equipment, industrial inductive heaters, and radio transmitters must be forced-air cooled in order to realize their full ratings (some are absolutely dependent on cooling). Figure 27-7 shows two methods for providing the needed cooling air. In Figure 27-7A we see the situation where a blower is mounted so that the airflow is di-

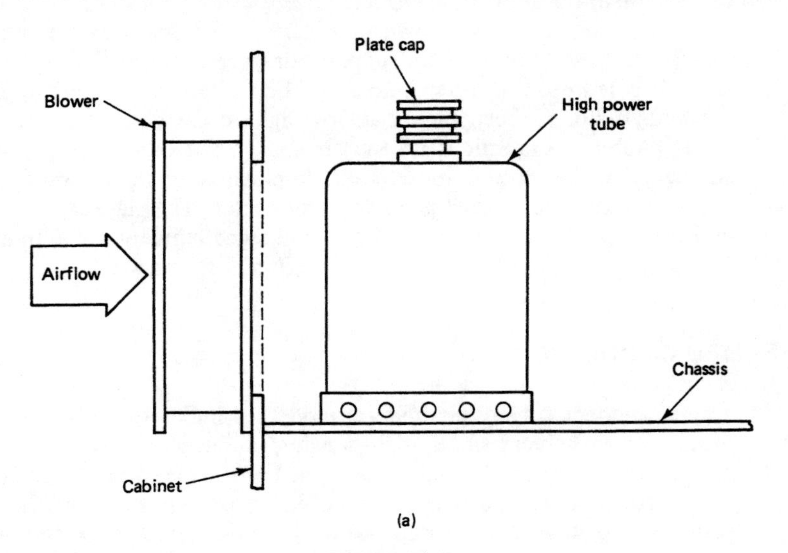

FIGURE 27-7

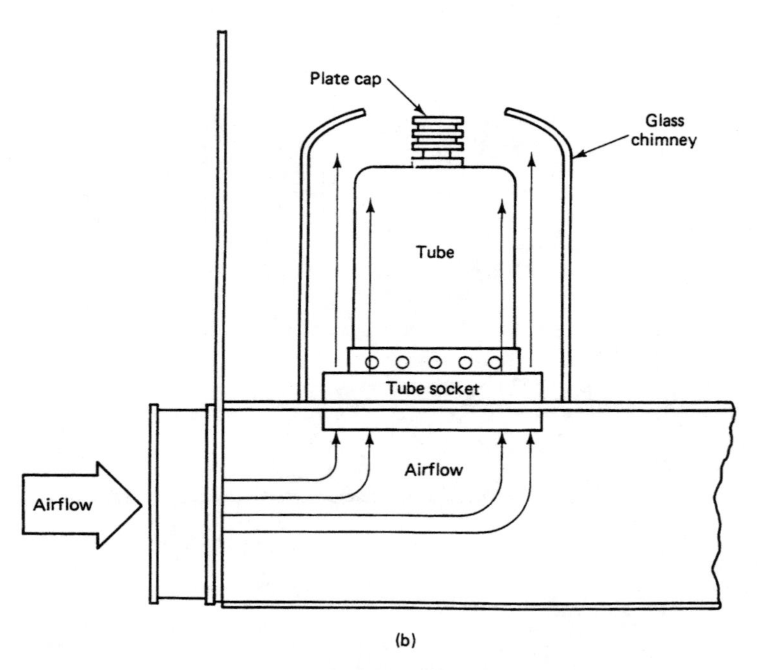

(b)

FIGURE 27-7 (continued)

rectly over the glass envelope. The fan may be mounted either exterior to the RF compartment (as shown) or inside.

The other method, shown in Figure 27-7B, assumes the use of "air system" tube sockets. A blower or fan supplies air to the bottom side of the socket, and the air is directed upward through holes in the socket and around the glass envelope. A "chimney" aids in keeping the airflow against the glass. Some air system sockets have plumbing connections for the air hose, while others are dependent upon pressurization of the lower compartment. In either case, the reason this socket is better is that the lead seals in the glass are kept cooler. The plate cap lead seal should also be kept cool, if possible. Toward this end some builders use a finned "heat-dissipating" plate cap to make electrical connection to the anode.

IC PRINTED CIRCUIT BOARDS

The component density possible on modern printed wiring boards (PWB) makes it possible to make very small, high-density, products such as modern radio communications equipment and digital computers. Unfortunately, as the number of IC devices on a card increases, so does the problem of cooling them off. In some cases, impingement airflow, as discussed earlier, is neither feasible nor desirable—but we still have to remove the heat. One solution is shown in Figure 27-8. This method uses a ladder heatsink built onto the board.

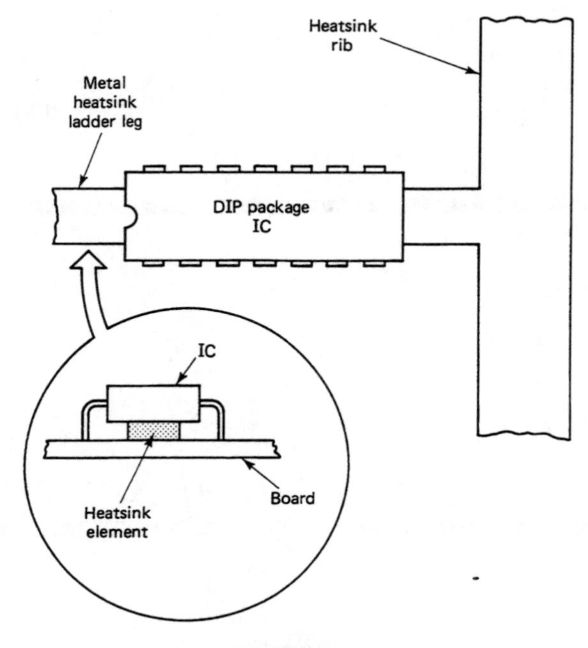

FIGURE 27-8

In Figure 27-8 a heavy metal "ladder" is run underneath each IC device (see inset), and is joined to a large heatsink bar on the card edge. Heat is removed from the IC area by conduction. In some cases, airflow can de directed across the card edge heatsinks. In this type of construction, we usually want to place the most heat-producing components as close as possible to the edges of the PWB where the heatsink bar is located.

CONCLUSION

Heat is the great destroyer of electronic components. If a piece of medical equipment runs too hot, then the result will be erratic operation, frequent breakdowns, and all the headaches that accompany low reliability. Although it is ordinarily unwise for professional servicers to custom modify equipment without expressly written instructions from the manufacturer, there are sometimes exceptions to this rule. An obviously overheating piece of equipment that can be modified with no adverse effects is a candidate for exception to the rule. The simple methods shown in this chapter will permit you to modify equipment to gain the longest and most reliable use possible for your customer (or employer if you are an in-house servicer).

28

Electrical Safety: Your Job!

Electrical and electronic equipment is inherently dangerous, and if not used according to some basic commonsense rules can result in injury or even death. The medical environment has some special problems regarding electrical safety because the normally protective skin of the patient is breached. There are two electrical safety situations to consider: *macroshock* and *microshock*. The former pertains to both patients and personnel, while the latter pertains specifically to patients.

Macroshock is the type of electrical shock to which all people are subject, and comes from direct contact with an electrical source. If you touch the 110-volt AC line while grounded, then a very painful and possibly fatal shock will occur. This is macroshock, and does not require wounds or other breaches of the skin.

Microshock is a more subtle form of electrical shock, and at one time it was not recognized. But increased use of electrical equipment in hospitals in the 1950s and 1960s led some authorities at the time (1970) to speculate that as many as 1200 people a year were being accidentally electrocuted in hospitals from tiny currents that went unnoticed by the medical staff. Microshock is electrical shock from minute currents that are too small to affect persons with intact skin, but will affect persons if they are introduced inside the body through a wound. We will deal with microshock in some detail later in this chapter.

In all forms of electrical shock a difference of electrical potential must exist between two points on the body. In other words, two points of contact must exist between the victim and the electrical source. That is why you sometimes see harmless "hair-raising" exhibits when a person touches an electrostatic high voltage (>200,000 volts) and their hair stands on end—but there is no shock. These potentials are monopolar with respect to the demonstrator, so no current flow exists. Similarly, some of the less than prudent electricians work circuits "hot" (that is, without turning off the power) in seeming safety because they take care to not ground themselves, or in any other way come between the hot wire and ground, or across two hot wires. Even so, it is bad practice that ought to be strongly discouraged.

In addition to electrical shock there are other safety concerns regarding electricity. One major problem is fire. Overloaded or defective electrical circuits can start a fire. Many residential, business, industrial, and health care facility fires every year are traced to faulty wiring or malfunctioning electrical equipment.

Electrical faults will also damage the equipment, the building, or other equipment. A short circuit that is not protected by a fuse may create more damage to the shorted equipment, and may also cause damage to the building wiring and electrical components. In some cases, a fire may result. When fuses and circuit breakers are either not used or defeated ("penny in the fuse box" syndrome), then a severe fire hazard exists and any damage at all to the equipment is most certainly increased.

Less recognized, but nonetheless possible, is the hazard of explosion from electrical faults. At least two mechanisms are found. First, an overloaded circuit or electrical component builds up internal pressure (often from gas released when the device is severely overheated) and ruptures spectacularly. Examples include high-power transformers and the main capacitors inside defibrillators.

The second mechanism of explosion is sparking in the presence of flammable gases or vapors. If an electrical circuit is disconnected while operating, or if certain faults exist, then a spark may result. If that spark occurs when flammable gases, oxygen (which isn't flammable, but acts that way because it violently promotes burning of other materials), or vapors (such as gasoline, certain waxes) are present, then a violent and dangerous explosion may result.

Besides the obvious danger of "shrapnel" from the casing of an exploding device, there is also the possibility of boiling oil splattering nearby personnel. There is a specific health danger regarding this oil in some cases. Certain older electrical capacitors and transformers were built using PCB oil as an internal coolant. *PCB oil is a carcinogen*. The importance of that statement cannot be underestimated: PCB is dangerous stuff! Although most PCB-bearing electrical devices are now out of service, it is possible that some are still around—especially in older equipment or buildings. Equipment to be especially suspicious of include elderly high-power electrosurgery machines (vacuum tube models, not spark-gap machines) and defibrillators. If one of these machines is found, then it is a good idea to have it checked by a competent technician or engineer to determine if the large, high-voltage capacitor(s) inside uses PCB oil as an insulating coolant or dielectric material. A PCB spill can close a building for a long period of time until a proper cleanup routine is completed.

Before discussing either form of electrical shock let's discuss the mechanism of electrical shock and the proper approach to dealing with a shock victim.

WHAT TO DO FOR AN ELECTRICAL SHOCK VICTIM

The usual mechanism of death for electrical shock is usually a phenomenon called *ventricular fibrillation* (V.Fib.). This is an arrhythmic heartbeat in which the heart merely quivers instead of beats. Unfortunately, V.Fib. is incapable of sustaining blood pumping effectiveness, so the victim dies within a few minutes unless someone trained in cardiopulmonary resuscitation (CPR) is nearby.

Before you can aid the victim of electrical shock, you must be sure that either the victim is away from the current or the current is turned off! Otherwise, *when you touch the victim in order to help him or her, then you will also become a victim!*

As soon as the victim is clear of the electrical current, initiate cardiopulmonary resucitation (CPR) and send for help. CPR will generally not bring the victim out of V.Fib. Rather, its function is to provide life support until properly equipped and trained medical personnel can be summoned. They will use a defibrillator to shock the victim's heart back into correct rhythm. They will also use drugs and intravenous (IV) solutions to reestablish the body's balance.

None of these actions can be performed by the untrained person. In fact, even CPR cannot be effectively performed by the untrained person. Everyone who works near, on, or around electrical or electronic equipment should learn CPR. In addition, teenage and adult family members should also learn CPR; after all, who is going to save *you* when the electrical accident occurs at home? The local Red Cross, the Heart Association, some community colleges, and most local hospitals can direct you to certified CPR courses. *It is impossible to learn CPR by watching medical shows on television,* so get trained by a knowledgeable instructor!

HOW MUCH CURRENT IS DANGEROUS OR FATAL?

The author worked in a hospital electronics laboratory. One day I overheard an intern claim that 110 volts AC from the wall socket is not dangerous because they told him in medical school that it's not the voltage that kills, it's the current. I asked him: "Doctor, have you ever heard of Ohm's law?" According to Ohm's law, the current is the quotient of voltage and resistance: $I = E/R$. Besides, a little statistic that the doctor apparently didn't know was that 110 volts AC from residential wall sockets is the most common cause of electrocution in the United States. In addition, medical studies reveal that the 50–60-Hz frequency used in AC power distribution almost worldwide is the most dangerous range of frequencies. Higher and lower AC frequencies are less dangerous (but not safe!) than 60-Hz AC.

According to medical experts who have studied electrical shock, the killing factor is *current density* in a certain area in the right atrium of the heart called the *sinoatrial node*. Any flow of current through the body that causes a high level of current to flow in that section of the heart can induce fatal V.Fib. In general, for limb-contact electrical shocks through intact skin (macroshock), the following rules of thumb are accepted:

1–5 mA	Level of perception
10 mA	Level of pain

100 mA	Severe muscular contraction
100–300 mA	Electrocution

Keep in mind that these figures are approximate and *are not to be taken as a guideline to an assumed risk!* Death can occur under certain circumstances with considerably lower levels of current. For example, when you are sweating, and are standing in salty or dirty water, the risk of electrocution escalates tremendously. In medical situations, the level of current that can kill is in the 20–150-microampere level because the current is induced directly into the body, which is essentially a "salt-water" environment (human skin has a resistance of 1000 to 20,000 ohms, internal tissue has a resistance of 50 ohms or less). Microshock, which is discussed presently, indicates that electrocution can occur at considerably lower current levels.

IS HIGH CURRENT DANGEROUS?

The author once attended a design review meeting for a high-power mobile transmitter such as the type used in ambulances and police cars. The engineer's specification called for insulation of low-voltage (28-V DC), high-current (30-amperes) DC power supply terminals. One of the engineers present sneered that was something like asking him to insulate the battery terminals of his car. Implied in that comment is that low current can't hurt you. There are two false premises to that opinion.

First, although low-voltage, high-current points rarely cause electrical shock, it is possible for dangerous shock to occur when the person has a very low electrical skin resistance (is very sweaty) or has an open wound. Although the case did not result in electrocution, one electronics technician injured himself severely when he cut himself on a +5-V DC, 30-ampere computer power supply terminal. A large amount of current flowed in his arm and caused severe pain and some physical damage to muscle tissue.

Second, the high current is extremely dangerous if you happen to be wearing jewelry! A two-way radio shop used 12-volt batteries and battery chargers for the troubleshooting bench supply for mobile service. A technician working on the battery rack dropped a wrench, and it fell onto the battery-making contact from (−) to (+) through his watchband. The large current turned the watchband red hot and gave him serious second- and third-degree burns on his wrist.

Don't ever assume that low-voltage, high-current power supplies are harmless!

MECHANISMS OF ELECTRICAL SHOCK

To raise our consciousness about how shock can occur in the workplace, let's take a look at certain scenarios of electrical shock that might occur to electronics service technicians. Figure 28-1 shows the direct approach to fatal electrical shock. You are grounded through conductive shoes and touch an electrically hot point. You need not be outdoors to be affected by this scenario. A concrete garage, shop, or basement

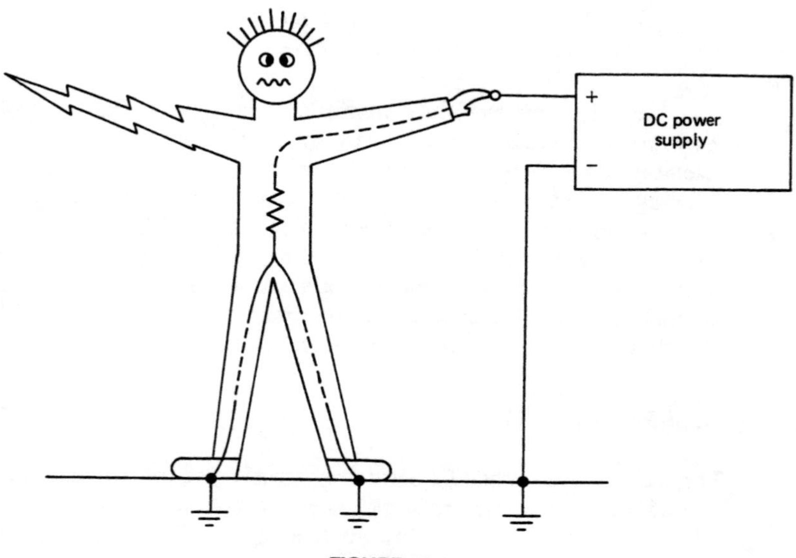

FIGURE 28-1

floor is a reasonably good conductor, as are wet leather and some forms of rubber shoe soles.

Figure 28-2 shows an indirect electric shock scenario that especially affects electronics workers. Consider the grounded instrument probe (in this case an oscilloscope). When you grasp that probe, you may be grounded through the 'scope shield and the power cord ground conductor. If you touch a "hot" point, then you will get shocked—*and maybe killed.*

A related scenario is shown in Figure 28-3. Here we have an AC/DC consumer appliance, such as a low-cost radio or TV set. Note that the oscilloscope probe ground is connected to the set ground, *which also happens to be on one side of the AC power line*. Everything is fine as long as the AC plug is oriented correctly in the wall and if the wall socket is wired correctly. But if you plug it into the wall receptacle backward, then there will be an *explosive short circuit* and possible electrocution of the operator.

This scenario is one reason why many hospitals ban patient-owned equipment.

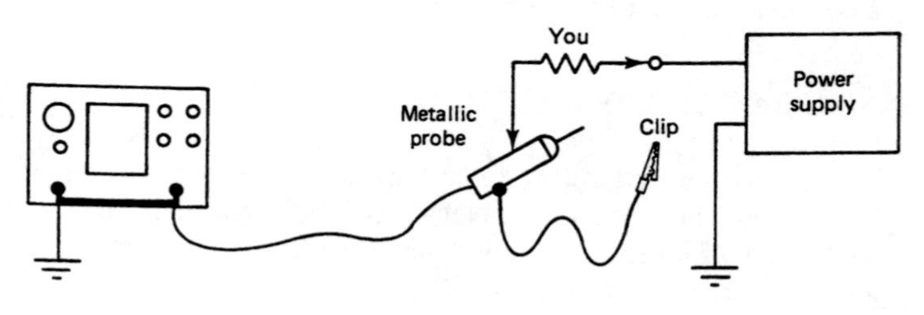

FIGURE 28-2

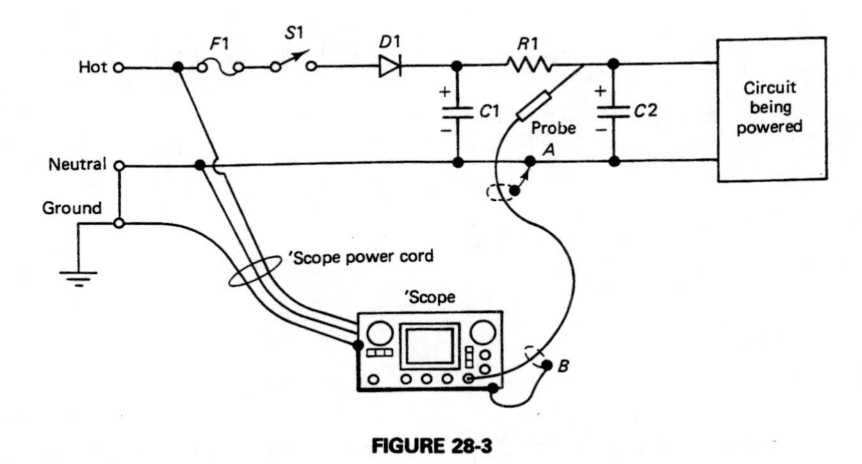

FIGURE 28-3

The medical environment is typically electrically grounded, while many consumer devices are AC/DC operated. These two environments may be benign in themselves, but are lethal when combined. Another reason why hospitals ban patient-owned equipment is the potential fire hazard which unregulated appliances represent.

Another scenario is the fatal antenna erection job. It is never good practice to erect an antenna near a power line! *Never*. Every year we hear stories of people electrocuted because (1) an antenna they were working on fell across the power lines, (2) they tried to toss a wire antenna over the power line in order to raise the antenna above the lines, or (3) a ladder they were using fell across the power lines. *Foolish!* These tactics will kill you. Incidentally, this reason is why OSHA-approved industrial ladders are made of wood or other nonconductive material and not of aluminum as are consumer ladders.

SOME CURES FOR THE PROBLEM

Figure 28-4 shows the schematic for the usual U.S. residential AC electrical system. Industrial electrical systems, such as used in hospitals are a bit different at the service entrance, but become much like Figure 28-4 when the power is distributed throughout the building. The power company distributes energy through high-voltage lines. When it arrives to a point a short distance from the customer, it is stepped down in a "pole pig" transformer to 220-volts AC center-tapped. The center-tap (CT) of the transformer secondary is grounded, and therein lies the root of the problem. The two ends of the 220-V AC secondary are brought into the building as a pair of 110-V AC hot lines. Tapping across the two hot lines produces a 220-V AC outlet; tapping from the ground line (that is, transformer CT) to either hot line produces a 110-V AC outlet.

The problem is that the electrical system in the hospital is *ground referenced*. The solution is to make the local (that is, in-room) electrical system nonground ref-

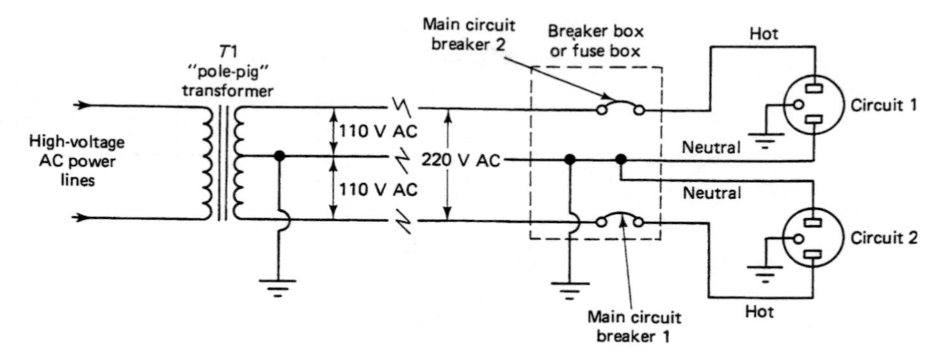

FIGURE 28-4

erenced (that is, *isolated*). This method is used in hospital operating rooms and in some intensive care units.

Figure 28-5 shows the wiring for such a system that can be used on repair benches to improve safety. Transformer T1 is one of two forms of isolation transformer: a 1:1 transformer gives a 110-V AC isolated (nonground-referenced) AC line from a 110-V AC standard line; a 2:1 transformer does the same thing from a 220-V AC line. A second transformer, operating from the secondary of the isolation transformer, gives you some control over the actual voltage available on the bench. The variable transformer is technically known as an *autotransformer* because it uses a common winding for both primary and secondary. One common brand of these devices is Variac®.

If you work on either radio transmitters or other high-power RF-producing devices such as electrosurgery machines, or work near such generators, then you might want to place an electromagnetic interference (EMI) filter in the line at the points marked *X*. The EMI filter is an LC-section that attenuates RF, but not the 60 Hz power.

The "MOV" is a *metal oxide varistor*. It is used to clip the amplitude of high-

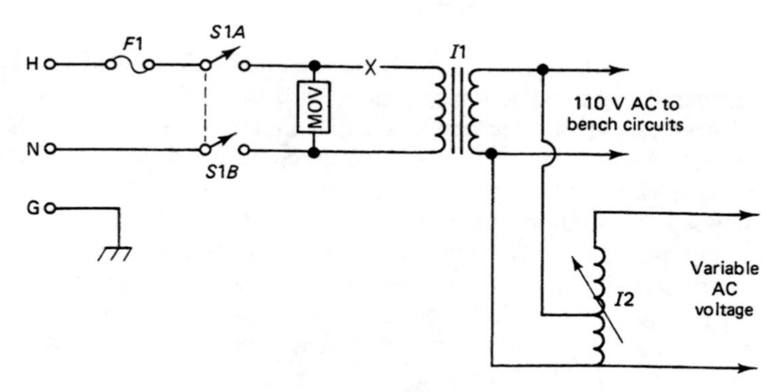

FIGURE 28-5

voltage line transients (100 microseconds or so) that could either damage or interfere with the operation of the equipment on the bench.

The circuit breaker or fuse is used to protect equipment on the bench, as well as the transformer. It is always placed in the hot line, or in both lines. Fuses and circuit breakers are never placed in the neutral line only. The switching shown in Figure 28-5 breaks both lines. I prefer this approach on the theory that hot and neutral lines can be reversed accidentally, and leave you in the position of breaking a neutral and leaving the hot line as alive as a hissing cobra. Figure 28-6A shows a shop-built line isolation transformer for use on a workbench. The transformer inside the box is a 1000-V AC model, so this box is capable of powering most workbenches used for biomedical instrumentation servicing. The output voltage is monitored from the front panel by a 0- to 150 VAC meter. The meter is not strictly necessary, but does serve to provide an indication of line voltage conditions (which becomes critical during summer brownout conditions).

A commercially available line isolation transformer is shown in Figure 28-6B. This model is especially useful for situations where computers and other digital electronic devices are used. In fact, it is likely that hospital and medical school organizations who own computers will find that they tend to "crash" or "bomb out" unpredictably. Those problems are often caused by problems with the AC line power and are significantly mitigated by this type of transformer. In the biomedical instrumentation laboratory, these transformers can also be used for powering the bench and thereby making it a safer working environment.

Isolation transformers are also sometimes used to allow outside equipment to

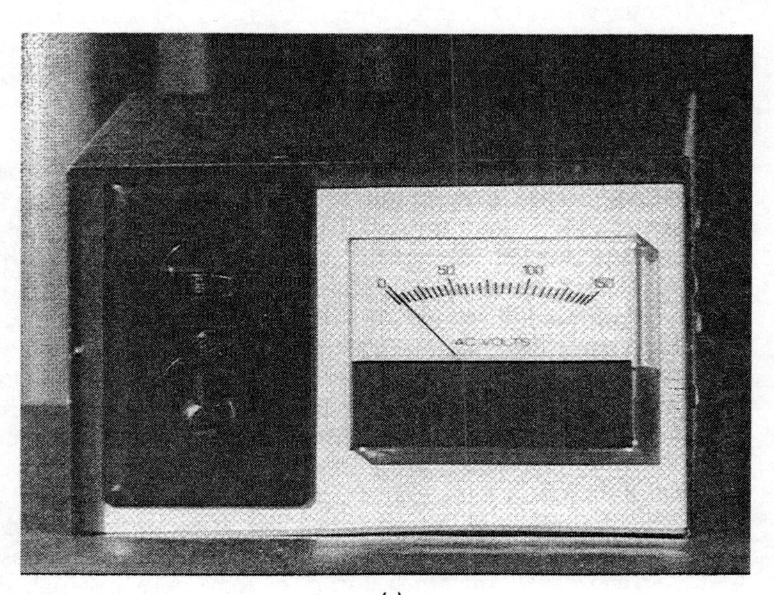

(a)

FIGURE 28-6

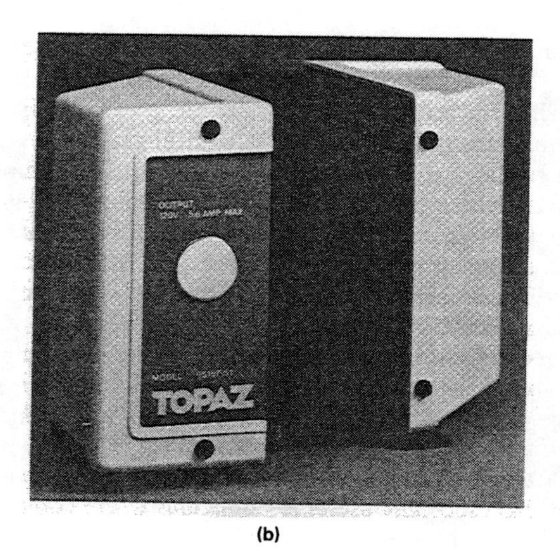

(b)

FIGURE 28-6 (continued)

be used in the hospital. Devices that were not manufactured especially for medical use are inherently unsafe in the medical environment because they do not perform to the same standards as medical devices. This problem is especially acute with two-wire electrical appliances such as small radios and other entertainment devices. An isolation transformer will make them safer. It is good policy to ban outside devices altogether.

SOME GENERAL ADVICE FOR SAFETY

There is only one way to ensure that the AC line won't shock you: *disconnect it*. Make it your practice *never* to work on equipment that has the plug inserted into the power outlet, *never*. Don't trust switches, fuses, circuit breakers, or other people. If someone were to hand you a pistol, claiming that it was unloaded, the first thing you'd do is check it yourself—the same advice also holds true for the electrical connection (which can kill you just as dead as a loaded and cocked pistol).

It is often advised that you work on high-voltage devices with your left hand in your pants pocket. That advice is based on the theory that the "left hand to either leg path" is supposedly the most deadly. Even if the physiology is correct, placing one hand in your pocket leaves you awkward and you are unable to work safely on the circuit with only one hand. It is better to use both hands, arrange it so that the work environment is safe, and use safe techniques.

What is a safe work environment? The power system should be isolated (as discussed). The floor should be insulated by a carpet, treated masonite, a plastic cover, a rubber mat, wooden planking, or some other material; the floor should always be well insulated and kept dry.

When working on high-voltage DC circuits, keep in mind that *capacitors store energy*. All filter capacitors must be discharged manually after the power is turned off. Also, *the capacitor must be discharged multiple times*. Even when a short circuit is placed across the capacitor terminals, not all of the energy is removed the first time. Some energy is stored in the dielectric even after the main charge is discharged.

MICROSHOCK: A PARTICULAR MEDICAL EQUIPMENT HAZARD

Microshock is a form of electrical shock that is almost unique to the medical environment. By definition, microshock is electrical shock from currents that are too small to be perceptible by persons whose skin is intact. Typically, microshock currents are those in the *microampere* (μA) range. Although some experts disagree on the specific level at which microshock occurs (20 μA to 140 μA are usually cited), it is clear that very-small 60-Hz AC currents can be extremely dangerous to patients in the medical environment under the right conditions. It is even possible for the medical and nursing staff to convey dangerous AC currents to the patient even though the same current is below the threshold of perception for themselves.

From where does this problem come? Figure 28-7 shows a generic piece of medical equipment connected to a patient. Typically, there is a power transformer (T1) supplying low-voltage AC (stepped down from 115 V AC) to the power supply and instrumentation circuits (as required). Although the wiring to the transformer is *insulated* from the chassis, it is not necessarily true that it is *isolated* from the chassis. Any time two electrical conductors, such as the power wiring and chassis of a piece of medical equipment, are in close proximity, there will be a certain amount of *capacitance* between them. This stray capacitance is shown as C_s in Figure 28-7. Capacitors will pass alternating current, so some small *AC leakage current* from the AC power lines passes to the chassis of the equipment.

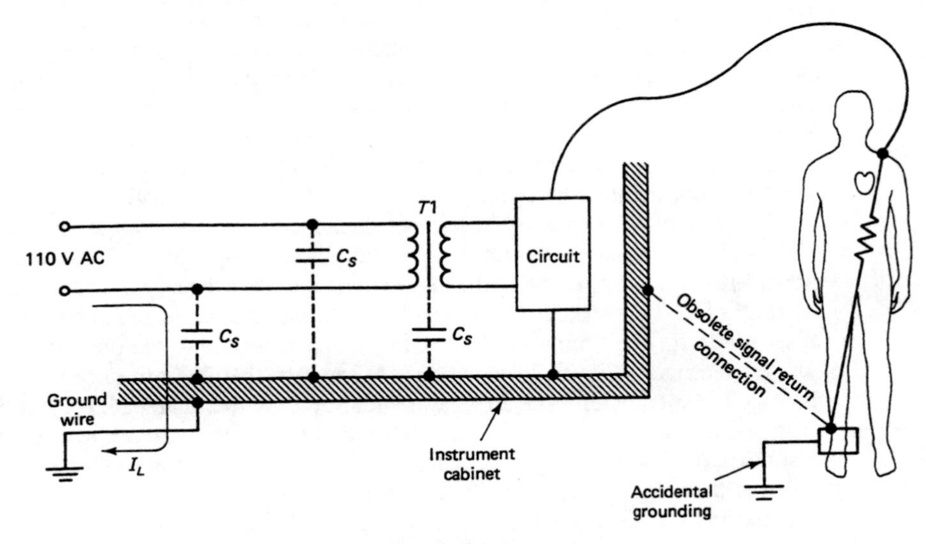

FIGURE 28-7

The level of leakage current depends upon the capacitive reactance of the capacitor and the applied AC voltage. For example, a 200-pF (picofarad) capacitance is not at all unusual between the power line wiring and chassis of an instrument or appliance. At a frequency of 60 Hz the capacitive reactance will be about 13 megohms. When 115 V AC is applied, the leakage current will be V/X_c, or about 8.8 μA. Normally, this current level is negligible. In some older equipment, or those that worked in the presence of electrosurgery machines, there was one or more capacitors between the power lines and ground. These capacitors, which may be part of an LC filter network, are used for the suppression of electromagnetic interference (EMI). These capacitors may have values from 0.001 μF to 0.1 μF, so under the same conditions may pass currents as high as 4 mA. This current is way above the microshock level and is within the threshold of perception range.

In Figure 28-7 the equipment cabinet or chassis is connected to ground through the "third wire" (usually green or green with a yellow tracer in U.S.-made equipment) in the AC power cord. The leakage current (I_L) can drain harmlessly to ground through this wire. But what happens when the ground wire breaks? Or what happens when the spring tension of the ground pin of the power receptacle fails to grip the power cord ground lug sufficiently tight to make a good contact? It is then that severe problems might arise.

Some older equipment (now considered obsolete, but still occasionally found in service) created a signal return path via a ground connection to the equipment chassis. Again, there is not particular problem because the leakage current can go off harmlessly to ground through the third wire in the AC power cord. But if the ground wire breaks, or is somehow defeated, then the alternative path is followed—*through the patient!* So how is the patient grounded in this case?

Even in more modern equipment, which isolates the patient signal lines (as is true in ECG amplifiers today), there might be an accidental grounding of the patient. In the hospital room the majority of the equipment and appliances (including the bed) are electrically grounded, so accidental grounding is not merely possible but nearly inevitable. Thus, a second possible path to ground exists through the patient and other devices when a device ground wire is broken. In modern equipment, the signal path does not go through the equipment chassis, but it is possible to make accidental contact with the equipment case itself to complete the path. It is here that the attending medical personnel can accidentally shock the patient.

Nearly two decades ago it was determined that 10 μA is the maximum permissible leakage current to a patient. How did this seemingly low value of current come about? It is known that the real problem is the current density in the *sinoatrial node* of the heart. This structure is a small natural pacemaker in the right atrium and is responsible for the timing of the heart rate. An experiment was done in which a dog was catheterized (Figure 28-8), and an AC current thereby introduced into the dog's heart via the catheter. The ECG was monitored as the current level was increased from zero. The point at which the dog's heart entered fatal ventricular fibrillation was 20 μA. The safety standard for humans was set arbitrarily (but not unreasonably) at half this amount, or 10 μA. Although some people have taken issue with the method of this experiment, and others feel that the standard is too conservative, the majority of the industry feels that the consequence to the patient if the critics are

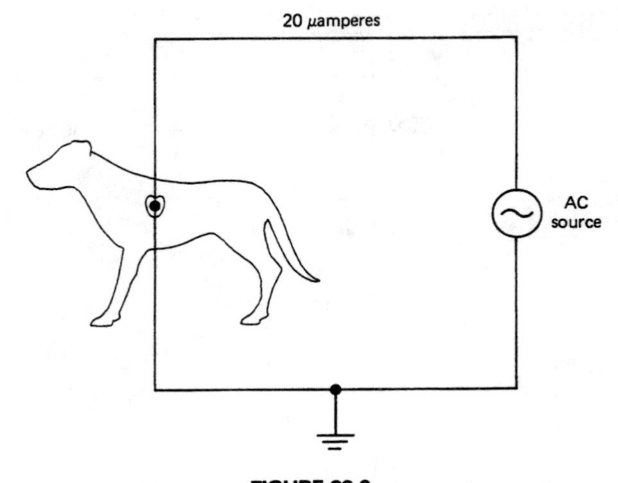

FIGURE 28-8

wrong is simply too great to opt for less than the most conservative standard: 10 μA therefore stands.

A good impedance value (for discussion sake) for an electrode on the surface of intact skin is about 10 Kohms. But when the skin is breached, and the electrode is introduced inside the body the impedance drops to a much lower value around 50 ohms. Thus, the internal resistance of the body is some 200 times lower than the external resistance. It therefore takes a lot less voltage to raise the current to a point above the 10 μA limit. Let's take a look at a scenario in which the current can be generated by tiny, inadvertent voltage drops between the power systems applied to two different pieces of equipment.

Figure 28-9 shows a situation in which two rooms are side by side. The electrical systems for the two rooms are directly tapped from the main hospital electrical system. As is standard practice, the lines to opposite sides of the room are taken from different branches in order to save wiring costs. Thus, the two outlets (A and B) are from different branches, but connect together at the main electrical system outside of the room. Also standard practice is to use the same branch feeder on either side of a wall dividing two rooms. Again, cost is the main consideration. In Figure 28-9 we see that outlets A and C are in different rooms, but are fed from the same branch circuit.

Assume that the two lines are approximately equal and have a resistance of 0.080 ohms (80 milliohms). Under normal conditions, there is a load of about 0.5 amperes on each line (typical for small monitors or other small instruments), so the voltage drops across the line resistances are equal, and on the order of 0.02 volts.

But suppose someone turns on a heavy appliances, such as a waxer or vacuum cleaner, in the unoccupied room. This appliance draws 4 amperes of current through outlet C from the same branch circuit as outlet A. The current in this branch is now 4.5 amperes, so the voltage drop is 1.62 volts. Thus, the two equipments in the

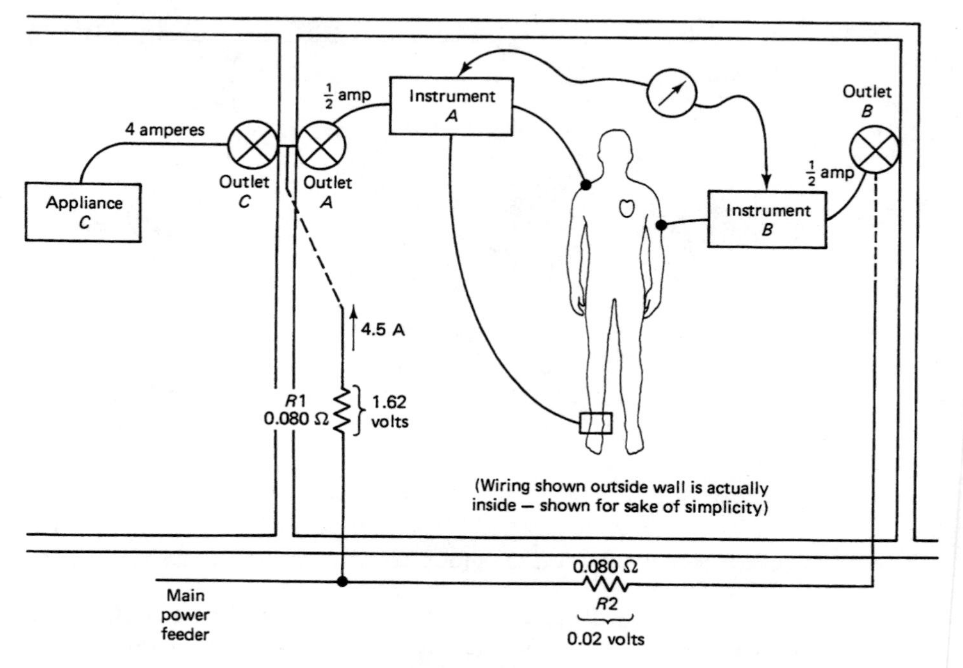

FIGURE 28-9

occupied room are at a potential difference of 1.62–0.02 or 1.6 volts. The current that will flow through the 50-ohm patient resistance from this voltage difference is 0.032 amperes. This current is equal to 32,000 μA, so is clearly considerably above the supposed safe value!

There are two general methods for reducing the danger from differential voltages in medical environments: *use an isolated electrical system* and *use an equipotential ground system*. The isolated system is similar in concept to the isolated power system created for the workbench earlier. Figure 28-10 shows a typical medical isolated power system, as is common in operating rooms and the trauma rooms of emergency departments. The main hospital electrical system uses the standard three-wire distribution system: *hot, neutral,* and *ground*. These wires are not sent to the room, but rather connect to an isolation transformer that feeds power into the room. All branch circuits in the room are fed from the secondary winding of this transformer.

Notice that the system of Figure 28-10 provides two safety mechanisms. First, the local room power system is isolated from the main hospital system through the transformer, so scenarios like that of Figure 28-9 cannot easily occur. Second, the two lines from the secondary of the transformer are *floating* above ground, so there is no ground-referenced system in the room. That eliminates the leakage current problem *if the isolation transformer is of good design and working properly*.

An *equipotential ground system* is shown in Figure 28-11. This method of protection is common in coronary care units (CCU) and intensive care units (ICU) of

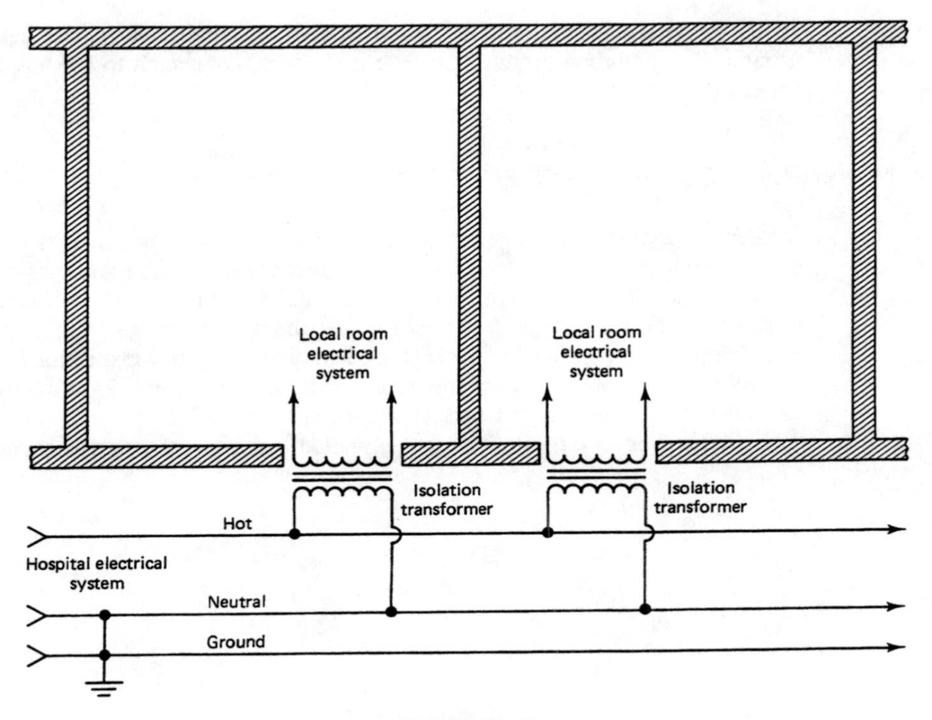

FIGURE 28-10

hospitals. In this case, we are using the normal hospital electrical system, but have provided redundant grounds. The heavy wires shown in Figure 28-11 are additional, external, grounds provided to back up the grounds in the power cord. There will be a common ground bus at the bedside (usually a large metal plate with special ground wire sockets on it) for these redundant grounds to connect. Every instrument, appli-

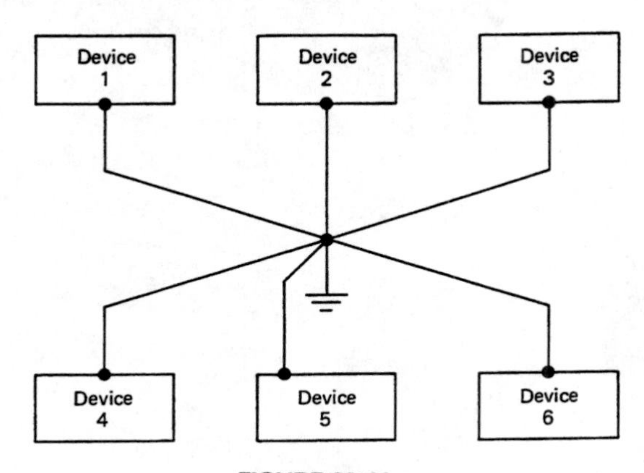

FIGURE 28-11

ance, or device, including the patient's bed, is connected to the equipotential ground. The common ground bus plate is, in turn, connected to the hospital power system ground bus.

MAINTENANCE OF A PROPER ELECTRICAL ENVIRONMENT

In order to maintain the integrity of the electrical power system, it is necessary to have a well-thought-out surveillance and preventative maintenance system. There should be regular checks (e.g., monthly) of AC leakage currents, as well as inspections of the power outlets in the rooms and the power cords of the equipment. A significant aid in making regular inspections, quality control inspections of repaired or calibrated equipment before it is returned to service, or doing troubleshooting, is an electrical system analyzer such as shown in Figure 28-12.

In addition to the correct instrumentation and tools, those responsible for elec-

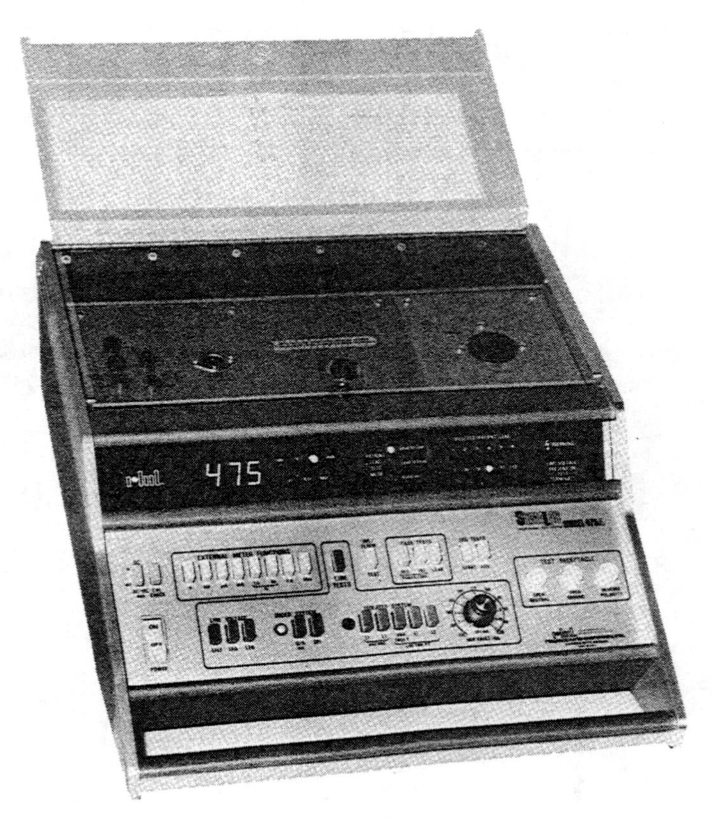

FIGURE 28-12

trical safety will need to know the latest JCAH regulations, AAMI and industry standards, the NFPA and Underwriter's standards, as well as local codes, laws, and health care facility regulations.

CONCLUSION

There is no such a thing as complete, failure-free safety system anywhere. This statement is especially true for electrical devices. But proper recognition of the mechanisms of danger and proper management of the risks will ensure that the environment is as safe as possible—and stays that way.

Index